FOURTEENTH EDITION

FIT&WELL

Core Concepts and Labs in Physical Fitness and Wellness

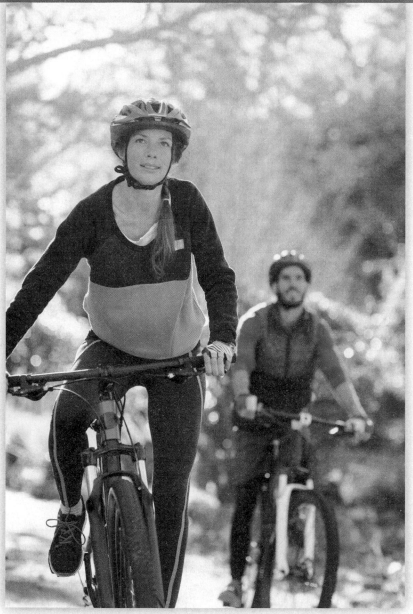

wavebreakmediamicro/123RF

Thomas D. Fahey
California State University, Chico

Paul M. Insel
Stanford University

Walton T. Roth
Stanford University

Claire E. Insel
*California Institute
of Human Nutrition*

Mc
Graw
Hill

FIT & WELL: CORE CONCEPTS AND LABS IN PHYSICAL FITNESS AND WELLNESS,
FOURTEENTH EDITION

Published by McGraw-Hill Education, 2 Penn Plaza, New York, NY 10121. Copyright ©2021 by McGraw-Hill
Education. All rights reserved. Printed in the United States of America. Previous editions ©2019, 2017, and
2015. No part of this publication may be reproduced or distributed in any form or by any means, or stored in
a database or retrieval system, without the prior written consent of McGraw-Hill Education, including, but
not limited to, in any network or other electronic storage or transmission, or broadcast for distance learning.

Some ancillaries, including electronic and print components, may not be available to customers outside the
United States.

This book is printed on acid-free paper.

1 2 3 4 5 6 7 8 9 LWI 24 23 22 21 20

ISBN 978-1-264-01308-1 (bound edition)
MHID 1-264-01308-6 (bound edition)
ISBN 978-1-260-26130-1 (loose-leaf edition)
MHID 1-260-26130-1 (loose-leaf edition)

Executive Portfolio Manager: *Claire Brantley*
Senior Product Developer: *Kirstan Price*
Senior Marketing Manager: *Meredith Leo*
Lead Content Project Manager: *Sandy Wille*
Senior Content Project Manager: *George Theofanopoulos*
Senior Buyer: *Sandy Ludovissy*
Design: *Egzon Shaqiri*
Senior Content Licensing Specialist: *Brianna Kirschbaum*
Cover Image: *Jacob Lund/Shutterstock*
Compositor: *Aptara®, Inc.*

All credits appearing on page or at the end of the book are considered to be an extension of the copyright page.

Library of Congress Cataloging-in-Publication Data

Names: Fahey, Thomas D. (Thomas Davin), 1947- author. | McGraw-Hill
    Education (Firm)
Title: Fit & well : core concepts and labs in physical fitness and wellness
    / Thomas D. Fahey, California State University, Chico, Paul M. Insel,
    Stanford University, Walton T. Roth, Stanford University, Claire E.
    Insel, California Institute of Human Nutrition.
Other titles: Fit and well
Description: Fourteenth Edition. | New York : McGraw-Hill Education, 2020.
Identifiers: LCCN 2019031552 (print) | LCCN 2019031553 (ebook) | ISBN
    9781260261301 (Spiral Bound) | ISBN 9781264013081 (Hardcover) | ISBN
    9781260696813 (eBook) | ISBN 9781260696868 (eBook other)
Subjects: LCSH: Physical fitness. | Health.
Classification: LCC GV481 .F26 2020 (print) | LCC GV481 (ebook) | DDC
    613.7/1–dc23
LC record available at https://lccn.loc.gov/2019031552
LC ebook record available at https://lccn.loc.gov/2019031553

2015033669

mheducation.com/highered

BRIEF CONTENTS

CONTENTS

12

13

14

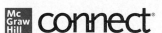 The Behavior Change Workbook and the laboratory activities are also found in an interactive format in Connect (connect.mheducation.com).

LEARN WITHOUT LIMITS

Mc Graw Hill connect®

McGraw-Hill Connect is a digital teaching and learning environment that improves performance over a variety of critical outcomes; it is easy to use, and it is proven effective. Connect® empowers students to achieve better outcomes by continually adapting to deliver precisely what they need, when they need it, and how they need it, so your class time is more engaging and effective. Connect for *Fit & Well* offers a wealth of interactive online content, including fitness and wellness labs and self-assessments, video activities on timely health topics and exercise techniques, a behavior change workbook, and practice quizzes with immediate feedback. The Connect eBook makes it easy for students to access their reading materials on smartphones and tablets; they can study on the go and don't need internet access to use it.

McGraw-Hill's **Application-Based Activities** are highly interactive, automatically graded, online learn-by-doing exercises that provide students the opportunity to assess their current fitness and wellness status and apply critical thinking skills to improve well-being. For this edition of *Fit & Well,* the Application-Based Activities include some of the most popular Lab Activities from the text as well as additional self-assessments. (The Lab Activities from the text also remain available in standard question bank format.)

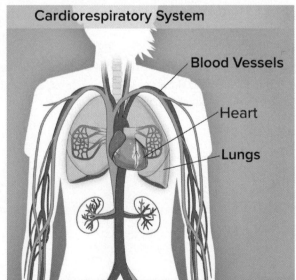

Cardiorespiratory System

Blood Vessels

Heart

Lungs

Expanded for this edition are assignable and assessable **Concept Clips,** which help students to master key personal health concepts. Using colorful animation and easy-to-understand audio narration, Concept Clips provide step-by-step presentations to promote student comprehension. Topics include the stages of change model, diabetes types and metabolism, changes to the Nutrition Facts label, the cardiorespiratory system, exercise program planning, and the stress response.

Also expanded are **NewsFlash** activities, which tie current news stories to key fitness and wellness concepts. After interacting with a contemporary news story, students are assessed on their understanding and their ability to make the connections between real-life events and course content. Examples of NewsFlash topics include dangers of sedentary time, colon cancer screening, and low-fat versus low-carb diets.

Finally, the Dietary Analysis Tool **NutritionCalc Plus** provides a suite of powerful dietary self-assessment tools that help students track their food intake and activity and analyze their diet and health goals. Students and instructors can trust the reliability of the ESHA database while interacting with a robust selection of reports. This tool is provided at no additional charge inside Connect for *Fit & Well.*

Mc Graw Hill SMARTBOOK®

Available within Connect, **SmartBook 2.0** makes study time as productive and efficient as possible by identifying and closing knowledge gaps. SmartBook identifies what an individual student knows and doesn't know based on the student's confidence level, responses to questions, and other factors. SmartBook continually adapts to an individual student's needs, creating a personalized learning experience for each student. SmartBook creates a more productive learning experience by focusing students on the concepts they need to study the most. Students spend less time on concepts they already understand and more time on those they don't. This ensures that every minute spent with SmartBook is returned to the student as the most value-added minute possible. The result? More confidence, better grades, and greater success. Find out more about the powerful personalized learning experience in SmartBook 2.0 at www.mheducation.com/highered/connect/smartbook.

New to this edition, SmartBook 2.0 is now available on all mobile smart devices. Just like the Connect eBook, SmartBook 2.0 is available in the ReadAnywhere app both online and offline. Read Anywhere includes the same functionality as the eBook offered in Connect with auto-sync across both platforms. SmartBook 2.0 was designed and developed for all students, including those learners with visual, auditory, and cognitive difficulties, or situations in which it's more convenient to read the book on a mobile device. Visit mheducation.com/ReadAnywhere to learn more.

PROVEN, SCIENCE-BASED CONTENT

The digital teaching and learning tools within Connect are built on the solid foundation of *Fit & Well*'s authoritative, science-based content. *Fit & Well* is written by experts who work and teach in the fields of exercise science, physical education, and health education. *Fit & Well* provides accurate, reliable current information on key health and fitness topics while also addressing issues related to mind-body health, diversity, research, and consumer health.

 Wellness in the Digital Age sections focus on the many fitness- and wellness-related devices and applications that are appearing every day.

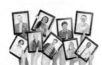 **Diversity Matters** features address the ways that our biological and cultural differences influence our health strengths, risks, and behaviors.

 Evidence for Exercise sections demonstrate that physical activity and exercise recommendations are based on solid scientific evidence.

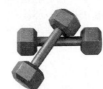 **Fitness Tips** and **Wellness** Tips catch students' attention and get them thinking about—and acting to improve—their fitness and wellness.

 Critical Consumer boxes help students navigate the numerous and diverse set of health-related products currently available.

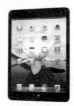 **Hands-on lab activities** give students the opportunity to assess their current level of fitness and wellness and to create their own individualized programs for improvement.

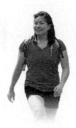 **Take Charge** features provide a wealth of practical advice for students on how to apply concepts from the text to their own lives.

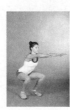 **Exercise photos and online videos** demonstrate how to correctly perform exercises described in the text.

CHAPTER-BY-CHAPTER CHANGES IN *FIT & WELL*, 14TH EDITION

UPDATES INFORMED BY STUDENT DATA

Changes to the 14th edition reflect new research findings, updated statistics, and current hot topics that impact students' fitness and wellness behaviors. Revisions were also guided by student performance data collected anonymously from the tens of thousands of students who have used SmartBook with *Fit & Well*. Because virtually every text paragraph is tied to several questions that students answer while using SmartBook, the specific concepts that students are having the most difficulty with can be pinpointed through empirical data.

Aggregated student performance data collected anonymously from SmartBook helps pinpoint concepts students find most challenging, guiding revisions to the text and Connect program.

Contemplation

52%
0:39
7337

People at this stage know they have a problem and intend to take action within six months. They acknowledge the benefits of behavior change but worry about the costs of changing. To be successful, people must believe that the benefits of change outweigh the costs. People in the contemplation stage wonder about possible courses of action but don't know how to proceed. There may also be specific barriers to change that appear too difficult to overcome.

Preparation

73%
0:24
4361

People at this stage plan to take action within a month or may already have begun to make small changes in their behavior. They may be engaging in their new, healthier behavior but not yet regularly or consistently. They may have created a plan for change but may be worried about failing.

Action

62%
0:36
15084

During the action stage, people outwardly modify their behavior and their environment. The action stage requires the greatest commitment of time and energy, and people in this stage are at risk for reverting to old, unhealthy patterns of behavior.

CHAPTER-BY-CHAPTER CHANGES

Chapter 1: Introduction to Wellness, Fitness, and Lifestyle Management

- Updated statistics on leading causes of death and the lifestyle factors that contribute to them
- Updated discussion of health insurance
- Updated review of the inverse relationship between longevity and physical activity, from the second edition of the *Physical Activity Guidelines for Americans*
- New information on *Healthy People 2030*

Chapter 2: Principles of Physical Fitness

- New and updated information on the 2018 second edition of the *Physical Activity Guidelines for Americans,* stressing the importance of regular physical activity for health and longevity and emphasizing that some physical activity is better than none
- Updated statistics and research on the role of exercise on health and longevity and on the benefits of endurance and resistance exercise for brain health and function

- Updated 2019 version of the *PAR-Q+ Physical Activity Readiness Questionnaire for Everyone* in Lab 2.1

Chapter 3: Cardiorespiratory Endurance

- New and updated information on the immediate and long-term effects of endurance exercise and on the role of endurance exercise in reducing risk for cancers of the colon, breast, bladder, endometrium, esophagus, lung, kidney, and stomach
- Clarification of the importance of endurance exercise for older adults
- Updated information on how resistance exercise stresses blood vessels and training techniques to reduce or eliminate related problems

Chapter 4: Muscular Strength and Endurance

- New Common Questions Answered focused on training at home and on muscle soreness and injury
- Updated statistics on muscular strength and power
- Updated coverage of strength training for older adults and on gender differences in strength

Chapter 5: Flexibility and Low-Back Health

- Updated statistics on the prevalence of osteoporosis and back pain
- Clarification of the importance of minimizing bedrest following the onset of acute back pain
- Updated resources and references for flexibility exercise training and preventing and treating back pain

Chapter 6: Body Composition

- Updated statistics on body composition and obesity
- New and updated information on the roles of exercise and diet in maintaining a healthy weight
- Updated resources and references for measuring body composition and preventing obesity

Chapter 7: Putting Together a Complete Fitness Program

- Updated information on popular exercise programming apps for smartphones
- Updated information on exercise program design for special populations

Chapter 8: Nutrition

- New section entitled "Planning and Budgeting for Healthy Eating"
- New and updated information on food and supplement labels, plant-based diets, and meatless burgers
- Updated discussion about nutritional recommendations for athletes
- Streamlined discussions of AMDRs, fats, fibers, and supplements

Chapter 9: Weight Management

- New presentation of three models related to weight management: energy balance, carbohydrate-insulin, and multi-factor models
- Updated discussion of the roles of diet and exercise in avoiding weight gain, losing weight, and maintaining weight loss
- New and updated sections on factors affecting RMR and appetite, including hormones and food choices
- New Common Question Answered focus on nuts as a healthy snack

Chapter 10: Stress Management and Sleep

- Updated discussion and illustrations of the stress response and symptoms of excess stress
- New discussions of Generation Z and loneliness
- Updated sections on sleep stages and sleep apnea
- New box entitled "Sleep and Learning"

Chapter 11: Cardiovascular Health and Diabetes

- Updated statistics and information on CVD types, recommendations for treatment of elevated cholesterol, and diabetes
- Updated information on blood pressure classification
- New illustration of the process of atherosclerosis

Chapter 12: Cancer

- New box entitled "Electronic Health Records"
- Updated statistics on cancer cases and deaths
- Updated recommendations on cancer screenings and HPV vaccination

Chapter 13: Substance Use and Misuse

- Updated statistics and information on nonmedical drug use among Americans, medical marijuana, rates of binge drinking, e-cigarettes, and rates of tobacco use among different population groups
- Updated examples of addictive behaviors
- Updated discussion of the opioid epidemic, including new figure showing increase in overdoses
- New sections on menthol cigarettes and thirdhand smoke

Chapter 14: Sexually Transmitted Infections

- Updated statistics on major STIs, HIV/AIDS, HIV transmission, and use of condoms by college students
- Updated information on HIV testing and HPV vaccination
- New information about *C. trachomatis* and syphilis

Chapter 15: Environmental Health

- Updated statistics on world population growth, components of solid waste, greenhouse emissions, and water shortages
- New information on the ozone layer, environmental tobacco smoke, and recycling

YOUR COURSE, YOUR WAY

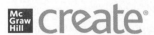

Craft your teaching resources to match the way you teach! With **McGraw-Hill Create**, you can easily rearrange chapters, combine material from other content sources, and quickly upload content you have written, such as your course syllabus or teaching notes. Find the content you need in Create by searching through thousands of leading McGraw-Hill textbooks and rights-secured third-party articles, cases, and readings. Create even allows you to personalize your book's appearance by selecting the cover and adding your name, school, and course information. Order a Create book and you'll receive a complimentary print review copy in three to five business days or a complimentary electronic review copy (eComp) via e-mail in minutes. Go to create.mheducation.com today and register to experience how McGraw-Hill Education Create® empowers you to teach your students your way.

TEGRITY: LECTURES 24/7

Tegrity in Connect is a tool that makes class time available 24/7 by automatically capturing every lecture. With a simple one-click start-and-stop process, you capture all computer screens and corresponding audio in a format that is easy to search, frame by frame. Students can replay any part of any class with easy-to-use, browser-based viewing on a PC, Mac, iPod, or other mobile device. Educators know that the more students can see, hear, and experience class resources, the better they learn. In fact, studies prove it. Tegrity's unique search feature helps students efficiently find what they need, when they need it, across an entire semester of class recordings. Help turn your students' study time into learning moments immediately supported by your lecture. With Tegrity, you also increase intent listening and class participation by easing students' concerns about note-taking. Using Tegrity in Connect will make it more likely you will see students' faces, not the tops of their heads.

TRUSTED SERVICE AND SUPPORT

- Connect integrates with your LMS to provide single sign-on and automatic syncing of grades. Integration with Blackboard®, D2L®, and Canvas also provides automatic syncing of the course calendar and assignment-level linking.
- Connect offers comprehensive service, support, and training throughout every phase of your implementation.
- If you're looking for some guidance on how to use Connect or want to learn tips and tricks from super users, you can find tutorials as you work. Our Digital Faculty Consultants and Student Ambassadors offer insight into how to achieve the results you want with Connect: www.mheducation.com/connect.

INSTRUCTOR RESOURCES

Instructor resources available through Connect for *Fit & Well* include a course integrator guide, test bank, image bank, and PowerPoint presentations for each chapter.

New to 14e is **Test Builder**, a cloud-based tool available within Connect that enables instructors to create tests that can be printed or administered within an LMS. Test Builder offers a modern, streamlined interface for easy content configuration that matches course needs, without requiring a download. It allows access to all test bank content from a title as well as robust filtering, scrambling, and layout options. Test Builder provides a secure interface for better protection of content and allows for just-in-time updates to flow directly into assessments.

ACKNOWLEDGMENTS

Fit & Well has benefited from the thoughtful commentary, expert knowledge, and helpful suggestions of many people. We are deeply grateful for their participation in the project.

Academic Advisors and Reviewers

Michael Bohne, *Utah Valley University*
Robert Bowen, *Truett McConnell University*
Ronnie Carda, *University of Wisconsin–Madison*
Barbara Coleman, *Northern Michigan University*
Tanya Crawford, *Treasure Valley Community College*
Karen Dennis, *Illinois State University*
Elizabeth Edwards, *James Madison University*
Nancy Estes, *Broward College*
Melissa Ferbert, *Missouri Western State University*
Robert Hess, *Community College of Baltimore County*

Terri Fleming, *Ivy Tech Community College*
Kyle Fogle, *Illinois Valley Community College*
Terry Folen, *Mt. Hood Community College*
John Jackson, *Pellissippi State Community College*
Karla Jones, *Central Piedmont Community College*
Justin Kraft, *Missouri Western State University*
Laura Marinaro, *Salisbury University*
Caryn Martin, *Anne Arundel Community College*
Keith McKelphin, *Montgomery College*
William Miller, *Concord University*
Jeannie Nieman, *Edmonds Community College*
Marnie Vanden Noven, *Belmont University*
Denise Penzkofer, *Pellissippi State Community College*
Shinya Takahashi, *University of Nebraska–Lincoln*
Kendra Zenisek, *Ball State University*

Introduction to Wellness, Fitness, and Lifestyle Management

LOOKING AHEAD...

After reading this chapter, you should be able to

- Describe the dimensions of wellness.

- Identify the major health and lifestyle problems in the United States today.

- Describe the behaviors that are part of a wellness lifestyle.

- Explain the steps in creating a behavior management plan.

- Evaluate some of the available sources of wellness information.

TEST YOUR KNOWLEDGE

1. Which of the following lifestyle factors is the leading preventable cause of death for Americans?
   a. excess alcohol consumption
   b. cigarette smoking
   c. obesity

2. The terms *health* and *wellness* mean the same thing. True or false?

3. A person's genetic makeup determines whether he or she will develop certain diseases (such as breast cancer), regardless of that person's health habits. True or false?

See answers on the next page.

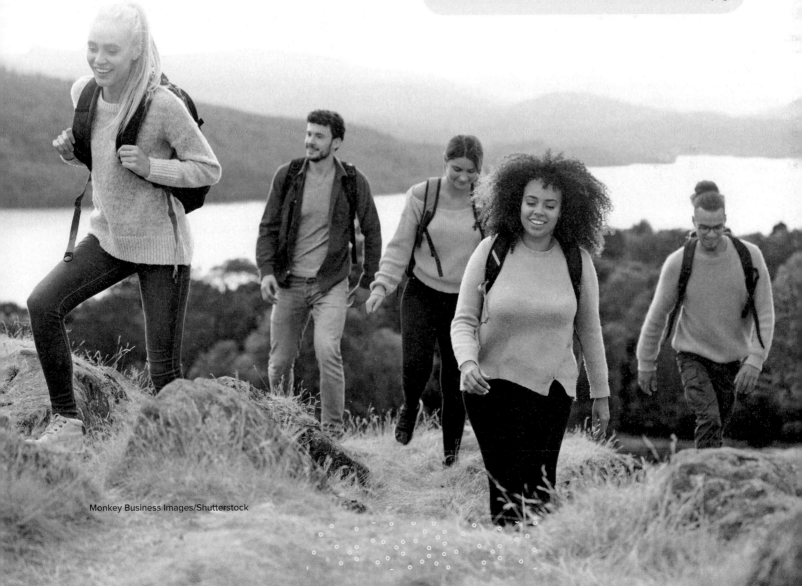

Monkey Business Images/Shutterstock

The next time you ask someone, "How are you?" and you get the automatic response "Fine," be grateful. If that person had told you how he or she actually felt—physically, emotionally, mentally—you might wish you had never asked. Your friend might be one of the too many people who live most of their lives feeling no better than just all right, or so-so, or downright miserable. Some do not even know what optimal wellness is. How many people do you know who feel great most of the time? Do you?

WELLNESS: NEW HEALTH GOALS

Generations of people have viewed health simply as the absence of disease, and that view largely prevails today. The word **health** typically refers to the overall condition of a person's body or mind and to the presence or absence of illness or injury. **Wellness** expands this idea of health to include our ability to achieve optimal health and vitality—to living life to its fullest. Although we use the terms *health* and *wellness* interchangeably in this book, they differ in two important ways:

- Health—or some aspects of it—can be determined or influenced by factors beyond your control, such as your genes, age, and family history. For example, a man with a family history of prostate cancer will have a higher-than-average risk for developing prostate cancer.

- Wellness is largely determined by the decisions you make about how you live. That same man can reduce his risk of cancer by eating sensibly, exercising, and having regular screening tests. Even if he develops the disease, he may still reduce its effects and live a rich, meaningful life. This means not only caring for himself physically, but also maintaining a positive outlook, keeping up his relationships with others, challenging himself intellectually, and nurturing other aspects of his life.

Wellness, therefore, involves making conscious decisions to control **risk factors** that contribute to disease or injury. Age and family history are risk factors you cannot control. Behaviors such as exercising, eating a healthy diet, and choosing not to smoke are well within your control.

The Dimensions of Wellness

The concept of wellness includes nine dimensions, all of which contribute to overall wellness. These dimensions are physical, emotional, intellectual, interpersonal, cultural, spiritual, environmental, financial, and occupational. The process of achieving wellness is continuing and dynamic, involving change and growth. Each dimension affects the others. Figure 1.1 lists

PHYSICAL WELLNESS	EMOTIONAL WELLNESS	INTELLECTUAL WELLNESS
• Eating well • Exercising • Avoiding harmful habits • Practicing safer sex • Recognizing symptoms of disease • Getting regular checkups • Avoiding injuries	• Optimism • Trust • Self-esteem • Self-acceptance • Self-confidence • Ability to understand and accept one's feelings • Ability to share feelings with others	• Openness to new ideas • Capacity to question • Ability to think critically • Motivation to master new skills • Sense of humor • Creativity • Curiosity • Lifelong learning
INTERPERSONAL WELLNESS	**CULTURAL WELLNESS**	**SPIRITUAL WELLNESS**
• Communication skills • Capacity for intimacy • Ability to establish and maintain satisfying relationships • Ability to cultivate a support system of friends and family	• Creating relationships with those who are different from you • Maintaining and valuing your own cultural identity • Avoiding stereotyping based on ethnicity, gender, religion, or sexual orientation	• Capacity for love • Compassion • Forgiveness • Altruism • Joy and fulfillment • Caring for others • Sense of meaning and purpose • Sense of belonging to something greater than oneself
ENVIRONMENTAL WELLNESS	**FINANCIAL WELLNESS**	**OCCUPATIONAL WELLNESS**
• Having abundant, clean natural resources • Maintaining sustainable development • Recycling whenever possible • Reducing pollution and waste	• Having a basic understanding of how money works • Living within one's means • Avoiding debt, especially for unnecessary items • Saving for the future and for emergencies	• Enjoying what you do • Feeling valued by your manager • Building satisfying relationships with coworkers • Taking advantage of opportunities to learn and be challenged

Figure 1.1 Qualities and behaviors associated with the dimensions of wellness.

specific qualities and behaviors associated with the nine dimensions of wellness. Ignoring any dimension of wellness can have harmful effects on your life. The following sections briefly introduce the dimensions of wellness. Lab 1.1 will help you learn what wellness means to you, what your wellness strengths and weaknesses are, and where you fall in each dimension on a continuum from low to high wellness.

Physical Wellness Your physical wellness includes not just your body's overall condition and the absence of disease, but also your fitness level and your ability to care for yourself. The higher your fitness level, the higher your level of physical wellness will be. Similarly, as you take better care of your own physical needs, you ensure greater physical wellness. The decisions you make now—and the habits you develop over your lifetime—will largely determine the length and quality of your life.

Emotional Wellness Your emotional wellness reflects your ability to understand and deal with your feelings. Emotional wellness involves attending to your own thoughts and feelings, monitoring your reactions, and identifying obstacles to emotional stability. *Self-acceptance* is your personal satisfaction with yourself, which might exclude society's expectations, whereas *self-esteem* relates to the way you think others perceive you. *Self-confidence* can be a part of both acceptance and esteem. Achieving this type of wellness means finding solutions to emotional problems, with professional help if necessary.

Intellectual Wellness Those who enjoy intellectual wellness continually challenge their minds. An active mind is essential to wellness because it detects problems and finds solutions. People who enjoy intellectual wellness never stop learning. They seek out and relish new experiences and challenges.

Interpersonal Wellness Satisfying and supportive relationships are important to physical and emotional wellness. Learning good communication skills, developing the capacity for intimacy, and cultivating a supportive network are all important to interpersonal (or social) wellness. Social wellness requires participating in and contributing to your community and to society.

Cultural Wellness Cultural wellness refers to the way you interact with others who are different from you in terms of ethnicity, religion, gender, sexual orientation, age, and customs (practices). It involves creating relationships with others and suspending judgment on others' behavior until you have lived with them or "walked in their shoes." It also includes accepting, valuing, and even celebrating the different cultural ways people interact in the world. The extent to which you value your own and others' cultural identities is one measure of cultural wellness.

Spiritual Wellness To enjoy spiritual wellness is to possess a set of guiding beliefs, principles, or values that give meaning

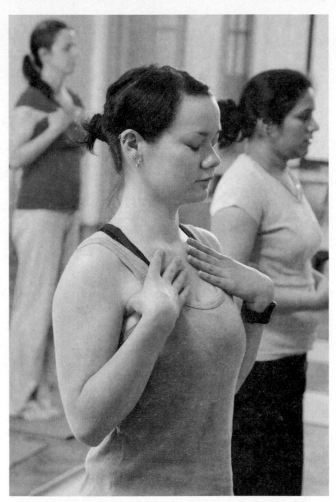

Wellness Tip Enhancing one dimension of wellness can have positive effects on others. For example, joining a meditation group can help you enhance your spiritual well-being, but it can also affect the emotional and interpersonal dimensions of wellness by enabling you to meet new people and develop new friendships.

Jonathan Goldberg/Alamy Stock Photo

and purpose to your life, especially in difficult times. The well person uses spirituality to focus on positive aspects of life and to fend off negative feelings such as cynicism, anger, and pessimism. Organized religions help many people develop spiritual health. Religion, however, is not the only source or form of spiritual wellness. Many people find meaning and purpose in their lives on their own—through nature, art, meditation, or good works—or with their loved ones.

TERMS

health The overall condition of body or mind and the presence or absence of illness or injury.

wellness Optimal health and vitality, encompassing all dimensions of well-being.

risk factor A condition that increases one's chances of disease or injury.

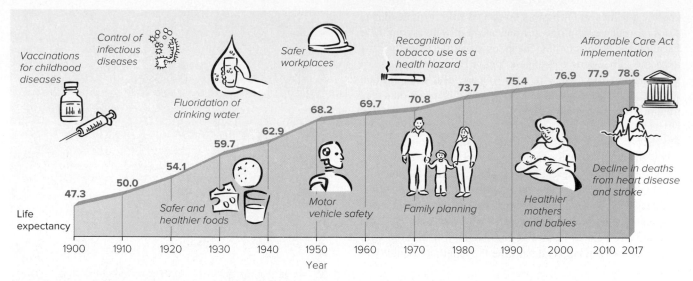

Figure 1.2 Public health and life expectancy of Americans from birth. Public health achievements during the 20th and 21st centuries are credited with adding more than 25 years to life expectancy for Americans, greatly improving quality of life, and dramatically reducing deaths from infectious diseases. Recent public health improvements include greater roadway safety, a steep decline in childhood lead poisoning, and an expansion of health insurance coverage. Still, in 2016 and 2017, U.S. life expectancy declined, especially for men. The overall decline is likely due to the opioid and obesity epidemics.

SOURCE: Murphy, S. L., et al. 2018. "Mortality in the United States, 2017." *NCHS Data Brief,* No. 328; Centers for Disease Control and Prevention. 1999. "Ten great public health achievements—United States, 1900–1999," *MMWR* 48(50): 1141.

Environmental Wellness Your environmental wellness is defined by the livability of your surroundings. Personal health depends on the health of the planet—from the safety of the food supply to the degree of violence in society. To improve your environmental wellness, you can learn about and protect yourself against hazards in your surroundings and work to make your world a cleaner, safer, and more beautiful place.

Financial Wellness Financial wellness refers to your ability to live within your means and manage your money in a way that gives you peace of mind. It includes balancing your income and expenses, staying out of debt, saving for the future, and understanding your emotions related to money. For more on this topic, see the box "Financial Wellness."

Occupational Wellness Occupational wellness refers to the level of happiness and fulfillment you gain through your work. High salaries and prestigious titles can be gratifying, but they alone do not bring about occupational wellness. Your occupational wellness depends on liking your work, feeling connected with others in the workplace, and feeling as though you're making a contribution. Another important aspect of occupational wellness is recognition from managers and colleagues.

New Opportunities for Taking Charge

In the 19th and early 20th centuries, Americans considered themselves lucky just to survive to adulthood. A boy born in 1850, for example, could expect to live only about 38 years, and a girl, 40 years. Many people died from common **infectious diseases**

(such as pneumonia, tuberculosis, or diarrhea) and poor environmental conditions (such as water pollution and poor sanitation).

By 2017, however, life expectancy nearly doubled, to 78.6 years (Figure 1.2). This increase in life span is due largely to the development of vaccines and antibiotics to fight infections, and to public health measures to improve living conditions. But even though life expectancy has increased, poor health limits most Americans' activities during the last 10–15% of their lives, resulting in some form of impaired life (Figure 1.3).

Today, a different set of diseases has emerged as our major health threat: Heart disease and cancer are now the top two leading

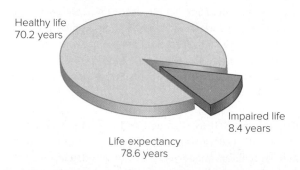

Figure 1.3 Quantity of life versus quality of life. Years of healthy life as a proportion of life expectancy in the U.S. population.
SOURCE: National Center for Health Statistics. 2016. *Healthy People 2020 Midcourse Review*, Hyattsville, MD.

infectious disease A disease that can spread from person to person, and which is caused by microorganisms such as bacteria and viruses. **TERMS**

Students feel less prepared to manage their money than to handle almost any other aspect of college life, according to a 2016 study of nearly 90,000 college students. They also express distress over their current and future financial decisions. Front and center in their minds is how to manage student loan debt. Financial wellness means having a healthy relationship with money.

Follow a Budget

A budget is a way of tracking where your money goes and making sure you're spending it on the things that are most important to you. Start by listing your monthly income and your expenditures. If you aren't sure where you spend your money, track your expenses for a few weeks or a month. Then organize them into categories, such as housing, food, transportation, entertainment, services, personal care, clothes, books and school supplies, health care, loan payments, and miscellaneous. Knowing where your money goes is the first step in achieving control of it.

Be Wary of Credit Cards

Students have easy access to credit but little training in finances. The percentage of students who have access to credit cards has increased from 28% in 2012 to 63% in 2016. This increase in credit card use has also correlated with an increase in paying credit card bills late, paying only the minimum amount, and having larger total outstanding credit balances.

Shifting away from using credit cards and toward using debit cards is a good strategy for staying out of debt. Familiarity with financial terminology helps as well. Basic financial literacy with using credit cards involves understanding terms like APR (annual percentage rate—the interest you're charged on your balance), credit limit (the maximum amount you can borrow), minimum monthly payment (the smallest payment your creditor will accept each month), grace period (the number of days you have to pay your bill before interest or penalties are charged), and over-the-limit and late fees (the amounts you'll be charged if you go over your credit limit or your payment is late).

Manage Your Debt and Get Politically Active

When it comes to student loans, having a personal plan for repayment can save time and money, reduce stress, and help you prepare for the future. Student loan debt in 2014 was almost four times the amount in 2000, surpassing $1.1 trillion. However, only about 10% of students feel they have all the information needed to pay off their loans. Work with your lender and make sure you know how to access your balance, when to start repayment, how to make payments, what your repayment plan options are, and what to do if you have trouble making payments. Information on managing federal student loans is available from https://studentaid.ed.gov/sa/.

Your student debt may reflect circumstances beyond your control. For example, financial aid programs may require students to hold down jobs while also maintaining certain grade point averages. Consider contacting policymakers and asking them to pass measures to help students in need. One suggestion is for the Free Application for Federal Student Aid (FAFSA) to take into account how much debt a family or student already has when determining how much aid to grant.

Start Saving

If you start saving early, the same miracle of compound interest that locks you into years of credit card debt can work to your benefit (for an online compound interest calculator, visit http://www.interestcalc.org). Experts recommend "paying yourself first" every month—that is, putting some money into savings before you start paying your bills, depending on what your budget allows. You may want to save for a large purchase, or you may even be looking ahead to retirement. If you work for a company with a 401(k) retirement plan, contribute as much as you can every pay period.

Become Financially Literate

Most Americans have not received basic financial training. For this reason, the U.S. government has established the Financial Literacy and Education Commission (MyMoney.gov) to help Americans learn how to save, invest, and manage money better. Developing lifelong financial skills should begin in early adulthood, during the college years, if not earlier, as money-management experience appears to have a more direct effect on financial knowledge than does education. For example, when tested on their basic financial literacy, students who had checking accounts had higher scores than those who did not.

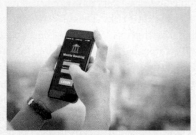

Panuwat Phimpha/Shutterstock

SOURCES: U.S. Financial Literacy and Education Commission, MyMoney.gov, 2013. (http://www.mymoney.gov); Xiao, J. J., N. Porto, and I. M. Mason. 2018. "Financial capability of student loan holders: Comparing college graduates, dropouts, and enrollees," *Working Paper*, University of Rhode Island (https://papers.ssrn.com/sol3/papers.cfm?abstract_id=3321898); EverFi, *Money Matters on Campus: Examining Financial Attitudes and Behaviors of Two-Year and Four-Year College Students.* (www.moneymattersoncampus.org).

Table 1.1 — Leading Causes of Death in the United States, 2017

RANK	CAUSE OF DEATH	NUMBER OF DEATHS	PERCENTAGE OF TOTAL DEATHS	LIFESTYLE FACTORS
1	Heart disease	647,457	23.0	D I S A O
2	Cancer	599,108	21.3	D I S A O
3	Accidents (unintentional injuries)	169,936	6.0	I S A
4	Chronic lower respiratory diseases	160,201	5.7	D I S O
5	Stroke	146,383	5.2	D I S A O
6	Alzheimer's disease	121,404	4.3	I S
7	Diabetes mellitus	83,564	3.0	D I S A O
8	Influenza and pneumonia	55,672	2.0	S A
9	Kidney disease	50,633	1.8	S A O
10	Intentional self-harm (suicide)	47,173	1.7	A
	All causes	2,813,503	100.0	

Key
D Diet plays a part
I Inactive lifestyle plays a part
S Smoking plays a part
A Excessive alcohol use plays a part
O Obesity is a contributing factor

NOTE: Although not among the overall top 10 causes of death, HIV/AIDS (5,611 deaths in 2017) is a major killer. In 2017, HIV/AIDS was the ninth leading cause of death for Americans aged 25–44 years.

SOURCE: Heron, M. 2019. "Deaths: Leading causes for 2017." *National Vital Statistics Reports* (68)6. Hyattsville, MD: National Center for Health Statistics.

causes of death for Americans (Table 1.1). While life expectancy has consistently increased each decade in the United States since 1850, the rate of improvement has slowed (and as of 2015 actually dropped for the first time in decades). A recent increase in deaths from heart disease, stroke, and diabetes may be linked to the obesity epidemic that began in the late 1970s. Medical treatments may be reaching their limits in treating heart disease and in preventing other early deaths related to obesity. Moreover, people are becoming obese at earlier ages, exposing them to the adverse effects of excess body fat over a longer period of time. Obesity and poor eating habits can lead to all the major **chronic diseases**.

The good news is that people have some control over whether they develop chronic diseases. Every day people can make choices that increase or decrease their risks. These **lifestyle choices** include decisions regarding smoking, diet, exercise, sleep, and alcohol use. Table 1.2 shows the estimated number of annual deaths tied to selected underlying causes. Because the cause of death is not always clearly attributable to a single factor, these numbers are rough estimates. But they give the idea that lifestyle choices contribute to many deaths. For example, the estimated 90,000 deaths due to alcohol include deaths due directly to alcohol poisoning as well as alcohol-related deaths from liver cancer and accidents. The need to make good choices is especially true for teens and young

adults. For Americans aged 15–24, for example, the leading cause of death is unintentional injuries (accidents), with the greatest number of deaths linked to car crashes (Table 1.3).

National Health

Wellness is a personal concern, but the U.S. government has financial and humanitarian interests in it, too. A healthy population is the nation's source of vitality, creativity, and wealth. Poor health drains the nation's resources and raises health care costs for all.

Health Insurance Options The Affordable Care Act (ACA), also called "Obamacare," was signed into law on March 23, 2010. It has remained in effect since that time, although certain provisions have been altered. Health insurance costs will likely increase as a result.

FINDING A PLAN Under the ACA, health insurance marketplaces, also called health exchanges, facilitate the purchase of health insurance at the state level. The health exchanges provide a selection of government-regulated health care plans that students and others may choose from. Those who are below income requirements are eligible for federal help with the premiums. Many employers and universities also offer health insurance to their employees and students. Small businesses and members of certain associations may also be able to purchase insurance through membership in a professional group.

BENEFITS TO COLLEGE STUDENTS The ACA permits young adults to stay on their parents' health insurance plans until age 26—even if they are married or have access to coverage through an employer. Students not on their parents' plans who do not want to purchase insurance through their schools can do so through a health insurance marketplace.

TERMS

chronic diseases A disease that develops and continues over a long period of time, such as heart disease or cancer.

lifestyle choice A conscious behavior that can increase or decrease a person's risk of disease or injury; such behaviors include decisions regarding smoking, eating a healthy diet, exercising, and using alcohol.

Table 1.2 Key Contributors to Death among Americans

	NUMBER OF DEATHS PER YEAR	PERCENTAGE OF TOTAL DEATHS PER YEAR
Tobacco	480,000+	17.5
Diet/activity patterns (obesity)	470,000	17.1
Microbial agents*	100,000	3.6
Alcohol consumption	90,000	3.3
Illicit drug use	70,000	2.6
Motor vehicles	39,000	1.4
Firearms	38,000	1.4
Sexual behavior**	11,000	0.4

*Microbial agents include bacterial and viral infections, such as influenza, pneumonia, and hepatitis. Infections transmitted sexually are counted in the "sexual behavior" category, including a proportion of deaths related to hepatitis, which can be transmitted both sexually and nonsexually.

**Estimated deaths linked to sexual behavior include those from cervical cancer (4,000) and sexually acquired HIV (6,000), hepatitis B (1,700), and hepatitis C (900). Because these infections can also be transmitted nonsexually, for example through needle sharing, only a proportion of the total deaths from these infections appears in this category. Averages of the rates of sexual transmission for different sexes and sexual orientations were taken as percentages of the number of total deaths.

SOURCES: Scholl, L., et al. 2019. "Drug and opioid-involved overdose deaths—United States, 2013–2017," *MMWR* 67(5152): 1419–1427; Centers for Disease Control and Prevention. 2019. *Leading Causes of Injury Deaths by Age Group Highlighting Unintentional Injury Deaths, United States—2017* (https://www.cdc.gov/injury/images/lc-charts/leading _causes_of_death_by_age_group_unintentional_2017_1100w850h.jpg); Centers for Disease Control and Prevention. 2019. *Smoking & Tobacco Use: Fast Facts.* (https://www.cdc.gov/tobacco/data_statistics/fact_sheets /fast_facts/index.htm); U.S. Department of Health & Human Services. 2018. *Viral Hepatitis* (https://www.cdc.gov/hepatitis); Xu, J., et al. 2018. "Deaths: Final data for 2016," *National Vital Statistics Reports* 67(5); Heron, M. 2019. "Deaths: Leading causes for 2017." *National Vital Statistics Reports* (68)6. Hyattsville, MD: National Center for Health Statistics.

Table 1.3 Leading Causes of Death among Americans Aged 15–24, 2017

RANK	CAUSE OF DEATH	NUMBER OF DEATHS	PERCENTAGE OF TOTAL DEATHS
1	Unintentional injuries (accidents)	13,441	42.0
	Motor vehicle	6,697	20.9
	Poisoning*	5,030	15.7
2	Suicide	6,252	19.5
3	Homicide	4,905	15.3
4	Cancer	1,374	4.3
5	Heart disease	913	2.9
	All causes	32,025	100.0

*Poisoning deaths in this age group are primarily due to drug and alcohol overdose.

SOURCE: Centers for Disease Control and Prevention. 2019. "10 leading causes of death by age group, United States, 2017." *Web-based Injury Statistics Query and Reporting System* (www.cdc.gov/injury/wisqars).

Young, healthy people may prefer to buy a "catastrophic" health plan. Such plans tend to have low premiums but require you to pay all medical costs up to a certain amount, usually several thousand dollars. This can be risky if you select a plan that does not cover the ACA's 10 essential benefits: preventive care, outpatient care, emergency services, hospitalization, maternity care, mental health and substance use treatment, prescription drugs, rehabilitative services and devices, lab services, preventive services and chronic disease management, and pediatric care. It's recommended that everyone select a plan that covers all of these important types of care.

Students whose income is below a certain level may qualify for Medicaid. Check with your state. Individuals with nonimmigrant status, which includes worker visas and student visas, qualify for insurance coverage through the exchanges. You can browse plans and apply for coverage at HealthCare.gov.

The Healthy People Initiative The national Healthy People initiative aims to prevent disease and improve Americans'

quality of life. Healthy People reports, published each decade since 1980, set national health goals based on 10-year agendas. *Healthy People 2030* is in development and proposes the eventual achievement of the following broad national health objectives:

- Eliminate preventable disease, disability, injury, and premature death.
- Achieve health equity, eliminate disparities, and improve health literacy.
- Create social, economic, and physical environments that promote good health for all.
- Promote healthy development and healthy behaviors across every stage of life.
- Engage leadership and the public to design effective health policies.

Continuing a trend set by *Healthy People 2020,* this initiative emphasizes the importance of factors that affect the health of individuals, demographic groups, or entire populations. These factors are social (including race and ethnicity, education level, or economic status) and environmental (including natural and human-made environments).

Examples of individual health-promotion goals from *Healthy People 2020,* along with estimated progress, appear in Table 1.4.

Behaviors That Contribute to Wellness

A lifestyle based on good choices and healthy behaviors maximizes quality of life. It helps people avoid disease, remain strong and fit, and maintain their physical and mental health as long as they live.

Be Physically Active The human body is designed to be active. It readily adapts to nearly any level of activity and exertion.

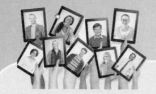

DIVERSITY MATTERS
Wellness Issues for Diverse Populations

We all need to exercise, eat well, manage stress, and cultivate positive relationships. Protecting ourselves from disease and injuries is important, too. But some of our differences—both as individuals and as members of groups—have important implications for wellness. These differences can be biological (determined genetically) or cultural (acquired as patterns of behavior through daily interactions with family, community, and society). Many health conditions are a function of biology and culture combined. You share patterns of influences with others; and information about groups can be useful in identifying areas that may be of concern to you and your family. Wellness-related differences among groups can be described in terms of a number of characteristics, including the following:

Sex and Gender. *Sex* represents the biological and physiological characteristics that define men, women, and intersex people. In contrast, *gender* refers to how people identify themselves and also the roles, behaviors, activities, and attributes that a given society considers appropriate. A person's gender is rooted in biology and physiology, but it is shaped by experience and environment—how society responds to individuals based on

their sex. Examples of gender-related characteristics that affect wellness include the higher rates of smoking and drinking found among men and the lower earnings found among women compared with men doing similar work. Although men are more biologically likely than women to suffer from certain diseases (a sex issue), men are less likely to visit their physicians for regular exams (a gender issue). Men have higher rates of death from injuries, suicide, and homicide, whereas women are at greater risk for Alzheimer's disease and depression. Men and women also differ in body composition and certain aspects of physical performance.

Race and Ethnicity. Although the concept of race is complex, with the number of people who identify themselves as biracial or multiracial growing, it is still useful to identify and track health risks among population groups. Some diseases are concentrated in certain gene pools, the result of each racial or ethnic group's relatively distinct history. Diabetes is more prevalent among individuals of Native American or Latino heritage, for example, and African Americans have higher rates of hypertension. Racial and ethnic groups may vary in their traditional diets; their family

and interpersonal relationships; their attitudes toward tobacco, alcohol, and other drugs; and their health beliefs and practices.

Income and Education. Of all the variables, inequalities in income and education are the most highly correlated to health status. Income and education are closely related, and groups with the highest poverty rates and least education have the worst health status. These Americans have higher rates of infant mortality, traumatic injury, violent death, and many diseases. They are more likely to eat poorly, be overweight, smoke, drink, and use drugs. They are exposed to more day-to-day stressors and have less access to health care services.

Disability. People with disabilities have activity limitations or need assistance due to a physical or mental impairment. About one in five people in the United States has some level of disability, and the rate is rising, especially among younger segments of the population. People with disabilities are more likely to be inactive and overweight. They report more days of depression than people without disabilities. Many also lack access to health care services.

Physical fitness is a set of physical attributes that allows the body to respond or adapt to the demands and stress of physical effort. The more we ask of our bodies, the stronger and more fit they become. When our bodies are not kept active, they deteriorate: Bones lose density, joints stiffen, muscles become weak, and cellular energy systems degenerate. To be truly well, human beings must be active.

Unfortunately, a **sedentary** lifestyle is common among Americans. According to the U.S. Department of Health and

| Table 1.4 | Progress toward *Healthy People* Targets |

OBJECTIVE	BASELINE (% MEETING GOAL IN 2008)	MOST RECENT PROGRESS (% MEETING GOAL IN 2016–17)	TARGET (% BY 2020)
Increase proportion of people with health insurance	83.2	89.3	100.0
Reduce proportion of adults with hypertension	29.9	29.5	26.9
Reduce proportion of obese adults	33.9	38.6	30.5
Reduce proportion of adults who drank excessively in past 30 days	28.2	27.2	25.4
Increase proportion of adults who meet federal guidelines for exercise	18.2	24.3	20.1
Reduce proportion of adults who use cigarettes	20.6	14.1	12.0

SOURCE: U.S. Department of Health and Human Services. *Healthy People 2020* data search (https://www.healthypeople.gov/2020/data-search/Search-the-Data).

- Increased endurance, strength, and flexibility
- Healthier muscles, bones, and joints
- Increased energy (calorie) expenditure
- Improved body composition
- More energy
- Improved ability to cope with stress
- Improved mood, higher self-esteem, and a greater sense of well-being
- Improved ability to fall asleep and sleep well

- Reduced risk of dying prematurely from all causes
- Reduced risk of developing and/or dying from heart disease, diabetes, high blood pressure, and colon cancer
- Reduced risk of becoming obese
- Reduced anxiety, tension, and depression
- Reduced risk of falls and fractures
- Reduced spending for health care

Figure 1.4 **Benefits of regular physical activity.**

Human Services, only 26% of men, 19% of women, and 20% of adolescents meet the federal physical activity guidelines (150 minutes or more per week of moderate aerobic exercise or 75 minutes per week of vigorous aerobic exercise). The older the adults, the less likely they are to meet the guidelines.

The benefits of physical activity are both physical and mental, immediate and long term (Figure 1.4). In the short term, being physically fit makes it easier to do everyday tasks, such as lifting; it provides reserve strength for emergencies; and it helps people look and feel good. In the long term, being physically fit confers protection against chronic diseases and lowers the risk of dying prematurely. (See the box "Does Being Physically Active Make a Difference in How Long You Live?") Physically active people are less likely to develop or die from heart disease, respiratory disease, high blood pressure, cancer, osteoporosis, and type 2 diabetes (the most common form of diabetes). As they get older, they may be able to avoid weight gain, muscle and bone loss, fatigue, and other problems associated with aging.

Choose a Healthy Diet In addition to being sedentary, many Americans have a diet that is too high in calories, unhealthy fats, and added sugars, as well as too low in fiber, complex carbohydrates, fruits, and vegetables. Like physical inactivity, this diet is linked to a number of chronic diseases. A healthy diet provides necessary nutrients and sufficient energy without also providing too much of the dietary substances linked to diseases.

Maintain a Healthy Body Weight Overweight and obesity are associated with a number of disabling and potentially fatal conditions and diseases, including heart disease, cancer, and type 2 diabetes. Researchers estimate that obesity kills between 112,000 and 500,000 Americans each year. Healthy body weight is an important part of wellness—but short-term

physical fitness A set of physical attributes that allows the body to respond or adapt to the demands and stress of physical effort.

sedentary Physically inactive; literally, "sitting."

TERMS

dieting is not part of fitness or wellness. Maintaining a healthy body weight requires a lifelong commitment to regular exercise, a healthy diet, and effective stress management.

Manage Stress Effectively Many people cope with stress by eating, drinking, or smoking too much. Others don't deal with it at all. In the short term, inappropriate stress management can lead to fatigue, sleep disturbances, and other symptoms. Over longer periods of time, poor stress management can lead to less efficient functioning of the immune system and increased susceptibility to disease. Learning to incorporate effective stress management techniques into daily life is an important part of a fit and well lifestyle.

Avoid Tobacco and Drug Use and Limit Alcohol Consumption Tobacco use is associated with 9 of the top 10 causes of death in the United States; personal tobacco use and secondhand smoke kill nearly 500,000 Americans each year, more than any other behavioral or environmental factor. In 2017, 14% of adult Americans described themselves as current smokers. Lung cancer is the most common cause of cancer death among both men and women and one of the leading causes of death overall. On average, the direct health care costs associated

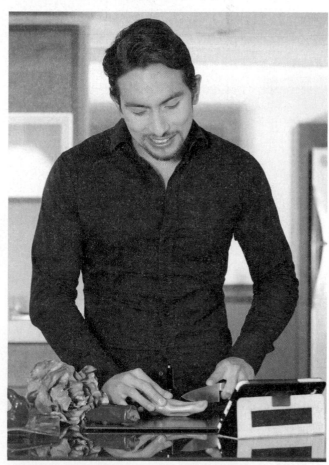

Wellness Tip In Table 1.1, notice how many causes of death are related to lifestyle. This is an excellent motivator for adopting healthy habits and staying in good condition. Maintaining physical fitness and a healthy diet can lead to a longer life. It's a fact!
Pablo Hidalgo/pxhidalgo/123RF

THE EVIDENCE FOR EXERCISE
Does Being Physically Active Make a Difference in How Long You Live?

How can we be sure that physical activity and exercise are good for our health? To answer this question, the U.S. Department of Health and Human Services asked a committee to review scientific literature. The committee's mission was to determine if enough evidence existed to warrant the government making physical activity recommendations to the public. The answer was yes. The committee's report, which summarized the scientific evidence for the health benefits of regular physical activity, formed the basis of the *Physical Activity Guidelines for Americans,* first released in 2008. The evidence was evaluated again in the lead-up to the release of the second edition of the guidelines in 2018.

The 2018 Physical Activity Guidelines Advisory Committee reviewed the link between moderate-to-vigorous physical activity and all-cause mortality (deaths from all causes). They looked at studies involving hundreds of thousands of people from all age groups and from different racial and ethnic groups. The data from these studies strongly support an *inverse relationship* between physical activity and all-cause mortality; that is, physically active people were less likely to die during the follow-up periods of the studies.

The review found that active people have about a 30% lower risk of dying compared with inactive people. These inverse associations were found not just for healthy adults but also for older adults (age 65 and older); for people with coronary artery disease, diabetes, or impaired mobility; and for people who were overweight or obese. Poor fitness and low physical activity levels were found to be better predictors of premature death than smoking, diabetes, or obesity. Based on the evidence, the committee determined that about 150 minutes (2.5 hours) of physical activity per week is enough to reduce all-cause mortality (see

Yellowdog/Cultura/Getty Images

Chapter 2 for more details). It appears that it is the overall volume of energy expended, no matter which kinds of activities are done, that makes a difference in risk of premature death.

The committee also looked at whether there is a *dose-response* relation between physical activity and all-cause mortality—that is, whether more activity reduces death rates even further. Again, the studies showed an inverse relation between these two variables. So, more activity above and beyond 150 minutes per week produces greater benefits. Surprisingly, for inactive people, benefits are seen at levels below 150 minutes per week. In fact, *any* increase in physical activity resulted in reduced risk of death. The 2018 *Physical Activity Guidelines* refer to this as the "some is better than none" message. A target of 150 minutes per week is recommended, but any level of activity below the target is encouraged for inactive people.

Looking more closely at this relationship, the committee found that the greatest risk reduction is seen at the lower end of the physical activity spectrum (30–90 minutes per week). In fact, sedentary people who become more active have the greatest potential for improving health and reducing the risk of premature death. Additional risk reduction occurs as physical activity increases, but at a slower rate. For example, people who engaged in physical activity 90 minutes per week had a 20% reduction in mortality risk compared with inactive people, and those who were active 150 minutes per week, as noted earlier, had a 30% reduction in risk. But to achieve a 40% reduction in mortality risk, study participants had to be physically active 420 minutes per week (7 hours).

A 2018 American Heart Association report projected that cardiovascular disease costs in the United States will exceed $1.1 trillion by 2035. Regular exercise reduces the risk of cardiovascular disease and related health problems such as hypertension, high cholesterol, and diabetes. The message from the research is clear: It doesn't matter what activity you choose or even how much time you can devote to it per week, as long as you get moving!

SOURCE: Benjamin, E. J., et al. 2018. "Heart disease and stroke statistics—2018 update: A report from the American Heart Association," *Circulation* 137: e67–e492; 2015 Dietary Guidelines Advisory Committee. 2015. *Scientific Report of the 2015 Dietary Guidelines Advisory Committee.* Washington, DC: U.S. Department of Health and Human Services; 2018 Physical Activity Guidelines Advisory Committee. 2018. *2018 Physical Activity Guidelines Advisory Committee Report.* Washington, DC: U.S. Department of Health and Human Services.

with smoking exceed $170 billion per year. If the cost of lost productivity from sickness, disability, and premature death is included, the total exceeds $300 billion.

Excessive alcohol consumption is linked to 8 of the top 10 causes of death and results in about 90,000 deaths a year in the United States. The social, economic, and medical costs of alcohol abuse are estimated at more than $250 billion per year. Alcohol or drug intoxication is an especially notable factor in the death and disability of young people, particularly through

unintentional injuries (such as drownings and car crashes caused by drunken driving) and violence.

Protect Yourself from Disease and Injury The most effective way of dealing with disease and injury is to prevent them. Many of the lifestyle strategies discussed here help protect you against chronic illnesses. In addition, you can take specific steps to avoid infectious diseases, particularly those that are sexually transmitted.

Take Other Steps toward Wellness Other important behaviors contribute to wellness, including these:

- *Developing meaningful relationships*—for example, learning to communicate and dealing with anger
- *Planning for successful aging*—for example, anticipating physical challenges and maintaining hobbies
- *Learning about the health care system*—for example, knowing what treatment options are available to you
- *Acting responsibly toward the environment*—for example, helping to reduce pollution and encouraging sustainable practices

Wellness Factors That Seem Outside Our Control

Heredity, the environment, and adequate health care are other important influences on health and wellness. These factors can interact in ways that raise or lower the quality of a person's life and the risk of developing particular diseases. For example, a sedentary lifestyle combined with a genetic predisposition for diabetes can greatly increase a person's risk of developing the disease. If such people also lack adequate health care, they are much more likely to suffer dangerous complications from diabetes.

But in many cases, behavior can tip the balance toward health even if heredity or environment is a negative factor. Breast cancer, for example, can run in families, but it is also associated with overweight and a sedentary lifestyle. A woman with a family history of breast cancer is less likely to die from the disease if she controls her weight, exercises, and has regular mammograms to help detect the disease in its early, most treatable stage.

College Students and Wellness

Each year, thousands of students lose productive academic time to activities causing stress and other physical and emotional health problems—some of which can continue for a lifetime. According to the Spring 2018 American College Health Association National College Health Assessment II, the following were commonly reported factors affecting academic performance:

- Stress (33.2% of students affected)
- Anxiety (26.5%)
- Sleep difficulties (21.8%)
- Depression (18.7%)
- Work (15.3%)
- Cold/flu/sore throat (16.1%)
- Concern for a troubled friend/family member (11.9%)
- Internet use/computer games (9.9%)

Each of these factors is related to one or more dimensions of wellness, and most can be influenced by choices students make daily. For example, there are many ways to manage stress: By reducing unhealthy choices, such as using alcohol to relax, and by increasing healthy choices, such as using time-management techniques, even busy students can reduce the impact of stress.

What about wellness choices in other areas? The American College Health Association survey found the following:

- Only 44.4% of sexually active students reported that they used a condom mostly or always during vaginal intercourse in the past 30 days.
- About 15.5% of students had seven or more drinks the last time they partied.
- About 11.0% of students used one or more prescription drugs that were not prescribed to them within the past year.
- About 7.5% of students smoked cigarettes, and 9.0% used e-cigarettes, at least once during the past month.

How do your daily wellness choices compare to those of other students?

Ask Yourself

QUESTIONS FOR CRITICAL THINKING AND REFLECTION

How often do you feel exuberant? Vital? Joyful? What makes you feel that way? Conversely, how often do you feel downhearted, de-energized, or depressed? What makes you feel that way? Have you ever thought about how you might increase experiences of vitality and decrease experiences of discouragement?

REACHING WELLNESS THROUGH LIFESTYLE MANAGEMENT

Moving in the direction of wellness means cultivating healthy behaviors and working to overcome unhealthy ones. This approach to lifestyle management is called **behavior change**. As you may already know from experience, changing an unhealthy habit, or a condition such as depression, can be harder than it sounds. When you embark on a behavior change plan, it may seem like too much work at first. But as you make progress, you will gain confidence in your ability to take charge of your life. You will also experience the benefits of wellness—more energy, greater vitality, deeper feelings of appreciation and curiosity, and a higher quality of life.

The rest of this chapter outlines a general process for changing unhealthy behaviors that is backed by research and has worked for many people. You will also find many specific strategies and tips for change. For additional support, work through the activities in the Behavior Change Workbook at the end of the text.

behavior change A lifestyle management process that involves cultivating healthy behaviors and working to overcome unhealthy ones.   **TERMS**

WELLNESS IN THE DIGITAL AGE
Quantify Yourself

You feel stressed and under the weather. How can you feel better? Do you have a habit you want to kick. Where to start?

People's increasing desire to track their moods, sleep, exercise, and diet patterns has brought about some 165,000 health-related apps and movements, like Quantified Self—a California-based company that promotes self-tracking tools among communities across the world. By giving you numerical data related to your daily behaviors, digital trackers provide objective feedback about what is going on with your health. The technology also helps you describe your behaviors to doctors and can be integrated with behavior change strategies learned through counseling. Here are three steps to making good use of technology for wellness:

1. **Monitor yourself.** How much are you smoking? Sleeping? Exercising? What are you eating? Digital trackers can help answer these questions for you. A wristband can record whether you are getting enough restful sleep. Your smartphone can tell you how many steps you took to get across campus.

2. **Analyze your data.** You've tracked your sleep, your blood pressure, and your steps. You've kept a journal related to your diet. You've taken your body measurements. What patterns do you notice? What time of day do you tend to need food? Cigarettes? Sleep? How do your patterns match up with your goals?

   Standard weight-loss apps allow users to input weight goals and monitor progress toward those goals; more sophisticated apps can analyze users' data and offer daily physical-activity goals, or help them establish a regular eating schedule. You can now find advice, education, e-mail reminders, alerts for lapses in progress, motivational messages, and journals to record and track negative emotion. Many weight-loss apps also link to social media for encouragement and social support, or rewarding games and challenges. Additional features can be critical; tracking alone isn't sufficient for successful behavior change. You need to apply change strategies such as those described later in the chapter.

3. **Extend the list of behaviors you'd like to change.** You can track more than just your diet and exercise habits with digital assistance. Electronic devices and smart programs are available to help with many aspects of wellness, including the following:

   - Stress management
   - Meditation and spirituality
   - Heart rate and respiration
   - Menstrual cycles
   - Family medical history
   - Journaling

With so many possibilities, how do you choose what to monitor? Start with one or two variables. The interactive labs at the end of each chapter focus on aspects of fitness and wellness to get you going. Also, you'll find a variety of digital devices and apps discussed in later chapters, in "Wellness in the Digital Age" boxes. You may find one or more apps (many of which are free) that appeal to you and can help you make progress toward your fitness and wellness goals.

SOURCES: IMS Institute for Healthcare Informatics. 2015. *IMS health study: Patient options expand as mobile healthcare apps address wellness and chronic disease treatment needs.* (http://www.imshealth.com/en/about-us/news/ims-health-study:-patient-options-expand-as-mobile-healthcare-apps-address-wellness-and-chronic-disease-treatment-needs); Schoeppe, S., et al. 2016. "Efficacy of interventions that use apps to improve diet, physical activity and sedentary behaviour: A systematic review," *International Journal of Behavioral Nutrition and Physical Activity* 13(127).

Getting Serious about Your Health

Before you can start changing a wellness-related behavior, you have to know that the behavior is problematic and that you *can* change it. To make good decisions, you need information about relevant topics and issues, including what resources are available to help you change.

Examine Your Current Health Habits Consider how your current lifestyle is affecting your health today. How will it affect your health in the future? Do you know which of your current habits enhance your health and which ones may be harmful? Begin your journey toward wellness with self-assessment: Think about your own behavior, complete the self-assessment in Lab 1.2, and talk with friends and family members about what they've noticed about your lifestyle and your health. Digital trackers can also help with your self-assessment; see the box "Quantify Yourself."

Choose a Target Behavior Changing any behavior can be demanding. This is why it's a good idea to start small, by choosing one behavior you want to change—called a **target behavior**—and working on it until you succeed. Your chances of success will be greater if your first goal is simple, such as resisting the urge to snack on junk food between classes. As you change one behavior, make your next goal a little more significant, and build on your success over time.

Learn about Your Target Behavior After you've chosen a target behavior, you need to learn its risks and benefits for you—both now and in the future. As a starting point, use this text and the resources listed in the For Further Exploration section at the end of each chapter;

target behavior An isolated behavior selected as the object of a behavior change program. **TERMS**

Surveys indicate that college students are smart about evaluating health information. They trust the health information they receive from health professionals and educators and are skeptical about popular information sources, such as magazine articles and websites.

How smart are you about evaluating health information? Here are some tips.

General Strategies

Whenever you encounter health-related information, take the following steps to make sure it is credible:

- **Go to the original source.** Media reports and social media posts often simplify the results of medical research. Find out for yourself what a study really reported, and determine whether it was based on good science. What type of study was it? Was it published in a recognized medical journal? Was it an animal study, or did it involve people? Did the study include a large number of people? What did the study's authors actually report?

- **Watch for misleading language.** Reports that tout "breakthroughs" or "dramatic proof" are probably hype. A study may state that a behavior "contributes to" or is "associated with" an outcome, but this does not prove a cause-and-effect relationship.

- **Distinguish between research reports and public health advice.** Do not change your behavior based on the results of a single report or study. If an agency such as the National Cancer Institute urges a behavior change, however, you should follow the advice. Large, publicly funded organizations issue such advice based on many studies, not a single report.

- **Remember that anecdotes are not facts.** A friend may tell you he lost weight on some new diet, but individual success stories do not mean the plan is truly safe or effective. Do any scientific studies back up the claims of the article?

- **Be skeptical.** If a report seems too good to be true, it probably is. Be wary of information contained in advertisements. An ad's goal is to sell a product, even if there is no need for it, and sometimes even if the product has not been proven to be safe or effective.

- **Make choices that are right for you.** Friends and family members can be a great source of ideas and inspiration, but you need to make health-related choices that work best for you.

Internet Resources

Online information sources pose special challenges. When reviewing a health-related website, ask these questions:

- **What is the source of the information?** Websites maintained by government agencies, professional associations, or established academic or medical institutions are likely to present trustworthy information. Many other groups and individuals post accurate information, but it is important to look at the qualifications of the people who are behind the site. (Check the home page or click the "About Us" link.) Verify information you get from social media by visiting the originating organization's website and evaluating the source.

- **How often is the site updated?** Look for sites that are updated frequently. Check the "last modified" date of any web page. Newer studies may contradict the results of earlier ones.

- **Is the site promotional?** Be wary of information from sites that sell specific products, use testimonials as evidence, appear to have a social or political agenda, or ask for money.

- **What do other sources say about a topic?** Be wary of claims and information that appear at only one site or come from a chat room, bulletin board, or blog. Do other authors cite the same studies as the ones in this article?

- **Does the site conform to any set of guidelines or criteria for quality and accuracy?** Look for sites that identify themselves as conforming to some code or set of principles, such as those set forth by the Health on the Net Foundation or the American Medical Association. Medical and health journals that have been peer reviewed (edited by experts in the field), and websites maintained by government agencies, professional associations, or established academic or medical institutions are most likely to present trustworthy information.

---

see the box "Evaluating Sources of Health Information" for additional guidelines. Ask these questions:

- How is your target behavior affecting your level of wellness today?

- Which diseases or conditions does this behavior place you at risk for?

- What effect would changing your behavior have on your health?

Find Help Have you identified a particularly challenging target behavior or mood—something like overuse of alcohol, binge eating, or depression—that interferes with your ability to function or places you at a serious health risk? You may need help to change behaviors or conditions that are too deeply rooted or too serious for self-management. Don't be discouraged by the seriousness or extent of the problem; many resources are available to help you solve it. On campus, the student health center or campus counseling center can provide assistance. To locate community resources, consult yellowpages.com, your physician, or the internet.

Building Motivation to Change

Knowledge is necessary for behavior change, but it isn't usually enough to make people act. Millions of people have sedentary lifestyles, for example, even though they know it's bad for their

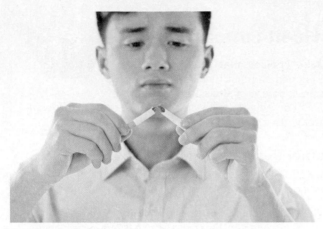

Wellness Tip Look for behavior-change support if you need it. Certain health behaviors are exceptionally difficult to change. Some people can quit smoking on their own; others get help from a smoking cessation program or a nicotine replacement product.

baona/iStock/Getty Images

health. To succeed at behavior change, you need to be motivated and to know that even though an active lifestyle may seem difficult, it may be required.

Examine the Pros and Cons of Change

Health behaviors have short-term and long-term benefits and costs. Consider the benefits and costs of an inactive lifestyle:

- *Short-term.* Such a lifestyle allows you more time to watch TV and hang out with friends, but it leaves you less fit and less able to participate in recreational activities.
- *Long-term.* This lifestyle increases the risk of heart disease, cancer, stroke, and premature death.

To successfully change your behavior, you must believe that the benefits of change outweigh the costs.

Carefully examine the pros and cons of continuing your current behavior and of changing to a healthier one. Focus on the effects that are most meaningful to you, including those tied to your personal identity and values. For example, engaging in regular physical activity and getting adequate sleep can support an image of yourself as an active person who is a good role model for others. To work toward being independent and taking control over your life, quitting smoking can be one way to eliminate a dependency. To complete your analysis, ask friends and family members about the effects of your behavior on them. For example, a younger sister may tell you that your smoking habit influenced her decision to take up smoking.

Although some people are motivated by long-term goals, such as avoiding a disease that may hit them in 30 years, most are more likely to be moved to action by shorter-term, more personal goals. Feeling better, doing better in school, improving at a sport, reducing stress, and increasing self-esteem are common, more immediate benefits of health behavior change. Many wellness behaviors are associated with immediate improvements in quality of life. For example, surveys of Americans have found that nonsmokers feel healthy and full of energy more days each month than do smokers, and they report fewer days of sadness and troubled sleep. The same is true when physically active people are compared with sedentary people. Over time, these types of differences add up to a substantially higher quality of life for people who engage in healthy behaviors.

Boost Self-Efficacy

When you start thinking about changing a health behavior, a big factor in your eventual success is whether you have confidence in yourself and in your ability to change. **Self-efficacy** refers to your belief in your ability to successfully take action and perform a specific task. Strategies for boosting self-efficacy include developing an internal locus of control, using visualization and self-talk, and getting encouragement from supportive people.

LOCUS OF CONTROL Who do you believe is controlling your life? Is it your parents, friends, or school? Is it "fate"? Or is it you? **Locus of control** refers to the figurative "place" a person designates as the source of responsibility for the events in his or her life. People who believe they are in control of their own lives are said to have an *internal locus of control*. Those who believe that factors beyond their control determine the course of their lives are said to have an *external locus of control*.

For lifestyle management, an internal locus of control is an advantage because it reinforces motivation and commitment. An external locus of control can sabotage efforts to change behavior. For example, if you believe that you are destined to die of breast cancer because your mother died from the disease, you may view screening mammograms as a waste of time. In contrast, if you believe that you can take action to reduce your risk of breast cancer in spite of hereditary factors, you will be motivated to follow guidelines for early detection of the disease.

If you find yourself attributing too much influence to outside forces, gather more information about your wellness-related behaviors. List all the ways that making lifestyle changes will improve your health. If you believe you'll succeed, and if you recognize that you are in charge of your life, you're on your way to wellness.

VISUALIZATION AND SELF-TALK One of the best ways to boost your confidence and self-efficacy is to visualize yourself successfully engaging in a new, healthier behavior. Imagine yourself going for an afternoon run three days a week or no longer smoking cigarettes. Also visualize yourself enjoying all the short-term and long-term benefits that your lifestyle change will bring. Create a new self-image: What will you and your life be like when you become a regular exerciser or a nonsmoker?

You can also use **self-talk**, the internal dialogue you carry on with yourself, to increase your confidence in your ability to

---

self-efficacy The belief in one's ability to take action and perform a specific task.

locus of control The figurative "place" a person designates as the source of responsibility for the events in his or her life.

self-talk A person's internal dialogue.

TERMS

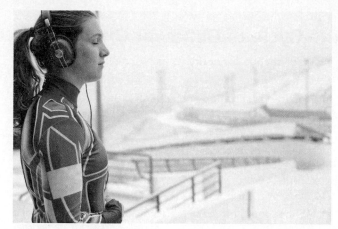

Fitness Tip Visualization is such a powerful technique that Olympic athletes learn how to harness it for peak performance. It works for average people, too. Set a small fitness goal, then imagine yourself doing it—as clearly and as often as you can. Visualization can help you believe in yourself, and belief can be a step toward success!

Hero Images Inc./Alamy Stock Photo

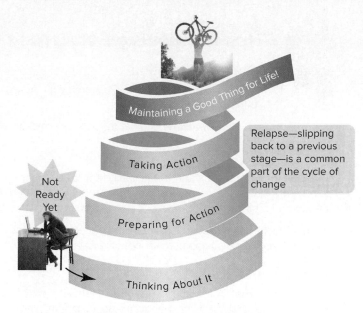

Figure 1.5   The stages of change: A spiral model.
SOURCE: Centers for Disease Control and Prevention. (n.d.). *PEP Guide: Personal Empowerment Plan for Improving Eating and Increasing Physical Activity.* Dallas, TX: The Cooper Institute.

(bike): Adam Brown/UpperCut Images/Getty Images; (desk): Ray Kachatorian/ The Image Bank/Getty Images

change. Counter any self-defeating patterns of thought with more positive or realistic thoughts: "I am a strong, capable person, and I can maintain my commitment to change." See Chapter 10 for more on self-talk.

ROLE MODELS AND OTHER SUPPORTIVE INDIVIDUALS
Social support can make a big difference in your level of motivation and your chances of success. Perhaps you know people who have reached the goal you are striving for; they could be role models or mentors, providing information and support for your efforts. Gain strength from their experiences, and tell yourself, "If they can do it, so can I." In addition, find a friend who wants to make the same changes you do and who can take a helpful role in your behavior change program. For example, an exercise partner can provide companionship and encouragement when you might be tempted to skip your workout.

Identify and Overcome Barriers to Change Don't let past failures at behavior change discourage you; they can be a great source of information you can use to boost your chances of future success. Make a list of the problems and challenges you faced in any previous behavior change attempts. To this list, add the short-term costs of behavior change that you identified in your analysis of the pros and cons of change. After you've listed these key barriers to change, develop a practical plan for overcoming each one. For example, if you always smoke when you're with certain friends, decide in advance how you will turn down the next cigarette you are offered.

Enhancing Your Readiness to Change

The transtheoretical, or "stages-of-change," model is an effective approach to lifestyle self-management. According to this model, you move through distinct stages as you work to change your target behavior. It is important to determine what stage you are in now so that you can choose appropriate strategies for progressing through the cycle of change (Figure 1.5). This approach can help you enhance your readiness and intention to change.

Precontemplation People at this stage do not think they have a problem and do not intend to change their behavior. They may be unaware of the risks associated with their behavior or may deny them. They may have tried unsuccessfully to change in the past and may now think the situation is hopeless. They may also blame other people or external factors for their problems. People in the precontemplation stage believe that there are more reasons or more important reasons not to change than there are reasons to change.

Contemplation People at this stage know they have a problem and intend to take action within six months. They acknowledge the benefits of behavior change but worry about the costs of changing or specific barriers that appear too difficult to overcome. To be successful, people must believe that the benefits of change outweigh the costs. People in the contemplation stage wonder about possible courses of action but don't know how to proceed.

Preparation People at this stage plan to take action within a month or may already have begun to make small changes in their behavior. They may be engaging in their new, healthier behavior but not yet regularly or consistently. They may have created a plan for change but may be worried about failing.

Precontemplation

- **Raise your awareness.** Research your target behavior and its effects.

- **Be self-aware.** Look at the mechanisms you use to resist change, such as denial or rationalization. Find ways to counteract these mechanisms.

- **Seek social support.** Friends and family members can help you identify target behaviors and understand their impact on the people around you.

- **Identify helpful resources.** These might include exercise classes or stress-management workshops offered by your school.

Contemplation

- **Keep a journal.** A record of your target behavior and the circumstances that elicit the behavior can help you plan a change program.

- **Do a cost-benefit analysis.** Identify the costs and benefits (both current and future) of maintaining your behavior and of changing it. Costs can be monetary, social, emotional, and so on.

- **Identify barriers to change.** Knowing these obstacles can help you overcome them.

- **Engage your emotions.** Watch movies or read books about people with your target behavior. Imagine what your life will be like if you don't change.

- **Create a new self-image.** Imagine what you'll be like after changing your target behavior. Try to think of yourself in new terms right now.

- **Think before you act.** Learn why you engage in the target behavior. Determine what "sets you off" and train yourself not to act reflexively.

Preparation

- **Create a plan.** Include a start date, goals, rewards, and specific steps you will take to change your behavior.

- **Make change a priority.** Create and sign a contract with yourself.

- **Practice visualization and self-talk.** These techniques can help prepare you mentally for challenging situations.

- **Take short steps.** Successfully practicing your new behavior for a short time—even a single day—can boost your confidence and motivation.

Action

- **Monitor your progress.** Keep up with your journal entries.

- **Change your environment.** Make changes that will discourage the target behavior—for example, getting rid of snack foods or not stocking the refrigerator with beer.

- **Find alternatives to your target behavior.** Make a list of things you can do to replace the behavior.

- **Reward yourself.** Rewards should be identified in your change plan. Give yourself lots of praise, and focus on your success.

- **Involve your friends.** Tell them you want to change, and ask for their help.

- **Don't get discouraged.** Real change is difficult.

Maintenance

- **Keep going.** Continue using the positive strategies that worked in earlier stages.

- **Be prepared for lapses.** Don't let slip-ups set you back.

- **Be a role model.** After you have successfully changed your behavior, you may be able to help someone else do the same thing.

If relapses keep occurring or if you can't seem to control them, you may need to return to a previous stage of the behavior change process. If this is necessary, reevaluate your goals and your strategy. A different or less stressful approach may help you avoid setbacks when you try again.

Action During the action stage, people outwardly modify their behavior and their environment. Although people in this stage are at risk for reverting to old, unhealthy patterns of behavior, they may also be reaping the rewards of a positive behavior change. The action stage requires the greatest commitment of time and energy.

Maintenance People at this stage have maintained their new, healthier lifestyle for at least six months. Lapses may have occurred, but people in maintenance have been successful in quickly reestablishing the desired behavior. The maintenance stage can last for months or years.

Termination People at the termination stage have exited the cycle of change and are no longer tempted to lapse back into their old behavior. They have a new self-image and total self-efficacy with regard to their target behavior. For ideas on changing stages, see the box "Tips for Moving Forward in the Cycle of Behavior Change."

Dealing with Relapse

People seldom progress through the stages of change in a straightforward, linear way. Rather, they tend to move to a new stage and then slip back to a previous stage before resuming their

| Date | November 5 | | | | Day | M | **TU** | W | TH | F | SA | SU | | | |

Time of day	M/S	Food eaten	Cals.	H	Where did you eat?	What else were you doing?	How did someone else influence you?	What made you want to eat what you did?	Emotions and feelings?	Thoughts and concerns?
7:30	M	1 C Crispix cereal 1/2 C skim milk coffee, black 1 C orange juice	110 40 — 120	3	home	looking at news headlines on my phone	alone	I always eat cereal in the morning	a little keyed up & worried	thinking about quiz in class today
10:30	S	1 apple	90	1	hall outside classroom	studying	alone	felt tired & wanted to wake up	tired	worried about next class
12:30	M	1 C chili 1 roll 1 pat butter 1 orange 2 oatmeal cookies 1 soda	290 120 35 60 120 150	2	campus food court	talking	eating w/ friends; we decided to eat at the food court	wanted to be part of group	excited and happy	interested in hearing everyone's plans for the weekend
	M/S = Meal or snack			H = Hunger rating (0–3)						

Figure 1.6 Sample health journal entries.

forward progress. Research suggests that most people make several attempts before they successfully change a behavior; four out of five people experience some degree of backsliding. For this reason, the stages of change are best conceptualized as a spiral in which people cycle back through previous stages but are further along in the process each time they renew their commitment.

If you experience a *lapse*—a single slip—or a *relapse*—a return to old habits—don't give up. Relapse can be demoralizing, but it is not the same as failure. Failure means stopping before you reach your goal and never changing your target behavior. During the early stages of the change process, it's a good idea to plan for relapse so that you can avoid guilt and self-blame and get back on track quickly. Follow these steps:

1. *Forgive yourself.* A single setback isn't the end of the world.

2. *Give yourself credit for the progress you have already made.* You can use that success as motivation to continue.

3. *Move on.* You can learn from a relapse and use that knowledge to deal with potential setbacks in the future.

Developing Skills for Change: Creating a Personalized Plan

Once you are committed to making a behavior change, it's time to develop the necessary skills to make that change successful. This includes setting goals, anticipating problems, finding rewards, and taking the following steps:

1. *Monitor your behavior and gather data.* Keep a record of your target behavior and the circumstances surrounding it. Record this information for at least a week or two. Keep your notes in a health journal or on your smartphone (see the sample journal entries in Figure 1.6). Record each occurrence of your behavior, noting the following:

   - What the activity was
   - When and where it happened
   - What you were doing
   - How you felt at that time

   If your goal is to start an exercise program, track your activities to determine how to make time for workouts.

2. *Analyze the data and identify patterns.* After you have collected data on the behavior, analyze the data to identify patterns. Note the connections between your feelings and such external cues as time of day, location, situation, and actions of others around you. When are you most likely to overeat? To skip a meal? What events trigger your appetite? For example, perhaps you overindulge in food and drink when you go to a particular restaurant or when you're with certain friends.

3. *Be "SMART" about setting goals.* If your goals are too challenging, you may have trouble making steady progress and may be more likely to give up altogether. If, for example, you are in poor physical condition, it will not make sense to set a goal of being ready to run a marathon within two months. If you set goals you can live with, it will be easier to stick with your behavior change plan and be successful.

   Following the SMART criteria, your behavior change goals should be

   - *Specific.* Avoid vague goals like "eat more fruits and vegetables." Instead, state your objectives in specific terms, such as "eat two cups of fruit and three cups of vegetables every day."

- *Measurable.* Recognize that your progress will be easier to track if your goals are quantifiable, so give your goal a number. You might measure your goal in terms of time (such as "walk briskly for 20 minutes a day"), distance ("run two miles, three days per week"), or some other amount ("drink eight glasses of water every day").

- *Attainable.* Set goals that are within your physical limits. For example, if you are a poor swimmer, you might not be able to meet a short-term fitness goal by swimming laps. Walking or biking might be better options.

- *Realistic.* Manage your expectations when you set goals. For example, long-time smokers may not be able to quit cold turkey. A more realistic approach might be to use nicotine replacement patches or gum for several weeks while getting help from a support group.

- *Time frame-specific.* Give yourself a reasonable amount of time to reach your goal, state the time frame in your behavior change plan, and set your agenda to meet the goal within the given time frame.

Using these criteria, sedentary people who want to improve their health and build fitness might set a goal of being able to run three miles in 30 minutes, to be achieved within a time frame of six months. To work toward that goal, they might set a number of smaller, intermediate goals that are easier to achieve. For example, the list of goals might look like this:

WEEK	FREQUENCY	ACTIVITY	DURATION (MINUTES)
1	3	Walk < 1 mile	10–15
2	3	Walk 1 mile	15–20
3	4	Walk 1–2 miles	20–25
4	4	Walk 2–3 miles	25–30
5–7	3–4	Walk/run 1 mile	15–20
21–24	4–5	Run 2–3 miles	25–30

You may not be able to meet these goals, but you never know until you try. As you work toward meeting your long-term goal, you may find it necessary to adjust your short-term goals. For example, you may find that you can start running sooner than you thought, or you may be able to run farther than you originally estimated. In such cases, you may want to make your goals more challenging. To stay motivated, however, some people may choose to make them easier.

For some goals and situations, it may make more sense to focus on something other than your outcome goal. If your goal involves a long-term lifestyle change, such as reaching a healthy weight, focus on developing healthy habits rather than targeting a specific weight loss. Your goal in this case might be exercising 30 minutes every day, reducing portion sizes, or eliminating late-night snacks.

4. *Devise a plan of action.* Develop a strategy that will support your efforts to change. Your plan of action should include the following steps:

- *Get what you need.* Identify resources that can help you. For example, you can join a community walking club or sign up for a smoking cessation program. You may also need to buy some new running shoes or nicotine replacement patches. Get the items you need right away; waiting can delay your progress.

- *Modify your environment.* If you have cues in your environment that trigger your target behavior, try to control them. For example, if you normally have alcohol at home, getting rid of it can help prevent you from indulging. If you usually study with a group of friends in an environment that allows smoking, move to a nonsmoking area. If you always buy a snack at a certain vending machine, change your route to avoid it.

- *Control related habits.* You may have habits that contribute to your target behavior; modifying these habits can help change the behavior. For example, if you usually plop down on the sofa while watching TV, try putting an exercise bike or yoga mat in front of the TV so that you can burn calories while watching.

- *Reward yourself.* Giving yourself instant, real rewards for good behavior will reinforce your efforts. Decide in advance what each one will be and how you will earn it. For example, you might treat yourself to a movie after a week of avoiding snacks. Make a list of items or events to use as rewards. They should be special to you and preferably unrelated to food or alcohol.

- *Involve the people around you.* Ask family and friends to help you with your plan. To help them respond appropriately to your needs, create a specific list of dos and don'ts. For example, ask them to support you when you set aside time to exercise or when you avoid second helpings at dinner.

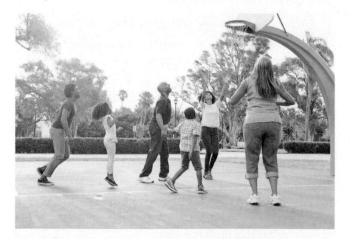

Wellness Tip Your environment contains powerful cues for both positive and negative lifestyle choices. The presence of parks and running/bike paths encourages physical activity, even in an urban setting. Examine your environment for cues that can support your behavior change efforts.

Monkey Business Images/Shutterstock

- *Plan for challenges.* Think about situations and people that might derail your program and develop ways to cope with them. For example, if you think it will be hard to stick to your usual exercise program during exams, schedule short bouts of physical activity (such as a brisk walk) as stress-reducing study breaks.

5. *Make a personal contract.* A serious personal contract—one that commits you to your word—can result in a higher chance of follow-through than a casual, offhand promise. Your contract can help prevent procrastination by specifying important dates and can also serve as a reminder of your personal commitment to change.

   Your contract should include a statement of your goal and your commitment to reaching it. The contract should also include details, such as the following:

   - The date you will start
   - The steps you will take to measure your progress
   - The strategies you plan to use to promote change
   - The date you expect to reach your final goal

   Have someone—preferably someone who will be actively helping you with your program—sign your contract as a witness.

Figure 1.7 shows a sample behavior change contract for someone committing to eating more fruit every day. A blank contract is included as Activity 8 in the Behavior Change Workbook at the end of this text.

Behavior Change Contract

1. I, [Tammy Lau], agree to
   [increase my consumption of fruit from 1 cup per week to 2 cups per day.]

2. I will begin on [10/5] and plan to reach my goal of
   [2 cups of fruit per day] by [12/7]

3. To reach my final goal, I have devised the following schedule of mini-goals. For each step in my program, I will give myself the reward listed.

I will begin to have ½ cup of fruit with breakfast	10/5	see movie
I will begin to have ½ cup of fruit with lunch	10/26	new video game
I will begin to substitute fruit juice for soda 1 time per day	11/16	concert

   My overall reward for reaching my goal will be [trip to beach]

4. I have gathered and analyzed data on my target behavior and have identified the following strategies for changing my behavior:
   [Keep the fridge stocked with easy-to-carry fruit. Pack fruit in my backpack every day. Buy lunch at place that serves fruit.]

5. I will use the following tools to monitor my progress toward my final goal:
   [Chart on fridge door
   Diet log app]

   I sign this contract as an indication of my personal commitment to reach my goal: [Tammy Lau] [9/28]

   I have recruited a helper who will witness my contract and [also increase his consumption of fruit; eat lunch with me twice a week.]
   [Eric March] [9/28]

Figure 1.7 A sample behavior change contract.

Putting Your Plan into Action

The starting date has arrived, and you are ready to put your plan into action. This stage requires commitment, the resolve to stick with the plan no matter what temptations you encounter. Remember all the reasons you have to make the change—and remember that *you* are the boss. Use all your strategies to make your plan work. Make sure your environment is change friendly, and get as much support and encouragement from others as possible. Keep track of your progress in your health journal, and give yourself regular rewards. Most important, congratulate yourself; notice how much better you look or feel, and feel good about how far you've come and how you've gained control of your behavior.

Staying with It

As you continue with your program, don't be surprised when you run up against obstacles; they're inevitable. In fact, it's a good idea to expect problems and give yourself time to step back, see how you're doing. Feel free to make some changes before going on. If your program is grinding to a halt, identify what is blocking your progress. It may come from one of the sources described in the following sections.

Social Influences Take a hard look at the reactions of the people you're counting on, and see if they're really supporting you. If they come up short, connect with others who will be more supportive. A related trap is trying to get your friends or family members to change *their* behaviors. The decision to make a major behavior change is something people come to only after intensive self-examination. You may be able to influence someone by tactfully providing facts or support, but that's all. Focus on yourself. When you succeed, you may become a role model for others.

Levels of Motivation and Commitment You won't make real progress until an inner drive prompts you to the stage of change at which you are ready to make a personal commitment to the goal. If commitment is your problem, you may need to wait until the behavior you're dealing with makes you unhappier or unhealthier; then your desire to change it will be stronger. Or you may find that changing your goal will inspire you to keep going. For more ideas, refer to Activity 9 in the Behavior Change Workbook.

Choice of Techniques and Level of Effort If your plan is not working as well as you thought it would, make changes where you're having the most trouble. If you've lagged on your running schedule, for example, maybe it's because you don't like running. An aerobics class might suit you better. Alternatively, you may not be trying hard enough. Plan to push toward your goal. If it were easy, you wouldn't need a plan.

Stress Barrier If you hit a wall in your program, look at the sources of stress in your life. If the stress is temporary, such as catching a cold or having a term paper due, you may want to wait until it passes before strengthening your efforts. If the stress is ongoing, find healthy ways to manage it (see Chapter 10). You may even want to make stress management your highest priority for behavior change.

Procrastinating, Rationalizing, and Blaming Be alert to games you might be playing with yourself, so you can stop them. Such games include the following:

- *Procrastinating.* If you tell yourself, "It's Friday already; I might as well wait until Monday to start," you're procrastinating. Break your plan into smaller steps that you can accomplish one day at a time.

- *Rationalizing.* If you tell yourself, "I wanted to go swimming today but wouldn't have had time to wash my hair afterward," you're making excuses.

- *Blaming.* If you tell yourself, "I couldn't exercise because Dave was hogging the elliptical trainer," you're blaming others for your own failure to follow through. Blaming is a way of taking focus off the real problem and denying responsibility for your own actions.

Being Fit and Well for Life

Your first attempts at making behavior changes may never go beyond the contemplation or preparation stage. But as you experience some success, you'll start to have more positive feelings about yourself. You may discover new physical activities and sports you enjoy, and you may encounter new situations and meet new people. Perhaps you'll surprise yourself by accomplishing things you didn't think were possible—breaking a long-standing nicotine habit, competing in a race, climbing a mountain, or developing a leaner body. Most of all, you'll discover the feeling of empowerment that comes from taking charge of your health. Being healthy takes effort, but the paybacks in energy and vitality are priceless.

Once you've started, don't stop. Assume that health improvement is forever. Take on the easier problems first, and then use what you learn to tackle more difficult problems later. When you feel challenged, remind yourself that you are creating a lifestyle that minimizes your health risks and maximizes your enjoyment of life. You can take charge of your health in a dramatic and meaningful way. *Fit & Well* will show you how.

Ask Yourself

QUESTIONS FOR CRITICAL THINKING AND REFLECTION

Think about the last time you made an unhealthy choice instead of a healthy one. How could you have changed the situation, the people in the situation, or your own thoughts, feelings, or intentions to avoid making that choice? What can you do in similar situations in the future to produce a different outcome?

✱ TIPS FOR TODAY AND THE FUTURE

You are in charge of your health. Many of the decisions you make every day have an impact on the quality of your life, both now and in the future.

RIGHT NOW YOU CAN
- Go for a 15-minute walk.
- Have a piece of fruit for a snack.
- Call a friend and arrange for a time to catch up with each other.
- Think about whether you have a health behavior you'd like to change. If you do, consider the elements of a behavior change strategy. For example, begin a mental list of the pros and cons of the behavior, or talk to someone who can support you in your attempts to change.

IN THE FUTURE YOU CAN
- Stay current on health and wellness news and issues.
- Participate in health awareness and promotion campaigns in your community—for example, support smoking restrictions in local venues.
- Be a role model for someone else who is working on a health behavior you have successfully changed.

SUMMARY

- Wellness is the ability to live life fully, with vitality and meaning. Wellness is dynamic and multidimensional; it incorporates physical, emotional, intellectual, interpersonal, cultural, spiritual, environmental, financial, and occupational dimensions.

- As chronic diseases have emerged as major health threats in the United States, people must recognize that they have greater control over and greater responsibility for their health than ever before.

- Behaviors that promote wellness include being physically active, choosing a healthy diet, maintaining a healthy body weight, managing stress effectively, avoiding tobacco and limiting alcohol use, and protecting yourself from disease and injury.

- Although heredity, environment, and health care all play roles in wellness and disease, behavior can change their negative effects.

- The national *Healthy People 2030* initiative aims to prevent disease and improve Americans' quality of life. To achieve this goal, it proposes broad national health objectives, emphasizing the importance of health determinants—factors that affect the health of individuals, demographic groups, or entire populations.

- To make lifestyle changes, you need information about yourself, your health habits, and available resources to help you change.

- You can increase your motivation for behavior change by examining the benefits and costs of change, boosting self-efficacy, and identifying and overcoming key barriers to change.

- The stages-of-change model describes six stages that people may move through as they try to change their behavior: precontemplation, contemplation, preparation, action, maintenance, and termination.

- A specific plan for change can be developed by (1) collecting and recording data on your behavior; (2) analyzing the data; (3) setting specific goals; (4) devising strategies for modifying the environment, rewarding yourself, and involving others; and (5) making a personal contract.

- To start and maintain a behavior change program, you need commitment, a well-developed and manageable plan, social support, and stress-management techniques. You will also benefit from monitoring the progress of your program and revising it as necessary.

FOR FURTHER EXPLORATION

Centers for Disease Control and Prevention (CDC). Through phone, fax, and the internet, the CDC provides a wide variety of health information.

http://www.cdc.gov

Federal Deposit Insurance Corporation: Money Smart. A free source of information, unaffiliated with commercial interests, that includes eight modules on topics such as "borrowing basics" and "paying for college and cars."

https://www.fdic.gov/consumers/consumer/moneysmart/

Federal Trade Commission: Consumer Information: Health & Fitness. Includes online brochures about a variety of consumer health topics, including fitness equipment, generic drugs, and fraudulent health claims.

https://www.consumer.ftc.gov/health

Healthfinder. A gateway to online publications, websites, support and self-help groups, and agencies and organizations that produce reliable health information.

http://www.healthfinder.gov

Health.gov. A portal for online information from a wide variety of federal agencies.

http://health.gov

Healthy Campus. The American College Health Association's introduction to the Healthy Campus program.

http://www.acha.org/HealthyCampus

Healthy People. Provides information on Healthy People objectives and priority areas.

http://www.healthypeople.gov

MedlinePlus. Provides links to news and reliable information about health from government agencies and professional associations; also includes a health encyclopedia and information on prescription and over-the-counter drugs.

https://medlineplus.gov/

National Health Information Center (NHIC). Puts consumers in touch with the organizations that are best able to provide answers to health-related questions.

http://www.health.gov/nhic/

National Institutes of Health (NIH). Provides information about all NIH activities as well as consumer publications, hotline information, and an A-to-Z listing of health issues with links to the appropriate NIH institute.

http://www.nih.gov

National Wellness Institute. Serves professionals and organizations that promote optimal health and wellness.

http://www.nationalwellness.org

Office of Minority Health. Promotes improved health among racial and ethnic minority populations.

http://minorityhealth.hhs.gov

Office on Women's Health. Provides information and answers to frequently asked questions.

http://www.womenshealth.gov

Quantified Self. Offers a forum for people interested in tracking their diet, sleep, and other behaviors and activities using technology.

http://quantifiedself.com

Surgeon General. Includes information on activities of the Surgeon General and the text of many key reports on such topics as tobacco use, physical activity, and mental health.

http://www.surgeongeneral.gov

World Health Organization (WHO). Provides information about health topics and issues affecting people around the world.

http://www.who.int/en

SELECTED BIBLIOGRAPHY

American Cancer Society. 2019. *Cancer Facts and Figures—2019*. Atlanta, GA: American Cancer Society (https://www.cancer.org/content/dam/cancer-org/research/cancer-facts-and-statistics/annual-cancer-facts-and-figures/2019/cancer-facts-and-figures-2019.pdf).

American College Health Association. 2018. *American College Health Association—National College Health Assessment II: Reference Group Executive Summary Spring 2018*. Silver Spring, MD: American College Health Association (https://www.acha.org/NCHA/ACHA-NCHA_Data/Publications_and_Reports/NCHA/Data/Reports_ACHA-NCHAIIc.aspx

American Heart Association. 2018. *Heart Disease and Stroke Statistics—2018 Update*. Dallas, TX: American Heart Association (https://www.ahajournals.org/doi/10.1161/CIR.0000000000000558).

Centers for Disease Control and Prevention. 2018. *Economic Trends in Tobacco* (https://www.cdc.gov/tobacco/data_statistics/fact_sheets/economics/econ_facts/index.htm).

Centers for Disease Control and Prevention. 2018. *HIV Surveillance Report* (https://www.cdc.gov/hiv/pdf/library/reports/surveillance/cdc-hiv-surveillance-report-2017-vol-29.pdf).

Centers for Disease Control and Prevention. 2018. *Racial and Ethnic Approaches to Community Health (REACH)* (http://www.cdc.gov/nccdphp/dch/programs/reach).

Centers for Medicare and Medicaid Services. 2018. *National Health Expenditure Data: Projections 2017-2026* (https://www.cms.gov/Research-Statistics-Data-and-Systems/Statistics-Trends-and-Reports/NationalHealthExpendData/NationalHealthAccountsProjected.html).

Flegal, K. M., et al. 2016. Prevalence and trends in obesity among U.S. adults, 2005-2014. *Journal of the American Medical Association* 315(21): 2284-2291.

Gentzke, A. S., et al. 2019. Vital signs: Tobacco product use among middle and high school students—United States, 2011-2018. *MMWR*. (http://dx.doi.org/10.15585/mmwr.mm6806e1).

Goldrick-Rab, S. 2016. *Paying the Price: College Costs, Financial Aid, and the Betrayal of the American Dream*. Chicago, IL: University of Chicago Press.

Hersi, M., et al. 2017. Risk factors associated with the onset and progression of Alzheimer's disease: A systematic review of the evidence. *NeuroToxicology* 61: 143-187.

Inoue, T., and Y. Tanaka. 2016. Hepatitis B virus and its sexually transmitted infection—an update. *Microbial Cell* 3(9): 420-437.

Jepsen, R., et al. 2015. Physical activity and quality of life in severely obese adults during a two-year lifestyle intervention programme. *Journal of Obesity* Article ID 314194 (https://www.hindawi.com/journals/jobe/2015/314194/).

Kaiser Family Foundation. 2017. *Key Facts About the Uninsured Population* (http://kff .org/uninsured/fact-sheet/key-facts-about-the-uninsured-population).

Keehan, S. P., et al. 2017. National health expenditure projections, 2016-25: Price increases, aging push sector to 20 percent of economy. *Health Affairs* 36(3): 553–563.

Kochanek, K. D., et al. 2018. "Deaths: Final data for 2016. *National Vital Statistics Reports* 67(5) (https://www.cdc.gov/nchs/data/nvsr/nvsr67/nvsr67_05.pdf).

Kovesdy, C. P., S. L. Furth, and C. Zoccali, on behalf of the World Kidney Day Steering Committee. 2017. Obesity and kidney disease: Hidden consequences of the epidemic. *Journal of Renal Care* 43(1): 3–10.

Morris, J. K., et al. 2017. Aerobic exercise for Alzheimer's disease: A randomized controlled pilot trial. *PLoS ONE* 12(2): e0170547.

National Center for Complementary and Integrative Health. 2018. *Finding and Evaluating Online Resources* (https://nccih.nih.gov/health/webresources).

National Center for Health Statistics. 2016. *Healthy People 2020 Midcourse Review*. Hyattsville, MD: National Center for Health Statistics (https://www.cdc.gov/nchs /healthy_people/hp2020/hp2020_midcourse_review.htm).

National Center for Health Statistics. 2017. *National Health Insurance Coverage: Early Release of Estimates from the National Health Interview Survey, 2016* (https://www .cdc.gov/nchs/data/nhis/earlyrelease/insur201705.pdf).

National Center for Health Statistics. 2018. *Health, United States, 2017: With Special Feature on Mortality*. Hyattsville, MD. National Center for Health Statistics (https://www.cdc.gov/nchs/data/hus/hus17.pdf).

National Institutes of Health. 2018. *Fact Sheet: Cervical Cancer* (https://report.nih.gov /nihfactsheets/viewfactsheet.aspx?csid=76).

National Kidney Foundation. 2018. *Smoking and Your Health* (https://www.kidney .org/atoz/content/smoking).

National Research Council, Institute of Medicine. 2015. *Measuring the Risks and Causes of Premature Death: Summary of Workshops* (p. 24). Washington, DC: National Academies Press (https://www.ncbi.nlm.nih.gov/pubmed/25834864).

Persky, S., et al. 2014. The role of weight, race, and health care experiences in care use among young men and women. *Obesity* 22(4): 1194–1200.

Petrides, J., et al. 2019. Lifestyle changes for disease prevention. *Primary Care* 46(1): 1–12.

Prochaska, J. O., J. C. Norcross, and C. C. DiClemente. 1995. *Changing for Good: The Revolutionary Program That Explains the Six Stages of Change and Teaches You How to Free Yourself from Bad Habits*. New York: Morrow.

Taksler, G., et al. 2017. "Resilience and Grit: Pursuing Organizational Change & Preventing Burnout in GIM." Research presented at The Society of General Internal Medicine 2017 Annual Meeting, April 19-22, 2017. Washington, DC.

Terrault, N. A., et al. 2013. Sexual transmission of hepatitis C virus among monogamous heterosexual couples: The HCV partners study. *Hepatology* 57(3): 881–889.

Tohme, R. A., and S. D. Holmberg. 2010. Is sexual contact a major mode of hepatitis C virus transmission? *Hepatology* 52(4): 1497–1505.

University of California, Berkeley. 2018. *Evaluating Web Pages: Techniques to Apply and Questions to Ask* (http://www.lib.berkeley.edu/TeachingLib/Guides/Internet /Evaluate.html).

U.S. Department of Health and Human Services. 2018. *Physical Activity Guidelines for Americans* (2nd ed.). Washington, DC: U.S. Department of Health and Human Services.

Wai, S. N., et al. 2017. Dietary patterns and clinical outcomes in chronic kidney disease: The CKD.QLD nutrition study. *Journal of Renal Nutrition* 27(3): 175–182.

Name _____ **Section** _____ **Date** _____

LAB 1.1 Your Wellness Profile

Consider how your lifestyle, attitudes, and characteristics relate to each of the dimensions of wellness. Fill in at least three strengths for each dimension (examples of strengths are listed with each dimension). Once you've completed your lists, choose what you believe are your five most important strengths and circle them.

Physical wellness: To maintain overall physical health and engage in appropriate physical activity (e.g., stamina, strength, flexibility, healthy body composition).

_____

_____

_____

Emotional wellness: To have a positive self-concept, deal constructively with your feelings, and develop positive qualities (e.g., optimism, trust, self-confidence, determination).

_____

_____

_____

Intellectual wellness: To pursue and retain knowledge, think critically about issues, make sound decisions, identify problems, and find solutions (e.g., common sense, creativity, curiosity).

_____

_____

_____

Interpersonal/social wellness: To develop and maintain meaningful relationships with a network of friends and family members, and to contribute to your community (e.g., friendly, good-natured, compassionate, supportive, good listener).

_____

_____

_____

Cultural wellness: To accept, value, and even celebrate personal and cultural differences (e.g., refuse to stereotype based on ethnicity, gender, religion, or sexual orientation; create relationships with those who are different from you; maintain and value your own cultural identity).

_____

_____

_____

Spiritual wellness: To develop a set of beliefs, principles, or values that gives meaning or purpose to your life; to develop faith in something beyond yourself (e.g., religious faith, service to others).

_____

_____

_____

Environmental wellness: To protect yourself from environmental hazards and to minimize the negative impact of your behavior on the environment (e.g., carpooling, recycling).

_____

_____

_____

Financial wellness: To be able to live within your means and manage your money in a way that gives you peace of mind (e.g., drawing up a budget, setting up a savings account).

_____

_____

_____

Occupational wellness: To gain a measure of happiness and fulfillment through your work (e.g., enjoy what you do, feel valued by your manager, build positive relationships with coworkers, take advantage of opportunities to learn and be challenged).

_____

_____

_____

LABORATORY ACTIVITIES

Next, think about where you fall on the wellness continuum for each of the dimensions of wellness. Indicate your placement for each—physical, emotional, intellectual, interpersonal/social, cultural, spiritual, environmental, financial, and occupational—by placing Xs on the continuum below.

| Low level of wellness | Physical, psychological, emotional symptoms | Change and growth | High level of wellness |

Based on both your current lifestyle and your goals for the future, what do you think your placement on the wellness continuum will be in 10 years? What new health behaviors will you have to adopt to achieve your goals? Which of your current behaviors will you need to change to maintain or improve your level of wellness in the future?

_____

_____

Does the description of wellness given in this chapter encompass everything you believe to be part of wellness for you? Write your own definition of wellness, including any additional dimensions that are important to you. Then rate your level of wellness based on your own definition.

_____

_____

Using Your Results

How did you score? Are you satisfied with your current level of wellness—overall and in each dimension? In which dimension(s) would you most like to increase your level of wellness?

_____

_____

What should you do next? As you consider possible target behaviors for a behavior change program, choose things that will maintain or increase your level of wellness in one of the dimensions you listed as an area of concern. Remember to consider health behaviors that may threaten your level of wellness in the future, such as smoking or eating a high-fat diet. List several possible target behaviors and the wellness dimensions that they influence.

Target behavior   **Wellness dimension**

1. _____   _____

2. _____   _____

3. _____   _____

For additional guidance in choosing a target behavior, complete the lifestyle self-assessment in Lab 1.2.

Name _____ Section _____ Date _____

LAB 1.2 Lifestyle Evaluation

How does your current lifestyle compare with the lifestyle recommended for wellness? For each question, choose the answer that best describes your behavior. Then add up your score for each section.

Exercise/Fitness

	Almost Always	Sometimes	Never
1. I engage in moderate exercise, such as brisk walking or swimming, for the equivalent of at least 150 minutes per week.	4	1	0
2. I do exercises to develop muscular strength and endurance at least twice a week.	2	1	0
3. I spend some of my leisure time participating in individual, family, or team activities, such as gardening, bowling, or softball.	2	1	0
4. I maintain a healthy body weight, avoiding overweight and underweight.	2	1	0

Exercise/Fitness Score: _____

Nutrition

	Almost Always	Sometimes	Never
1. I eat a variety of foods each day, including seven or more servings of fruits and/or vegetables.	3	1	0
2. I limit the amount of saturated and trans fat in my diet.	3	1	0
3. I avoid skipping meals.	2	1	0
4. I limit the amount of salt and added sugars I eat.	2	1	0

Nutrition Score: _____

Tobacco and Nicotine

	Almost Always	Sometimes	Never
1. I avoid smoking cigarettes.	4	1	0
2. I avoid using pipes, cigars, and e-cigarettes.	2	1	0
3. I avoid spit tobacco.	2	1	0
4. I limit my exposure to environmental tobacco smoke.	2	1	0

Tobacco Use Score: _____

Alcohol and Drugs

	Almost Always	Sometimes	Never
1. I avoid alcohol, or I drink no more than one (women) or two (men) drinks a day.	4	1	0
2. I avoid using alcohol or other drugs as a way of handling stressful situations or the problems in my life.	2	1	0
3. I am careful not to drink alcohol when taking medications (such as cold or allergy medications) or when pregnant.	2	1	0
4. I read and follow the label directions when using prescribed and over-the-counter drugs.	2	1	0

Alcohol and Drugs Score: _____

Emotional Health

	Almost Always	Sometimes	Never
1. I enjoy being a student, and I have a job or do other work that I enjoy.	2	1	0
2. I find it easy to relax and express my feelings freely.	2	1	0
3. I manage stress well.	2	1	0
4. I have close friends, relatives, or others whom I can talk to about personal matters and call on for help when needed.	2	1	0
5. I participate in group activities (such as community or church organizations) or hobbies that I enjoy.	2	1	0

Emotional Health Score: _____

LABORATORY ACTIVITIES

	Almost Always	Sometimes	Never
Safety			
1. I wear a safety belt while riding in a car.	2	1	0
2. I avoid driving while under the influence of alcohol or other drugs.	2	1	0
3. I obey traffic rules and the speed limit when driving.	2	1	0
4. I read and follow instructions on the labels of potentially harmful products or substances, such as household cleaners, poisons, and electrical appliances.	2	1	0
5. I avoid using a cell phone while driving.	2	1	0

Safety Score: _____

	Almost Always	Sometimes	Never
Disease Prevention			
1. I know the warning signs of cancer, heart attack, and stroke.	2	1	0
2. I avoid overexposure to the sun and use sunscreen.	2	1	0
3. I get recommended medical screening tests (such as blood pressure and cholesterol checks and Pap tests), immunizations, and booster shots.	2	1	0
4. I do not share needles to inject drugs.	2	1	0
5. I am not sexually active, *or* I have sex with only one mutually faithful, uninfected partner, *or* I always engage in safer sex (using condoms).	2	1	0

Disease Prevention Score: _____

Scores of 9 and 10 Excellent! Your answers show that you are aware of the importance of this area to your health. More important, you are putting your knowledge to work for you by practicing good health habits. As long as you continue to do so, this area should not pose a serious health risk.

Scores of 6 to 8 Your health practices in this area are good, but there is room for improvement.

Scores of 3 to 5 Your health risks are showing.

Scores of 0 to 2 You may be taking serious and unnecessary risks with your health.

Using Your Results

How did you score? In which areas did you score the lowest? Are you satisfied with your scores in each area? In which areas would you most like to improve your scores?

_____

_____

What should you do next? To improve your scores, look closely at any item to which you answered "sometimes" or "never." Identify and list at least three possible targets for a health behavior change program. (If you are aware of other risky health behaviors you currently engage in, but that were not covered by this assessment, you may include those in your list.) For each item on your list, identify your current "stage of change" and one strategy you could adopt to move forward (see the section "Enhancing Your Readiness to Change"). Possible strategies might include obtaining information about the behavior, completing an analysis of the pros and cons of change, or beginning a written record of your target behavior.

Behavior	**Stage**	**Strategy**
1. _____	_____	_____
2. _____	_____	_____
3. _____	_____	_____

SOURCE: Adapted from *Healthstyle: A Self-Test*, developed by the U.S. Public Health Service. The behaviors covered in this test are recommended for most Americans, but some may not apply to people with certain chronic diseases or disabilities or to pregnant women, who may require special advice from their physician.

Design elements: Evidence for Exercise box (shoes and stethoscope): Vstock LLC/Tetra Images/Getty Images; Take Charge box (lady walking): VisualCommunications/E+/Getty Images; Critical Consumer box (man): Sam74100/iStock/Getty Images; Diversity Matters box (holding devices): Robert Churchill/iStockphoto/Rawpixel Ltd/Getty Images; Wellness in the Digital Age box (Smart Watch): Hong Li/DigitalVision/Getty Images

Principles of Physical Fitness

LOOKING AHEAD...

After reading this chapter, you should be able to

- Describe how much physical activity is recommended for developing health and fitness.

- Identify the components of physical fitness and the way each component affects wellness.

- Explain the goal and basic principles of physical training.

- Describe the principles involved in designing a well-rounded exercise program.

- List the steps for making an exercise program safe, effective, and successful.

TEST YOUR KNOWLEDGE

1. To improve your health, you must exercise vigorously for at least 30 minutes straight, 5 or more days per week. True or false?

2. Which of the following activities uses about 150 calories?
   a. washing a car for 45–60 minutes
   b. shooting a basketball for 30 minutes
   c. jumping rope for 15 minutes
   d. all three

3. Regular exercise can make a person smarter. True or false?

See answers on the next page.

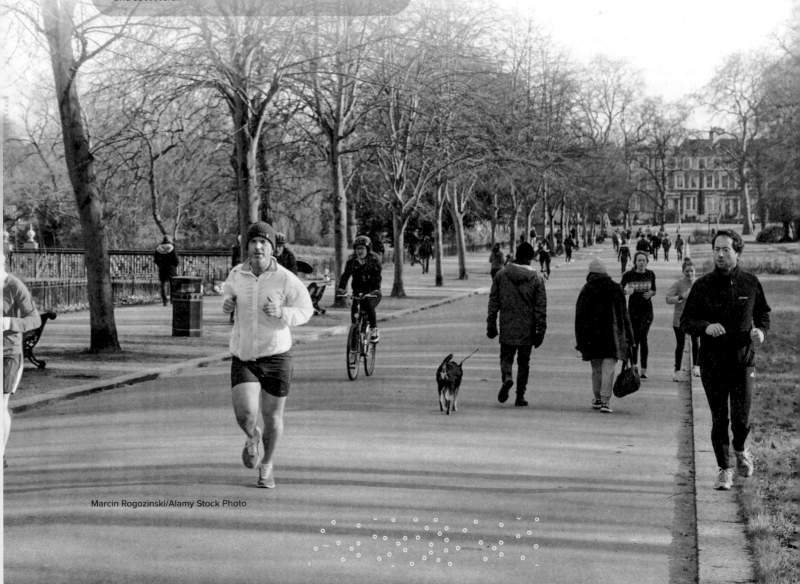

Marcin Rogozinski/Alamy Stock Photo

Any list of the benefits of physical activity is impressive. Although people vary greatly in physical fitness and performance ability, the benefits of regular physical activity are available to everyone. Much of the increased health benefits from exercise occurs when going from no activity (sedentary) to some moderate-intensity activity (Figure 2.1). Further health benefits occur when exercising harder or longer. The relative risk of death from all causes and the risk of heart disease decrease by as much as 65% when comparing the least and most active men and women. In Figure 2.1, relative risk of death refers to the risk of death per year of sedentary people compared to people in various activity levels.

This chapter provides an overview of physical fitness. It explains how both lifestyle physical activity and more formal exercise programs contribute to wellness. It also describes the components of fitness, the basic principles of physical training, and the essential elements of a well-rounded exercise program. Chapters 3, 4, 5, and 6 provide in-depth looks at the elements of a fitness program; Chapter 7 puts these elements together in a complete, personalized program.

PHYSICAL ACTIVITY AND EXERCISE FOR HEALTH AND FITNESS

Almost any physical activity promotes health. Try to be more active during the day, regardless of whether you can fit in a formal workout. Short periods of intense exercise do not compensate for hours of inactivity. So try to get up and move around each hour when studying, working on the computer, or watching TV (see the box "Move More, Sit Less"). Physical activity and exercise are points along a continuum.

Physical Activity on a Continuum

Physical activity is movement that is carried out by the skeletal muscles and requires energy. Different physical activities can vary by ease or intensity. Standing up or walking down a hallway requires little energy or effort, but each is a higher level of activity than sitting or lying down. More intense sustained activities, such as cycling five miles or running in a race, require considerably more effort.

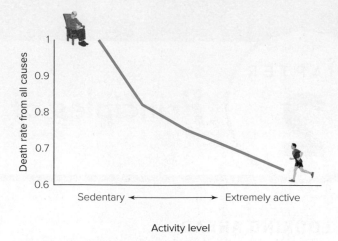

Figure 2.1 Exercise promotes longevity. The risk of death each year from all causes decreases with increased amounts and intensities of weekly physical activity.

SOURCES: Adapted from a composite of 12 studies involving over 300,000 men and women. 2018 Physical Activity Guidelines Advisory Committee. 2018. *2018 Physical Activity Guidelines Advisory Committee Scientific Report.* Washington, DC: U.S. Department of Health and Human Services; Schnohr, P., et al. 2015. "Dose of jogging and long-term mortality: the Copenhagen City Heart Study," *Journal American College of Cardiology* 65(5): 411–419.

Exercise refers to planned, structured, repetitive movement intended specifically to improve or maintain physical fitness. As discussed in Chapter 1, physical fitness is a set of physical attributes that allows the body to respond or adapt to the demands and stress of physical effort—to perform moderate to vigorous levels of physical activity without becoming overly tired. Levels of fitness depend on such physiological factors as the heart's ability to pump blood and the energy-generating capacity of the cells. These factors in turn depend both on *genetics*—a person's inborn potential for physical fitness—and *behavior*—getting enough physical activity to stress the body and cause long-term physiological changes.

Physical activity is essential to health and confers wide-ranging health benefits, but exercise is necessary to significantly improve physical fitness. This important distinction between physical activity, which improves health and wellness, and exercise, which improves fitness, is a key concept in understanding the guidelines discussed in this section.

Increasing Physical Activity to Improve Health and Wellness According to the U.S. Surgeon General's Office, "Engaging in regular physical activity is one of the most important things that people of all ages can do to improve their health." Physical activity is central to the national prevention strategy to improve health by promoting community design to support active lifestyles, encouraging exercise in young people, providing safe and accessible places for sports and exercise, and supporting physical activity in the workplace. The U.S. Department of Health and Human Services, American College of Sports Medicine, the American Heart Association, and the Surgeon General's Office have made specific exercise recommendations for promoting health. Their reports stress the importance of

A regular exercise program provides huge wellness benefits, but it does not cancel out all the negative effects of too much sitting during the day. Advances in technology promote sedentary behavior; we can now work or study at a desk, watch TV or play video games in our leisure time, order takeout and delivery for meals, and shop and bank online. To avoid the negative health effects of too little daily activity, you may need a plan to reduce your sitting time. Try some of these strategies:

- Stand up and/or walk when you are on work or personal phone calls, in a meeting or study session, or on a coffee break.

- Take the stairs whenever and wherever you can; walk up and down escalators instead of just riding them.

- At work, walk to a coworker's desk rather than e-mailing or calling; take the long route to the restroom; and take a walk break whenever you take a coffee or snack break. Drink plenty of water so that you'll have to take frequent restroom breaks.

- Set reminders to get up and move: Use commercial breaks while watching TV; at work or while using a digital device, use the clock function on your computer or phone to make sure you don't sit for longer than an hour at a time.

- Engage in active chores and leisure activities.

- Track your sedentary time to get a baseline, and then continue monitoring to note any improvements. You can also use a fitness tracker such as the Fitbit or step counter to track your general activity level or to set reminders to get up and move after sitting for a particular length of time.

regular physical activity and emphasize that some physical activity is better than none. They also present evidence that regular activity promotes health and prevents premature death and a variety of diseases (see Figure 2.1). The reports include these key guidelines for adults:

- For substantial health benefits, adults should do at least 150 minutes (2 hours and 30 minutes) a week of moderate-intensity aerobic physical activity, or 75 minutes (1 hour and 15 minutes) a week of vigorous-intensity aerobic physical activity, or an equivalent combination of moderate- and vigorous-intensity aerobic activity. As a rule of thumb for calculating a weekly total, 1 minute of vigorous-intensity activity is the equivalent of 2 minutes of moderate-intensity activity. Any amount of moderate- to vigorous-intensity activity contributes to these goals.

- For additional and more extensive health benefits, adults should increase their aerobic physical activity to 300 minutes (5 hours) a week of moderate-intensity activity, or 150 minutes a week of vigorous-intensity activity, or an equivalent combination of moderate- and vigorous-intensity activity. Adults can enjoy additional health benefits by engaging in physical activity beyond this amount. The Health and Retirement Study—a long-term study of older adults sponsored by the National Institute on Aging—found that people who exercised vigorously had a lower death rate than those who exercised at moderate intensities or did no physical activity. After 16 years, the survival rate was 84% in those doing vigorous exercise, 78% in those doing moderate-intensity physical activity, and only 65% in those doing no physical activity.

- Adults should also do muscle-strengthening activities, such as moderate- or high-intensity weight training or body weight exercise involving all major muscle groups on two or more days a week. These activities provide additional health benefits—for example, they prevent muscle loss and falls in older adults.

- Everyone should avoid inactivity. Spend less time in front of a television or computer screen because such inactivity decreases metabolic health, contributes to a sedentary lifestyle, and increases the risk of obesity.

The reports state that physical activity benefits people of all ages and of all racial and ethnic groups, including people with disabilities. The reports emphasize that the benefits of activity outweigh the dangers. These levels of physical activity promote health and wellness by lowering the risk of high blood pressure, stroke, heart disease, type 2 diabetes, colon cancer, and osteoporosis and by reducing feelings of mild to moderate depression and anxiety.

What is moderate physical activity? Activities such as brisk walking, dancing, swimming, cycling, and yard work can all count toward the daily total. A moderate amount of activity uses about 150 **calories** of energy and causes a noticeable increase in heart rate, such as would occur with a brisk walk. Examples of activities that use about 150 calories in 15–60 minutes are shown in Figure 2.2. You can burn the same number of calories by doing a lower-intensity activity for a longer time or a higher-intensity activity for a shorter time. People are most likely to participate in physical activities they enjoy, such as dancing.

In contrast to moderate-intensity activity, *vigorous* physical activity—such as jogging—causes rapid breathing and a

physical activity Body movement that is carried out by the skeletal muscles and requires energy. **TERMS**

exercise Planned, structured, repetitive movement intended to improve or maintain physical fitness.

calorie The commonly used term for *kilocalorie,* which is a measure of energy equal to the amount of heat it takes to raise the temperature of 1 liter of water 1°C. One kilocalorie contains 1,000 calories, but the familiar term *calorie* is often used for the larger energy unit, including on food labels.

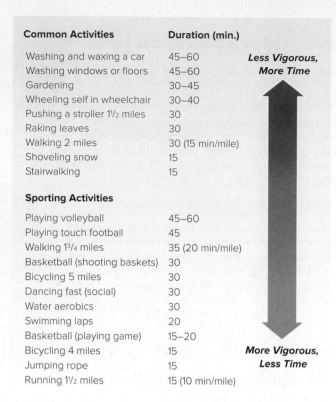

Common Activities	Duration (min.)	
Washing and waxing a car	45–60	**Less Vigorous, More Time**
Washing windows or floors	45–60	
Gardening	30–45	
Wheeling self in wheelchair	30–40	
Pushing a stroller 1½ miles	30	
Raking leaves	30	
Walking 2 miles	30 (15 min/mile)	
Shoveling snow	15	
Stairwalking	15	
Sporting Activities		
Playing volleyball	45–60	
Playing touch football	45	
Walking 1¾ miles	35 (20 min/mile)	
Basketball (shooting baskets)	30	
Bicycling 5 miles	30	
Dancing fast (social)	30	
Water aerobics	30	
Swimming laps	20	
Basketball (playing game)	15–20	
Bicycling 4 miles	15	
Jumping rope	15	**More Vigorous, Less Time**
Running 1½ miles	15 (10 min/mile)	

Figure 2.2 Examples of moderate-intensity physical activity. Each example uses about 150 calories.

SOURCE: National Heart, Lung, and Blood Institute, *Why Is Exercise Important?* (www .nhlbi.nih.gov/health/public/heart/obesity/lose_wt/physical/htm; September 1, 2015).

substantial increase in heart rate (Table 2.1). Physical activity and exercise recommendations for promoting general health, fitness, and weight management are shown in Table 2.2.

The daily total of physical activity can be accumulated in multiple bouts of 10 or more minutes per day—for example, two 10-minute bike rides to and from class and a brisk 10-minute walk to the store. In this lifestyle approach to physical activity, people can choose activities that they find enjoyable and that fit into their daily routine; everyday tasks at school, work, and home can be structured to contribute to the daily activity total. If Americans who are currently sedentary were to increase their lifestyle physical activity to 30 minutes per day, both public health and their individual well-being would benefit enormously (see the box "Exercise Is Good for Your Brain").

Increasing Physical Activity to Manage Weight

Because two-thirds of Americans are overweight, the U.S. Department of Health and Human Services has also published physical activity guidelines focusing on weight management. These guidelines recognize that for people who need to prevent weight gain, lose weight, or maintain weight loss, 150–300 minutes per week of physical activity may not be enough. Instead, they recommend up to 90 minutes of physical activity per day. Unfortunately, exercise alone will seldom promote long-term weight loss; but exercise has many health benefits, even in the absence of substantial weight loss.

Exercising to Improve Physical Fitness As men-

tioned earlier, moderate physical activity confers significant health and wellness benefits, especially for those who are

Table 2.1	Examples of Moderate- and Vigorous-Intensity Exercise

MODERATE-INTENSITY ACTIVITY

Uses 3.5–7 calories per minute and causes your breathing and heart rate to increase but still allows for comfortable conversation:

- Actively playing with children or pets
- Archery
- Ballroom dancing
- Bicycling or stationary bike, moderate pace
- Downhill skiing, moderate intensity
- Figure skating, recreational
- Fly fishing or walking along stream
- Gardening or yard work, moderate pace
- Golf
- Hiking, leisurely pace
- Horseback riding, recreational
- Housework, moderate intensity
- Skateboarding
- Softball
- Using stair-climber, elliptical trainer, or rowing machine, moderate pace
- Table tennis
- Tennis, doubles
- Walking at a moderate pace: walking to school or work, walking for pleasure
- Water aerobics
- Waxing the car
- Weight training and bodybuilding
- Yoga

VIGOROUS-INTENSITY ACTIVITY

Uses more than 7 calories per minute and increases your heart and breathing rates considerably. These exercises cause larger increases in physical fitness:

- Group exercise: high-impact step aerobics, aerobic dance
- Backpacking
- Basketball, recreational
- Bicycling, high intensity
- Calisthenics, vigorous: jumping jacks, burpees, air squats
- Circuit weight training
- Cross-country skiing or snowshoeing
- Cross-training, such as CrossFit
- Downhill skiing, vigorous intensity
- Football, recreational
- Gardening or yard work, shoveling heavy snow, digging ditches
- Hand cycling
- Horseback riding, galloping or jumping
- In line skating
- Interval training: running, elliptical trainer, swimming, cycling
- Jogging
- Kayaking, whitewater
- Pushing a car
- Running up stairs
- Soccer, recreational
- Tennis, singles
- Wheelchair wheeling training

SOURCE: Centers for Disease Control and Prevention. 2015. *General Physical Activities Defined by Level of Intensity.* (http://www.cdc.gov/nccdphp/dnpa/ physical/pdf/PA_Intensity_table_2_1.pdf).

Table 2.2	Physical Activity and Exercise Recommendations for Promoting General Health, Fitness, and Weight Management

GOAL	RECOMMENDATION
General health	Perform moderate-intensity aerobic physical activity for at least 150 minutes per week (30 minutes 5 times per week) or 75 minutes of vigorous-intensity physical activity per week (25 minutes 3 times per week). Also, be more active in your daily life: Walk instead of driving, take the stairs instead of the elevator, and watch less television.
Increased health benefits	Exercise at moderate intensity for 300 minutes per week or at vigorous intensity for 150 minutes per week.
Achieve or maintain weight loss	Exercise moderately for 60–90 minutes per day on most days of the week.
Muscle strength and endurance	Perform 1 or more sets of resistance exercises that work the major muscle groups for 8–12 repetitions (10–15 reps for older adults) on at least two nonconsecutive days per week. Examples include weight training and exercises that use body weight as resistance (such as core-stabilizing exercises, pull-ups, push-ups, lunges, and squats).
Flexibility	Perform range-of-motion (stretching) exercises at least two or three days per week. Hold each stretch for 10–30 seconds.
Neuromuscular training	Older adults should do balance training at least two or three days per week. Examples include yoga, tai chi, and balance exercises (standing on one foot, step-ups, and walking lunges). These exercises are beneficial for young and middle-aged adults, as well.

SOURCES: American College of Sports Medicine. 2017. *ACSM's Guidelines for Exercise Testing and Prescription,* 10th ed. Philadelphia: Wolters Kluwer; Garber, C. E., et al. 2011. "Quantity and quality of exercise for developing and maintaining cardiorespiratory, musculoskeletal, and neuromotor fitness in apparently healthy adults: Guidance for prescribing exercise," *Medicine and Science in Sports and Exercise* 43(7): 1334–1359; 2018 Physical Activity Guidelines Advisory Committee. 2018. *2018 Physical Activity Guidelines Advisory Committee Scientific Report.* Washington, DC: U.S. Department of Health and Human Services.

currently sedentary and become moderately active. However, people can obtain even greater health and wellness benefits by increasing the duration and intensity of physical activity. With increased activity, they will see more improvements in quality of life and greater reductions in disease and mortality risk.

More vigorous activity, as in a structured, systematic exercise program, also improves physical fitness. Moderate physical activity alone is not enough. Physical fitness requires more intense movement that poses a substantially greater challenge to the body. The American College of Sports Medicine has issued guidelines for creating a formal exercise program that will develop physical fitness. These guidelines are described in detail later in the chapter.

How Much Physical Activity Is Enough?

Some experts believe that people get most of the health benefits of physical activity simply by becoming more active over the course of the day; the amount of activity needed depends on an individual's health status and goals. Other experts believe that leisure-time physical activity is not enough; they argue that people should exercise long enough and intensely enough to improve the body's capacity for exercise—that is, to improve physical fitness. There is probably some truth in both of these positions.

Regular physical activity, regardless of the intensity, makes you healthier and can help protect you from many chronic diseases. Although you get many of the health benefits of exercise by being more active, you obtain even more benefits when you are physically fit. In addition to long-term health benefits, fitness also contributes significantly to quality of life. Fitness can give you freedom to move your body the way you want. Fit people have more energy and better body control. They can enjoy a more active lifestyle than their more sedentary counterparts. Even if you don't like sports, you need physical energy and stamina in your daily life and

for many non-sport leisure activities, such as visiting museums, playing with children, and gardening.

Where does this leave you? Most experts agree that some physical activity is better than none, but that more—as long as it does not result in injury—is better than some. To set a personal goal for physical activity and exercise, consider your current activity level, your health status, and your overall goals. At the very least, strive to become more active and do 30 minutes of moderate-intensity activity at least five days per week. Choose to be active whenever you can. If weight management is a concern for you, begin by achieving the goal of 30 minutes of activity per day and then try to raise your activity level further, to 60–90 minutes per day or more. For even better health and well-being, participate in a structured exercise program that develops physical fitness. Any increase in physical activity will contribute to your health and well-being, now and in the future.

COMPONENTS OF PHYSICAL FITNESS

Some components of fitness relate to specific skill activities, such as tennis and skiing, and others to general health. **Health-related fitness** includes the following components:

- Cardiorespiratory endurance
- Muscular strength
- Muscular endurance
- Flexibility
- Body composition

health-related fitness Physical capacities that contribute to health: cardiorespiratory endurance, muscular strength, muscular endurance, flexibility, and body composition. TERMS

THE EVIDENCE FOR EXERCISE
Exercise Is Good for Your Brain

Some scientists call exercise the new "brain food." Studies show that even moderate physical activity can improve brain health and function and may delay the decline in cognitive function that occurs for many people as they age. Regular physical activity has these positive effects on the brain:

- Endurance and resistance exercise improve cognitive function—the brain's ability to learn, remember, think, and reason. Exercising before an exam might boost your score.

- Exercise can help overcome the negative effects of a poor diet on brain health.

- Exercise promotes the creation of new nerve cells (neurons) throughout the nervous system. By promoting this process (called *neurogenesis*), exercise provides protection against injury and degenerative conditions that destroy neurons. Physical activity is less effective for promoting brain health when exercising in polluted air.

- Exercise enhances the nervous system's *plasticity*—its ability to change and adapt. In the brain, spinal cord, and nerves, this can mean developing new pathways for transmitting sensory information or motor commands.

- Exercise has a protective effect on the brain as people age, helping to delay or even prevent the onset of neurodegenerative disorders such as Alzheimer's disease. Exercise can reduce age-related shrinkage of the hippocampus, a brain structure involved in memory, learning, and emotions.

- Exercise reduces anxiety—a consistent finding independent of culture, gender, age, education, and socioeconomic status. It promotes the release of endorphins, which in turn promotes feelings of well-being and prevents depression.

Although most people consider brain health to be a concern for the elderly, it is vital to wellness throughout life. For this reason, many studies on exercise and brain health include children as well as older adults. Exercise improves health and well-being in people with disorders such as cerebral palsy, multiple sclerosis, and developmental disabilities.

Along with the brain's physical health, mental health is enhanced by exercise. Even modest activity, such as taking a

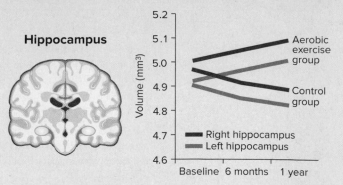

Hippocampus

In a study of older adults, aerobic exercise training increased the volume of the hippocampus, effectively reversing age-related loss of volume by 1 to 2 years.

SOURCE: Erickson, K. I., et al. 2011. "Exercise training increases size of hippocampus and improves memory," *Proceedings of the National Academy of Sciences 108*(7), 3017–3022. Reprinted with permission.

daily walk, can help combat a variety of mental health disorders and improve mood.

It's hard to understate the impact of physical and mental disorders related to brain health. According to the Alzheimer's Association, 5.3 million Americans currently suffer from Alzheimer's disease, and the number is increasing by 70 people per second. People with depression, anxiety, or other mental disorders are more likely to suffer from chronic physical conditions. Taken together, these and other brain-related disorders cost untold millions of dollars in health care costs and lost productivity, as well as thousands of years of productive lifetime lost.

So, for your brain—as well as your muscles, bones, and heart—start creating your exercise program soon. You'll be healthier, and you may even feel a little smarter.

SOURCES: 2018 Physical Activity Guidelines Advisory Committee. 2018. *2018 Physical Activity Guidelines Advisory Committee Scientific Report.* Washington, DC: U.S. Department of Health and Human Services; Stubbs, B., et al. 2015. "Physical activity and anxiety," *Journal Affective Disorders* 208, 545–552; Erickson, K. I., et al. 2011. "Exercise training increases size of hippocampus and improves memory," *Proceedings of the National Academy of Sciences* 108(7): 3017–3022; Szuhany, K. L., et al. 2015. "A meta-analytic review of the effects of exercise on brain-derived neurotrophic factor," *Journal of Psychiatric Research* 60, 56–64.

Health-related fitness helps you withstand physical challenges and protects you from diseases.

Cardiorespiratory Endurance

Cardiorespiratory endurance is the ability to perform prolonged, large-muscle, dynamic exercise at moderate to high levels of intensity. It depends on such factors as the ability of the lungs to deliver **oxygen** from the environment to the bloodstream, the capacity of the heart to pump blood, the ability of the nervous system and blood vessels to regulate blood flow, and the

capability of the cells' chemical systems to use oxygen and process fuels for exercise and rest.

TERMS

cardiorespiratory endurance The ability of the body to perform prolonged, large-muscle, dynamic exercise at moderate to high levels of intensity.

oxygen An element that makes up 20.8% of the atmosphere that is bound to a second oxygen atom in the environment. It is critical for generating usable energy in the body and is an important component of carbohydrates, fats, and proteins.

When cardiorespiratory fitness is low, the heart has to work hard during normal daily activities and may not be able to work hard enough to sustain high-intensity physical activity in an emergency. As cardiorespiratory fitness improves, related physical functions also improve:

- The heart pumps more blood per heartbeat.
- The ability to consume oxygen due to adaptations in the heart, circulation, and tissues improves.
- Breathing volume decreases during daily activities and submaximal exercising—that is, when exercising at less than full intensity.
- Resting heart rate slows.
- Blood volume increases.
- Blood supply to tissues improves.
- The body can cool itself better.
- Blood vessels become more pliable.
- Resting blood pressure decreases.
- Metabolism in skeletal muscle is enhanced, which improves fuel use.
- The level of antioxidant chemicals in the body increases and oxidative stress decreases. During metabolism, the body naturally produces chemicals called free radicals (oxidative stress) that cause cell damage. Exercise training increases the production of antioxidants that help neutralize free radicals.

A healthy heart can better withstand the strains of everyday life, the stress of occasional emergencies, and the wear and tear of time.

Cardiovascular endurance training also improves the functioning of the body's chemical systems, particularly in the muscles and liver. These changes enhance the body's ability to derive energy from food, allow the body to perform more exercise with less effort, increase sensitivity to insulin, and prevent type 2 diabetes. Exercise reduces blood vessel inflammation, which is linked to coronary artery disease, heart attack, and stroke. Exercise helps maintain normal levels of water and electrolytes in the cells, which in turn preserves muscle cell function and delays fatigue.

Physically fit people also have healthier, more resilient genes. Exercise preserves gene structures called telomeres, which form the ends of the DNA strands and hold them together. Over time the telomeres shorten, reducing their effectiveness, which triggers illness and death. Exercise helps to keep them from getting too short.

Cardiorespiratory endurance is a central component of health-related fitness because heart and lung function is so essential to overall good health. A person can't live long or well without a healthy heart or healthy lungs. Poor cardiorespiratory fitness is linked with heart disease, type 2 diabetes, colon cancer, stroke, depression, and anxiety. A moderate level of cardiorespiratory fitness can help compensate for certain health risks, including excess body fat: People who have higher levels of body fat but who otherwise are fit have been found to have lower death rates than those who are lean but have low cardiorespiratory fitness.

You can develop cardiorespiratory endurance through activities that involve continuous, rhythmic movements of large-muscle groups, such as the legs. Such activities include walking, jogging, cycling, and group aerobics.

? Ask Yourself

QUESTIONS FOR CRITICAL THINKING AND REFLECTION

Does your current lifestyle include enough physical activity—30 minutes of moderate-intensity activity five or more days a week—to support health and wellness? Does your lifestyle go beyond this level to include enough vigorous physical activity and exercise to build physical fitness? What changes could you make in your lifestyle to develop physical fitness?

Muscular Strength

Muscular strength is the ability of a muscle to exert force in a single maximum effort. It depends on such factors as the size of muscle cells and the ability of nerves to activate muscle cells. **Relative strength** is the maximum force exerted relative to body weight, body size, and muscle size. Strong muscles are important for everyday activities, such as climbing stairs, as well as for emergency situations. They help keep the skeleton in proper alignment, preventing back and leg pain and providing the support necessary

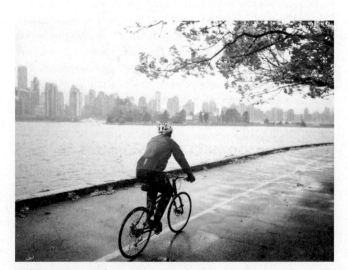

Fitness Tip Cardiorespiratory endurance is a key component of health-related fitness. Like studying, you'll be more likely to exercise if you set aside blocks of time for it and make it part of your daily routine. Schedule your workouts, make them a priority, and include alternatives to account for things such as bad weather and vacations.

John P Kelly/The Image Bank/Getty Images

muscular strength The ability of a muscle to exert force in a single maximum effort.

relative strength The maximum force exerted, relative to body weight, body size, and muscle size.

TERMS

for good posture. Muscular strength has obvious importance in recreational activities. Strong people can hit a tennis ball harder, kick a soccer ball farther, and ride a bicycle uphill more easily.

Muscle tissue is an important element of overall body composition. Greater muscle mass means faster energy use and a higher rate of **metabolism**, and the sum of all the vital processes by which food energy and nutrients are made available to and used by the body. Greater muscle mass reduces markers of oxidative stress and maintains mitochondria (the "powerhouses" of the cell); both of these benefits are important for metabolic health and long life. Training to build muscular strength can also help people manage stress and boost their self-confidence.

Maintaining strength and muscle mass is vital for healthy aging. Stronger people live longer. Older people tend to experience a decrease in both number and size of muscle cells, a condition called *sarcopenia*. Many of the remaining muscle cells become slower, and some become nonfunctional because they lose their attachment to the nervous system. Strength training (also known as *resistance training* or *weight training*) increases antioxidant enzymes and lowers oxidative stress. It also helps maintain muscle mass and function and possibly helps decrease the risk of osteoporosis (bone loss) in older people, greatly enhancing their quality of life and preventing life-threatening injuries.

Muscular Endurance

Muscular endurance is the ability to resist fatigue and sustain a given level of muscle tension—that is, to hold a muscle contraction for a long time or to contract a muscle over and over again. It depends on such factors as the size of muscle cells, the ability of muscles to store fuel, blood supply, and the metabolic capacity of muscles.

Muscular endurance is important for good posture and for injury prevention. For example, if abdominal and back muscles cannot support and stabilize the spine correctly when you sit or stand for long periods, the chances of low back pain and back injury are increased. Good muscular endurance in the trunk muscles is more important than muscular strength for preventing back pain. Muscular endurance helps people cope with daily physical demands and enhances performance in sports and work.

Flexibility

Flexibility is the ability to move the joints through their full ranges of motion. It depends on joint structure, the length and elasticity of connective tissue, and nervous system activity. Flexible, pain-free joints are important for good health and well-being. Inactivity causes the joints to become stiffer with age. Stiffness, in turn, often causes people to assume unnatural body postures that can stress joints and muscles. Stretching exercises can help ensure a healthy range of motion for all major joints.

Body Composition

Body composition refers to the proportion of fat and **fat-free mass** (muscle, bone, and water) in the body. Healthy body composition involves a high proportion of fat-free mass and an acceptably low level of body fat, adjusted for age and gender. A person with excessive body fat—especially excess fat in the abdomen—is more likely to experience health problems, including heart disease, insulin resistance, high blood pressure, stroke, joint problems, type 2 diabetes, gallbladder disease, blood vessel inflammation, some types of cancer, back pain, and premature death.

The best way to lose fat is through a lifestyle that includes a sensible diet and exercise. The best way to add muscle mass is through strength training. Large changes in body composition are not necessary to improve health; even a small increase in physical activity and a small decrease in body fat can lead to substantial health improvements.

Somatotype, or body build, affects a person's choice of exercise. *Endomorphs* are round and pear-shaped. They often excel at weight lifting and weight-supported aerobic exercises such as swimming or cycling. Conversely, they might find distance running difficult and painful. *Mesomorphs* are lean and muscular and usually excel at almost any kind of physical activity or sport. *Ectomorphs* are thin and linear. Their light frame helps them succeed in activities such as distance running and ballet. No matter what body type you have, you can benefit from some form of physical activity.

Skill (Neuromuscular)–Related Components of Fitness

In addition to the five health-related components of physical fitness, the ability to perform a particular sport or activity may depend on **skill (neuromuscular)–related fitness**. Neuromuscular refers to the complex control of muscles and movement by the brain and spinal column. The components of skill-related fitness include the following:

- *Speed*—the ability to perform a movement in a short period of time
- *Power*—the ability to exert force rapidly, based on a combination of strength and speed

---

TERMS

metabolism The sum of all the vital processes by which food energy and nutrients are made available to and used by the body.

muscular endurance The ability of a muscle to remain contracted or to contract repeatedly for a long period of time.

flexibility The ability to move joints through their full ranges of motion.

body composition The proportion of fat and fat-free mass (muscle, bone, and water) in the body.

fat-free mass The nonfat component of the human body, consisting of skeletal muscle, bone, and water.

somatotype A body-type classification system that describes people as predominantly muscular (mesomorph), tall and thin (ectomorph), or round and heavy (endomorph).

skill (neuromuscular)–related fitness Physical capacities that contribute to performance in a sport or an activity, including speed, power, agility, balance, coordination, and reaction time; neuromuscular fitness refers specifically to maintaining performance levels of balance, agility, and coordination through the control of muscles and movement by the brain and spinal column.

- *Agility*—the ability to change the position of the body quickly and accurately
- *Balance*—the ability to maintain equilibrium while moving or while stationary
- *Coordination*—the ability to perform motor tasks accurately and smoothly using body movements and the senses
- *Reaction and movement time*—the ability to respond and react quickly to a stimulus

Skill-related fitness tends to be sport-specific and is best developed through practice. For example, playing basketball can develop the speed, coordination, and agility needed to engage in the sport. Participating in sports is fun, can help build fitness, and contributes to other areas of wellness. Young adults often find it easier to exercise regularly when they participate in sports and activities they enjoy, such as dancing, tennis, snowboarding, or basketball.

While not considered a health-related fitness component, neuromuscular fitness is important for healthy aging. Older adults are at risk for life-threatening falls, and development of neuromuscular fitness can reduce the risk of falls. Neuromuscular training activities such as yoga and tai chi are recommended for older adults.

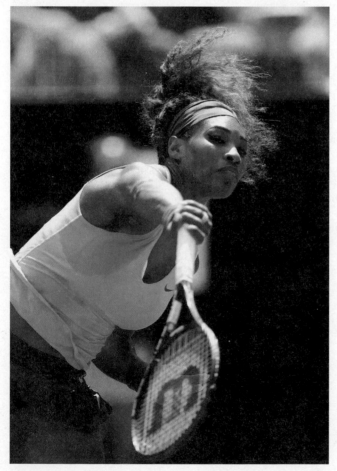

Fitness Tip You don't need to develop the skills of a professional athlete to participate in sports, but boosting sport-specific skills such as speed, power, coordination, and reaction time can make participating in sports more fun. And if you enjoy yourself, you are more likely to stick with the activity!

Clive Mason/Getty Images

PRINCIPLES OF PHYSICAL TRAINING: ADAPTATION TO STRESS

The human body is very adaptable. The greater the demands made on it, the more it adjusts to meet those demands. Over time, immediate, short-term adjustments (**adaptations**) translate into long-term changes and improvements. When breathing and heart rate increase during exercise, for example, the heart gradually develops the ability to pump more blood with each beat. Then, during exercise, it doesn't have to beat as fast to meet the cells' demands for oxygen. The goal of **physical training** is to produce these long-term changes and improvements in the body's functioning and fitness. Although people differ in the maximum levels of physical fitness and performance they can achieve through training, the wellness benefits of exercise are available to everyone (see the box "Fitness and Disability").

Particular types and amounts of exercise are most effective in developing the various components of fitness. To put together an effective exercise program, you should first understand the basic principles of physical training, including:

- Specificity
- Progressive overload
- Reversibility
- Individual differences

All of these rest on the larger principle of adaptation.

Specificity—Adapting to Type of Training

To develop a particular fitness component, you must perform exercises designed specifically for that component. This is the principle of **specificity**. Weight training, for example, develops muscular strength but is less effective for developing cardiorespiratory endurance or flexibility. Specificity also applies to the skill-related fitness components (to improve at tennis, you must practice tennis) and to the different parts of the body (to develop stronger arms, you must exercise your arms). A well-rounded exercise program includes exercises geared to each component of fitness, to different parts of the body, and to specific activities or sports.

Sports science pioneer Franklin Henry from the University of California, Berkeley, developed the principle of specificity of training. His studies showed that a specific movement performed at a specific speed develops a unique skill. Motor-control studies have shown that practice reinforces motor patterns in the brain that are

adaptation The physiological changes that occur with exercise training.

TERMS

physical training The performance of different types of activities that cause the body to adapt and improve its level of fitness.

specificity The training principle that developing a particular fitness component requires performing exercises specifically designed for that component.

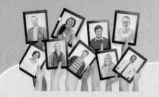

DIVERSITY MATTERS
Fitness and Disability

Physical fitness and athletic achievement are not limited to the able-bodied. People with disabilities can also attain high levels of fitness and performance. Elite athletes compete in the Paralympics, the premier event for athletes with disabilities held in the same year and city as the Olympics. The performance of these skilled athletes makes it clear that people with disabilities can be active, healthy, and extraordinarily fit. Just like able-bodied athletes, athletes with disabilities strive for excellence and can serve as role models.

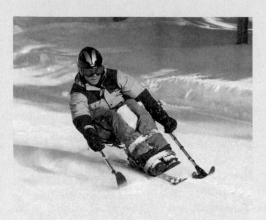

Boomer Jerritt/All Canada Photos/Getty Images

According to the U.S. Census Bureau, about 57 million Americans have some type of chronic disability. Some disabilities are the result of injury, such as spinal cord injuries sustained in car crashes or war. Other disabilities result from illness, such as the blindness that sometimes occurs as a complication of diabetes or the joint stiffness that accompanies arthritis. And some disabilities are present at birth, as in the case of congenital limb deformities or cerebral palsy.

Exercise and physical activity are as important for people with disabilities as for able-bodied individuals—if not more important. Being active helps prevent secondary conditions that may result from prolonged inactivity, such as circulatory or muscular problems. Currently, about 19% of people with disabilities engage in regular moderate-intensity activity.

People with disabilities don't have to be elite athletes to participate in sports and lead an active life. Some health clubs, fitness centers, city recreation centers, and universities offer activities and events geared for people of all ages and types of disabilities. They may have modified aerobics classes, special weight-training machines, classes for mild exercise in warm water, and other activities adapted for people with disabilities. Popular sports and recreational activities include adapted horseback riding, golf, swimming, and skiing. Competitive sports are also available—for example, there are wheelchair versions of billiards, tennis, weight lifting, hockey, and basketball, as well as sports for people with hearing, visual, or mental impairments. For those who prefer to get their exercise at home, special videos are geared to individuals who use wheelchairs or to those with arthritis, hearing impairments, metabolic diseases, or many other disabilities.

The U.S. Department of Education's Office for Civil Rights has issued guidelines for providing equal opportunities for sports and exercise to students with disabilities. Schools and universities must make reasonable modifications to ensure that students with disabilities have equal access to sports and physical education.

If you have a disability and want to be more active, check with your physician about what's appropriate for you. Contact your local community center, university, YMCA/YWCA, hospital, independent living center, or fitness center to locate facilities. Look for a facility with experienced personnel and appropriate adaptive equipment. For specialized videos, check with hospitals and health associations that address specific disabilities, such as the Arthritis Foundation.

specific to a given movement. In other words, there is no general coordination, agility, balance, and accuracy. The balance required in skiing is different from the balance required to stand on one foot or do tricks on a skateboard. Each requires its own specific training.

Progressive Overload—Adapting to the Amount of Training and the FITT-VP Principle

The body adapts to the demands placed on it. When the body is stressed by a greater-than-normal amount or intensity of exercise, the body adapts and improves fitness. The amount of new activity added above a person's usual level of activity is known as *overload*. When this stress is increased progressively, fitness continues to improve. This is the training principle of **progressive overload.**

The amount of overload is important. Too little exercise will have no effect on fitness (although it may improve health); too much may cause injury and problems with the body's immune or endocrine (hormone) systems. The point at which exercise becomes excessive is highly individual; it occurs at a much higher level in an Olympic athlete than in a sedentary person. For every type of exercise, there is a training threshold at which fitness benefits begin to occur, a zone within which maximum fitness benefits occur, and an upper limit of safe training.

The exercise needed to improve fitness depends on the individual's current level of fitness, the person's genetically determined capacity to adapt to training, his or her fitness goals, and the component being developed. A novice, for example, might

progressive overload   The training principle that progressively increasing amounts of stress on the body causes adaptation that improves fitness.

TERMS

experience fitness benefits from jogging a mile in 10 minutes, but this level of exercise would not benefit a trained distance runner. Beginners should start at the lower end of the fitness benefit zone; fitter individuals will make more rapid gains by exercising at the higher end of the fitness benefit zone. Progressive overload is critical. Performing the same exercise during every training session will maintain fitness but will not increase it because the training stress is below the threshold required to produce adaptation. Fitness increases only if overload increases.

The overload needed to maintain or improve a particular level of fitness for a particular fitness component is determined through six dimensions, represented by the acronym FITT-VP:

- *Frequency*—how often
- *Intensity*—how hard or how fast
- *Time*—how long (duration)
- *Type*—mode of activity
- *Volume*—how much (frequency × intensity × time)
- *Progression*—how a program advances over time

Chapters 3, 4, and 5 show you how to apply the FITT-VP principle to exercise programs for cardiorespiratory endurance, muscular strength and endurance, and flexibility, respectively.

Frequency Developing fitness requires regular exercise. Optimum exercise frequency, expressed in number of days per week, varies with the component being developed and the individual's fitness goals. For most people, a frequency of three to five days per week for cardiorespiratory endurance exercise and two or more days per week for resistance and flexibility training are appropriate for a general fitness program.

An important consideration in determining appropriate exercise frequency is recovery time. The time required to recover from exercise is highly individual and depends on factors such as training experience, age, and intensity of training. For example, 24 hours of rest between highly intense workouts involving heavy weights or track sprints is not usually enough recovery time for safe and effective training. Intense workouts need to be spaced out during the week to allow for sufficient recovery time. But you can exercise every day if your program consists of moderate-intensity walking or cycling. Learn to "listen to your body" to get enough rest between workouts. Chapters 3, 4, and 5 provide more detailed information about training techniques and recovery periods for workouts focused on different fitness components.

Intensity Fitness benefits occur when a person exercises harder than his or her normal level of activity. The appropriate exercise intensity varies with each fitness component. To develop cardiorespiratory endurance, for example, you must raise your heart rate above normal; you might do that by walking, swimming, or cycling faster. To develop muscular strength, you must lift a heavier weight than normal. To develop flexibility, you must stretch muscles beyond their normal length.

Time (Duration) Fitness benefits occur when you exercise for an extended period. For cardiorespiratory endurance exercise, 20–60 minutes per exercise session is recommended. Exercise can take place in a single session or in several sessions of 10 or more minutes. The greater the intensity of exercise, the less time needed to obtain fitness benefits. For high-intensity exercise, such as running, 20–30 minutes is appropriate. For moderate-intensity exercise, such as walking, 45–60 minutes may be needed. High-intensity exercise poses a greater risk of injury than low-intensity exercise, so if you are a nonathletic adult, first emphasize low- to moderate-intensity activity of longer duration.

To build muscular strength, muscular endurance, and flexibility, similar time is advisable, but training for these health components is more commonly organized in terms of a specific number of *repetitions* of a particular exercise. For resistance training, for example, a recommended program includes one or more sets of 8–12 repetitions of 8–10 different exercises that work the major muscle groups. Older adults should do 10–15 repetitions per set with lighter weights.

Type (Mode of Activity) The exercise in which you should engage varies with each fitness component and with your personal fitness goals. To develop cardiorespiratory endurance, you need to engage in continuous activities involving large-muscle groups—walking, jogging, cycling, or swimming, for example. Resistance exercises develop muscular strength and endurance, and stretching exercises build flexibility. The frequency, intensity, and time of the exercise will be different for each type of activity. (See the section "Designing Your Own Exercise Program" for more on choosing appropriate activities for your fitness program.)

Volume Volume is the product of frequency, intensity, and time—the FIT of exercise. For endurance exercise, average adults should strive to expend at least 1,000 calories per week in

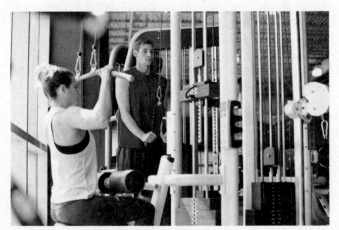

Fitness Tip Progressive overload is important because the body adapts to overload by becoming more fit. This is true even if your starting level of fitness is low. At the gym, don't be intimidated by people who seem to be in better shape than you are. Remember: They got in shape by focusing on themselves, not by worrying about what other people thought about them.

Hero Images/Getty Images

exercise, which is the equivalent of about 150 minutes per week of moderate-intensity exercise. This same volume of exercise can be accomplished in a shorter or longer time frame, depending on the FIT variables. For example, 75 minutes of vigorous-intensity exercise will also burn about 1,000 calories. Volume also applies to other fitness components: In weight training, lifting 10 pounds for 3 sets of 10 repetitions produces a total volume of 300 pounds ($10 \times 3 \times 10$); lifting 20 pounds in the same workout increases the volume to 600 pounds.

Progression Fitness levels off as the body adapts to exercise training, so you need to gradually increase overload over time to improve fitness. How quickly you adapt to training depends on your genetic makeup and the effort you put into your training program. To avoid injury, progress by slowly increasing the volume of exercise; for example, add 5 minutes to your jogging workout or add 10 pounds for a weight training exercise. Don't increase frequency, intensity, and time all at once. With each increase, make sure you can maintain your program before moving forward. Don't overtrain: Excessive exercise can cause injury and fatigue.

Reversibility—Adapting to a Reduction in Training

Fitness is a reversible adaptation. The body adjusts to lower levels of physical activity the same way it adjusts to higher levels. This is the principle of **reversibility**. When a person stops exercising, up to 50% of fitness improvements are lost within two months. However, not all fitness levels reverse at the same rate. Strength fitness is very resilient, so a person can maintain strength fitness by doing resistance exercise as infrequently as once a week. In contrast, cardiovascular and cellular fitness reverse themselves more quickly—sometimes within just a few days or weeks. If you must temporarily reduce the frequency or duration of your training, you can maintain much of your fitness improvement by keeping the intensity of your workouts constant.

Individual Differences—Limits on Adaptability

Anyone watching the Olympics can see that, from a physical standpoint, we are not all created equal. There are large individual differences in our ability to improve fitness, achieve a desirable body composition, and learn and perform sports skills. Some people are able to run longer distances, lift more weight, or kick a soccer ball more skillfully than others will ever be able to, no matter how much they train. People respond to training at different rates, so a program that works for one person may not be right for another person.

> **reversibility** The training principle that fitness improvements are lost when demands on the body are lowered.
>
> **TERMS**

There are limits on the adaptability—the potential for improvement—of any human body. The body's ability to transport and use oxygen, for example, can be improved by only about 5–30% through training. An endurance athlete must therefore inherit a large metabolic capacity to reach competitive performance levels. In the past few years, scientists have identified specific genes that influence body fat, strength, and endurance. For example, more than 800 genes are associated with endurance performance, and 100 of those determine individual differences in exercise capacity. However, physical training improves fitness regardless of heredity. The average person's body can improve enough to achieve reasonable fitness goals.

DESIGNING YOUR OWN EXERCISE PROGRAM

Physical training works best when you have a plan. A plan helps you make gradual but steady progress toward your goals. First, determine that exercise is safe for you (or your family members); then assess how fit you are, decide what your goals are, and choose the right activities to help you get there.

Getting Medical Clearance

Participating in exercise and sports is usually a wonderful experience that improves wellness in both the short and the long term. In rare instances, however, vigorous exertion is associated with sudden death. It may seem difficult to understand that although regular exercise protects people from heart disease, exercise also increases the risk of sudden death for some.

Exercise and Cardiac Risk Overall, the risk of death from exercise is small—and people are much safer exercising than engaging in many other common activities, including driving a car. One study of joggers found one death for every 396,000 hours of jogging; another study of men involved in a variety of physical activities found one death per 1.5 million hours of exercise.

In people under age 35, congenital heart defects (heart abnormalities present at birth) are the most common cause of exercise-related sudden death. In nearly all other cases, coronary artery disease is responsible. In this condition, fat and other substances build up in the arteries that supply blood to the heart. Death can result if an artery becomes blocked or if the heart's rhythm and pumping action are disrupted. Exercise, particularly intense exercise, may trigger a heart attack in someone with underlying heart disease. The riskiest scenario may involve the middle-aged or older individual who suddenly begins participating in a vigorous sport or activity after being sedentary for a long time. Engaging in very vigorous exercise over the long term can also be risky for some individuals, due to the stress on the cardiovascular system. For example, a study of joggers in Denmark found the lowest mortality rate among those who jogged a moderate amount (2–3 workouts for a total of 60–150 minutes per week); higher rates of death were found among non-joggers and those who jogged at a very intense level and/or for long distances (even moderate jogging is high-intensity exercise). Viral, bacterial, and fungal infections can also cause heart muscle inflammation and sudden death, so don't exercise when you have a fever or flu.

Where does this leave you? Overall, exercise has enough benefits that make up for a slightly increased risk of sudden death—in healthy people as well as those with heart disease. Active people who stop exercising can expect their heart attack risk to increase by 300%. The risk of heart-related sudden death in middle-aged and older adults is lowest in people who exercise approximately 150 minutes per week—the activity level recommended by the U.S. Department of Health and Human Services.

Medical Clearance Recommendations People of any age who are not at high risk for serious health problems can safely exercise at a moderate intensity (60% or less of maximum heart rate) without a prior medical evaluation (see Chapter 3 for a discussion of maximum heart rate). Likewise, if you are male and under 40 or female and under 50 and in good health, vigorous exercise is probably safe for you. If you do not fit into these age groups, or if you have health problems—especially high blood pressure, heart disease, muscle or joint problems, or obesity—see your physician before starting a vigorous exercise program. The Physical Activity Readiness Questionnaire for Everyone (PAR-Q+) can help evaluate exercise safety; it is included in Lab 2.1. Completing it should alert you to any potential problems you may have. If a physician isn't sure whether exercise is safe for you, she or he may recommend an **exercise stress test** or a **graded exercise test (GXT)** to see whether you show symptoms of heart disease during exercise. For most people, however, it's far safer to exercise than to remain sedentary.

Assessing Yourself

The first step in creating a successful fitness program is to assess your current level of physical activity and fitness for each of the five health-related fitness components. The results of the assessment tests will help you set specific fitness goals and plan your fitness program. Lab 2.3 gives you the opportunity to assess your current overall level of activity and determine if it is appropriate. Assessment tests in Chapters 3, 4, 5, and 6 will help you evaluate your cardiorespiratory endurance, muscular strength, muscular endurance, flexibility, and body composition.

Setting Goals

The ultimate general goal of every health-related fitness program is the same—wellness that lasts a lifetime. That lifelong goal might include the specific goals of walking 30–60 minutes every day or doing a few calisthenic exercises every morning. Whatever your specific goals, they must be important enough to you to keep you motivated. Most sports psychologists believe that setting and achieving goals is the most effective way to stay motivated about exercise. (Refer to Chapter 1 for more on goal setting, as well as

Common Questions Answered at the end of this chapter.) After you complete the assessment tests in Chapters 3, 4, 5, and 6, you will be able to set goals directly related to each fitness component, such as working toward a three-mile jog or doing 20 push-ups. First, though, think carefully about your overall goals, and be clear about why you are starting a program.

Choosing Activities for a Balanced Program

An ideal fitness program combines a physically active lifestyle with systematic exercise to develop and maintain physical fitness. This overall program is shown in the physical activity pyramid in Figure 2.3. If you are currently sedentary, your goal should be to focus on activities at the bottom of the pyramid and gradually increase the amount of moderate-intensity physical activity in your daily life. Appropriate activities include walking briskly, climbing stairs, doing yard work, and washing your car. You don't have to exercise vigorously, but you should experience a moderate increase in your heart and breathing rates. As described earlier, your activity time can be broken up into small blocks over the course of a day.

The next two levels of the pyramid illustrate parts of a formal exercise program. The principles of this program are consistent with those of the American College of Sports Medicine (ACSM), the professional organization for people involved in sports medicine and exercise science. The ACSM has established guidelines for creating an exercise program that will develop physical fitness (Table 2.3). A balanced program includes activities to develop all the health-related components of fitness:

• *Cardiorespiratory endurance* is developed by continuous rhythmic movements of large-muscle groups in activities such as walking, jogging, cycling, swimming, aerobic dance, and other forms of group exercise. High-intensity interval training (HIIT)—short bouts of high-intensity exercise followed by rest—builds endurance quickly, improves blood sugar control and blood pressure, and reduces body fat. Another advantage of HIIT is it takes less time than traditional endurance training. The disadvantage is it can be painful and uncomfortable. The safety of HIIT has not been determined.

Choose activities that you enjoy and that are convenient. Popular choices are in line skating, skiing, dancing, cycling, and backpacking. Start-and-stop activities such as tennis, racquetball, and soccer can also develop cardiorespiratory endurance if your skill level is sufficient to enable periods of continuous play. Training for cardiorespiratory endurance is discussed in Chapter 3.

exercise stress test A test usually administered on a treadmill or cycle ergometer using an electrocardiogram (EKG or ECG) to analyze changes in electrical activity in the heart during exercise; used to determine if any heart disease is present and to assess current fitness level.

graded exercise test (GXT) An exercise test that starts at an easy intensity and progresses to maximum capacity.

TERMS

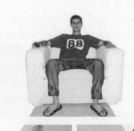

Sedentary Activities
Watching television, surfing the Internet, talking on a landline.

Limit Your Sedentary Activities

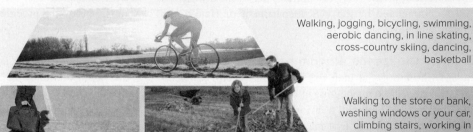

Strength Training
2–3 nonconsecutive days per week (all major muscle groups)
Bicep curls, push-ups, abdominal curls, bench press, calf raises

Flexibility Training
At least 2–3 days per week, ideally 5–7 days per week (all major joints)
Calf stretch, side lunge, step stretch, hurdler stretch

Cardiorespiratory Endurance Exercise
3–5 days per week (20–60 minutes per day)

Walking, jogging, bicycling, swimming, aerobic dancing, in line skating, cross-country skiing, dancing, basketball

Moderate-Intensity Physical Activity
150–300 minutes per week; for weight loss or prevention of weight regain following weight loss, 60–90 minutes per day

Walking to the store or bank, washing windows or your car, climbing stairs, working in your yard, walking your dog, cleaning your room

Figure 2.3   Physical activity pyramid.

George Doyle/Stockbyte/Getty Images; Ryan McVay/Photodisc/Getty Images; Photo taken by Shirlee Stevens; Westend61/Getty Images; Gioele Mottarlini/Shutterstock; UpperCut Images/Alamy Stock Photo

Table 2.3	**ACSM Exercise Recommendations for Fitness Development in Healthy Adults**
	EXERCISE TO DEVELOP AND MAINTAIN CARDIORESPIRATORY ENDURANCE AND BODY COMPOSITION

EXERCISE TO DEVELOP AND MAINTAIN CARDIORESPIRATORY ENDURANCE AND BODY COMPOSITION

Frequency of training	At least five days per week for moderate-intensity exercise and at least three days per week for vigorous-intensity exercise.
Intensity of training	55/65-90% of maximum heart rate or 40/50-85% of heart rate reserve or oxygen uptake reserve. (Reserve refers to the difference between resting and maximum values of heart rate or oxygen consumption.) The lower-intensity values (55-64% of maximum heart rate and 40-49% of heart rate reserve plus rest) are most applicable to unfit individuals. For average individuals, intensities of 70-85% of maximum heart rate or 60-80% of heart rate reserve plus rest are appropriate. Well-trained people can train at near maximum intensities. These methods increase exercise intensity within the limits of each person's reserve capacity.
Time (duration) of training	20-60 total minutes per day of continuous or intermittent (in sessions lasting 10 or more minutes) aerobic activity. Duration depends on the intensity of activity; thus, low-intensity activity should be conducted over a longer period of time (30 minutes or more). Low- to moderate-intensity activity of longer duration is recommended for nonathletic adults.
Type (mode) of activity	Any activity that uses large-muscle groups, can be maintained continuously, and is rhythmic and aerobic in nature—for example, walking-hiking, running-jogging, bicycling, cross-country skiing, aerobic dancing and other forms of group exercise, rope-skipping, rowing, stair-climbing, swimming, skating, and endurance game activities.
Volume	Expend the equivalent of at least 1,000 calories per week, which is equivalent to about 150 minutes per week of moderate-intensity exercise.
Progression	Adjust frequency, intensity, and/or time until you reach your goal.

EXERCISE TO DEVELOP AND MAINTAIN MUSCULAR STRENGTH AND ENDURANCE, FLEXIBILITY, AND BODY COMPOSITION

Resistance training	One set of 8-10 exercises that condition the major muscle groups, performed two to three days per week. Most people should complete 8-12 repetitions of each exercise to the point of fatigue; practicing other repetition ranges (e.g., 3-5 or 12-15) also builds strength and endurance; for older and frailer people (approximately 50-60 and older), 10-15 repetitions with a lighter weight may be more appropriate. Multiple-set regimens will provide greater benefits if time allows. Any mode of exercise that is comfortable throughout the full range of motion is appropriate (e.g., free weights, kettlebells, calisthenics, elastic bands, or weight machines).
Flexibility training	Static stretches, performed for the major muscle groups at least two to three days per week, ideally daily. Stretch to the point of tightness, holding each stretch for 10-30 seconds; perform 2-4 repetitions of each stretch, for a total of 60 seconds of stretching time for each exercise.

*Chapter 3 provides instructions for calculating target heart rate intensity for cardiorespiratory endurance exercise.

SOURCES: American College of Sports Medicine. 2017. *ACSM's Guidelines for Exercise Testing and Prescription,* 10th ed. Philadelphia: Wolters Kluwer; Garber, C. E., et al. 2011. "Quantity and quality of exercise for developing and maintaining cardiorespiratory, musculoskeletal, and neuromotor fitness in apparently healthy adults: Guidance for prescribing exercise," *Medicine and Science in Sports and Exercise* 43(7): 1334–1359.

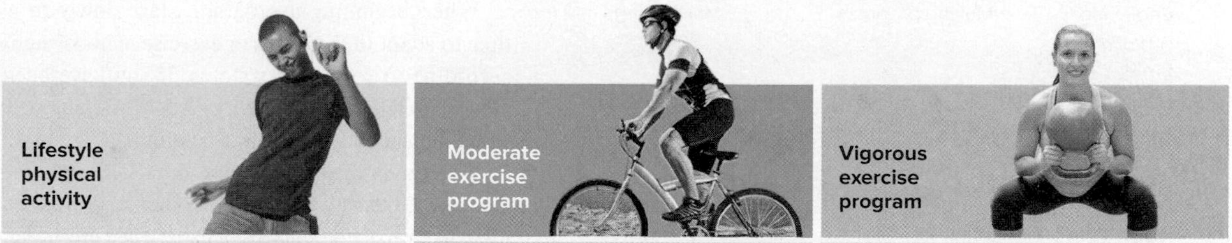

	Lifestyle physical activity	Moderate exercise program	Vigorous exercise program
Description	Moderate physical activity (150 minutes per week; muscle-strengthening exercises 2 or more days per week)	Cardiorespiratory endurance exercise (20–60 minutes, 3–5 days per week); strength training (2–3 nonconsecutive days per week); and stretching exercises (2 or more days per week)	Cardiorespiratory endurance exercise (20–60 minutes, 3–5 days per week); interval training; strength training (3–4 nonconsecutive days per week); and stretching exercises (5–7 days per week)
Sample activities or program	• Walking to and from work, 15 minutes each way • Cycling to and from class, 10 minutes each way • Doing yard work for 30 minutes • Dancing (fast) for 30 minutes • Playing basketball for 20 minutes • Muscle exercises such as push-ups, squats, or back exercises	• Jogging for 30 minutes, 3 days per week • Weight training, 1 set of 8 exercises, 2 days per week • Stretching exercises, 3 days per week	• Running for 45 minutes, 3 days per week • Intervals, running 400 m at high effort, 4 sets, 2 days per week • Weight training, 3 sets of 10 exercises, 3 days per week • Stretching exercises, 6 days per week
Health and fitness benefits	Better blood cholesterol levels, reduced body fat, better control of blood pressure, improved metabolic health, and enhanced glucose metabolism; improved quality of life; reduced risk of some chronic diseases Greater amounts of activity can help prevent weight gain and promote weight loss	All the benefits of lifestyle physical activity, plus improved physical fitness (increased cardiorespiratory endurance, muscular strength and endurance, and flexibility) and even greater improvements in health and quality of life and reductions in chronic disease risk	All the benefits of lifestyle physical activity and a moderate exercise program, with greater increases in fitness and somewhat greater reductions in chronic disease risk Participating in a vigorous exercise program may increase risk of injury and overtraining

Figure 2.4   Health and fitness benefits of different amounts of physical activity and exercise.

Rubberball Productions/Photodisc/Getty Images; Ljupco Smokovski/123RF; Juriah Mosin/Alamy Stock Photo

• *Muscular strength and endurance* can be developed through resistance training—training with weights or performing calisthenics such as push-ups, planks, and curl-ups. Training for muscular strength and endurance is discussed in Chapter 4.

• *Flexibility* is developed by stretching the major muscle groups regularly and with proper technique. Flexibility is discussed in Chapter 5.

• *Healthy body composition* can be developed through a sensible diet and a program of regular exercise. Cardiorespiratory endurance exercise is best for reducing body fat; resistance training builds muscle mass, which, to a small extent, helps increase metabolism. Body composition is discussed in Chapter 6.

Chapter 7 contains guidelines to help you choose activities and put together a complete exercise program that will suit your goals and preferences. (Refer to Figure 2.4 for a summary of the health and fitness benefits of different levels of physical activity and exercise programs.)

What about the tip of the activity pyramid? Although sedentary activities are often unavoidable—attending class, studying, working in an office, and so on—many people *choose* inactivity over activity during their leisure time. During sedentary activities, periodically stand, perform air squats, or walk around the room—even if only for a few minutes. Change sedentary patterns by becoming more active whenever you can.

Guidelines for Training

The following guidelines will make your exercise program more effective and successful.

Train the Way You Want Your Body to Change

Stress your body so that it adapts in the desired manner. To have a more muscular build, lift weights. To be more flexible, do stretching exercises. To improve performance in a particular sport, practice that sport or its movements.

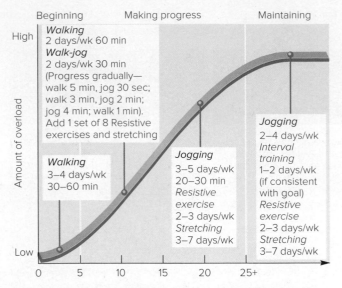

Beginning	Making progress	Maintaining

High

Walking
2 days/wk 60 min
Walk-jog
2 days/wk 30 min
(Progress gradually—
walk 5 min, jog 30 sec;
walk 3 min, jog 2 min;
jog 4 min; walk 1 min).
Add 1 set of 8 Resistive
exercises and stretching

Walking
3–4 days/wk
30–60 min

Jogging
3–5 days/wk
20–30 min
*Resistive
exercise*
2–3 days/wk
Stretching
3–7 days/wk

Jogging
2–4 days/wk
*Interval
training*
1–2 days/wk
(if consistent
with goal)
*Resistive
exercise*
2–3 days/wk
Stretching
3–7 days/wk

Low

Amount of overload

0   5   10   15   20   25+

Time since beginning an exercise program (in weeks)

Figure 2.5 Progression of an exercise program. This figure shows how you can increase the amount of overload gradually in a walking and running program. Begin with slow walking for several weeks and gradually pick up the pace. Gradually introduce short periods of running during your walks, progressively running farther and walking less until you can run continuously. Add interval training after four to six weeks of jogging—if you want to reach higher levels of fitness. Regardless of the activity and the exercise program, begin slowly and progress gradually. After you achieve the desired level of fitness, you can maintain it by exercising three to five days a week.

SOURCE: Progression data from American College of Sports Medicine. 2018. *ACSM's Guidelines for Exercise Testing and Prescription,* 10th ed. Philadelphia: Wolters Kluwer/Lippincott Williams & Wilkins Health.

Train Regularly Consistency is the key to improving fitness. Fitness improvements are lost if too much time passes between exercise sessions. When you can't follow your regular routine, do something physical—for example, squat with rocks or soup cans, sprint in place for 20 seconds, or train at a local gym for an hour when on vacation or traveling for business. Lab 2.2, Overcoming Barriers to Being Active, will help develop strategies for exercising regularly.

Start Slowly, and Get in Shape Gradually As Figure 2.5 shows, an exercise program can be divided into three phases:

- *Beginning phase.* The body adjusts to the new type and level of activity.

- *Progress phase.* Fitness increases.

- *Maintenance phase.* The targeted level of fitness is sustained over the long term.

When beginning a program, start slowly to give your body time to adapt to the stress of exercise. Choose activities carefully according to your fitness status. If you have been sedentary or are overweight, try an activity such as walking or swimming that won't jar the body or strain the joints.

As you progress, increase duration and frequency before increasing intensity. If you train too much or too intensely, you are more likely to suffer injuries or experience **overtraining**, a condition characterized by lack of energy, aching muscles and joints, depressed immune function, and decreased physical performance. Injuries and overtraining slow an exercise program and impede motivation. The goal is not to get in shape as quickly as possible but to gradually become and then remain physically fit.

Warm Up before Exercise Warming up can decrease your chances of injury by helping your body gradually progress from rest to activity. A good warm-up can increase muscle temperature, reduce joint stiffness, bathe the joint surfaces in lubricating fluid, and increase blood flow to the muscles, including the heart. Some studies suggest that warming up may also enhance muscle metabolism and mentally prepare you for a workout.

A warm-up should include low-intensity, whole-body movements similar to those used in the activity. For example, runners may walk and jog slowly prior to running at full speed. A tennis player might hit forehands and backhands at a low intensity before playing a vigorous set of tennis. A warm-up is not the same as a stretching workout. For safety and effectiveness, it is best to stretch *after* an endurance or strength training workout, when muscles are warm—and not as part of a warm-up. (Appropriate and effective warm-ups are discussed in greater detail in Chapters 3, 4, 5, and 6.)

Cool Down after Exercise During exercise, as much as 90% of circulating blood is directed to the muscles and skin, up from as little as 20% during rest. If you stop moving

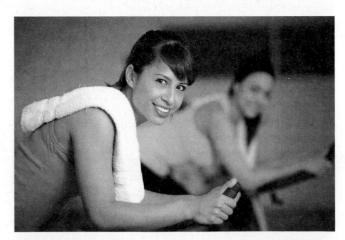

Wellness Tip Moderation is important, especially if you're just starting to get physically active. Work at a pace that's comfortable and enjoyable, with a goal of making gradual improvements. This will help you get into the habit of being active and will help you avoid burnout.

JoseGirarte/E+/Getty Images

suddenly after exercise, the amount of blood returning to your heart and brain may be insufficient, and you may experience dizziness, a drop in blood pressure, or other problems. Cooling down at the end of a workout helps safely restore circulation to its normal resting condition. So, after you exercise, cool down before you sit or lie down or jump into the shower. Cool down by continuing to move at a slow pace—walking for 5–10 minutes, for example, as your heart and breathing rate and blood pressure slowly return to normal. At the end of the cool-down period, do stretching exercises while your muscles are still warm. Cool down longer after intense exercise sessions.

Exercise Safely Physical activity can cause injury or even death if you don't consider safety. For example, you should always do the following:

- Wear a helmet when biking, skiing, or rock climbing.

- Wear eye protection when playing racquetball or squash.

- Wear bright clothing or safety lights when exercising on a public street.

- Walk or run with a partner when exercising on a deserted track or in a park.

- Give vehicles plenty of leeway, even when you have the right of way.

- In the weight room, be aware of people exercising near you, use spotters and collars when appropriate, and don't use broken equipment.

- Always use good technique. Don't put your back or joints at risk trying to lift weights or perform physical skills beyond your ability.

Overloading your muscles and joints can lead to serious injury, so train within your capacity. Use high-quality equipment and keep it in good repair. Report broken gym equipment to the health club manager or physical education instructor. (See Appendix A for more information on personal safety.)

Listen to Your Body and Get Adequate Rest Rest can be as important as exercise for improving fitness. Fitness reflects an adaptation to the stress of exercise. Building fitness involves a series of exercise stresses, recuperation, and adaptation leading to improved fitness, followed by further stresses. Build rest into your training program, and don't exercise if it doesn't feel right. Sometimes you need a few days of rest to recover enough to train with the intensity required for improving fitness. Getting enough sleep is an important part of the recovery process. On the other hand, don't train sporadically, either. If you listen to your body and it always tells you to rest, you won't make any progress.

Cycle the Volume and Intensity of Your Workouts To add enjoyment and variety to your program and to further improve fitness, don't train at the same intensity during every workout. Train intensely on some days and train lightly on others. Proper management of workout intensity is a key to improving physical fitness. Use cycle training, also known as *periodization,* to provide enough recovery for intense training: By training lightly one workout, you can train harder the next. However, take care to increase the volume and intensity of your program gradually—never more than 10% per week.

Vary Your Activities Change your exercise program from time to time to keep things fresh and help develop a higher degree of fitness. The body adapts quickly to an exercise stress, such as walking, cycling, or swimming. Gains in fitness in a particular activity become more difficult with time. Varying the exercises in your program allows you to adapt to many types of exercise and develops fitness in a variety of activities (see the box "Vary Your Activities"). Changing activities may also help reduce your risk of injury. This is a central principle in cross-training exercise techniques such as CrossFit. CrossFit is a commercial exercise program that uses a variety of training methods to improve fitness, including running, swimming, climbing, gymnastics, functional training, Olympic weight lifting, kettlebells, rope-climbing, and calisthenics.

Train with a Partner People who train together can motivate and encourage each other through rough spots and help each other develop proper exercise techniques. Training with a partner can make exercising seem easier and more fun. It can also help you keep motivated and on track. A commitment to a friend is a powerful motivator. If you can afford it, you may benefit from a certified personal trainer who can give you instruction in exercise techniques and help provide motivation.

Train Your Mind Becoming fit requires commitment, discipline, and patience. These qualities come from understanding the importance of exercise and setting clear and reachable goals. Use the lifestyle management techniques discussed in Chapter 1 to keep your program on track. Learning about the science behind a healthy lifestyle helps keep your program relevant.

Fuel Your Activity Appropriately Good nutritional choices can help you recover from a bout of exercise and get you ready for your next workout. Consume adequate fluids to stay hydrated as well as enough calories to support your exercise program without gaining body fat. Nutrition for exercise is discussed in greater detail in Chapters 3 and 8.

Have Fun You are more likely to stick with an exercise program if it's fun. Choose a variety of activities that you enjoy. Some people like to play competitive sports, such as tennis, golf, or volleyball. Competition can boost motivation, but remember: Sports are competitive, whereas training for fitness is not. Other people like more solitary activities, such as jogging, walking, or swimming. Still others like high-skill individual sports, such as snowboarding, surfing, or skateboarding. Many activities can help you get fit, so choose the ones you enjoy. You can also boost your enjoyment and build your social support network by exercising with friends and family.

Track Your Progress Monitoring the progress of your program can help keep you motivated and on track. Depending on the activities you've included in your program, you may track different measures of your program—minutes of jogging, miles of cycling, laps of swimming, number of push-ups, amount of weight lifted, and so on. If your program focuses on increasing daily physical activity, consider using an inexpensive step counter or exercise GPS app to monitor the number of steps you take each day. (See Lab 2.3 for more information on setting goals and monitoring activity with a digital tracker; see the box "Digital Workout Aids" for an introduction to products and apps that can help you track your progress.) Specific examples of program monitoring can be found in the labs for Chapters 3, 4, and 5.

Get Help and Advice If You Need It One of the best places to get help starting an exercise program is an exercise class. If you join a health club or fitness center, follow the guidelines in the box "Choosing a Fitness Center." There, expert instructors can help you learn the basics of training and answer your questions. Make sure the instructor is certified by a recognized professional organization and/or has formal training in exercise physiology. Read articles by credible experts in fitness magazines (such as *Fitness Rx for Women* and *Fitness Rx for Men*). Many of these magazines include articles by leading experts in exercise science written at a layperson's level.

A qualified personal trainer can also help you get started in an exercise program or a new form of training. Make sure this person has proper qualifications, such as certification by the ACSM, National Strength and Conditioning Association (NSCA), or International Sports Sciences Association (ISSA). Don't seek out a person for advice simply because he or she looks fit. UCLA researchers found that 60% of the personal trainers in their study couldn't pass a basic exam on training methods, exercise physiology, or biomechanics. Trainers who performed best had college degrees in exercise physiology, physical education, or physical therapy. So choose your trainer carefully and don't get caught up with fads or appearances.

Keep Your Exercise Program in Perspective As important as physical fitness is, it is only part of a well-rounded life. You need time for work and school, family and friends, relaxation and hobbies. Some people become over involved in exercise and neglect other parts of their lives. They think of themselves as runners, dancers, swimmers, or triathletes rather than as people who happen to participate in those activities. Balance and moderation are key ingredients of a fit and well life.

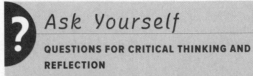

? Ask Yourself

QUESTIONS FOR CRITICAL THINKING AND REFLECTION

If you were to start planning a fitness program, what would be your three most important long-term goals? What would you set as short-term goals? What rewards would be meaningful to you?

When you're just beginning physical activity, you can wind up with a lot of questions. How many miles did I walk? How many kettlebell swings did I do, and how explosively did I do them? How many minutes did I run? When your mind is completely focused on just *doing* an activity, it's easy to lose count of time, distance, and reps. But it's important to keep track of these things: Move too little and you will see little progress; move too much and you risk injury or burnout. Either outcome is bad news for your exercise program.

Luckily, we live in a digital age, and the fitness industry is providing an ever-growing array of high-tech tools and apps that can track your progress for you. If you like to walk or run, cell phone apps can track your distance, or the number of steps you take, and give you a detailed map of where you ran, biked, or skied. Advanced trackers can even record any hills you encounter during your workout. Heart rate monitors can help you reach and maintain the right exercise intensity. Accelerometers can measure your power output, or explosiveness, during weight lifting. If calisthenics are your choice, there are gaming systems and smartphone apps that work for specific exercises to count reps, assess your form, and challenge you to push yourself harder.

Smartphone apps, such as Coach's Eye, Hudl Technique, and Dartfish, can help you analyze your golf swing or tennis forehand in slow motion. The programs even make it possible to gauge your progress by comparing technique videos during different phases of your program (e.g., tennis technique during week 1 versus week 10).

In choosing a digital tracker, keep the following in mind:

- Consider your fitness goals and how you plan to monitor and evaluate the progress of your program.

- Look for the features you need; don't pay extra for capabilities you won't use.

- Try out a tracker before you buy it; make sure it fits and that you find it easy to use.

- Confirm that any tracker or analysis app is compatible with your smartphone or computer.

Remember, a tracker works only when you use it!

TIPS FOR TODAY AND THE FUTURE

Physical activity and exercise offer benefits in nearly every area of wellness. Even a low to moderate level of activity provides valuable health benefits. The important thing is to get moving!

RIGHT NOW YOU CAN

- Look at your calendar for the rest of the week and write in some physical activity—such as walking, running, biking, skating, swimming, hiking, or playing Frisbee—on as many days as you can. Schedule the activity for a specific time and stick to it.
- Call a friend and invite her or him to plan a regular exercise program with you.
- Download a pedometer app on your phone and keep track of your daily activity.

IN THE FUTURE YOU CAN

- Schedule a session with a qualified personal trainer who can evaluate your fitness level and help you set personalized fitness goals.
- Create seasonal workout programs for the spring, summer, fall, and winter. Develop programs that are varied but consistent with your overall fitness goals.

SUMMARY

- Moderate daily physical activity contributes substantially to good health. Even without a formal, vigorous exercise program, you can get many of the same health benefits just by becoming more physically active.

- If you are already active, you benefit even more by increasing the intensity or duration of your activities.

- The five components of physical fitness most important for health are cardiorespiratory endurance, muscular strength, muscular endurance, flexibility, and body composition.

- Physical training produces long-term improvements in the body's functioning through exercise. All training involves adaptation to physical stress.

- According to the principle of specificity, bodies change specifically in response to the training received.

- Bodies also adapt to progressive overload. The overload needed to maintain or improve a particular level of fitness for a particular fitness component is determined through six dimensions, represented by the acronym FITT-VP: frequency, intensity, time, type, volume, and progression.

- Bodies adjust to lower levels of activity by losing fitness, a principle known as reversibility. To counter the effects of reversibility, keep training at the same intensity, even if you have to reduce the number or length of sessions.

- According to the principle of individual differences, people vary in the maximum level of fitness they can achieve and in the rate of change they can expect from an exercise program.

- When designing an exercise program, determine if you need medical clearance, assess your current level of fitness, set realistic goals, and choose activities that develop all the components of fitness.

- Train regularly, get in shape gradually, warm up and cool down, maintain a structured but flexible program, get enough rest, exercise safely, vary activities, consider training with a partner or personal trainer, train your mind, eat sensibly, have fun, monitor your progress, and keep exercise in perspective.

CRITICAL CONSUMER
Choosing a Fitness Center

Fitness centers can provide you with many benefits—motivation and companionship are among the most important. A fitness center may also offer expert instruction and supervision as well as access to better equipment than you could afford on your own. All fitness centers, however, are not of the same overall quality, and every fitness center is not for every person. If you're thinking of joining a fitness center, here are some guidelines to help you choose a club that's right for you.

Convenience

- Look for an established facility that's within 10–15 minutes of your home or work. If it's farther away, your chances of sticking to an exercise regimen diminish.

- Visit the facility during the times you would normally exercise. Is there adequate parking? Will you have easy access to equipment and classes?

- What child care services are available, and how are they supervised?

Atmosphere

- Look around to see if there are other members who are your age and at about your fitness level. Some clubs cater to a certain age group or lifestyle, such as hard-core bodybuilders or weight lifters.

- Observe how the members dress. Will you fit in, or will you be uncomfortable?

- Observe the staff. Are they easy to identify? Are they friendly, professional, and helpful?

- Check to see that the facility is clean, including showers and lockers. Make sure the facility is climate controlled, well ventilated, and well lit.

Safety

- Find out if the facility offers some type of preactivity screening in addition to basic fitness testing that includes cardiovascular screening.

- Determine if personnel are trained in CPR and if there is emergency equipment such as automated external defibrillators (AEDs) on the premises. An AED can help someone in cardiac arrest.

- Ask if at least one staff member on each shift is trained in first aid.

Trained Personnel

- Determine if the personal trainers and fitness instructors are certified by a recognized professional association such as the ACSM, Aerobics and Fitness Association of America (AFAA), National Strength and Conditioning Association (NSCA), or International Sport Sciences Association (ISSA). All personal trainers are not equal; over 100 organizations certify trainers, and few of these require much formal training.

- Find out if the club has a trained exercise physiologist on staff, such as someone with a degree in exercise physiology,

kinesiology, or exercise science. If the facility offers nutritional counseling, it should employ someone who is a registered dietitian or has similar formal training.

- Ask how much experience the instructors have. Ideally, trainers should have both academic preparation and practical experience.

Cost

- Buy only what you need and can afford. To use only workout equipment, you may not need a club with racquetball courts and saunas.

- Check the contract. Choose the one that covers the shortest time possible, especially if it's your first fitness club experience. Don't feel pressured to sign a long-term contract.

- Make sure the contract permits you to extend your membership if you have a prolonged illness or go on vacation. Some clubs have exchange agreements that allow you to train in other cities while on vacation or business.

- Try out the club. Ask for a free trial workout, or a one-day pass, or an inexpensive one- or two-week trial membership.

- Find out whether there is an extra charge for the particular services you want. Get any special offers in writing.

Effectiveness

- Tour the facility. Does it offer what the brochure says it does? Does it offer the activities and equipment you want?

- Check the equipment. A good club will have treadmills, bikes, stair-climbers, resistance machines, and weights. Make sure these machines are up to date and well maintained.

- Find out if new members get a formal orientation and instruction on how to safely use the equipment. Will a staff member help you develop a program that is appropriate for your current fitness level and goals?

- Make sure the facility is certified. Look for the displayed names ACSM, American Council on Exercise (ACE), AFAA, or International Health, Racquet, and Sportsclub Association (IHRSA).

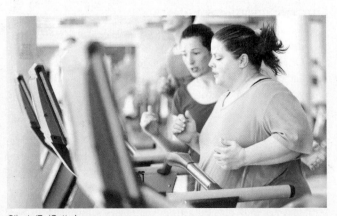

Gilaxia/E+/Getty Images

COMMON QUESTIONS ANSWERED

Q I have asthma. Is it OK for me to start an exercise program?

A Probably, but you should see your doctor before you start exercising, especially if you have been sedentary up to this point. Your personal physician can advise you on the type of exercise program that is best for you, given the severity of your condition, and how to avoid suffering exercise-related asthma attacks.

Q What should my fitness goals be?

A Begin by thinking about your general overall goals—the benefits you want to obtain by increasing your activity level and/or beginning a formal exercise program. Examples of long-term goals include reducing your risk of chronic diseases, increasing your energy level, and maintaining a healthy body weight.

To help shape your fitness program, you need to set specific, short-term goals based on measurable factors. These specific goals should be an extension of your overall goals—the specific changes to your current activity and exercise habits needed to achieve your general goals. In setting short-term goals, be sure to use the SMART criteria described in Chapter 1. As noted there, your goals should be Specific, Measurable, Attainable, Realistic, and Time frame–specific (SMART).

You need information about your current levels of physical activity and physical fitness to set appropriate goals. The labs in this chapter will help you determine your physical activity level—for example, how many minutes per day you engage in moderate or vigorous activity or how many daily steps you take. Using this information, you can set goals for lifestyle physical activity to help you meet your overall goals. For example, if your general long-term goals are to reduce the risk of chronic disease and prevent weight gain, the Dietary Guidelines recommend 60 minutes of moderate physical activity daily. If you currently engage in 30 minutes of moderate activity daily, then your behavior change goal would be to add 30 minutes of daily physical activity (or an equivalent number of additional daily steps—about 3,500–4,000); your time frame for the change might be 8–12 weeks.

Labs in Chapters 3, 4, 5, and 6 provide opportunities to assess your fitness status for all the health-related components of fitness. The results of these assessments can guide you in setting specific fitness goals. For instance, if the labs in Chapter 4 indicate that you have good muscular strength and endurance in your lower body but poor strength and endurance in your upper body, then setting a specific goal for improving upper-body muscle fitness would be an appropriate goal—increasing the number of push-ups you can do from 22 to 30, for example. Chapters 3–6 include additional advice for setting appropriate goals.

After you start your behavior change program, you may discover that your goals aren't quite appropriate; perhaps you were overly optimistic, or maybe you set the bar too low. There are limits to the amount of fitness you can achieve, but within the limits of your genes, health status, and motivation, you can make significant improvements in fitness. Adjust your goals as needed.

Q Should I follow my exercise program if I'm sick?

A If you have a mild head cold or feel one coming on, it is probably okay to exercise moderately. Just begin slowly and see how you feel. However, if you have symptoms of a more serious illness—fever, swollen glands, nausea, extreme tiredness, muscle aches—wait until you have recovered fully before resuming your exercise program. Continuing to exercise while suffering from an illness more serious than a cold can compromise your recovery and may even be dangerous.

FOR FURTHER EXPLORATION

American College of Sports Medicine (ACSM). The principal professional organization for sports medicine and exercise science. Provides brochures, publications, and videos.

http://www.acsm.org

American Council on Exercise (ACE). Promotes exercise and fitness; the website features fact sheets on many consumer topics, including choosing shoes, cross-training, and steroids.

http://www.acefitness.org

American Heart Association: Walking 101. Provides practical advice about walking for people of all fitness levels.

http://www.heart.org/HEARTORG/HealthyLiving/PhysicalActivity/Walking-101_UCM_461766_Article.jsp

CDC Physical Activity Information. Provides information on the benefits of physical activity and suggestions for incorporating moderate physical activity into daily life.

http://www.cdc.gov/physicalactivity

Disabled Sports USA. Provides sports and recreation services to people with physical or mobility disorders.

http://www.disabledsportsusa.org

Health and Retirement Study. A website describing a study of 20,000 people begun in 1992 at the University of Michigan and updated every two years. Included is an extensive reference list of published studies.

hrsonline.isr.umich.edu.

International Health, Racquet, and Sportsclub Association (IHRSA): Health Clubs. Provides guidelines for choosing a health or fitness facility and links to clubs that belong to IHRSA.

http://www.healthclubs.com

National Academy of Kinesiology. Promotes the study and application of physical activity through publications and professional meetings.

http://nationalacademyofkinesiology.org

International Sports Sciences Association (ISSA). Trains and certifies personal trainers.

http://www.issaonline.com

MedlinePlus: Exercise and Physical Fitness. Provides links to news and reliable information about fitness and exercise from government agencies and professional associations.

https://medlineplus.gov/exerciseandphysicalfitness.html

President's Council on Fitness, Sports and Nutrition. Provides information on programs and publications, including fitness guides and fact sheets.

http://www.fitness.gov

https://www.hhs.gov/fitness

Shape America: Society of Health and Physical Educators. A professional organization for health and physical educators.

http://www.shapeamerica.org

Shape Up America! A nonprofit organization that provides information and resources on exercise, nutrition, and weight loss.

http://www.shapeupus.org

StrongFirst. A school of strength, directed by kettlebell master Pavel Tsatsouline, that teaches men and women how to reach high levels of strength and fitness without interfering with work, school, family, or sport. The program offers clinics and web-based information.

http://www.strongfirst.com

SELECTED BIBLIOGRAPHY

Alzheimer's Association. 2016. *2016 Alzheimer's Disease Facts and Figures.* Chicago: Alzheimer's Association.

American College of Sports Medicine. 2011. *ACSM's Complete Guide to Fitness & Health.* Champaign, IL: Human Kinetics.

American College of Sports Medicine. 2011. The recommended quantity and quality of exercise for developing and maintaining cardiorespiratory and muscular fitness, and flexibility in healthy adults. ACSM position stand. *Medicine and Science in Sports and Exercise* 43(7): 1334–1359.

American College of Sports Medicine. 2012. *ACSM's Health/Fitness Facility Standards and Guidelines,* 4th ed. Champaign, IL: Human Kinetics.

American College of Sports Medicine. 2014. *ACSM's Resource Manual for Guidelines for Exercise Testing and Prescription,* 7th ed. Philadelphia, PA: Wolters Kluwer/ Lippincott Williams & Wilkins Health.

American College of Sports Medicine. 2018. *ACSM's Guidelines for Exercise Testing and Prescription,* 10th ed. Philadelphia, PA: Wolters Kluwer.

American Heart Association. 2017. *Cardiovascular disease: a costly burden for America. Projections through 2035.* Washington, DC: American Heart Association.

Bangsbo, J., et al. 2019. Copenhagen consensus statement 2019: Physical activity and ageing. *British Journal of Sports Medicine.* In press.

Biswas, A., et al. 2015. Sedentary time and its association with risk for disease incidence, mortality, and hospitalization in adults: A systematic review and meta-analysis. *Annals of Internal Medicine* 162(2): 123–132.

Bouchard, C., et al. 2015. Personalized preventive medicine: Genetics and the response to regular exercise in preventive interventions. *Progress in Cardiovascular Diseases* 57(4): 337–346.

Bos, I., et al. 2013. Subclinical effects of aerobic training in urban environment. *Medicine and Science in Sports and Exercise* 45(3): 439–447.

Casazza, K., et al. 2013. Myths, presumptions, and facts about obesity. *New England Journal of Medicine* 368(5): 446–454.

Centers for Disease Control and Prevention. 2014. *State Indicator Report on Physical Activity, 2014.* Atlanta, GA: U.S. Department of Health and Human Services.

Dietary Guidelines Advisory Committee. 2015. *Scientific Report of the 2015 Dietary Advisory Committee.* Washington, DC: U.S. Department of Agriculture, Agricultural Research Service.

Donnelly, J. E., et al. 2009. Appropriate physical activity intervention strategies for weight loss and prevention of weight regain for adults (ACSM position stand). *Medicine and Science in Sports and Exercise* 41(2): 459–471.

Ekblom-Bak, E., et al. 2014. The importance of non-exercise physical activity for cardiovascular health and longevity. *British Journal of Sports Medicine* 48(3): 233–238.

Fahey, T., and M. Fahey. 2014. Nutrition, physical activity, and the obesity epidemic: Issues, policies, and solutions (1960s–present). In T. Oliver (Ed.), *The Guide to U.S. Health and Health Care Policy,* pp. 363–374. New York, NY, DWJ Books.

Fontes, E. B., et al. 2015. Brain activity and perceived exertion during cycling exercise: An fMRI study. *British Journal of Sports Medicine* 49(8): 556–560.

Gordon, B. A., et al. 2016. Physical activity intensity can be accurately monitored by smartphone global positioning system "app." *European Journal of Sport Science* 16(5): 624–631.

Hampton, T. 2016. Experts ponder whether too much exercise can compromise cardiovascular health and longevity. *Circulation* 134: 833–834.

Howley, E., and D. Thompson. 2012. *Fitness Professional's Handbook,* 6th ed. Champaign, IL: Human Kinetics.

John, D. 2013. *Intervention: Course Correction for the Athlete and Trainer.* Santa Cruz, CA: On Target.

Katz, P. P., and R. Pate. 2016. Exercise as medicine. *Annals of Internal Medicine.* 165(12): 880–881.

Leifer, E. S., et al. 2016. Adverse cardiovascular response to aerobic exercise training: is this a concern. *Medicine and Science in Sports and Exercise* 48(1): 20–25.

McArdle, W. D., et al. 2014. *Exercise Physiology: Nutrition, Energy, and Human Performance.* Philadelphia, PA: Wolters Kluwer.

Park, S. Y., et al. 2016. Exercise training improves vascular mitochondrial function. *American Journal of Physiology: Heart and Circulatory Physiology* 310(7): H821–H829.

Pate, R., and D. Buchner. 2014. *Implementing Physical Activity Strategies.* Champaign, IL: Human Kinetics.

Physical Activity Guidelines Advisory Committee. 2008. *Physical Activity Guidelines Advisory Committee Report, 2008.* Washington, DC: U.S. Department of Health and Human Services.

Physical Activity Guidelines Advisory Committee. 2018. *Physical Activity Guidelines Advisory Committee Scientific Report, 2018.* Washington, DC: U.S. Department of Health and Human Services.

Puterman, E., et al. 2015. Determinants of telomere attrition over 1 year in healthy older women: Stress and health behaviors matter. *Molecular Psychiatry* 20(4): 529–535.

Rivera-Torres, S., et al. 2019. Adherence to exercise programs in older adults: Informative report. *Gerontology Geriatric Medicine* 5: 1–10.

Ross, R. E., et al. 2019. High-intensity aerobic exercise acutely increases brain-derived neurotrophic factor. *Medicine and Science in Sports and Exercise.* In press.

Song, J., et al. 2017. Do inactive older adults who increase physical activity experience less disability: Evidence from the osteoarthritis initiative. *Journal of Clinical Rheumatology* 23(1): 26–32.

Szuhany, K. L., et al. 2015. A meta-analytic review of the effects of exercise on brain-derived neurotrophic factor. *Journal of Psychiatric Research* 60: 56–64.

Thompson, W. R. 2016. Worldwide survey of fitness: Trends for 2017. *ACSM's Health & Fitness Journal* 20(6): 8–17.

U.S. Department of Health and Human Services. 1996. *Physical Activity and Health: A Report of the Surgeon General.* Atlanta, GA: U.S. Department of Health and Human Services.

U.S. Department of Health and Human Services. 2008. *Physical Activity Guidelines for Americans.* Washington, DC: U.S. Department of Health and Human Services.

U.S. Department of Health and Human Services. 2010. *The Surgeon General's Vision for a Healthy and Fit Nation.* Rockville, MD: U.S. Department of Health and Human Services, Office of the Surgeon General.

U.S. Department of Health and Human Services. 2013. *Physical Activity Guidelines for Americans Midcourse Report.* Washington, DC: U.S. Department of Health and Human Services.

U.S. Department of Health and Human Services. 2018. *Physical Activity Guidelines for Americans,* 2nd ed. Washington, DC: U.S. Department of Health and Human Services.

Wilke, J., et al. 2019. Acute effects of resistance exercise on cognitive function in healthy adults: A systematic review with multilevel meta-analysis. *Sports Medicine.* Published online.

Zhu, W., and N. Owen. 2018. *Sedentary Behavior and Health: Concepts, Assessments, and Interventions.* Champaign, IL: Human Kinetics.

Name _____ Section _____ Date _____

LAB 2.1   Safety of Exercise Participation: PAR-Q+

2019 PAR-Q+

The Physical Activity Readiness Questionnaire for Everyone

The health benefits of regular physical activity are clear; more people should engage in physical activity every day of the week. Participating in physical activity is very safe for MOST people. This questionnaire will tell you whether it is necessary for you to seek further advice from your doctor OR a qualified exercise professional before becoming more physically active.

GENERAL HEALTH QUESTIONS

Please read the 7 questions below carefully and answer each one honestly: check YES or NO.	YES	NO
1) Has your doctor ever said that you have a heart condition ☐ OR high blood pressure ☐?	☐	☐
2) Do you feel pain in your chest at rest, during your daily activities of living, **OR** when you do physical activity?	☐	☐
3) Do you lose balance because of dizziness **OR** have you lost consciousness in the last 12 months? Please answer **NO** if your dizziness was associated with over-breathing (including during vigorous exercise).	☐	☐
4) Have you ever been diagnosed with another chronic medical condition (other than heart disease or high blood pressure)? **PLEASE LIST CONDITION(S) HERE:** _____	☐	☐
5) Are you currently taking prescribed medications for a chronic medical condition? **PLEASE LIST CONDITION(S) AND MEDICATIONS HERE:** _____	☐	☐
6) Do you currently have (or have had within the past 12 months) a bone, joint, or soft tissue (muscle, ligament, or tendon) problem that could be made worse by becoming more physically active? Please answer **NO** if you had a problem in the past, but it **does not limit your current ability** to be physically active. **PLEASE LIST CONDITION(S) HERE:** _____	☐	☐
7) Has your doctor ever said that you should only do medically supervised physical activity?	☐	☐

✔ **If you answered NO to all of the questions above, you are cleared for physical activity.**
Please sign the PARTICIPANT DECLARATION. You do not need to complete Pages 2 and 3.

▶ Start becoming much more physically active – start slowly and build up gradually.

▶ Follow International Physical Activity Guidelines for your age (www.who.int/dietphysicalactivity/en/).

▶ You may take part in a health and fitness appraisal.

▶ If you are over the age of 45 yr and NOT accustomed to regular vigorous to maximal effort exercise, consult a qualified exercise professional before engaging in this intensity of exercise.

▶ If you have any further questions, contact a qualified exercise professional.

PARTICIPANT DECLARATION
If you are less than the legal age required for consent or require the assent of a care provider, your parent, guardian or care provider must also sign this form.

I, the undersigned, have read, understood to my full satisfaction and completed this questionnaire. I acknowledge that this physical activity clearance is valid for a maximum of 12 months from the date it is completed and becomes invalid if my condition changes. I also acknowledge that the community/fitness center may retain a copy of this form for its records. In these instances, it will maintain the confidentiality of the same, complying with applicable law.

NAME _____ DATE _____

SIGNATURE _____ WITNESS _____

SIGNATURE OF PARENT/GUARDIAN/CARE PROVIDER _____

⬢ **If you answered YES to one or more of the questions above, COMPLETE PAGES 2 AND 3.**

⚠ **Delay becoming more active if:**

✔ You have a temporary illness such as a cold or fever; it is best to wait until you feel better.

✔ You are pregnant - talk to your health care practitioner, your physician, a qualified exercise professional, and/or complete the ePARmed-X+ at **www.eparmedx.com** before becoming more physically active.

✔ Your health changes - answer the questions on Pages 2 and 3 of this document and/or talk to your doctor or a qualified exercise professional before continuing with any physical activity program.

Copyright © 2019 PAR-Q+ Collaboration 1 / 4
11-01-2018

SOURCE: Warburton, D. E. R., V. Jamnik, S. S. D. Bredin, R. J. Shephard, and N. Gledhill. The 2019 Physical Activity Readiness Questionnaire for Everyone (PARQ+) and electronic Physical Activity Readiness Medical Examination (ePARmedX+). ©2019 PARQ+ Collaboration. Used with permission.

2019 PAR-Q+

FOLLOW-UP QUESTIONS ABOUT YOUR MEDICAL CONDITION(S)

1. Do you have Arthritis, Osteoporosis, or Back Problems?

If the above condition(s) is/are present, answer questions 1a-1c   If **NO** ☐ go to question 2

1a.	Do you have difficulty controlling your condition with medications or other physician-prescribed therapies? (Answer **NO** if you are not currently taking medications or other treatments)	YES ☐ NO ☐
1b.	Do you have joint problems causing pain, a recent fracture or fracture caused by osteoporosis or cancer, displaced vertebra (e.g., spondylolisthesis), and/or spondylolysis/pars defect (a crack in the bony ring on the back of the spinal column)?	YES ☐ NO ☐
1c.	Have you had steroid injections or taken steroid tablets regularly for more than 3 months?	YES ☐ NO ☐

2. Do you currently have Cancer of any kind?

If the above condition(s) is/are present, answer questions 2a-2b   If **NO** ☐ go to question 3

2a.	Does your cancer diagnosis include any of the following types: lung/bronchogenic, multiple myeloma (cancer of plasma cells), head, and/or neck?	YES ☐ NO ☐
2b.	Are you currently receiving cancer therapy (such as chemotherapy or radiotherapy)?	YES ☐ NO ☐

3. Do you have a Heart or Cardiovascular Condition? This includes Coronary Artery Disease, Heart Failure, Diagnosed Abnormality of Heart Rhythm

If the above condition(s) is/are present, answer questions 3a-3d   If **NO** ☐ go to question 4

3a.	Do you have difficulty controlling your condition with medications or other physician-prescribed therapies? (Answer **NO** if you are not currently taking medications or other treatments)	YES ☐ NO ☐
3b.	Do you have an irregular heart beat that requires medical management? (e.g., atrial fibrillation, premature ventricular contraction)	YES ☐ NO ☐
3c.	Do you have chronic heart failure?	YES ☐ NO ☐
3d.	Do you have diagnosed coronary artery (cardiovascular) disease and have not participated in regular physical activity in the last 2 months?	YES ☐ NO ☐

4. Do you have High Blood Pressure?

If the above condition(s) is/are present, answer questions 4a-4b   If **NO** ☐ go to question 5

4a.	Do you have difficulty controlling your condition with medications or other physician-prescribed therapies? (Answer **NO** if you are not currently taking medications or other treatments)	YES ☐ NO ☐
4b.	Do you have a resting blood pressure equal to or greater than 160/90 mmHg with or without medication? (Answer **YES** if you do not know your resting blood pressure)	YES ☐ NO ☐

5. Do you have any Metabolic Conditions? This includes Type 1 Diabetes, Type 2 Diabetes, Pre-Diabetes

If the above condition(s) is/are present, answer questions 5a-5e   If **NO** ☐ go to question 6

5a.	Do you often have difficulty controlling your blood sugar levels with foods, medications, or other physician-prescribed therapies?	YES ☐ NO ☐
5b.	Do you often suffer from signs and symptoms of low blood sugar (hypoglycemia) following exercise and/or during activities of daily living? Signs of hypoglycemia may include shakiness, nervousness, unusual irritability, abnormal sweating, dizziness or light-headedness, mental confusion, difficulty speaking, weakness, or sleepiness.	YES ☐ NO ☐
5c.	Do you have any signs or symptoms of diabetes complications such as heart or vascular disease and/or complications affecting your eyes, kidneys, **OR** the sensation in your toes and feet?	YES ☐ NO ☐
5d.	Do you have other metabolic conditions (such as current pregnancy-related diabetes, chronic kidney disease, or liver problems)?	YES ☐ NO ☐
5e.	Are you planning to engage in what for you is unusually high (or vigorous) intensity exercise in the near future?	YES ☐ NO ☐

2019 PAR-Q+

6. **Do you have any Mental Health Problems or Learning Difficulties?** This includes Alzheimer's, Dementia, Depression, Anxiety Disorder, Eating Disorder, Psychotic Disorder, Intellectual Disability, Down Syndrome

If the above condition(s) is/are present, answer questions 6a-6b   If **NO** ☐ go to question 7

6a. Do you have difficulty controlling your condition with medications or other physician-prescribed therapies? (Answer **NO** if you are not currently taking medications or other treatments)   YES ☐ NO ☐

6b. Do you have Down Syndrome **AND** back problems affecting nerves or muscles?   YES ☐ NO ☐

7. **Do you have a Respiratory Disease?** This includes Chronic Obstructive Pulmonary Disease, Asthma, Pulmonary High Blood Pressure

If the above condition(s) is/are present, answer questions 7a-7d   If **NO** ☐ go to question 8

7a. Do you have difficulty controlling your condition with medications or other physician-prescribed therapies? (Answer **NO** if you are not currently taking medications or other treatments)   YES ☐ NO ☐

7b. Has your doctor ever said your blood oxygen level is low at rest or during exercise and/or that you require supplemental oxygen therapy?   YES ☐ NO ☐

7c. If asthmatic, do you currently have symptoms of chest tightness, wheezing, laboured breathing, consistent cough (more than 2 days/week), or have you used your rescue medication more than twice in the last week?   YES ☐ NO ☐

7d. Has your doctor ever said you have high blood pressure in the blood vessels of your lungs?   YES ☐ NO ☐

8. **Do you have a Spinal Cord Injury?** This includes Tetraplegia and Paraplegia

If the above condition(s) is/are present, answer questions 8a-8c   If **NO** ☐ go to question 9

8a. Do you have difficulty controlling your condition with medications or other physician-prescribed therapies? (Answer **NO** if you are not currently taking medications or other treatments)   YES ☐ NO ☐

8b. Do you commonly exhibit low resting blood pressure significant enough to cause dizziness, light-headedness, and/or fainting?   YES ☐ NO ☐

8c. Has your physician indicated that you exhibit sudden bouts of high blood pressure (known as Autonomic Dysreflexia)?   YES ☐ NO ☐

9. **Have you had a Stroke?** This includes Transient Ischemic Attack (TIA) or Cerebrovascular Event

If the above condition(s) is/are present, answer questions 9a-9c   If **NO** ☐ go to question 10

9a. Do you have difficulty controlling your condition with medications or other physician-prescribed therapies? (Answer NO if you are not currently taking medications or other treatments)   YES ☐ NO ☐

9b. Do you have any impairment in walking or mobility?   YES ☐ NO ☐

9c. Have you experienced a stroke or impairment in nerves or muscles in the past 6 months?   YES ☐ NO ☐

10. **Do you have any other medical condition not listed above or do you have two or more medical conditions?**

If you have other medical conditions, answer questions 10a-10c   If **NO** ☐ read the Page 4 recommendations

10a. Have you experienced a blackout, fainted, or lost consciousness as a result of a head injury within the last 12 months **OR** have you had a diagnosed concussion within the last 12 months?   YES ☐ NO ☐

10b. Do you have a medical condition that is not listed (such as epilepsy, neurological conditions, kidney problems)?   YES ☐ NO ☐

10c. Do you currently live with two or more medical conditions?   YES ☐ NO ☐

PLEASE LIST YOUR MEDICAL CONDITION(S) AND ANY RELATED MEDICATIONS HERE: _____

_____

GO to Page 4 for recommendations about your current medical condition(s) and sign the PARTICIPANT DECLARATION.

2019 PAR-Q+

☑ If you answered NO to all of the FOLLOW-UP questions (pgs. 2-3) about your medical condition, you are ready to become more physically active - sign the PARTICIPANT DECLARATION below:

▶ It is advised that you consult a qualified exercise professional to help you develop a safe and effective physical activity plan to meet your health needs.

▶ You are encouraged to start slowly and build up gradually - 20 to 60 minutes of low to moderate intensity exercise, 3-5 days per week including aerobic and muscle strengthening exercises.

▶ As you progress, you should aim to accumulate 150 minutes or more of moderate intensity physical activity per week.

▶ If you are over the age of 45 yr and **NOT** accustomed to regular vigorous to maximal effort exercise, consult a qualified exercise professional before engaging in this intensity of exercise.

⬢ If you answered YES to one or more of the follow-up questions about your medical condition:

You should seek further information before becoming more physically active or engaging in a fitness appraisal. You should complete the specially designed online screening and exercise recommendations program - the **ePARmed-X+ at www.eparmedx.com** and/or visit a qualified exercise professional to work through the ePARmed-X+ and for further information.

⚠ Delay becoming more active if:

✓ You have a temporary illness such as a cold or fever; it is best to wait until you feel better.

✓ You are pregnant - talk to your health care practitioner, your physician, a qualified exercise professional, and/or complete the ePARmed-X+ **at www.eparmedx.com** before becoming more physically active.

✓ Your health changes - talk to your doctor or qualified exercise professional before continuing with any physical activity program.

● You are encouraged to photocopy the PAR-Q+. You must use the entire questionnaire and NO changes are permitted.
● The authors, the PAR-Q+ Collaboration, partner organizations, and their agents assume no liability for persons who undertake physical activity and/or make use of the PAR-Q+ or ePARmed-X+. If in doubt after completing the questionnaire, consult your doctor prior to physical activity.

PARTICIPANT DECLARATION

● All persons who have completed the PAR-Q+ please read and sign the declaration below.

● If you are less than the legal age required for consent or require the assent of a care provider, your parent, guardian or care provider must also sign this form.

I, the undersigned, have read, understood to my full satisfaction and completed this questionnaire. I acknowledge that this physical activity clearance is valid for a maximum of 12 months from the date it is completed and becomes invalid if my condition changes. I also acknowledge that the community/fitness center may retain a copy of this form for records. In these instances, it will maintain the confidentiality of the same, complying with applicable law.

NAME _____   DATE _____

SIGNATURE _____   WITNESS _____

SIGNATURE OF PARENT/GUARDIAN/CARE PROVIDER _____

---------- For more information, please contact ----------
www.eparmedx.com
Email: eparmedx@gmail.com

Citation for PAR-Q+
Warburton DER, Jamnik VK, Bredin SSD, and Gledhill N on behalf of the PAR-Q+ Collaboration. The Physical Activity Readiness Questionnaire for Everyone (PAR-Q+) and Electronic Physical Activity Readiness Medical Examination (ePARmed-X+). Health & Fitness Journal of Canada 4(2):3-23, 2011.

Key References
1. Jamnik VK, Warburton DER, Makarski J, McKenzie DC, Shephard RJ, Stone J, and Gledhill N. Enhancing the effectiveness of clearance for physical activity participation; background and overall process. APNM 36(S1):S3-S13, 2011.
2. Warburton DER, Gledhill N, Jamnik VK, Bredin SSD, McKenzie DC, Stone J, Charlesworth S, and Shephard RJ. Evidence-based risk assessment and recommendations for physical activity clearance; Consensus Document. APNM 36(S1):S266-s298, 2011.
3. Chisholm DM, Collis ML, Kulak LL, Davenport W, and Gruber N. Physical activity readiness. British Columbia Medical Journal. 1975;17:375-378.
4. Thomas S, Reading J, and Shephard RJ. Revision of the Physical Activity Readiness Questionnaire (PAR-Q). Canadian Journal of Sport Science 1992;17:4 338-345.

The PAR-Q+ was created using the evidence-based AGREE process (1) by the PAR-Q+ Collaboration chaired by Dr. Darren E. R. Warburton with Dr. Norman Gledhill, Dr. Veronica Jamnik, and Dr. Donald C. McKenzie (2). Production of this document has been made possible through financial contributions from the Public Health Agency of Canada and the BC Ministry of Health Services. The views expressed herein do not necessarily represent the views of the Public Health Agency of Canada or the BC Ministry of Health Services.

Name _____ **Section** _____ **Date** _____

LAB 2.2   Overcoming Barriers to Being Active

Barriers to Being Active Quiz

Directions: People give the following reasons to describe why they do not get as much physical activity as they think they should. Please read each statement and circle the number that describes how likely you are to say each of these statements.

How likely are you to say this?	Very likely	Somewhat likely	Somewhat unlikely	Very unlikely
1. My day is so busy now, I just don't think I can make the time to include physical activity in my regular schedule.	3	2	1	0
2. None of my family members or friends like to do anything active, so I don't have a chance to exercise.	3	2	1	0
3. I'm just too tired after work to get any exercise.	3	2	1	0
4. I've been thinking about getting more exercise, but I just can't seem to get started.	3	2	1	0
5. I'm getting older, so exercise can be risky.	3	2	1	0
6. I don't get enough exercise because I have never learned the skills for any sport.	3	2	1	0
7. I don't have access to jogging trails, swimming pools, bike paths, etc.	3	2	1	0
8. Physical activity takes too much time away from other commitments—like work, family, etc.	3	2	1	0
9. I'm embarrassed about how I will look when I exercise with others.	3	2	1	0
10. I don't get enough sleep as it is. I just couldn't get up early or stay up late to get some exercise.	3	2	1	0
11. It's easier for me to find excuses not to exercise than to go out and do something.	3	2	1	0
12. I know of too many people who have hurt themselves by overdoing it with exercise.	3	2	1	0
13. I really can't see learning a new sport at my age.	3	2	1	0
14. It's just too expensive. You have to take a class or join a club or buy the right equipment.	3	2	1	0
15. My free times during the day are too short to include exercise.	3	2	1	0
16. My usual social activities with family or friends do not include physical activity.	3	2	1	0
17. I'm too tired during the week, and I need the weekend to catch up on my rest.	3	2	1	0
18. I want to get more exercise, but I just can't seem to make myself stick to anything.	3	2	1	0
19. I'm afraid I might injure myself or have a heart attack.	3	2	1	0
20. I'm not good enough at any physical activity to make it fun.	3	2	1	0
21. If we had exercise facilities and showers at work, then I would be more likely to exercise.	3	2	1	0

LABORATORY ACTIVITIES

Scoring

- Enter the circled numbers in the spaces provided, putting the number for statement 1 on line 1, statement 2 on line 2, and so on.

- Add the three scores on each line. Your barriers to physical activity fall into one or more of seven categories: lack of time, social influences, lack of energy, lack of willpower, fear of injury, lack of skill, and lack of resources. A score of 5 or above in any category shows that this is an important barrier for you to overcome.

1	+	8	+	15	= Lack of time
2	+	9	+	16	= Social influences
3	+	10	+	17	= Lack of energy
4	+	11	+	18	= Lack of willpower
5	+	12	+	19	= Fear of injury
6	+	13	+	20	= Lack of skill
7	+	14	+	21	= Lack of resources

Using Your Results

How did you score? How many key barriers did you identify? Are they what you expected?

What should you do next? For your key barriers, try the strategies listed on the following pages and/or develop additional strategies that work for you. Check off any strategy that you try.

Suggestions for Overcoming Physical Activity Barriers

Lack of Time

_____ Identify available time slots. Monitor your daily activities for one week. Identify at least three 30-minute time slots you could use for physical activity.

_____ Add physical activity to your daily routine. For example, walk or ride your bike to work or shopping, organize social activities around physical activity, walk the dog, exercise while you watch TV, park farther from your destination.

_____ Make time for physical activity. For example, walk, jog, or swim during your lunch hour, or take fitness breaks instead of coffee breaks.

_____ Select activities requiring minimal time, such as walking, jogging, or stair climbing.

_____ Other: _____

Social Influences

_____ Explain your interest in physical activity to friends and family. Ask them to support your efforts.

_____ Invite friends and family members to exercise with you. Plan social activities involving exercise.

_____ Develop new friendships with physically active people. Join a group, such as the YMCA or a hiking club.

_____ Other: _____

Lack of Energy

_____ Schedule physical activity for times in the day or week when you feel energetic.

_____ Convince yourself that if you give it a chance, exercise will increase your energy level. Then try it.

_____ Other: _____

Lack of Willpower

_____ Plan ahead. Make physical activity a regular part of your daily or weekly schedule and write it on your calendar.

_____ Invite a friend to exercise with you on a regular basis and write it on *both* your calendars.

_____ Join an exercise group or class.

_____ Other: _____

Fear of Injury

_____ Learn how to warm up and cool down to prevent injury.

_____ Learn how to exercise appropriately considering your age, fitness level, skill level, and health status.

_____ Choose activities involving minimal risk.

_____ Other: _____

Lack of Skill

_____Select activities requiring no new skills, such as walking, jogging, or stair-climbing.

_____Exercise with friends who are at the same skill level as you are.

_____Find a friend who is willing to teach you some new skills.

_____Take a class to develop new skills.

_____Other: _____

Lack of Resources

_____ Select activities that require minimal facilities or equipment, such as walking, jogging, jumping rope, or calisthenics.

_____ Identify inexpensive, convenient resources available in your community (community education programs, park and recreation programs, worksite programs, etc.).

_____ Other: _____

LABORATORY ACTIVITIES

Are any of the following additional barriers important for you? If so, try some of the strategies listed here or invent your own.

Weather Conditions

_____ Develop a set of regular activities that are always available regardless of weather (indoor cycling, aerobic dance, indoor swimming, calisthenics, stair-climbing, rope-skipping, mall-walking, dancing, gymnasium games, etc.).

_____ Look at outdoor activities that depend on weather conditions (cross-country skiing, outdoor swimming, outdoor tennis, etc.) as "bonuses"—extra activities possible when weather and circumstances permit.

_____ Other: _____

Travel

_____ Put a jump rope in your suitcase and jump rope.

_____ Walk the halls and climb the stairs in hotels.

_____ Stay in places with swimming pools or exercise facilities.

_____ Join the YMCA or YWCA (ask about reciprocal membership agreements).

_____ Visit the local shopping mall and walk for half an hour or more.

_____ Bring a personal music player loaded with your favorite workout music.

_____ Other: _____

Family Obligations

_____ Trade babysitting time with a friend, neighbor, or family member who also has small children.

_____ Exercise _with_ the kids–go for a walk together, play tag or other running games, or get an aerobic dance or exercise DVD for kids (there are several on the market) and exercise together. You can spend time together and still get your exercise.

_____ Hire a babysitter and look at the cost as a worthwhile investment in your physical and mental health.

_____ Jump rope, do calisthenics, ride a stationary bicycle, or use other home gymnasium equipment while the kids watch TV or when they are sleeping.

_____ Try to exercise when the kids are not around (e.g., during school hours or their nap time).

_____ Other: _____

Retirement Years

_____ Look on your retirement as an opportunity to become more active instead of less. Spend more time gardening, walking the dog, and playing with your grandchildren. Children with short legs and grandparents with slower gaits are often great walking partners.

_____ Learn a new skill you've always been interested in, such as ballroom dancing, square dancing, or swimming.

_____ Now that you have the time, make regular physical activity a part of every day. Go for a walk every morning or every evening before dinner. Treat yourself to an exercycle and ride every day during a favorite TV show.

_____ Other: _____

SOURCE: Adapted from CDC Division of Nutrition and Physical Activity. 2010. _Promoting Physical Activity: A Guide for Community Action,_ 2nd ed. Champaign, IL: Human Kinetics.

Name _____ Section _____ Date _____

LAB 2.3 Using a Fitness Tracker or Smartphone Exercise App to Measure Physical Activity

How physically active are you? Would you be more motivated to increase daily physical activity if you had an easy way to monitor your level of activity? If so, consider a smartphone exercise app or fitness tracker to measure your daily physical activity. Smartphone exercise apps use sensors that accurately measure exercise time, distance, peak speed, average speed, step count, and flights of stairs climbed per day. These apps are either low cost or free.

Determine Your Baseline

Wear the fitness tracker or use your smartphone fitness app for a week to obtain a baseline average daily number of steps.

	M	T	W	Th	F	Sa	Su	Average
Steps								
Distance								
Flights of Stairs								

Set Goals

Set an appropriate goal for increasing exercise time, steps, or flights of stairs. The goal of 60 minutes of activity or 10,000 steps per day is widely recommended, but your personal goal should reflect your baseline level of steps. For example, if your current daily steps are far below 10,000, a goal of walking 2,000 additional steps each day might be appropriate. If you are already close to 10,000 steps per day, choose a higher goal. Also consider the following guidelines from health experts:

- To reduce the risk of chronic disease, aim to accumulate at least 150 minutes of moderate physical activity per week.
- To help manage body weight and prevent gradual, unhealthy weight gain, engage in 60 minutes of moderate- to vigorous-intensity activity on most days of the week.
- To sustain weight loss, engage daily in at least 60–90 minutes of moderate-intensity physical activity.

To help gauge how close you are to meeting these time-based physical activity goals, you might walk for 10–15 minutes while wearing your fitness tracker or smartphone to determine how many steps correspond with the time-based goals.

Once you have set your overall goal, break it down into several steps. For example, if your goal is to increase daily steps by 2,000, set mini-goals of increasing daily steps by 500, allowing two weeks to reach each mini-goal. Smaller goals are easier to achieve and can help keep you motivated and on track. Having several interim goals also gives you the opportunity to reward yourself more frequently. Note your goals here:

Mini-goal 1: _____ Target date: _____ Reward: _____
Mini-goal 2: _____ Target date: _____ Reward: _____
Mini-goal 3: _____ Target date: _____ Reward: _____
Overall goal: _____ Target date: _____ Reward: _____

Develop Strategies for Increasing Steps, Exercise Time, and Flights of Stairs

What can you do to become more active? The possibilities include walking when you do errands, getting off one stop from your destination on public transportation, parking an extra block or two away from your destination, and doing at least one chore every day that requires physical activity. If weather or neighborhood safety is an issue, look for alternative locations to walk. For example, find an indoor gym or shopping mall or even a long hallway. Check out locations that are near or on the way to your campus, workplace, or residence. If you think walking indoors will be dull, walk with friends or family members or wear headphones (if safe) and listen to music or audiobooks.

Are there any days of the week for which your baseline steps are particularly low and/or it will be especially difficult because of your schedule to increase your number of steps? Be sure to develop specific strategies for difficult situations.

List at least five strategies for increasing daily steps, exercise time, or stair flights climbed:

_____   _____

_____   _____

_____   _____

Track Your Progress

Based on the goals you set, fill in the goal portion of the progress chart with your target average daily steps for each week. Then carry your smartphone or fitness tracker every day and note your total daily steps, exercise time, and flights of stairs climbed. Track your progress toward each mini-goal and your final goal. Every few weeks, stop and evaluate your progress. If needed, adjust your plan and develop additional strategies for increasing steps. In addition to the chart in this worksheet, you might also want to graph your daily steps to provide a visual reminder of how you are progressing toward your goals. Make as many copies of this chart as you need.

Week	Goal	M	Tu	W	Th	F	Sa	Su	Average
1									
2									
3									
4									

Weeks 1–4 Progress Checkup

How close are you to meeting your goal? How do you feel about your program and your progress?

If needed, describe changes to your plan and additional strategies for increasing total physical activity:

Week	Goal	M	Tu	W	Th	F	Sa	Su	Average
5									
6									
7									
8									

Weeks 5–8 Progress Checkup

How close are you to meeting your goal? How do you feel about your program and your progress?

If needed, describe changes to your plan and additional strategies for increasing total physical activity:

Week	Goal	M	Tu	W	Th	F	Sa	Su	Average
9									
10									
11									
12									

Weeks 9–12 Progress Checkup

How close are you to meeting your goal? How do you feel about your program and your progress?

If needed, describe changes to your plan and additional strategies for increasing total physical activity.

Design elements: Evidence for Exercise box (shoes and stethoscope): Vstock LLC/Tetra Images/Getty Images; Take Charge box (lady walking): VisualCommunications/E+/Getty Images; Critical Consumer box (man): Sam74100/iStock/Getty Images; Diversity Matters box (holding devices): Robert Churchill/iStockphoto/Rawpixel Ltd/Getty Images; Wellness in the Digital Age box (Smart Watch): Hong Li/DigitalVision/Getty Images

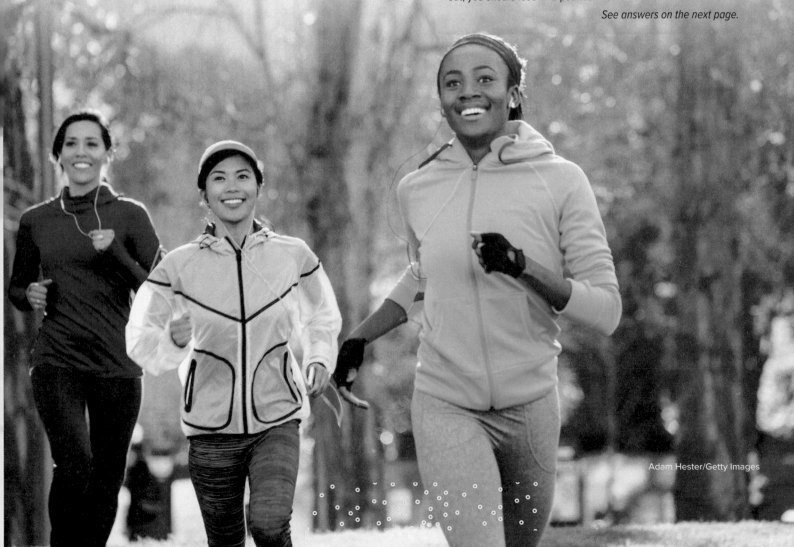

CHAPTER 3

Cardiorespiratory Endurance

LOOKING AHEAD...

After reading this chapter, you should be able to

- Describe how the body produces the energy it needs for exercise.

- List the major effects and benefits of cardiorespiratory endurance exercise.

- Explain how cardiorespiratory endurance is measured and assessed.

- Describe how frequency, intensity, time (duration), type of exercise, volume, and progression (FITT-VP) affect the development of cardiorespiratory endurance.

- Explain the best ways to prevent and treat common exercise injuries.

TEST YOUR KNOWLEDGE

1. Compared to sedentary people, those who engage in regular moderate endurance exercise are likely to
   a. have fewer colds.
   b. be less anxious and depressed.
   c. fall asleep more quickly and sleep better.
   d. be more alert and creative.
   e. all four

2. About how much blood does the heart pump each minute during maximum-intensity aerobic exercise?
   a. 5 quarts
   b. 10 quarts
   c. 20 quarts

3. During an effective 30-minute cardiorespiratory endurance work-out, you should lose 1–2 pounds. True or false?

See answers on the next page.

Adam Hester/Getty Images

Cardiorespiratory endurance—the ability of the body to perform prolonged, large-muscle, dynamic exercise at moderate to high levels of intensity—is a key health-related component of fitness. As explained in Chapter 2, a healthy cardiorespiratory system is essential to high levels of fitness and wellness.

This chapter reviews the short- and long-term effects and benefits of cardiorespiratory endurance exercise. It then describes several tests commonly used to assess cardiorespiratory fitness. Finally, it provides guidelines for creating your own cardiorespiratory endurance training program—one that is geared to your current level of fitness and built around activities you enjoy.

BASIC PHYSIOLOGY OF CARDIORESPIRATORY ENDURANCE EXERCISE

A basic understanding of the body processes involved in cardiorespiratory endurance exercise can help you design a safe and effective fitness program.

The Cardiorespiratory System

The **cardiorespiratory system** consists of the heart, the blood vessels, and the respiratory system (the lungs) (Figure 3.1). The cardiorespiratory system circulates blood through the body, transporting oxygen, nutrients, and other key substances to the organs and tissues that need them. It also carries away waste products so that they can be used or expelled.

The Heart The heart is a four-chambered, fist-sized muscle located just beneath the sternum (breastbone) (Figure 3.2). It pumps oxygen-poor blood to the lungs and delivers oxygen-rich blood to the rest of the body. Blood travels through two separate circulatory systems: The right side of the heart pumps blood to the lungs through **pulmonary circulation**, and the left side pumps blood through the rest of the body in **systemic circulation**.

The path of blood flow through the heart and cardiorespiratory system is illustrated in Figure 3.2. Refer to that illustration as you trace these steps:

1. Waste-laden, oxygen-poor blood travels through large vessels, called **venae cavae**, into the heart's right upper chamber, or **atrium**.

2. After the right atrium fills, it contracts and pumps blood into the heart's right lower chamber, or **ventricle**.

3. When the right ventricle is full, it contracts and pumps blood through the pulmonary artery into the lungs.

4. In the lungs, blood picks up oxygen and discards **carbon dioxide**. Oxygen moves from the lungs to the blood and carbon dioxide moves from the blood to the lungs by a process called **diffusion**. During exercise, you breathe faster to promote diffusion of these gases.

Answers (Test Your Knowledge)

1. **e. All four.** Endurance exercise has many immediate benefits that affect all the dimensions of wellness and improve overall quality of life.

2. **c.** During exercise, cardiac output increases to 20 or more quarts per minute, compared to about 5 quarts per minute at rest.

3. **False.** Any weight loss during an exercise session is due to fluid loss that needs to be replaced to prevent dehydration and enhance performance. It is best to drink enough during exercise to match fluid lost as sweat; weigh yourself before and after a workout to make sure you are drinking enough.

ventricle; the **pulmonary valve** allows blood flow from the right ventricle to the lungs; the **mitral valve** allows blood flow from the left atrium to the left ventricle; and the **aortic valve** allows blood flow into the aorta.

The period of the heart's contraction is called **systole**; the period of relaxation is called **diastole**. During systole, the atria contract first, pumping blood into the ventricles. A fraction of a second later, the ventricles contract, pumping blood to the lungs and the body. During diastole, blood flows into the heart.

Blood pressure, the force exerted by blood on the walls of the blood vessels, is created by the pumping action of the heart. Blood pressure is greater during systole than during diastole. A person weighing 150 pounds has about 5 quarts of blood, which are circulated about once every minute at rest. Hypertension (high blood pressure) is a major risk factor for heart and kidney disease (see Table 11.1).

The heartbeat—the split-second sequence of contractions of the heart's four chambers—is controlled by nerve impulses. These signals originate in a bundle of specialized cells in the right atrium called the *pacemaker,* or *sinoatrial (SA) node.* The heart produces nerve impulses at a steady rate—unless it is speeded up or slowed down by the brain in response to stimuli such as exercise.

The Blood Vessels Blood vessels are classified by size and function. **Veins** carry blood to the heart. **Arteries** carry it away from the heart. Veins have thin walls, but arteries have thick elastic walls that enable them to expand and relax with the volume of blood being pumped through them.

The blood vessels are lined with **endothelial cells** that secrete **nitric oxide**—a chemical messenger regulating blood flow. Inflammation, physical inactivity, poor diet, smoking, high blood pressure, or insulin resistance can promote blood vessel disease and interfere with nitric oxide secretion, which has a wide range of negative effects ranging from erectile dysfunction to heart disease. Regular physical activity helps maintain healthy blood vessels and normal nitric oxide metabolism.

After leaving the heart, the aorta branches into smaller and smaller vessels. The smallest arteries branch still further into

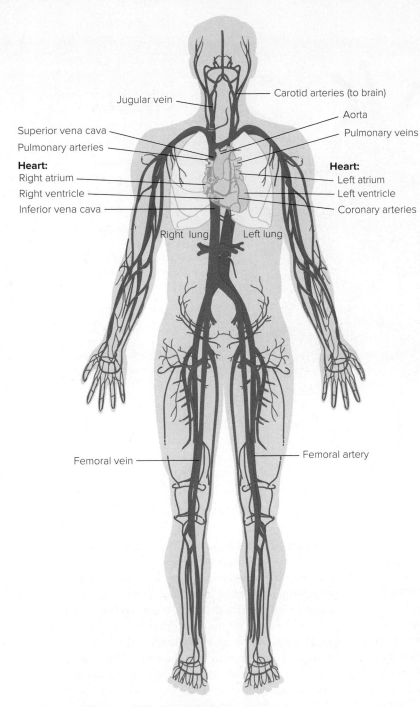

Jugular vein — — Carotid arteries (to brain)
— Aorta
Superior vena cava — — Pulmonary veins
Pulmonary arteries —
Heart:
Right atrium —
Right ventricle — **Heart:**
Inferior vena cava — — Left atrium
— Left ventricle
— Coronary arteries
Right lung   Left lung

Femoral vein — — Femoral artery

Figure 3.1   The cardiorespiratory system.

5. The cleaned, oxygenated blood flows from the lungs through the pulmonary veins into the heart's left atrium.

6. After the left atrium fills, it contracts and pumps blood into the left ventricle.

7. When the left ventricle is full, it pumps blood through the **aorta**—the body's largest artery—for distribution to the rest of the body's blood vessels.

The heart has four valves that prevent blood backflow and keep blood moving in the right direction: the **tricuspid valve** opens to allow blood flow from the right atrium to right

veins   Vessels that carry blood to the heart.   **TERMS**

arteries   Vessels that carry blood away from the heart.

endothelial cells   Cells lining the blood vessels.

nitric oxide   A gas released by the endothelial cells to promote blood flow. The capacity of these cells to release nitric oxide is an important marker of good health.

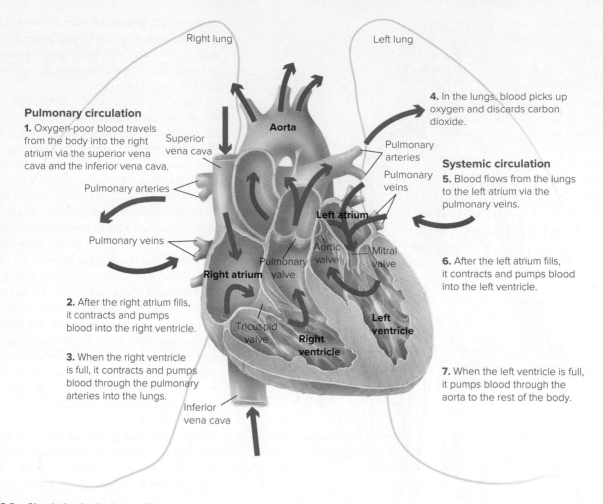

Pulmonary circulation

1. Oxygen-poor blood travels from the body into the right atrium via the superior vena cava and the inferior vena cava.

2. After the right atrium fills, it contracts and pumps blood into the right ventricle.

3. When the right ventricle is full, it contracts and pumps blood through the pulmonary arteries into the lungs.

4. In the lungs, blood picks up oxygen and discards carbon dioxide.

Systemic circulation

5. Blood flows from the lungs to the left atrium via the pulmonary veins.

6. After the left atrium fills, it contracts and pumps blood into the left ventricle.

7. When the left ventricle is full, it pumps blood through the aorta to the rest of the body.

Right lung | Left lung | Aorta | Superior vena cava | Pulmonary arteries | Pulmonary veins | Right atrium | Pulmonary valve | Tricuspid valve | Right ventricle | Inferior vena cava | Pulmonary arteries | Pulmonary veins | Left atrium | Aortic valve | Mitral valve | Left ventricle

Figure 3.2   Circulation in the heart. Blue arrows indicate oxygen-poor blood; red arrows indicate oxygen-rich blood.

capillaries, tiny vessels only one cell thick. The capillaries deliver oxygen and nutrient-rich blood to the tissues and pick up oxygen-poor, waste-laden blood. From the capillaries, this blood empties into small veins (*venules*) and then into larger veins that return it to the heart to repeat the cycle.

Blood pumped through the heart doesn't reach the heart's own cells, so the organ has its own network of blood vessels called the **coronary arteries**. Two large vessels, the right and left coronary arteries, branch off the aorta and supply the heart muscle with oxygenated blood. (The coronary arteries are shown in Figure 3.1). The fit-and-well lifestyle helps prevent coronary artery disease.

TERMS

capillaries Very small blood vessels that distribute blood to all parts of the body.

coronary arteries A pair of large blood vessels that branch off the aorta and supply the heart muscle with oxygenated blood.

respiratory system The lungs, air passages, and breathing muscles; supplies oxygen to the body and removes carbon dioxide.

alveoli Tiny air sacs in the lungs that allow the exchange of oxygen and carbon dioxide between the lungs and blood.

The Respiratory System The **respiratory system** supplies oxygen to the body, carries off carbon dioxide—a waste product of body processes—and helps regulate acid produced during metabolism. Air passes in and out of the lungs as a result of pressure changes brought about by the contraction and relaxation of the diaphragm and rib muscles. As air is inhaled, it passes through the nasal passages, throat, larynx, trachea (windpipe), and bronchi into the lungs. The lungs consist of many branching tubes that end in tiny, thin-walled air sacs called **alveoli**.

Carbon dioxide and oxygen are exchanged between alveoli and capillaries in the lungs. Carbon dioxide passes from blood cells into the alveoli, where it is carried up and out of the lungs (exhaled). Oxygen from inhaled air is passed from the alveoli into blood cells; these oxygen-rich blood cells then return to the heart and are pumped throughout the body. Oxygen is an important component of the body's energy-producing system, so the cardiorespiratory system's ability to pick up and deliver oxygen is critical for the functioning of the body.

The Cardiorespiratory System at Rest and during Exercise At rest and during light activity, the cardiorespiratory system functions at a fairly steady pace. Your heart beats at a rate of about 50–90 beats per minute, and you take about

12-20 breaths per minute. A typical resting blood pressure in a healthy adult, measured in millimeters of mercury, is 120 systolic and 80 diastolic (120/80 mmHg).

During exercise, the demands on the cardiorespiratory system increase. Body cells, particularly working muscles, need to obtain more oxygen and fuel and to eliminate more waste products. To meet these demands, your body makes the following changes:

- Heart rate increases, up to 170–210 beats per minute during intense exercise.

- The heart's **stroke volume** increases, meaning that the heart pumps out more blood with each beat.

- The heart pumps and circulates more blood per minute as a result of the faster heart rate and greater stroke volume. During exercise, this **cardiac output** increases to 20 or more quarts per minute, compared to about 5 quarts per minute at rest.

- Blood flow changes, so as much as 85–90% of the blood may be delivered to working muscles. At rest, about 15–20% of blood is distributed to the skeletal muscles.

- Systolic blood pressure increases, while diastolic blood pressure holds steady or declines slightly. A typical exercise blood pressure might be 175/65. Diastolic pressure is particularly important during exercise because the blood flow to the coronary arteries that supply the heart muscle is greatest during the relaxation phase of the cardiac cycle.

- To oxygenate this increased blood flow, you take deeper breaths and breathe faster, up to 40–60 breaths per minute.

All of these changes are controlled and coordinated by special centers in the brain, which use the nervous system and chemical messengers to control the process.

Energy Production

Metabolism is the sum of all the chemical processes necessary to maintain the body. Energy is required to fuel vital body functions—to build and break down tissue, contract muscles, conduct nerve impulses, regulate body temperature, and so on.

The rate at which your body uses energy—its **metabolic rate**—depends on your level of activity. At rest, you have a low metabolic rate; if you begin to walk, your metabolic rate increases. If you jog, your metabolic rate may increase more than 800% above its resting level. Olympic-caliber distance runners can increase their metabolic rate by 2,000% or more.

Energy from Food The body converts chemical energy from food into substances that cells can use as fuel. These fuels can be used immediately or stored for later use. The body's ability to store fuel is critical, because if all the energy from food were released immediately, much of it would be wasted.

The three classes of energy-containing nutrients in food are carbohydrates (sugar, wheat flour, honey), fats (meat, nuts, fried foods), and proteins (seafood, poultry, dairy food). During digestion, most carbohydrates are broken down into the simple sugar **glucose**. Some glucose circulates in the blood ("blood sugar"), where it can be used as a quick source of fuel to produce energy.

Glucose may also be converted to **glycogen** and stored mainly in the liver and muscles. If glycogen stores are full and the body's immediate need for energy is met, the remaining glucose is converted to fat and stored in the body's fatty tissues. Excess energy from fat in the diet is also stored as body fat. Protein in the diet is used primarily to build new tissue, but it can be broken down for energy or incorporated into fat stores. Glucose, glycogen, and fat are important fuels for the production of energy in the cells; protein is a significant energy source only when other fuels are lacking. (See Chapter 8 for more on the roles of carbohydrate, fat, and protein in the body.)

ATP: The Energy "Currency" of Cells The basic form of energy used by cells is **adenosine triphosphate**, or ATP. When a cell needs energy, it breaks down ATP, a process that releases energy in the only form the cell can use directly. Cells store a small amount of ATP; when they need more, they create it through chemical reactions that utilize the body's stored fuels—glucose, glycogen, and fat. When you exercise, your cells need to produce more energy. Consequently, your body mobilizes its stores of fuel to increase ATP production. The mitochondria of cells produce the most ATP. A high mitochondrial capacity is critical for endurance performance, health, and longevity.

Exercise and the Three Energy Systems

The muscles in your body use three energy systems to create ATP and fuel cellular activity. These systems use different fuels and chemical processes and perform different, specific functions during exercise (Table 3.1).

The Immediate Energy System The **immediate ("explosive") energy system** provides energy rapidly but for only a short period of time. It is used to fuel activities that last for about 10 or fewer seconds—such as weight lifting and shot-putting or in daily life just rising from a chair or picking up a bag of groceries. The fuels for this energy system include existing

---

TERMS

stroke volume The amount of blood the heart pumps with each beat.

cardiac output The volume of blood pumped by the heart per minute via heart rate and stroke volume.

metabolic rate The rate at which the body uses energy.

glucose A simple sugar circulating in the blood that can be used by cells to fuel adenosine triphosphate (ATP) production.

glycogen A complex carbohydrate stored principally in the liver and skeletal muscles; the major fuel source during most forms of intense exercise. Glycogen is the storage form of glucose.

adenosine triphosphate (ATP) The energy source for cellular processes.

immediate ("explosive") energy system The system that supplies very short bursts of energy to muscle cells through the breakdown of cellular stores of ATP and creatine phosphate (CP).

Table 3.1   Characteristics of the Body's Energy Systems

| | ENERGY SYSTEM* | | |
	IMMEDIATE	NONOXIDATIVE	OXIDATIVE
DURATION OF ACTIVITY FOR WHICH SYSTEM PREDOMINATES	0–10 seconds	10 seconds–2 minutes	>2 minutes
INTENSITY OF ACTIVITY FOR WHICH SYSTEM PREDOMINATES	High	High	Low to moderately high
RATE OF ATP PRODUCTION	Immediate, very rapid	Rapid	Slower, but prolonged
FUEL	Adenosine triphosphate (ATP), creatine phosphate (CP)	Muscle stores of glucose and glycogen	Body stores of glycogen, glucose, fat, and protein
OXYGEN USED?	No	No	Yes
SAMPLE ACTIVITIES	Weight lifting, picking up a bag of groceries	400-meter run, running up several flights of stairs	1500-meter run, 30-minute walk, standing in line for a long time

*For most activities, all three systems contribute to energy production; the duration and intensity of the activity determine which system predominates.

SOURCE: Brooks, G. A., et al. 2005. *Exercise Physiology: Human Bioenergetics and Its Applications*, 4th ed. New York: McGraw-Hill.

cellular ATP stores and **creatine phosphate** (CP), a chemical that cells can use to make ATP. CP levels deplete rapidly during exercise, so the maximum capacity of this energy system is reached within a few seconds. Cells must then switch to the other energy systems to restore levels of ATP and CP. (Without adequate ATP, muscles will stiffen and become unusable.)

The Nonoxidative Energy System The **nonoxidative (anaerobic) energy system** is used at the start of an exercise session and for high-intensity activities lasting for about 10 seconds to 2 minutes, such as the 400-meter run. During daily activities, this system may be called on to help you run to catch a bus or

creatine phosphate   A high-energy compound used to resynthesize ATP that is particularly important during high-intensity exercise.

nonoxidative (anaerobic) energy system   The system that supplies energy to muscle cells for highly intense exercise of short duration by breaking down muscle stores of glucose and glycogen; called the *anaerobic system* because chemical reactions take place without oxygen and produce lactic acid.

anaerobic   Occurring in the absence of oxygen.

lactic acid   A metabolic acid resulting from the metabolism of glucose and glycogen. It is broken down in the body into lactate and hydrogen ions as soon as it is produced.

lactate   Lactate is lactic acid without the acid. In the body, lactic acid immediately gets rid of the acid (hydrogen ion, H^+), so the body produces and uses lactate at rest and during exercise.

oxidative (aerobic) energy system   The system that supplies energy to cells for long periods of activity through the breakdown of glucose, glycogen, and fats; called the *aerobic system* because its chemical reactions require oxygen.

aerobic   Dependent on the presence of oxygen.

mitochondria   Cell structures that convert the energy in food to a form the body can use.

TERMS

dash up several flights of stairs. The nonoxidative energy system creates ATP by breaking down glucose and glycogen. This system doesn't require oxygen, which is why it is sometimes referred to as the **anaerobic** system. This system's capacity to produce energy is limited, but it can generate a great deal of ATP in a short period of time. For this reason, it is the most important energy system for very intense exercise.

The nonoxidative energy system has two key limitations. First, the body's supply of glucose and glycogen is limited. If these are depleted, a person may experience fatigue, dizziness, and impaired judgment. (The brain and nervous system rely on carbohydrates as fuel.) Second, the rapid metabolism caused by this energy system increases hydrogen and potassium ions that interfere with metabolism and muscle contraction and cause fatigue. During heavy exercise, such as sprinting, large increases in hydrogen and potassium ions cause muscles to fatigue rapidly.

The anaerobic energy system also creates metabolic acids. Fortunately, exercise training increases the body's ability to cope with metabolic acids. Improved fitness allows you to exercise at higher intensities before the abrupt buildup of metabolic acids—a point that scientists call the *lactate threshold*. One metabolic acid, called **lactic acid**, is often linked to fatigue during intense exercise. Lactic acid does not last long in blood. It breaks down into **lactate** and hydrogen ions (acid) as soon as it is produced. Lactate is an important fuel at rest and during exercise. Training improves the ability to use lactate as fuel.

The Oxidative Energy System The **oxidative (aerobic) energy system** operates during any physical activity that lasts longer than about two minutes, such as distance running, swimming, hiking, or even just standing in line. The oxidative system requires oxygen to generate ATP, which is why it is considered an **aerobic** system. The oxidative system cannot produce energy as quickly as the other two systems, but it can supply energy for much longer periods of time. It is the source of our energy during most daily activities.

In the oxidative energy system, ATP production takes place in cellular structures called **mitochondria**. Because mitochondria can use carbohydrates (glucose and glycogen) or fats to produce ATP, the body's stores of fuel for this system are much greater than those for the other two energy systems. The actual fuel used depends on the intensity and duration of exercise and on the fitness status of the individual. Carbohydrates are favored during more intense exercise (more than 65% of maximum capacity); fats are used for mild, low-intensity activities. During a prolonged exercise session, carbohydrates are the predominant fuel at the start of the workout, but fat utilization increases over time. Fit individuals use a greater proportion of fat as fuel because increased fitness allows people to do activities at lower intensities. This is an important adaptation because glycogen depletion is one of the limiting factors for the oxidative energy system. By being able to use more fat as fuel, a fit individual can exercise for a longer time before glycogen is depleted and muscles become fatigued. Aerobic exercise and high-intensity interval training increase the number and capacity of mitochondria. Increased mitochondrial capacity is the most important benefit of exercise. Mitochondrial health and fitness are linked to a reduced risk of disease and increased longevity.

Oxygen is another factor limiting exercise capacity. The oxygen requirement of this energy system is proportional to the intensity of exercise. As intensity increases, so does oxygen consumption. The body's ability to increase oxygen use is limited; this limit, known as **maximal oxygen consumption**, or $\dot{V}O_{2max}$, refers to the highest rate of oxygen consumption an individual is capable of during maximum physical effort. It is expressed in milliliters of oxygen per kilogram of body weight per minute or as liters per minute. In the symbol, the V stands for volume, the dot over the V means per minute, the O_2 stands for oxygen, and the max means maximum. $\dot{V}O_{2max}$ determines how intensely a person can perform endurance exercise and for how long, and it is considered the best overall measure of the capacity of the cardiorespiratory system. (The assessment tests described later in the chapter are designed to help you evaluate your $\dot{V}O_{2max}$).

The Energy Systems in Combination Your body typically uses all three energy systems when you exercise. The intensity and duration of the activity determine which system predominates. For example, when you play tennis, you use the immediate energy system when hitting the ball, but you replenish cellular energy stores by using the nonoxidative and oxidative systems. When cycling, the oxidative system predominates. However, if you must suddenly exercise intensely—by riding up a steep hill, for example—the other systems become important because the oxidative system is unable to supply ATP fast enough to sustain high-intensity effort.

Physical Fitness and Energy Production Physically fit people can increase their metabolic rate substantially, generating the energy needed for powerful or sustained exercise. People who are not fit cannot respond to exercise in the same way. Their bodies are less capable of delivering oxygen and fuel to exercising muscles, they can't burn as many calories during or after exercise, and they are less able to cope with lactate and other substances produced during intense physical activity that contribute to fatigue. Because of this, they become fatigued more rapidly; their legs hurt and they breathe heavily walking up a flight of stairs, for example. Regular physical training can substantially improve the body's ability to produce energy and meet the challenges of increased physical activity.

In designing an exercise program, focus on the energy system most important to your goals. Because improving the functioning of the cardiorespiratory system is critical to overall wellness, endurance exercise that utilizes the oxidative energy system—activities performed at moderate to high intensities for a prolonged duration—is a key component of any health-related fitness program.

BENEFITS OF CARDIORESPIRATORY ENDURANCE EXERCISE

Cardiorespiratory endurance exercise helps the body become more efficient and better able to cope with physical challenges. It also lowers risk for many chronic diseases.

Improved Cardiorespiratory Functioning

Earlier, this chapter described some of the major changes that occur in the cardiorespiratory system when you exercise, such as increases in cardiac output and blood pressure, breathing rate, and blood flow to the skeletal muscles. In the short term, all these changes help the body respond to the challenge of exercise. When performed regularly, endurance exercise also leads to permanent adaptation in the cardiorespiratory system (Figure 3.3). This improvement reduces the effort required to perform everyday tasks and enables the body to respond to physical challenges. This, in a nutshell, is what it means to be physically fit.

Endurance exercise enhances the heart's health by doing the following:

- Maintaining or increasing the heart's own blood and oxygen supply.
- Improving the heart muscle's function, enabling the heart to pump more blood per beat. This improved function keeps the heart rate lower both at rest and during exercise. The

? Ask Yourself

QUESTIONS FOR CRITICAL THINKING AND REFLECTION

When you think about the types of physical activity you engage in during your typical day or week, which ones use the immediate energy system? The nonoxidative energy system? The oxidative energy system? How can you increase activities that use the oxidative energy system?

maximal oxygen consumption ($\dot{V}O_{2max}$) The **TERMS** highest rate of oxygen consumption an individual is capable of during maximum physical effort, reflecting the body's ability to transport and use oxygen; measured in milliliters of oxygen used per kilogram of body weight per minute.

resting heart rate of a fit person is often 10–20 beats per minute lower than that of an unfit person. This translates into as many as 10 million fewer beats in the course of a year.

- Strengthening the heart's contractions.
- Increasing the heart's cavity size (in young adults).
- Increasing blood volume, enabling the heart to push more blood into the circulatory system during each contraction (larger stroke volume). Increased blood volume also improves temperature regulation, which reduces the load on the heart.
- Reducing blood pressure.
- Reducing blood cholesterol and triglycerides and increasing HDL (good cholesterol), which reduces the risk of coronary artery disease.

- Stabilizing the electrical activity of the heart, which protects against **cardiac arrest**.

Improved Cellular Metabolism

Regular endurance exercise improves the body's metabolism, down to the cellular level, enhancing your ability to produce and use energy efficiently. Cardiorespiratory training improves metabolism by doing the following (see Figure 3.3):

- Increasing the number of capillaries in the muscles. Additional capillaries supply the muscles with more fuel and oxygen and more quickly eliminate waste products. Greater capillary density also helps heal injuries and reduce muscle aches.

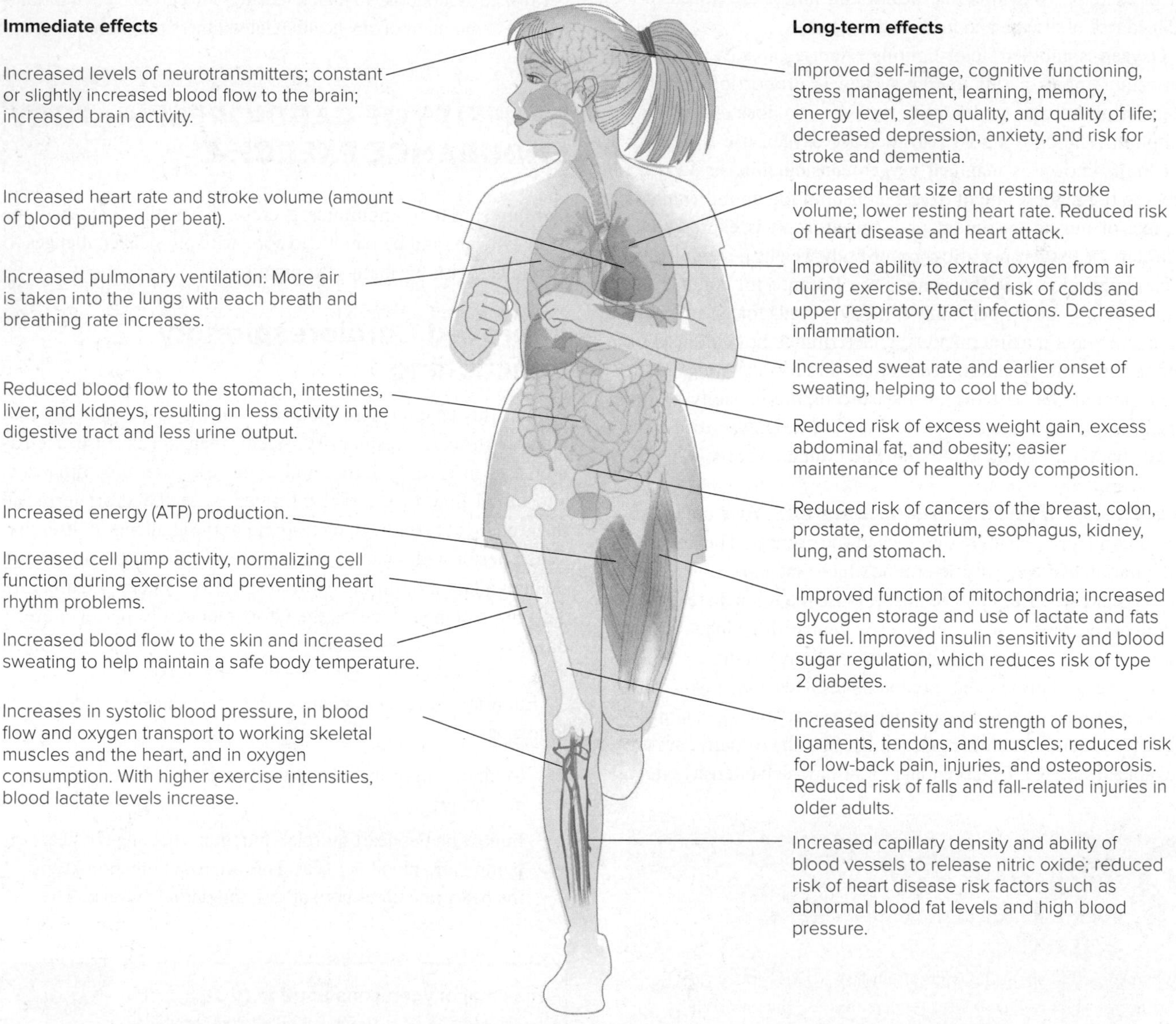

Immediate effects

Increased levels of neurotransmitters; constant or slightly increased blood flow to the brain; increased brain activity.

Increased heart rate and stroke volume (amount of blood pumped per beat).

Increased pulmonary ventilation: More air is taken into the lungs with each breath and breathing rate increases.

Reduced blood flow to the stomach, intestines, liver, and kidneys, resulting in less activity in the digestive tract and less urine output.

Increased energy (ATP) production.

Increased cell pump activity, normalizing cell function during exercise and preventing heart rhythm problems.

Increased blood flow to the skin and increased sweating to help maintain a safe body temperature.

Increases in systolic blood pressure, in blood flow and oxygen transport to working skeletal muscles and the heart, and in oxygen consumption. With higher exercise intensities, blood lactate levels increase.

Long-term effects

Improved self-image, cognitive functioning, stress management, learning, memory, energy level, sleep quality, and quality of life; decreased depression, anxiety, and risk for stroke and dementia.

Increased heart size and resting stroke volume; lower resting heart rate. Reduced risk of heart disease and heart attack.

Improved ability to extract oxygen from air during exercise. Reduced risk of colds and upper respiratory tract infections. Decreased inflammation.

Increased sweat rate and earlier onset of sweating, helping to cool the body.

Reduced risk of excess weight gain, excess abdominal fat, and obesity; easier maintenance of healthy body composition.

Reduced risk of cancers of the breast, colon, prostate, endometrium, esophagus, kidney, lung, and stomach.

Improved function of mitochondria; increased glycogen storage and use of lactate and fats as fuel. Improved insulin sensitivity and blood sugar regulation, which reduces risk of type 2 diabetes.

Increased density and strength of bones, ligaments, tendons, and muscles; reduced risk for low-back pain, injuries, and osteoporosis. Reduced risk of falls and fall-related injuries in older adults.

Increased capillary density and ability of blood vessels to release nitric oxide; reduced risk of heart disease risk factors such as abnormal blood fat levels and high blood pressure.

Figure 3.3 Immediate and long-term effects of regular cardiorespiratory endurance exercise. When endurance exercise is performed regularly, short-term changes in the body develop into permanent adaptations; these include improved ability to exercise, reduced risk of many chronic diseases, and improved psychological and emotional well-being. Regular endurance exercise is associated with a reduced death rate from all causes and increased longevity.

- Training muscles to make the most of oxygen and fuel so they work more efficiently.

- Increasing the size and number of mitochondria in muscle and brain cells, increasing the cells' energy capacity.

- Preventing glycogen depletion and increasing the muscles' ability to use lactate and fat as fuels.

- Increasing the activity of cell pumps for sodium, potassium, and calcium, which normalizes cell function and prevents fatigue and abnormal heart rhythms.

Regular exercise may also help protect cells from chemical damage caused by agents called *free radicals.* (See Chapter 8 for details on free radicals and the special enzymes the body uses to fight them.)

Fitness programs that best develop metabolic efficiency include both long-duration, moderately intense endurance exercise and brief periods of more intense effort. For example, climbing a small hill while jogging or cycling introduces the kind of intense exercise that leads to more efficient use of lactate and fats.

Reduced Risk of Chronic Disease

Regular endurance exercise lowers your risk of many chronic, disabling diseases. It can also help people with those diseases improve their health (see the box "Benefits of Exercise for Older Adults"). The most significant health benefits occur when someone who is sedentary becomes moderately active.

Cardiovascular Diseases Sedentary living is a key contributor to cardiovascular disease (CVD). CVD is a general category that encompasses several diseases of the heart and blood vessels, including coronary heart disease (which can cause heart attacks), stroke, and high blood pressure (see the box "Combine Aerobic Exercise with Strength Training"). Sedentary people are significantly more likely to die of CVD than are fit individuals.

Cardiorespiratory endurance exercise lowers your risk of CVD by doing the following:

- Promoting a healthy balance of fats in the blood. High concentrations of blood fats such as cholesterol and triglycerides are linked to CVD. Exercise raises levels of "good cholesterol" (high-density lipoproteins, or HDL) and may lower levels of "bad cholesterol" (low-density lipoproteins, or LDL).

- Reducing high blood pressure, which is a contributing factor to several kinds of CVD.

- Boosting **cell pump** activity (sodium-potassium and calcium pumps) that help maintain internal cellular health.

- Enhancing the capacity of cell mitochondria.

- Enhancing the function of the cells that line the arteries (endothelial cells).

- Reducing chronic inflammation.

- Preventing obesity and type 2 diabetes, both of which contribute to CVD.

Details on various types of CVD, their associated risk factors, and a lifestyle that can reduce your risk for developing CVD are discussed in Chapter 11.

Cancer Regular moderate- to vigorous-intensity exercise reduces the risk of cancer of the colon, breast, bladder, endometrium (lining of the uterus), esophagus, lung, kidney, and stomach. (See Chapter 12 for more information on various types of cancer.)

Type 2 Diabetes Regular exercise helps prevent type 2 diabetes, the most common form of diabetes. Physical activity is also an important part of treating the disease. Obesity is a key risk factor for diabetes, and exercise helps keep body fat at healthy levels. But even without fat loss, exercise improves control of blood sugar levels in many people with diabetes. Exercise metabolizes (burns) excess sugar and makes cells more sensitive to the hormone insulin, which helps regulate blood sugar levels. (See Chapter 11 for more on diabetes and insulin resistance.)

Osteoporosis A special benefit of exercise, especially for women, is protection against osteoporosis, a disease that results in loss of bone density and strength. Weight-bearing exercise—particularly weight training—helps build bone during the teens and 20s and maintain bone mass in later years. People with denser bones can better endure the bone loss that occurs with aging. With stronger bones and muscles and better balance, fit people are less likely to experience debilitating falls and bone fractures. (See Chapter 8 for more on osteoporosis.)

Inflammation **Inflammation** is the body's response to tissue and cell damage (from injury, high blood pressure, or intense exercise), environmental poisons (e.g., cigarette smoke), or poor metabolic health (high blood fats, poor blood sugar control). Acute inflammation is a short-term response to exercise and is an important way that the body improves physical fitness. For example, short-term inflammation triggers increased muscle protein synthesis, which promotes muscle fitness and recovery from exercise. Chronic inflammation, on the other hand, is a prolonged, abnormal process that causes tissue breakdown and diseases such as atherosclerosis, cancer, and rheumatoid arthritis.

Although exercise increases acute inflammation during and shortly after a workout, it reduces chronic levels of inflammation—if the training program is not too severe. For example, practicing

cardiac arrest   Malfunctioning of the heart, in which it suddenly stops beating due to "electrical" problems in the heart cells.   **TERMS**

cell pump   Structures in cell walls that work to maintain normal cell levels of sodium, potassium, and calcium. Exercise training increases the activity of these pumps, which helps prevent fatigue.

inflammation   The body's response to tissue and cell damage, environmental poisons, or poor metabolic health.

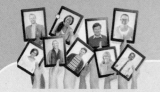

DIVERSITY MATTERS
Benefits of Exercise for Older Adults

Most aspects of physiological functioning peak when people are about 30 years old, then decline at a rate of about 0.5–1.0% per year. This decline in physical capacity occurs because of decreases in maximal oxygen consumption, cardiac output, muscular strength, fat-free mass, joint mobility, and other factors. Regular exercise slows the rate of decline and promotes both longevity and improved quality of life.

Regular endurance exercise can improve maximal oxygen consumption in older adults by up to 15–30%—the same improvement seen in young adults. Masters athletes in their 70s have aerobic capacities equivalent to those of sedentary 20 year olds.

At any age, endurance training can improve cardiorespiratory functioning, cellular metabolism, body composition, and psychological and emotional well-being. Older adults who exercise regularly have better balance and greater bone density and are less likely than

their sedentary peers to suffer injuries because of falls. Endurance and interval training also increase the cell mitochondria (powerhouses of the cell), a factor linked to increased longevity. Regular endurance training substantially reduces the risk of many chronic and disabling diseases, including heart disease, cancer, diabetes, osteoporosis, and dementia.

Other forms of exercise training are also beneficial for older adults. Resistance training, a safe and effective way to build strength and fat-free mass, helps people remain independent as they age. Older adults gain strength quickly, which improves performance in everyday tasks such as climbing stairs and carrying groceries. Flexibility exercises can improve the ranges of motion in joints, another aid in helping people maintain functional independence as they age.

It's never too late to begin an exercise program. In 2017, 105-year-old French cyclist Robert Marchand set

a masters world record by riding 22.5 kilometers (14 miles) in one hour. He didn't start competitive cycling until he was 68. Most older adults can participate in moderate walking and strengthening and stretching exercises, and modified programs can be created for people with chronic conditions and other special health concerns. The wellness benefits of exercise are available to people of all ages and levels of ability.

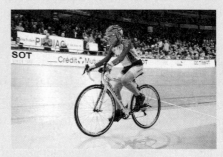

105-year-old cyclist Robert Marchand

Nolwenn Le Gouic/Icon Sport/Getty Images

---

endurance training three to five days a week will reduce inflammation, particularly when accompanied by weight and fat loss. Training excessively, such as running a marathon several times a month or doing severe cross-training workouts five to seven days per week, will cause overtraining and chronic inflammation. We could call this the Goldilocks effect: The training program should not be too much or too little; it should be just right.

Deaths from All Causes Physically active people have a reduced risk of dying prematurely from all causes, with the greatest benefits found for people with the highest levels of physical activity and fitness (Figure 3.4). Physical inactivity is a predictor of premature death and is as important a risk factor as smoking, high blood pressure, obesity, and diabetes.

Better Control of Body Fat

Too much body fat is linked to a variety of health problems, including cardiovascular disease, cancer, and type 2 diabetes. Healthy body composition can be difficult to achieve and maintain—especially for someone who is sedentary—because a diet that contains all essential nutrients can be relatively high in calories. Excess calories are stored in the body as fat. Regular exercise increases daily calorie expenditure, which

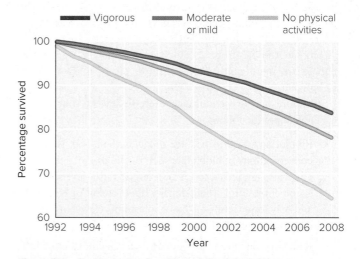

Figure 3.4 Survival rates for older adults doing vigorous, moderate, or no exercise, 1992–2008. The Health and Retirement Study—a long-term study of older adults—found that people who exercised vigorously over a 16-year period (1992–2008) had a lower death rate than those who exercised at moderate intensities or did no physical activity. After 16 years, the survival rate was 84% for those doing vigorous exercise, 78% for those doing moderate-intensity physical activity, and only 65% for those doing no physical activity. Exercising longer or more intensely reduces the risk of dying prematurely from a variety of causes.

SOURCE: Wen, M., et al. 2014. "Physical activity and mortality among middle-aged and older adults in the United States," *Journal Physical Activity & Health* 11(2): 303–312.

Emphasizing one aspect of fitness at the expense of others may be a special concern for those exercising with weights who don't do enough cardiorespiratory conditioning. Although exercise experts universally agree that resistance training is beneficial for a variety of reasons (as detailed in Chapter 4), it also has a downside.

Large population studies have tracked the impact of weight training exercises on the cardiovascular system to discover if it helps or harms the heart and blood vessels. These studies have shown that intense strength training poses short- and long-term risks to the cardiovascular system—especially to arterial health:

• Weight training promotes short-term stiffness of the blood vessels, which could promote hypertension (high blood pressure) over time and increase the load on the heart.

• Lifting weights (especially heavy weights) causes extreme short-term boosts in blood pressure; blood pressure can reach 480/350 mmHg during heavy lifting. Over the long term, sharp elevations in blood pressure can damage arteries, even if each pressure increase lasts only a few seconds.

• Weight training places stress on the endothelial cells that line blood vessels. Because these cells secrete nitric oxide (a chemical messenger involved in a variety of bodily functions), this stress can contribute to a wide range of negative effects, from erectile dysfunction to heart disease.

A variety of studies have shown that the best way to offset cardiovascular stress caused by strength training is to do cardiorespiratory endurance exercise (such as brisk walking or using an elliptical machine) immediately after a weight training session. Groundbreaking Japanese research showed that following resistance training with aerobic exercise prevents the stiffening of blood vessels and its associated damage. In this eight-week study, participants did aerobics before lifting weights, after lifting weights, or not at all. The group that did aerobics *after* weight training saw the greatest positive impact. Participants who lifted weights after aerobics saw no improvement in the health of their blood vessels.

Strength training promotes endurance fitness by improving nervous control of the muscles, increasing type IIa motor units (muscle fibers with a blend of strength and endurance capacity), and increasing tendon strength. These changes increase muscle strength and the rate of force development, enhance the economy of movement, and increase the speed with which blood cells travel through the muscles.

The bottom line of all this research? Both resistance training and cardiorespiratory exercise are good for you, if you do them in the right order. So, when you plan your workouts, do 15–60 minutes of aerobic exercise after each weight training session.

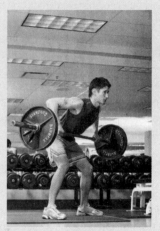

SOURCES: Kingsley, J. D., et al. 2016. "Arterial stiffness and autonomic modulation after free-weight resistance exercise in resistance trained individuals," *Journal of Strength Conditioning Research* 30(12): 3373 3380; Tagawa, K., et al. 2018. "Effects of resistance training on arterial compliance and plasma endothelin-1," *Physiological Research* 67: S155–S166; Okamoto, T. M., et al. 2007. "Combined aerobic and resistance training and vascular function: Effect of aerobic exercise before and after resistance training," *Journal of Applied Physiology* 103(5): 1655–1661.

Paul Burns/Digital Vision/Getty Images

means that a healthy diet is less likely to lead to weight gain. Endurance exercise burns calories directly and, if intense enough, continues to do so by raising resting metabolic rate for several hours following an exercise session. A higher metabolic rate makes it easier for a person to maintain a healthy weight or to lose weight. However, exercise alone cannot ensure a healthy body composition. As described in Chapters 6 and 9, you will lose more weight more rapidly and keep it off longer if you decrease your calorie intake and boost your calorie expenditure through exercise.

Improved Immune Function

Exercise can have either positive or negative effects on the **immune system**, the physiological processes that protect us from diseases such as colds, bacterial infections, and even cancer. Moderate endurance exercise boosts immune function, whereas overtraining (excessive training) depresses it, at least temporarily. Physically fit people get fewer colds and upper respiratory tract infections than people who are not fit.

Exercise affects immune function by influencing levels of specialized cells and chemicals involved in the immune response. As discussed in Chapter 2, physically active people also have healthier, more resilient genes, which promotes immunity. Exercise preserves the telomeres, which form the ends of the DNA strands and holds them together. Without exercise, the telomeres shorten over time, eventually reducing the effectiveness of the immune system. Besides getting regular moderate exercise, you can further strengthen your immune system by eating a well-balanced diet, managing stress, and getting seven to eight hours of sleep every night.

immune system The physiological processes that protect us from diseases such as colds, bacterial infections, and even cancer.

TERMS

Improved Psychological and Emotional Well-Being

Most people who participate in regular endurance exercise experience social, psychological, and emotional benefits. Skill mastery and self-control enhance one's self-image. Recreational sports provide an opportunity to socialize, have fun, and strive to excel. Endurance exercise lessens anxiety, depression, stress, anger, and hostility, thereby improving mood while boosting cardiovascular health. Regular exercise also improves sleep.

ASSESSING CARDIORESPIRATORY FITNESS

The body's ability to maintain a level of exertion (exercise) for an extended time is a direct reflection of cardiorespiratory fitness. One's level of fitness is determined by the body's ability to take up, distribute, and use oxygen during physical activity. The best quantitative measure of cardiorespiratory endurance is maximal oxygen consumption, expressed as $\dot{V}O_{2max}$, oxygen the body uses when a person reaches his or her maximum ability to supply oxygen during exercise. Maximal oxygen consumption can be measured precisely in an exercise physiology laboratory through analysis of the air a person inhales and exhales when exercising to a level of exhaustion (maximum intensity). This procedure can be expensive and time consuming, however, making it impractical for the average person.

Choosing an Assessment Test

Several simple assessment tests provide reasonably good estimates of maximal oxygen consumption (within 10–15% of the results of a laboratory test). Four commonly used assessments are the following:

- *The 1-Mile Walk Test.* This test measures the amount of time it takes you to complete 1 mile of brisk walking and your heart rate at the end of your walk. A fast time and a low heart rate indicate a high level of cardiorespiratory endurance.

- *The 3-Minute Step Test.* In the step test, you step continually at a steady rate for 3 minutes and then monitor your heart rate during recovery. The rate at which the pulse returns to normal is a good measure of cardiorespiratory capacity; heart rate remains lower and recovers faster in people who are more physically fit.

- *The 1.5-Mile Run-Walk Test.* Oxygen consumption increases with speed in distance running, so a fast time on this test indicates high maximal oxygen consumption.

- *The Beep Test.* This test predicting maximal oxygen consumption is excellent for people who are physically fit and wish to measure their capacity for high-intensity exercise, such as sprints. A prerecorded series of "beeps" (tones) sound off at faster and faster intervals. Your task is to keep up with the beeps during the exercise.

Lab 3.1 provides detailed instructions for each of these tests. An additional assessment, the 12-Minute Swim Test, is also provided.

To assess yourself, choose a method based on your access to equipment, your current physical condition, and your own preference.

Don't take these tests without checking with your physician if you are ill or have any of the risk factors for exercise discussed in Chapter 2 and Lab 2.1.

Monitoring Your Heart Rate

Each time your heart contracts, it pumps blood into your arteries. You can measure your heart rate—the number of heart contractions per minute—by using a heart rate monitor or counting your pulse beats. Modern heart rate monitors are inexpensive and fairly accurate. Several companies make heart rate monitor apps that are used with smartphones to measure heart rate, distances, route maps, running or cycling speed, calories burned, and even the electrical activity of the heart as it beats, which is what an electrocardiogram (ECG, or EKG) does. Counting your pulse is the traditional method of measuring heart rate. Each contraction of the heart produces a surge of blood that causes a pulse you can feel by holding your fingers against an artery. Heart rate is a good way to monitor exercise intensity during a workout. (Intensity is described in more detail in the next section.)

The radial artery in the wrist is the most common site to measure pulse rate (Figure 3.5). To take your pulse, press your index and middle fingers gently on the correct site. You may have to shift position several times to find the best place to feel your pulse. A good technique is to bend your fingers slightly and take your pulse with the tops of your fingers where you have many nerve endings. Don't use your thumb to check your pulse; it has a pulse of its own that can confuse your count.

Heart rates are usually assessed in beats per minute (bpm). But counting your pulse for an entire minute isn't practical when you're exercising. And because heart rate slows rapidly when you stop exercising, a full minute's worth of counting can give inaccurate results. It's best to do a shorter count—15 seconds—and then multiply the result by 4 to get your heart rate in beats per minute. (You can also use a heart rate monitor to check your

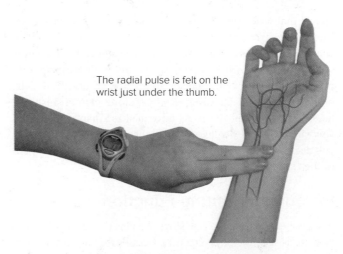

The radial pulse is felt on the wrist just under the thumb.

Figure 3.5 Checking your pulse. Take your pulse at the radial artery in the wrist.

Photo taken by Robin Mouat

Technology has transformed the market for trackers and monitors. It is difficult to keep up with the latest exercise monitors designed as stand-alone units, smartphone apps, and GPS accessories. A heart rate monitor is an electronic device that checks the user's pulse, either continuously or on demand. These devices make it easy to monitor your heart rate before, during, and after exercise. Some include global positioning system (GPS) receivers that help you track the distance you walk, run, or bike. Wearable fitness trackers, made by Apple, Fitbit, Polar, Timex, Mio, and Garmin, among others, measure distance and steps covered, calories burned, and exercise intensity. Most studies show that the heart rate monitors are highly accurate, but the calorie counters are less so. However, the activity trackers are excellent motivators and provide a relative benchmark from one workout to the next.

Fitness Trackers

High-tech monitors and phone apps such as the Nike + FuelBand, Cyclemeter, Nike + Sensor, and Adidas miCoach track daily activities including running and walking and sports like basketball. They track steps taken, distance covered, and calories burned. Fitness trackers allow you to keep track of your progress, compete against other people, and meet challenges.

Wearable Heart Rate Monitors

Heart rate monitors use either a chest strap that measures the electrical activity of the heart or an optical sensor worn on the wrist that measures heart rate by detecting changes in wrist blood flow. Chest-strap monitors are more accurate, but wrist monitors are more convenient. A wide variety of monitors are available, many at modest cost.

Monitors in Gym Equipment

Many pieces of workout equipment—including newer-model treadmills, stationary bikes, and elliptical trainers—feature built-in heart rate monitors. The monitor is usually mounted into the device's handles. To check your heart rate while working out, simply grip the handles in the appropriate place; within a few seconds, your heart rate will appear on the device's console.

Other Features

Heart rate monitors can do more than just check your pulse. Most can also tell you the following:

- Highest and lowest heart rate during a session
- Average heart rate

- Target heart rate range, based on your age, weight, and other factors
- Time spent within the target range
- Number of calories burned during a session

Some monitors can upload their data to a computer so information can be stored and analyzed. The analytical software can help you track your progress over a period of time or a number of workouts. AliveCor is an Apple Watch–compatible phone app that can produce a medical-quality ECG and store it or send it to a physician by e-mail. Monitors with GPS provide an accurate estimate of distance traveled during a workout or over an entire day.

Choosing and Using Monitors

Heart rate monitors are useful if close tracking of heart rate is important in your program. They offer several advantages:

- They are fairly accurate, and they reduce the risk of mistakes when checking your own pulse. (*Note:* Chest-strap monitors are considered more accurate than strapless models. If you use a monitor built in to gym equipment, its accuracy will depend on how well the device is maintained.)
- They are easy to use, although a sophisticated, multifunction monitor may take some time to master.
- They do the monitoring for you, so you don't have to worry about checking your own pulse.

When shopping for a heart rate, fitness tracker, phone app, or exercise GPS monitor, do your homework. Quality, reliability, and warranties vary. Ask personal trainers in your area for their recommendations, and look for independent product reviews and comparison accuracy tests in consumer magazines or online. Remember that the vast majority of devices on the market are for general, and not medical, use; only a few have been formally evaluated and approved by the U.S. Food and Drug Administration (FDA) as accurate enough for medical purposes.

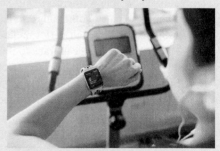
Kanut Srinin/Shutterstock

---

pulse. See the box "Fitness Trackers, Heart Rate Monitors, and GPS Devices" for more information.)

Interpreting Your Score

After you've completed one or more of the assessment tests, use the table under "Rating Your Cardiovascular Fitness" in Lab 3.1 to determine your current level of cardiorespiratory fitness.

As you interpret your score, remember that field tests of cardiorespiratory fitness are not precise scientific measurements and have up to a 10–15% margin of error.

You can use the assessment tests to monitor the progress of your fitness program by retesting yourself from time to time. Always compare scores for the *same* test: Your scores on different tests may vary considerably because of differences in skill and motivation and quirks in the tests themselves.

DEVELOPING A CARDIORESPIRATORY ENDURANCE PROGRAM

Cardiorespiratory endurance exercises are best for developing the type of fitness associated with good health, so they should serve as the focus of your exercise program. To create a successful endurance exercise program, follow these guidelines:

- Set realistic goals.
- Set your starting frequency, intensity, and duration of exercise at appropriate levels.
- Choose suitable activities.
- Warm up and cool down.
- Adjust your program as your fitness improves.

Setting Goals

You can use the results of cardiorespiratory fitness assessment tests to set a specific oxygen consumption goal for your cardiorespiratory endurance program. Your goal should be high enough to ensure a healthy cardiorespiratory system, but not so high that it will be impossible to achieve. Scores in the fair and good ranges for maximal oxygen consumption suggest good fitness; scores in the excellent and superior ranges indicate a high standard of physical performance.

Through endurance training, an individual may be able to improve maximal oxygen consumption $\dot{V}O_{2max}$ by about 10–30%. The amount of improvement possible depends on genetics, age, health status, and initial fitness level. People who start at a very low fitness level can improve by a greater percentage than elite athletes because the latter are already at a much higher fitness level, one that may approach their genetic physical limits. If you are tracking $\dot{V}O_{2max}$ by using the field tests described in this chapter, you may be able to increase your score by more than 30% due to improvements in other physical factors, such as muscle power, which can affect your performance on the tests.

Other physical factors you can track to monitor progress are resting heart rate—your heart rate at complete rest—and blood pressure, measured in the morning before you get out of bed and move around. Resting heart rate may decrease by as much as 10–15 beats per minute and resting systolic and diastolic blood pressure by 5 mmHg in response to endurance training. These changes may be noticeable after only about four to six weeks of training.

You may want to set other types of goals for your fitness program. For example, if you walk, jog, or cycle as part of your fitness program, you may want to set a time or distance goal—working up to walking 5 miles in one session, completing a 4-mile run in 28 minutes, or cycling a total of 35 miles per week. A more modest goal might be to achieve the recommendation of the U.S. Department of Health and Human Services and American College of Sports Medicine (ACSM) of 150 minutes per week of moderate-intensity physical activity. Although it's best to base your program on "SMART" goals (those that are specific, measurable, attainable, realistic, and time frame–specific), you may also want to set more qualitative goals, such as becoming more energetic, sleeping better, and improving the fit of your clothes.

Applying the FITT-VP Principle

As described in Chapter 2, you can use the acronym FITT-VP to set key parameters of your fitness program: Frequency, Intensity, Time (duration), Type of activity, Volume, and Progression.

Frequency of Training Accumulating at least 150 minutes per week of moderate-intensity physical activity (or at least 75 minutes per week of vigorous physical activity) is enough to promote health. Most experts recommend that people exercise three to five days per week to build cardiorespiratory endurance. Training more than five days per week can lead to injury and isn't necessary for the typical person on an exercise program designed to promote wellness. It is safe to do moderate-intensity activity such as walking and gardening every day. Training fewer than three days per week makes it difficult to improve your fitness (unless exercise intensity is very high) or to lose weight through exercise. Remember, however, that some exercise is better than none.

Intensity of Training Intensity is the most important factor for increasing aerobic fitness. You must exercise intensely enough to stress your body so that fitness improves. Four methods of monitoring exercise intensity are described in the following sections; choose the method that works best for you. Be sure to make adjustments in your intensity levels for environmental or individual factors. For example, on a hot and humid day or on your first day back to your program after an illness, you should decrease your intensity level.

TARGET HEART RATE ZONE   One of the best ways to monitor the intensity of cardiorespiratory endurance exercise is to measure your heart rate (calculated in beats per minute). It isn't necessary to exercise at your maximum heart rate to improve

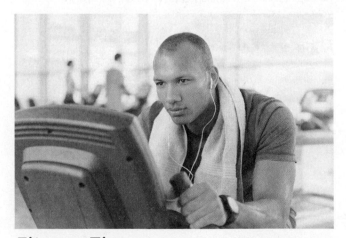

Fitness Tip Listen to fast-paced music for a better workout! In a recent study, students rode a stationary bike while listening to music at different tempos. The subjects rode harder when listening to faster music and performed less exercise in response to slower music.
Newco500/123RF

maximal oxygen consumption. Fitness adaptations occur at lower heart rates with a much lower risk of injury.

According to the ACSM, your **target heart rate zone**—the range of rates at which you should exercise to experience cardiorespiratory benefits—is between 65% and 90% of your maximum heart rate. To calculate your target heart rate zone, follow these steps:

1. Estimate your maximum heart rate (MHR) by subtracting your age from 220, or have it measured precisely by undergoing an exercise stress test in a doctor's office, hospital, or sports medicine lab. (*Note:* The formula to estimate MHR carries an error of about ±10-15 bpm and can be very inaccurate for some people, particularly older adults and young children. If your exercise heart rate seems inaccurate—that is, exercise within your target zone seems either too easy or too difficult—then use the perceived exertion method described in the next section, or have your MHR measured precisely.) You can get a reasonable estimate of maximal heart rate by exercising at maximal intensities on a stationary bike, treadmill, or elliptical trainer that has a built-in heart rate monitor. This method is not recommended unless you are physically fit and accustomed to intense exercise.

2. Multiply your MHR by 65% and 90% to calculate your target heart rate zone. Very unfit people should use 55% of MHR for their training threshold. For example, a 19 year old would calculate her target heart rate zone as follows:

$$MHR = 220 - 19 = 201 \text{ bpm}$$

$$65\% \text{ training intensity} = 0.65 \times 201 = 131 \text{ bpm}$$

$$90\% \text{ training intensity} = 0.90 \times 201 = 181 \text{ bpm}$$

To gain fitness benefits, the young woman in our example would have to exercise at an intensity that raises her heart rate to between 131 and 181 bpm.

An alternative method for calculating target heart rate zone uses **heart rate reserve**, the difference between maximum heart rate and resting heart rate. Using this method, target heart rate is equal to resting heart rate plus between 50% (40% for very unfit people) and 85% of heart rate reserve. Although some people (particularly those with very low levels of fitness) will obtain more accurate results using this more complex method, both methods provide reasonable estimates of an appropriate target heart rate zone. Lab 3.2 gives formulas for both methods of calculating target heart rate.

If you have been sedentary, start by exercising at the lower end of your target heart rate zone (65% of maximum heart rate or 50% of heart rate reserve) for at least four to six weeks. Exercising closer to the top of the range can cause fast and significant gains in maximal oxygen consumption, but you may increase your risk of injury and overtraining. You *can* achieve significant health benefits by exercising at the bottom of your target zone, so don't feel pressure to exercise at an unnecessarily intense level. If you exercise at a lower intensity, you can increase the duration or frequency of training to obtain as much benefit to your health, as long as you are above the 65% training threshold. For people with a very low initial level of fitness, a lower training intensity of 55-64% of maximum heart rate or 40-49% of heart rate reserve may be sufficient to achieve improvements

| Table 3.2 | Target Heart Rate Zone and 15-Second Counts |

AGE (years)	TARGET HEART RATE ZONE (bpm)*	15-SECOND COUNT (beats)
20–24	127–180	32–45
25–29	124–176	31–44
30–34	121–171	30–43
35–39	118–167	30–42
40–44	114–162	29–41
45–49	111–158	28–40
50–54	108–153	27–38
55–59	105–149	26–37
60–64	101–144	25–36
65+	97–140	24–35

*Target heart rates lower than those shown here are appropriate for individuals with a very low initial level of fitness. Ranges are based on the following formula: target heart rate = 0.65 to 0.90 of maximum heart rate, assuming maximum heart rate = 220 − age.

in maximal oxygen consumption, especially at the start of an exercise program. Intensities of 70-85% of maximum heart rate are appropriate for individuals with an average level of fitness.

By monitoring your heart rate, you will always know if you are working hard enough to improve, not hard enough, or too hard. As your program progresses and your fitness improves, you will need to jog, cycle, or walk faster to reach your target heart rate zone. To monitor your heart rate during exercise, use a heart rate monitor or count your pulse while you're still moving or immediately after you stop exercising. Count beats for 15 seconds, then multiply that number by 4 to see if your heart rate is in your target zone. Table 3.2 shows target heart rate ranges and 15-second counts based on the maximum heart rate formula.

METS One way scientists describe fitness is in terms of the capacity to increase metabolism (energy usage level) above rest. Scientists use METs to measure the metabolic cost of an exercise. One **MET** represents the body's resting metabolic rate—that is, the energy or calorie requirement of the body at rest. Exercise intensity is expressed in multiples of resting metabolic rate. For example, an exercise intensity of 2 METs is twice the resting metabolic rate.

METs are used to describe exercise intensities for occupational activities and exercise programs. Exercise intensities of

---

target heart rate zone   The range of heart **TERMS** rates that should be reached and maintained during cardiorespiratory endurance exercise to obtain optimal training effects.

heart rate reserve   The difference between maximum heart rate and resting heart rate; used in one method for calculating target heart rate zone.

MET   A unit of measure that represents the body's resting metabolic rate—that is, the energy requirement of the body at rest.

Table 3.3	Approximate MET and Energy Costs of Selected Activities for a 154-Pound Person	
ACTIVITY	METs	ENERGY COST (CALORIES PER MINUTE)
Rest	1	1.2
Light housework	2–4	2.4–4.8
Bowling	2–4	2.5–5
Walking	2–7	2.5–8.5
Archery	3–4	3.7–5
Dancing	3–7	3.7–8.5
Activity-promoting video game	3–7	3.7–8.5
Hiking	3–7	3.7–8.5
Horseback riding	3–8	3.7–10
Fishing (fly, stream)	4–6	5–7.5
Circuit training	4–8	5–10
Basketball (recreational)	4–9	5–11
Cycling	4–10	5–12
In-line skating	5–8	6–10
Skiing (downhill)	5–8	6–10
Swimming	5–9	6–11
Tennis	5–9	6–11
Rock climbing	5–10	6–12
Scuba diving	5–10	6–12
Rowing machine	5–12	6–15
Skiing (cross-country)	6–12	7.5–15
Jogging	8–12	10–15

NOTE: Intensity varies greatly with effort, skill, and motivation.

SOURCE: American College of Sports Medicine. 2018. *ACSM's Guidelines for Exercise Testing and Prescription*, 10th ed. Philadelphia: Wolters Kluwer/ Lippincott Williams & Wilkins Health; Ainsworth B. E., et al. 2011. *The Compendium of Physical Activities Tracking Guide*. (https://sites.google.com /site/compendiumofphysicalactivities/home)

RATING	DEFINITION
0	Nothing at all
0.5	Very, very easy
1	Very easy
2	Easy
3	Moderate
4	Somewhat hard
5	Hard
6	
7	Very hard
8	
9	Very, very hard
10	Impossible

Figure 3.6 Ratings of perceived exertion (RPE).
Experienced exercisers may use this subjective scale to estimate how near they are to their target heart rate zone.
SOURCE: Borg, G. 1990. "Psychophysical scaling with applications in physical work and the perception of exertion," *Scandinavian Journal of Work and Environmental Health* 16(suppl 1): 55–58.

Photo credits, top to bottom: Tyler Olson/iStockphoto/Getty Images; Diane Collins and Jordan Hollender/Digital Vision/Getty Images; Peathegee Inc/ Blend Images LLC

less than 3–4 METs are considered low. Household chores and most industrial jobs fall into this category. Exercise at these intensities does not improve fitness for most people, but it will improve fitness for people with low physical capacities. Activities that increase metabolism by 3–7 METs are classified as moderate-intensity exercises and are suitable for most people beginning an exercise program. Vigorous exercise increases metabolic rate by 8–12 METs. Fast running or cycling, as well as intense play in sports like racquetball, can place people in this category. Table 3.3 lists the MET ratings for various activities.

METs are intended to be only an approximation of exercise intensity. Skill, body weight, body fat, and environment affect the accuracy of METs. As a practical matter, however, we can disregard these limitations. METs are a good way to express exercise intensity because this system is easy for people to remember and apply.

RATINGS OF PERCEIVED EXERTION Another way to monitor intensity is to monitor your perceived level of exertion. Repeated pulse counting during exercise can become a nuisance if it

interferes with the activity. As your exercise program progresses, you will probably become familiar with the amount of exertion required to raise your heart rate to target levels. In other words, you will know how you feel when you have exercised intensely enough. If this is the case, you can use the scale of **ratings of perceived exertion (RPE)** shown in Figure 3.6 to monitor the intensity of your exercise session without checking your pulse.

To use the RPE scale, select a rating that corresponds to your subjective perception of how hard you are exercising when you are training in your target heart rate zone. If your target zone is about 135–155 bpm, exercise intensely enough to raise your heart rate to that level, and then associate a rating—for example, "somewhat hard" or "hard" (4 or 5)—with how hard you feel you are working. To reach and maintain a similar

ratings of perceived exertion (RPE) A system of monitoring exercise intensity by assigning a number to the subjective perception of target intensity. **TERMS**

Table 3.4 — Estimating Exercise Intensity

METHOD	MODERATE INTENSITY	VIGOROUS INTENSITY
Target heart rate (maximum heart rate method)	55–69%	70–90%
Target heart rate (heart rate reserve method)	40–59%	60–85%
METs	3–7 METs	8–12 METs
Ratings of perceived exertion	4–5 (somewhat hard)	5–8 (hard to very hard)
Talk test	Speech with some difficulty	Speech limited to short phrases

intensity in future workouts, exercise hard enough to reach what you feel is the same level of exertion. You should periodically check your RPE against your target heart rate zone to make sure it's correct. RPE is an accurate means of monitoring exercise intensity, and you may find it easier and more convenient than pulse counting.

TALK TEST   Another easy method of monitoring exercise exertion—in particular, to prevent overly intense exercise—is the talk test. Although your breathing rate will increase during moderate-intensity cardiorespiratory endurance exercise, you should not work out so intensely that you cannot communicate. Speech is limited to short phrases during vigorous-intensity exercise. The talk test is an effective gauge of intensity for many types of activities.

Table 3.4 provides a quick reference to each of the methods of estimating exercise intensity discussed here.

Time (Duration) of Training

A total duration of 20–60 minutes per day is recommended; exercise can take place in a single session or in multiple sessions lasting 10 or more minutes. The total duration of exercise depends on its intensity. To improve cardiorespiratory endurance during a low- to moderate-intensity activity such as walking or slow swimming, you should exercise for 30–60 minutes. For high-intensity exercise performed at the top of your target heart rate zone, a duration of 20 minutes is sufficient.

Some studies have shown that 5–10 minutes of extremely intense exercise (greater than 90% of maximal oxygen consumption) improves cardiorespiratory endurance. However, training at high intensity, particularly during high-impact activities, increases the risk of injury. Also, if you experience discomfort in high-intensity exercise, you are more likely to discontinue your exercise program. Longer-duration, low- to moderate-intensity activities generally result in more gradual gains in maximal oxygen consumption. In planning your program, start with less vigorous activities and gradually increase intensity.

Type of Activity

Cardiorespiratory endurance exercises include activities that involve the rhythmic use of large-muscle groups for an extended period of time, such as jogging, walking, cycling, aerobic dancing and other forms of group exercise, cross-country skiing, and swimming. Start-and-stop sports, such as tennis and racquetball, also qualify if you have enough skill to play continuously and intensely enough to raise your heart rate to target levels. Other important considerations are access to facilities, expense, equipment, and the time required to achieve an adequate skill level and workout.

Volume of Activity

Training volume is the product of frequency, intensity, and time. Increasing volume is the best way to improve fitness. Excessive volume, however, can lead to injury and overtraining. Activity trackers can help you gauge and monitor your progress. They can also help quantify your program in total energy expenditure in terms of calories (**calories per session**, week, month, and/or year) and **MET-minutes** (exercise intensity in METs times minutes of exercise). Exercise volume for cardiorespiratory endurance can be estimated using several different measures; each of the following is approximately equivalent:

- 150 minutes per week of moderate intensity activity
- Calories: 1,000 calories per week in moderate intensity exercise
- MET-minutes: 500 to 1,000 MET-mins per week
- Steps: 5,400 to 7,900 steps or more per day; for accuracy, combine step counts with recommend time (duration) of exercise

For most adults, this training volume for endurance exercise is associated with health and longevity benefits. A lower volume is appropriate for someone who is just starting an exercise program, while a higher volume may be needed for weight management.

Progression

The rate of progression depends on your goals, fitness, health, age, and adaptation to training. For general health, most benefits occur at moderate training intensities for about 150 minutes per week. Higher levels of fitness require more intense training programs. Increasing intensity is most important for increasing fitness, while increasing time and frequency can promote a healthy body composition by increasing overall energy expenditure with moderate-intensity activity.

Motivation determines your adherence to an exercise program. Highly motivated people are willing to put up with the high levels of discomfort that accompany intense training programs. Less motivated people often stop exercising if the program is too intense or uncomfortable.

TERMS

calories per session   The energy expenditure of an exercise session expressed in calories; as described earlier, in common usage *calories* represents the larger energy unit *kilocalories*.

MET-minute   A measure of training volume equal to exercise intensity expressed in METs times the total exercise time (METs × time).

Fitness determines your capacity to improve. Untrained people make rapid gains, whereas highly fit people improve more slowly. Genetics also determine how fast you will improve. People vary in their response to identical training programs. Finally, health and age influence your adaptability and capacity for training progression.

Warming Up and Cooling Down

As we saw in Chapter 2, it's important to warm up before every session of cardiorespiratory endurance exercise and to cool down afterward. Because the body's muscles work better when their temperature is slightly above resting level, warming up enhances performance and decreases the chance of injury. It gives the body time to redirect blood to active muscles and the heart time to adapt to increased demands. Warming up also helps spread protective fluid throughout the joints, preventing injury to their surfaces.

A warm-up session should include low-intensity, whole-body movements similar to those in the activity that will follow, such as walking slowly before beginning a brisk walk. An active warm-up of 5–10 minutes is adequate for most types of exercise. However, warm-up time will depend on your level of fitness, experience, and individual preferences.

What about stretching as part of a warm-up? Performing *static* stretches—those in which you move a joint to the end of the range of motion and hold the position—as part of your preexercise warm-up has not been found to prevent injury and has little or no effect on postexercise muscle soreness. Static stretching before exercise may also adversely affect strength, power, balance, reaction time, and movement time. (Stretching may interfere with muscle and joint receptors that are used in the performance of sport and movement skills.) For these reasons, it is often recommended that static stretches be performed at the end of your workout, after your cool-down but while your muscles are still warm and your joints are lubricated. On the flip side, *dynamic* stretches—those involving continuous movement of joints through a range of motion—can be an appropriate part of a warm-up. Slow and controlled movements such as walking lunges, heel kicks, and arm circles can raise muscle temperature while moving joints through their range of motion. (See Chapter 5 for a detailed discussion of stretching and flexibility exercises.)

Cooling down after exercise is important for returning the body to a nonexercising state. A cool-down helps maintain blood flow to the heart and brain and redirects blood from working muscles to other areas of the body. This helps prevent a large drop in blood pressure, dizziness, and other potential cardiovascular complications. A cool-down, consisting of 5–10 minutes of reduced activity, should follow every workout to allow heart rate, breathing, and circulation to return to normal. Decrease the intensity of exercise gradually during your cool-down. For example, following a running workout, begin your cool-down by jogging at half speed for 30 seconds to a minute; then do several minutes of walking, reducing your speed slowly. A good rule of thumb is to cool down at least until your heart rate drops below 100 bpm.

The general pattern of a safe and successful workout for cardiorespiratory fitness is illustrated in Figure 3.7.

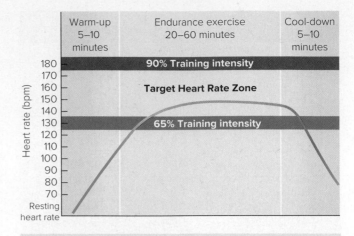

Frequency: 3–5 days per week

Intensity: 55/65–90% of maximum heart rate, 40/50–85% of heart rate reserve plus resting heart rate, or an RPE rating of about 4–8 (lower intensities—55–64% of maximum heart rate and 40–49% of heart rate reserve—are applicable to people who are quite unfit; for average individuals, intensities of 70–85% of maximum heart rate are appropriate)

Time (duration): 20–60 minutes (one session or multiple sessions lasting 10 or more minutes)

Type of activity: Cardiorespiratory endurance exercises, such as walking, jogging, biking, swimming, cross-country skiing, and rope skipping

Volume of activity: Equivalent to 150 minutes or 1,000 or more calories per week of moderate-intensity activity, consistent with individual fitness status and goals

Progression: Gradually increase volume (frequency, intensity, and/or time) over time, as appropriate for goals, fitness status, age, and adaptability

Figure 3.7   The FITT-VP principle for a cardiorespiratory endurance program. Longer-duration exercise at lower intensities can often be as beneficial for promoting health as shorter-duration, high-intensity exercise.

Building Cardiorespiratory Fitness

Building fitness is as much an art as a science. Your fitness improves when you overload your body. However, you must increase the frequency, intensity, and duration of exercise carefully to avoid injury and overtraining.

General Program Progression   For the initial stage of your program, which may last anywhere from three to six weeks, exercise at the low end of your target heart rate zone. Begin with a frequency of three or four days per week, and choose a duration appropriate for your fitness level: 12–15 minutes if you are very unfit, 20 minutes if you are sedentary but otherwise healthy, and 30–40 minutes if you are an experienced exerciser. Use this stage of your program to allow both your body and your schedule to adjust to your new exercise routine. When you can exercise at the upper levels of frequency (four or five days per week) and duration (30–40 minutes) without excessive fatigue or muscle soreness, you are ready to progress.

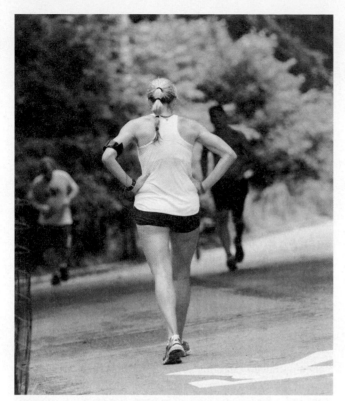

Fitness Tip Make warming up and cooling down a part of your exercise routine. Starting an exercise activity with a low-intensity version and slowing down gradually at the end helps your body adapt to being more active, protects you from certain injuries, and may make the health benefits of exercise last longer.

keepics/Alamy Stock Photo

Table 3.5	Sample Progression for an Endurance Program		
STAGE/WEEK	FREQUENCY (days/week)	INTENSITY* (beats/minute)	TIME (duration in minutes)
Initial stage			
1	3	120–130	15–20
2	3	120–130	20–25
3	4	130–145	20–25
4	4	130–145	25–30
Improvement stage			
5–7	3–4	145–160	25–30
8–10	3–4	145–160	30–35
11–13	3–4	150–165	30–35
14–16	4–5	150–165	30–35
17–20	4–5	160–180	35–40
21–24	4–5	160–180	35–40
Maintenance stage			
25+	3–5	160–180	20–60

*The target heart rates shown here are based on calculations for a healthy 20 year old with a resting heart rate of 60 bpm; the program progresses from an initial target heart rate of 50% to a maintenance range of 70–85% of heart rate reserve.

SOURCE: American College of Sports Medicine. 2018. *ACSM's Guidelines for Exercise Testing and Prescription*, 10th ed. Philadelphia: Wolters Kluwer/Lippincott Williams & Wilkins Health.

The next phase of your program is the improvement stage, lasting from four to six months. During this phase, slowly and gradually increase the amount of overload until you reach your target level of fitness (see the sample training progression in Table 3.5). Take care not to increase overload too quickly. It is usually best to avoid increasing both intensity and duration during the same session or increasing all three training variables (frequency, intensity, and duration) in one week. Increasing duration in increments of 5–10 minutes every two or three weeks is usually appropriate. Signs that you are increasing overload too quickly include muscle aches and pains, lack of usual interest in exercise, extreme fatigue, and inability to complete a workout. Keep an exercise log or training diary to monitor your workouts and progress; use a tracking app, spreadsheet, or paper journal—whatever works best for you.

Interval Training You will not improve your fitness indefinitely. The more fit you become, the harder you must work to improve. Few exercise techniques are more effective at improving fitness rapidly than *high-intensity interval training (HIIT)*—a series of very brief, high-intensity exercise sessions interspersed with short rest periods. The four components of interval training are distance, repetition, intensity, and rest, defined as follows:

- *Distance* refers to either the distance or the time of the exercise interval.
- *Repetition* is the number of times the exercise is repeated.

- *Intensity* is the speed at which the exercise is performed.
- *Rest* is the time spent recovering between exercises.

You can use interval training in your favorite aerobic exercises. In fact, the type of exercise you select is not important as long as you exercise at a high intensity and rest 3–5 minutes between repetitions. HIIT training can even be used to help develop sports skills. For example, a runner might do 4–8 repetitions of 200-meter sprints at near-maximum effort. A tennis player might practice volleys against a wall as fast as possible for 4–8 repetitions lasting 30 seconds each. A swimmer might swim 4–8 repetitions of 50 meters at 100% effort.

If you add HIIT to your exercise program, do not practice interval training more than three days per week. Intervals are exhausting and easily lead to injury. Let your body tell you how many days you can tolerate. If you become overly tired after doing interval training three days per week, cut back to two days. If you feel good, try increasing the intensity or number of intervals (but not the number of days per week) and see what happens. As with any kind of exercise program, begin HIIT training slowly and progress conservatively. Although HIIT training produces substantial fitness improvements, it is best to integrate it into your total exercise program.

PROS Canadian researchers found that practicing HIIT for 3 minutes per week (exercise, not counting rest, warm-up, and cool-down) for 12 weeks produced the same changes in cardiorespiratory fitness, blood sugar regulation, and skeletal muscle mitochondria as training continuously for 150 minutes per week at a moderate intensity. Each workout consisted of three 20-second maximum sprints on a stationary bike, interspersed with 2 minutes of light exercise. Continuous exercise involved 50 minutes of moderate-intensity exercise (70% of maximal heart rate), three times per week. Both programs involved a 2-minute warm-up and 3-minute cool-down. This study (and over 50 others) showed the value of HIIT for building aerobic capacity and endurance.

CONS High-intensity interval training appears to be safe and effective in the short term, but there are concerns about the long-term safety and effectiveness of this type of training, so consider these issues:

- High-intensity training could be dangerous for some people. A physician might be reluctant to give certain patients the green light for HIIT.

- Always warm up with several minutes of low-intensity exercise before practicing HIIT. High-intensity exercise without a warm-up can cause cardiac arrhythmias (abnormal heart rhythms), even in healthy people.

- HIIT might trigger overuse injuries in unfit people, so it is essential to start gradually, especially for someone at a low level of fitness. Exercise at submaximal intensities for at least four to six weeks before starting HIIT. Cut back on interval training or rest if you feel overly fatigued or develop overly sore joints or muscles.

Other types of high-intensity training may combine intervals with other types of exercises and training techniques; see the box "High-Intensity Conditioning Programs."

Maintaining Cardiorespiratory Fitness

There are limits to the level of fitness you can achieve, and if you increase intensity and duration indefinitely, you are likely to become injured or overtrained. After an improvement stage of four to six months, you may reach your goal of an acceptable level of fitness. You can then maintain fitness by continuing to exercise at the same intensity at least three nonconsecutive days every week. If you stop exercising, you lose your gains in fitness fairly rapidly. If you take time off for any reason, start your program again at a lower level and rebuild your fitness in a slow and systematic way.

When you reach the maintenance stage, you may want to set new goals for your program and make some adjustments to maintain your motivation. For example, you might set a new goal of participating in a local 5K race. Or you might add new buddies to your program, or mix up your exercise sessions by working out in a new setting. Adding variety to your program can be

Fitness Tip High-intensity interval training can be an effective technique for boosting fitness. For a runner, HIIT might be half a dozen 200-meter sprints one to three times a week. If you decide to try HIIT, be sure to start slowly, progress gradually, and listen to your body to avoid injury

Imagesourceprem/123RF

a helpful strategy. Engaging in multiple types of endurance activities, an approach known as **cross-training**, can help boost enjoyment and prevent some types of injuries. For example, someone who has been jogging five days a week may change her program so that she jogs three days a week, plays tennis one day a week, and goes for a bike ride one day a week.

Although all these activities build endurance, alternating between them reduces the strain on specific joints and muscles. Varying your activities also offers new physical and mental challenges that can keep your fitness program fresh and fun.

EXERCISE SAFETY AND INJURY PREVENTION

Exercising safely and preventing injuries are two important challenges for people who engage in cardiorespiratory endurance exercise. This section provides basic safety guidelines that can be applied to a variety of fitness activities. Chapters 4 and 5 include additional advice specific to strength training and flexibility training.

Hot Weather and Heat Stress

Human beings require a relatively constant body temperature to survive. A change of just a few degrees can quickly lead to distress and even death. If you lose too much water or if your body temperature gets too high, you may suffer from heat stress. Problems associated with heat stress include dehydration, heat cramps, heat exhaustion, and heatstroke.

When it is hot, exercise safety depends on the body's ability to dissipate heat and maintain blood flow to active muscles. The body releases heat from exercise through the evaporation of sweat. This process cools the skin and the blood circulating near the body's surface. Sweating is an efficient process as long

cross-training Training in two or more sports or types of exercises in order to produce more diverse fitness.

TERMS

In recent years, high-intensity power-based "extreme" conditioning programs, such as CrossFit, Gym Jones, and Insanity, have grown in popularity. The programs typically incorporate a range of activity types and may include high-intensity aerobic exercise, interval training, free-weight exercises, and gymnastics moves. The programs may be geared toward developing whole-body fitness, limiting workout time by utilizing short but high-intensity sessions, and/or adding a competitive aspect to fitness training.

CrossFit is a popular example of a high-intensity program that emphasizes use of broad and constantly changing training stimuli. It includes activities designed to develop not only cardiorespiratory endurance but also strength, power, speed, coordination, ability, balance, and accuracy. Workouts are short and intense but should be tailored to an individual's current fitness level and age. They may include aerobic activities such as running and rope-skipping, plus whole-body strength training activities such as power lifts, plyometrics, sled pulls, and kettlebell exercises. Do not attempt these rigorous training programs without thorough instruction in technical weight lifting and gymnastic exercises, and always use good technique.

These sample workouts provide a flavor of this type of high-intensity training.

Sample Workouts

Complete three circuits (series) of the activities, but do not exceed 20—30 minutes for the workout. Break the exercises into sets if you cannot complete all the repetitions (e.g., 20 pull-ups). Record your time. Train as hard and as fast as you can while maintaining good technique. Select a weight that allows you to complete the reps in the sets. (Principles of resistance exercise are described in Chapter 4.) Change the exercises with every workout.

Workout 1

40 push-ups

10 standing long jumps

40 squats with hands on your hips

20 dumbbell or kettlebell swings

Skip rope rapidly for 3 minutes

Rest 3 minutes; repeat circuit 2 more times

Workout 2

20 pull-ups

20 dumbbell thrusters (front squat with barbell or dumbbells, then immediately perform an overhead press)

20 overhead squats

10 kettlebell snatches (10 for each arm)

2 minutes spinning on bike while standing, maximum intensity

Rest 3 minutes; repeat circuit 2 more times

Cautions and Guidelines

High-intensity training programs have their critics, who point to the increased risk of severe injury and lack of concern for the principle of specificity (training the way you want your body to adapt) with this type of training. Good technique is essential: The emphasis on speed and intensity can make it difficult to achieve good technique, but performing high-speed free-weight exercises such as cleans and squats improperly can lead to severe injury.

Performing high-speed, high-repetition sit-ups or squats often pushes muscles and joints to failure, causing severe knee or back injury or muscle destruction (rhabdomyolysis or "rhabdo"). Until recently, physicians encountered rhabdo only after extreme trauma from automobile accidents. These days, rhabdo may become more common because of the popularity of "feel the burn" high-intensity training programs. Biomechanical studies suggest that high-speed sit-ups and squats can damage the spine. The benefits of high levels of fitness are counterbalanced by the risk of injury.

Despite the potential risks of high-intensity training, it can be a suitable option for fit individuals who enjoy and are motivated by varied, high-intensity workouts that require little time or equipment. If you are considering this type of training, note the following:

- Follow general guidelines for medical clearance for exercise (see Chapter 2).

- Use good form and safety equipment for all exercises and activities; do not sacrifice form for speed, number of repetitions, or any other goal.

- Drink plenty of water and avoid exercise in hot and humid environments.

- Don't push yourself beyond the limits of your strength or conditioning level. Monitor yourself for signs of overtraining (unusual fatigue or muscle soreness), injuries, and rhabdomyolysis (severe muscle pain or weakness; dark red or cola-colored urine).

- Get advice from a qualified professional; when choosing a class, fitness facility, or trainer, follow the guidelines presented in Chapter 2.

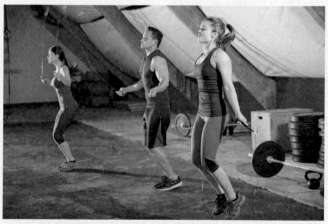

Antonio Diaz/123RF

SOURCES: Aune, K. T., and J. M. Powers. 2017. "Injuries in an extreme conditioning program," *Sports Health* 9(1): 52–58; Heinrich, K. M. 2014. "High-intensity compared to moderate-intensity training for exercise initiation, enjoyment, adherence, and intentions: An intervention study," *BMC Public Health* 14: 789.

as the air is relatively dry. As humidity increases, however, the sweating mechanism becomes less efficient because extra moisture in the air inhibits the evaporation of sweat from the skin. This is why it takes longer to cool down in humid weather than in dry weather.

You can avoid significant heat stress by staying fit, avoiding overly intense or prolonged exercise for which you are not prepared, drinking adequate fluids before and during exercise, and wearing clothes that allow heat to dissipate.

Dehydration Your body needs water to carry out many chemical reactions and to regulate body temperature. Sweating during exercise depletes your body's water supply and can lead to **dehydration**, excessive loss of body fluids, if fluids aren't replaced. Although dehydration is most common in hot weather, it can occur even in comfortable temperatures if fluid intake is insufficient.

Dehydration increases body temperature and decreases sweat rate, plasma volume, cardiac output, maximal oxygen consumption, exercise capacity, muscular strength, and stores of liver glycogen. You may begin to feel thirsty when you have a fluid deficit greater than about 1% of total body weight.

Drinking fluids before and during exercise is important to prevent dehydration and enhance performance. As a general rule, drink 16–20 ounces (about 2 cups) of fluid four hours before exercise, and 8–12 ounces 15 minutes immediately before exercise. During exercise lasting less than 60 minutes, drink 3–8 ounces of water every 15–20 minutes. Consume a sports drink with electrolytes every 15–20 minutes when exercising longer than 60 minutes.

Don't drink more than one quart of water per hour. Very rarely, active people consume too much water and develop *hyponatremia (water intoxication),* a condition that can cause lung congestion, muscle weakness, nervous system problems, and even death. Following the guidelines presented here can help prevent this condition.

To determine if you're drinking enough fluid, weigh yourself before and after an exercise session; any weight loss is due to fluid loss that needs to be replaced. Urine color is a good marker of hydration (Figure 3.8). A dark color means that you might be dehydrated. Diet and supplements can affect urine color, which affects the accuracy of the test.

Bring a water bottle when you exercise so that you can replace your fluids while they're being depleted. For exercise sessions lasting less than 60 minutes, cool water is an excellent fluid replacement. For longer workouts, choose sports drinks containing water and small amounts of electrolytes (sodium, potassium, and magnesium) and simple carbohydrates ("sugar," usually in the form of sucrose, glucose, lactate, or glucose polymers). Electrolytes, which are lost from the body in sweat, are important because they help regulate the balance of fluids in body cells and the bloodstream. The carbohydrates in typical sports drinks are rapidly digestible, which enables them to help maintain blood glucose levels. Choose a beverage with no more than eight grams of simple carbohydrate per 100 milliliters of fluid. Nonfat milk and chocolate milk, for those who can tolerate dairy products, are excellent fluid replacement beverages because they

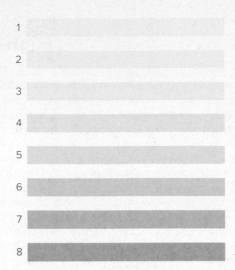

Figure 3.8   Urine chart to assess hydration. A large amount of light-colored urine means you are well hydrated. The darker the color, the more dehydrated you are. Vitamins and some foods can make urine darker.

SOURCE: American College of Sports Medicine. 2011. *Selecting and Effectively Using Hydration for Fitness.* Indianapolis: American College of Sports Medicine.

promote long-term hydration. See Chapter 8 for more on diet and fluid recommendations for active people.

Heat Cramps Involuntary cramping and spasms in the muscle groups used during exercise are sometimes called **heat cramps**. Although depletion of sodium and potassium from the muscles is involved with the problem, the primary cause of cramps is muscle fatigue. Children are particularly susceptible to heat cramps, but the condition can also occur in adults, even those who are fit. The best treatment for heat cramps is a combination of gentle stretching, replacement of fluid and electrolytes, and rest.

Heat Exhaustion Symptoms of **heat exhaustion** include the following:

- Rapid, weak pulse
- Low blood pressure
- Headache
- Faintness, weakness, dizziness
- Profuse sweating
- Pale face
- Psychological disorientation (in some cases)
- Normal or slightly elevated core body temperature

TERMS

dehydration   Excessive loss of body fluids.

heat cramps   Sudden muscle spasms and pain associated with intense exercise in hot weather.

heat exhaustion   Heat illness resulting from exertion in hot weather.

Heat exhaustion occurs when an insufficient amount of blood returns to the heart because so much of the body's blood volume is being directed to working muscles (for exercise) and to the skin (for cooling). Treatment for heat exhaustion includes resting in a cool area, removing excess clothing, applying cool or damp towels to the body, and drinking fluids. An affected individual should rest for the remainder of the day and drink plenty of fluids for the next 24 hours.

Heatstroke **Heatstroke** is a major medical emergency resulting from the failure of the brain's temperature regulatory center. The body does not sweat enough, and body temperature rises dramatically to extremely dangerous levels. In addition to high body temperature, symptoms can include the following:

- Hot, flushed skin (dry or sweaty), red face
- Chills, shivering
- Very high or very low blood pressure
- Confusion, erratic behavior
- Convulsions, loss of consciousness

A heatstroke victim should be cooled as rapidly as possible and immediately transported to a hospital. To lower body temperature, get out of the heat, remove excess clothing, drink cold fluids, and apply cool or damp towels to the body or immerse the body in cold water. People experiencing heatstroke during exercise may still be sweating.

Cold Weather

In extremely cold conditions, problems can occur if a person's body temperature drops or if particular parts of the body are exposed. If the body's ability to warm itself through shivering or exercise can't keep pace with heat loss, the core body temperature begins to drop. This condition, known as **hypothermia**, depresses the central nervous system, resulting in sleepiness and a lower metabolic rate. As metabolic rate drops, body temperature declines even further, and coma and death can result. The risk of hypothermia is particularly severe in cold water.

Frostbite—the freezing of body tissues—is another potential danger of exercise in extremely cold conditions. Frostbite most commonly occurs in exposed body parts like earlobes, fingers, and the nose. It can cause permanent circulatory damage; its symptoms are numbness, pale color, and lack of sensation to cold in the affected areas. Both hypothermia and frostbite require immediate medical treatment.

To exercise safely in cold conditions, don't stay out in very cold temperatures for too long. Take both the temperature and the wind into account when planning your exercise session. Frostbite is possible within 30 minutes in calm conditions when the temperature is colder than −5°F, or in windy conditions (30 mph or more) if the temperature is below 10°F. **Wind chill** values that reflect a combination of the temperature and the wind speed are available as part of a local weather forecast and from the National Weather Service (http://www.weather.gov).

Appropriate clothing provides insulation and helps trap warm air next to the skin. Dress in layers so that you can remove them as you warm up and can put them back on if you get cold. A substantial amount of heat loss comes from the head and neck, so keep these areas covered. In subfreezing temperatures, protect the areas of your body most susceptible to frostbite—fingers, toes, ears, nose, and cheeks—with warm socks, mittens or gloves, and a cap, hood, or ski mask. Wear clothing that breathes and will wick moisture away from your skin to avoid being cooled or overheated by trapped perspiration. Many types of comfortable, lightweight clothing that provide good insulation are available. It's also important in cold conditions to warm up thoroughly and to drink plenty of fluids.

Poor Air Quality

Air pollution can decrease exercise performance and negatively affect health, particularly if you smoke or have respiratory problems such as asthma, bronchitis, or emphysema. The effects of smog are worse during exercise than at rest because air enters the lungs faster. Polluted air may also contain carbon monoxide, which displaces oxygen in the blood and reduces the amount of oxygen available to working muscles. One study found that exercise in polluted air could decrease lung function to the same extent as heavy smoking. Another study found that training in a polluted environment counteracted the normally beneficial effects of exercise on the brain. Symptoms of exercising in poor air quality include eye and throat irritations, difficulty breathing, and possibly headache and malaise.

Do not exercise outdoors during a smog alert or if air quality is very poor. If you have any type of cardiorespiratory difficulty, you should take particular care to avoid exertion outdoors in poor air quality. You can avoid some smog and air pollution by exercising in indoor facilities, in parks, near water (riverbanks, lakeshores, and ocean beaches), or in residential areas with less traffic. Air quality is also usually better in the early morning and late evening, before and after the commute hours.

Exercise Injuries

Most injuries are annoying rather than serious or permanent. However, an injury that isn't cared for properly can escalate into a chronic problem, sometimes serious enough to permanently curtail the activity. It's important to learn how to deal with

---

TERMS

heatstroke A severe and often fatal heat illness characterized by significantly elevated core body temperature.

hypothermia Low body temperature due to exposure to cold conditions.

frostbite Freezing of body tissues characterized by pallor, numbness, and a loss of cold sensation.

wind chill A measure of how cold it feels based on the rate of heat loss from exposed skin caused by cold and wind.

Table 3.6   Care of Common Exercise Injuries and Discomforts

INJURY	SYMPTOMS	TREATMENT
Blister	Accumulation of fluid in one spot under the skin	Don't pop or drain it unless it interferes too much with your daily activities. If it does pop, clean the area with antiseptic and cover with a bandage. Do not remove the skin covering the blister.
Bruise (contusion)	Pain, swelling, and discoloration	R-I-C-E: rest, ice, compression, elevation.
Fracture and/or dislocation	Pain, swelling, tenderness, loss of function, and deformity	Seek medical attention, immobilize the affected area, and apply cold.
Joint sprain	Pain, tenderness, swelling, discoloration, and loss of function	R-I-C-E; apply heat when swelling has disappeared. Stretch and strengthen affected area.
Muscle cramp	Painful, spasmodic muscle contractions	Gently stretch for 15–30 seconds at a time and/or massage the cramped area. Drink fluids and increase dietary salt intake if exercising in hot weather.
Muscle soreness or stiffness	Pain and tenderness in the affected muscle	Stretch the affected muscle gently; exercise at a low intensity; apply heat. Nonsteroidal anti-inflammatory drugs, such as ibuprofen, help some people.
Muscle strain	Pain, tenderness, swelling, and loss of strength in the affected muscle	R-I-C-E; apply heat when swelling has disappeared. Stretch and strengthen the affected area.
Plantar fasciitis	Pain and tenderness in the connective tissue on the bottom of the foot	Apply ice, take nonsteroidal anti-inflammatory drugs, and stretch. Wear night splints when sleeping.
Shin splint	Pain and tenderness on the front of the lower leg; sometimes also pain in the calf muscle	Rest; apply ice to the affected area several times a day and before exercise; wrap with tape for support. Stretch and strengthen muscles in the lower legs. Purchase good-quality footwear and run on soft surfaces.
Side stitch	Pain on the side of the abdomen	Stretch the arm on the affected side as high as possible; if that doesn't help, try bending forward while tightening the abdominal muscles.
Tendinitis	Pain, swelling, and tenderness of the affected area	R-I-C-E; apply heat when swelling has disappeared. Stretch and strengthen the affected area.

injuries so that they don't derail your fitness program. Strategies for the care of common exercise injuries and discomforts appear in Table 3.6; some general guidelines are given in the following sections.

When to Call a Physician Some injuries require medical attention. Consult a physician for the following:

- Head and eye injuries
- Possible ligament injuries
- Broken bones
- Internal disorders: chest pain, fainting, elevated body temperature, intolerance to hot weather

Also seek medical attention for ostensibly minor injuries that do not get better within a reasonable amount of time. You may need to modify your exercise program for a few weeks to allow an injury to heal.

Managing Minor Exercise Injuries For minor cuts and scrapes, stop the bleeding and clean the wound. Treat injuries to soft tissue (muscles and joints) with the R-I-C-E principle: rest, ice, compression, and elevation.

- *Rest:* Stop using the injured area when you experience pain. Avoid any activity that causes pain.

- *Ice:* Apply ice to the injured area to reduce swelling and alleviate pain. Apply ice immediately for 10–20 minutes, and repeat every few hours for pain. Let the injured part return to normal temperature between icings, and do not apply ice to one area for over 20 minutes. An easy method for applying ice is to freeze water in a paper cup, peel some of the paper away, and rub the exposed ice on the injured area. If the injured area is large, you can surround it with several bags of crushed ice or ice cubes, or bags of frozen vegetables. Place a thin towel between the bag and your skin. If you use a cold gel pack, limit application time to 10 minutes. Some experts recommend regular icing for up to about 6 hours after an injury, while others suggest continuing as long as swelling persists.

- *Compression:* Wrap the injured area firmly with an elastic or compression bandage between icings. If the area throbs or begins to change color, the bandage may be wrapped too tightly. Do not sleep with the wrap on.

- *Elevation:* Raise the injured area above heart level to decrease the blood supply and reduce swelling. When lying down, use pillows, books, or a low chair or stool to raise the injured area.

Some experts recommend also taking an over-the-counter medication, such as aspirin, ibuprofen, or naproxen, the day

- Reduce the initial inflammation using the R-I-C-E principle (see text).

- After 36–48 hours, apply heat *if the swelling has disappeared completely.* Immerse the affected area in warm water or apply warm compresses, a hot water bottle, or a heating pad. As soon as it's comfortable, begin moving the affected joints slowly. If you feel pain, or if the injured area swells again, reduce the movement. Continue gently stretching and moving the affected area until you have regained normal range of motion.

- Gradually exercise the injured area to build strength and endurance. Depending on the injury, weight training, walking, and resistance training can all be effective.

- Gradually reintroduce the stress of an activity until you can return to full intensity. Don't progress too rapidly or you'll re-injure yourself. Before returning to full exercise participation, you should have a full range of motion in your joints, normal strength and balance among your muscles, normal coordinated patterns of movement (with no injury compensation movements, such as limping), and little or no pain.

---

after the injury, to decrease inflammation. To rehabilitate your body, follow the steps in the box "Rehabilitation Following a Minor Athletic Injury."

Preventing Injuries The best method for dealing with exercise injuries is to prevent them. If you choose activities for your program carefully and follow the training guidelines described here and in Chapter 2, you should be able to avoid most types of injuries. Important guidelines for preventing athletic injuries include the following:

- Train regularly and stay in condition.
- Gradually increase the frequency, intensity, or duration of your workouts.
- Avoid or minimize high-impact activities such as running; alternate them with low-impact activities such as swimming or cycling.
- Get proper rest between exercise sessions.
- Drink plenty of fluids.
- Warm up thoroughly before you exercise and cool down afterward.
- Achieve and maintain a normal range of motion in your joints.
- Use proper body mechanics when lifting objects or executing sports skills.
- Don't exercise when you are ill or overtrained.
- Use proper equipment, particularly shoes, and choose an appropriate exercise surface. If you exercise on a grass field, soft track, or wooden floor, you are less likely to be injured than on concrete or a hard track. (For information on athletic shoes, see the box "Choosing Exercise Footwear.")
- Don't return to your normal exercise program until any athletic injuries have healed. Restart your program at a lower intensity and gradually increase the amount of overload.

SUMMARY

- The cardiorespiratory system consists of the heart, blood vessels, and respiratory system; it picks up and transports oxygen, nutrients, and waste products.

- The body takes chemical energy from food and uses it to produce ATP and fuel cellular activities. ATP is stored in the body's cells as the basic form of energy.

- During exercise, the body supplies ATP and fuels cellular activities by combining three energy systems: immediate, for short periods of

Footwear is perhaps the most important item of equipment for almost any activity. Shoes protect and support your feet and improve your traction. When you jump or run, you place as much as six times more force on your feet than when you stand still. Shoes can help cushion against the stress this additional force places on your lower legs, preventing injuries. Some athletic shoes are also designed to help prevent ankle rollover, another common source of injury.

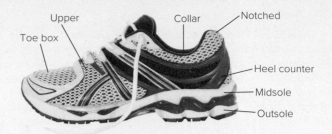

chictype/E+/Getty Images

General Guidelines

When choosing athletic shoes, first consider the activity you've chosen for your exercise program. Shoes appropriate for different activities have very different characteristics. Foot type is another important consideration. If your feet tend to roll inward excessively, you may need shoes with additional stability features on the inner side of the shoe to counteract this movement. If your feet tend to roll outward excessively, you may need highly flexible and cushioned shoes that promote foot motion. Most women will get a better fit if they choose shoes specifically designed for women's feet rather than downsized versions of men's shoes.

Successful Shopping

For successful shoe shopping, remember the following strategies:

- Shop late in the day or, ideally, following a workout. Your foot size increases over the course of the day and after exercise.

- Wear socks like those you plan to wear during exercise.

- Try on both shoes and wear them for 10 or more minutes. Try walking on a noncarpeted surface. Approximate the movements of your activity: walk, jog, run, jump, and so on.

  - Check the fit and style carefully:

  - Is the toe box roomy enough? Your toes will spread out when your foot hits the ground or when you push off. There should be at least one thumb's width of space from the longest toe to the end of the toe box.

  - Do the shoes have enough cushioning? Do your feet feel supported when you bounce up and down? Try bouncing on your toes and on your heels.

- Do your heels fit snugly into the shoe? Do they stay put when you walk, or do they slide up?

- Are the arches of your feet right on top of the shoes' arch supports?

- Do the shoes feel stable when you twist and turn on the balls of your feet? Try twisting from side to side while standing on one foot.

- Do you feel any pressure points?

- If you exercise at dawn or dusk, choose shoes with reflective sections for added visibility and safety.

- Replace athletic shoes about every three months or 300–500 miles of jogging or walking.

Barefoot Shoes or Minimalist Footwear

Two-thirds of runners experience an injury every year. Humans have evolved to run, so some scientists blame running shoes for the high injury rate. Most runners strike heel first when using heavily padded running shoes. Barefoot runners strike the ground with their forefoot (at least they're supposed to), which better uses the shock absorbing capacity of the skeleton. Some researchers speculate that using "minimalist" footwear allows people to run more naturally, which should cut down on the injury rate. Other research suggests that traditional running shoes provide a physiological advantage that makes running easier. We need more research to determine whether barefoot running is safe and viable or just the latest running fad.

activity; nonoxidative (anaerobic), for intense activity; and oxidative (aerobic), for prolonged activity. Which energy system predominates depends on the duration and intensity of the activity.

- Cardiorespiratory endurance exercise improves cardiorespiratory functioning and cellular metabolism; it reduces the risk of chronic diseases such as heart disease, cancer, type 2 diabetes, obesity, and osteoporosis; and it improves immune function and psychological and emotional well-being.

- Cardiorespiratory fitness is measured by determining how well the cardiorespiratory system transports and uses oxygen. The upper limit of this measure, called maximal oxygen consumption, or $\dot{V}O_{2max}$, can be measured precisely in a laboratory, or it can be estimated reasonably well through self-assessment tests.

- To create a successful exercise program, set realistic goals, choose suitable activities, begin slowly, and always warm up and cool down. As fitness improves, exercise more often, harder, and/or longer. Program design should consider the FITT-VP principle: **F**requency, **I**ntensity, **T**ime, **T**ype, **V**olume, and **P**rogression.

- Intensity of training can be measured through target heart rate zone, ratings of perceived exertion, METs, or the talk test.

COMMON QUESTIONS ANSWERED

Q Do I need a special diet for my endurance exercise program?

A No. For most people, a nutritionally balanced diet contains all the energy and nutrients needed to sustain an exercise program. Don't waste your money on unnecessary supplements. (Chapter 8 provides detailed information about putting together a healthy diet.)

Q How can I measure how far I walk or run?

A The simplest way to measure distance is with a GPS-based phone app, which measures your distance, speed, and change in elevation. You can also use a pedometer, which counts your steps. Although stride length varies among individuals, 2,000 steps typically equals about one mile, and 10,000 steps equals about five miles. To track your distance and your progress using a phone app or pedometer, follow the guidelines in Lab 2.3.

Q How can I avoid being so sore when I start an exercise program?

A Postexercise muscle soreness is caused by muscle injury followed by muscle inflammation. Muscles get stronger and larger in response to muscle tension and injury. However, excessive injury can delay progress. The best approach is to begin conservatively with low-volume, low-intensity workouts, and gradually increase the intensity of the exercise sessions. If you are currently sedentary, begin with 5–10 minutes of exercise and gradually increase the distance and speed you walk, run, cycle, or swim.

Q Is it okay to do cardiorespiratory endurance exercise while menstruating?

A Yes. There is no evidence that exercise during menstruation is unhealthy or that it has negative effects on performance. If you have headaches, backaches, and abdominal pain during menstruation, you may not feel like exercising. For some women, exercise helps relieve these symptoms. Listen to your body and exercise at whatever intensity is comfortable for you.

Q Will high altitude affect my ability to exercise?

A At high altitude (above 1,500 meters, or about 4,900 feet), there is less oxygen available in the air than at lower altitude. High altitude doesn't affect anaerobic exercise, such as stretching and weight lifting, but it does affect aerobic activities—that is, any type of cardiovascular endurance exercise—because the heart and lungs have to work harder, even when the body is at rest, to deliver enough oxygen to body cells. The increased cardiovascular strain of exercise at high altitude reduces endurance. To play it safe when at high altitude, avoid heavy exercise—at least for the first few days—and drink plenty of water. And don't expect to reach your normal lower-altitude exercise capacity.

• With careful attention to fluid intake, clothing, duration of exercise, and exercise intensity, endurance training can be safe in hot and cold weather conditions.

• Serious injuries require medical attention. Application of the R-I-C-E principle (rest, ice, compression, elevation) is appropriate for treating many types of muscle or joint injuries.

FOR FURTHER EXPLORATION

American Academy of Orthopaedic Surgeons: Sports Injuries & Prevention. Provides fact sheets on many fitness and sports topics, including how to begin a program, how to choose equipment, and how to prevent and treat many types of injuries.

http://orthoinfo.aaos.org/menus/sports.cfm

American Cancer Society: Eat Healthy and Get Active. Provides tools for managing an exercise program and discusses the links between cancer and lifestyle, including the importance of physical activity in preventing some cancers.

https://www.cancer.org/healthy/eat-healthy-get-active.html

American Heart Association: Exercise and Fitness. Provides information on cardiovascular health and disease, including the role of exercise in maintaining heart health and exercise tips for people of all ages.

https://www.heart.org/en/healthy-living/fitness

Centers for Disease Control and Prevention: Physical Activity for Everyone. Explains the latest government recommendations on exercise and physical activity and provides strategies for getting the appropriate type and amount of exercise.

https://www.cdc.gov/physicalactivity/

CrossFit Journal. A fitness, health, and lifestyle publication dedicated to the improvement of athletic performance, with new articles published daily and an archive of articles, videos, and audio files covering exercise technique, nutrition, injuries and rehab, equipment, coaching, and more.

http://journal.crossfit.com/

Exercise Is Medicine. A global health initiative managed by the American College of Sports Medicine that promotes physical activity for the treatment and prevention of many diseases.

http://www.exerciseismedicine.org/

Runner's World Online. Contains a wide variety of information about running, including tips for beginning runners, advice about training, and a shoe buyer's guide.

http://www.runnersworld.com

Weight-control Information Network: Walking. An online fact sheet that explains the benefits of walking for exercise, tips for starting a walking program, and techniques for getting the most from walking workouts.

https://www.niddk.nih.gov/health-information/weight-management/walking-step-right-direction

Women's Sports Foundation. Provides information and links about training and about many specific sports activities.

http://www.womenssportsfoundation.org

SELECTED BIBLIOGRAPHY

American College of Sports Medicine. 2014. *ACSM's Resource Manual for Guidelines for Exercise Testing and Prescription,* 7th ed. Philadelphia: Lippincott Williams and Wilkins.

American College of Sports Medicine. 2019. *ACSM's Health/Fitness Facility Standards and Guidelines,* 5th ed. Champaign, Ill: Human Kinetics.

American College of Sports Medicine. 2018. *ACSM's Guidelines for Exercise Testing and Prescription,* 10th ed. Philadelphia: Wolters Kluwer.

Brooks, G. A., et al. 2005. *Exercise Physiology: Human Bioenergetics and Its Applications,* 4th ed. New York: McGraw-Hill.

Chou, C. H., et al. 2019. High-intensity interval training enhances mitochondrial bioenergetics of platelets in patients with heart failure. *International Journal Cardiology* 274: 214–220.

Clausen, J. S. R., et al. 2018. Midlife cardiorespiratory fitness and the long-term risk of mortality: 46 years of follow-up. *Journal American College of Cardiology* 72(9): 987–995.

Dimitrov, S., Hulteng, E., and S. Hong. 2017. Inflammation and exercise: Inhibition of monocytic intracellular TNF production by acute exercise via β2-adrenergic activation. *Brain, Behavior, and Immunity* 61: 60–68.

Farrell, S. W., et al. 2018. The relationship between cardiorespiratory fitness and Montreal cognitive assessment scores in older adults. *Gerontology* 64(5): 440–445.

Fenesi, B., et al. 2017. Physical exercise moderates the relationship of apolipoprotein E (APOE) genotype and dementia risk: A population-based study. *Journal of Alzheimer's Disease* 56(1): 297–303.

Garber, C. E., et al. 2011. Quantity and quality of exercise for developing and maintaining cardiorespiratory, musculoskeletal, and neuromotor fitness in apparently healthy adults: Guidance for prescribing exercise. *Medicine and Science in Sport and Exercise* 43(7): 1334–1359.

Garcia-Hermoso, A., et al. 2018. Muscular strength as a predictor of all-cause mortality in an apparently healthy population: A systematic review and meta-analysis of data from approximately 2 million men and women. *Archives Physical Medicine Rehabilitation* 99(10): 2100–2113, e2105.

Gebel, K., et al. 2015. Effect of moderate to vigorous physical activity on all-cause mortality in middle-aged and older Australians. *Journal of the American Medical Association Internal Medicine* 175(6): 970–977.

Imboden, M. T., et al. 2018. Cardiorespiratory fitness and mortality in healthy men and women. *Journal American College Cardiology* 72(19): 2283–2292.

John, U., et al. 2018. Health risk behavior patterns in a national adult population survey. *International Journal Environmental Research Public Health* 15(5).

Kim, Y., et al. 2018. The combination of cardiorespiratory fitness and muscle strength, and mortality risk. *European Journal Epidemiology* 33(10): 953–964.

Lavie, C. J., et al. 2019. Sedentary behavior, exercise, and cardiovascular health. *Circulation Research* 124(5): 799–815.

Liu-Ambrose, T., et al. 2018. Physical activity for brain health in older adults. *Applied Physiology Nutrition Metabolism* 43(11): 1105–1112.

Mandsager, K., et al. 2018. Association of cardiorespiratory fitness with long-term mortality among adults undergoing exercise treadmill testing. *JAMA Network Open* 1(6): e183605.

Physical Activity Guidelines Advisory Committee. 2008. *Physical Activity Guidelines Advisory Committee Report, 2008.* Washington, DC: U.S. Department of Health and Human Services.

Rivera-Torres, S., et al. 2019. Adherence to exercise programs in older adults: Informative report. *Gerontology Geriatric Medicine* 5: 1–10.

Schnohr, P., et al. 2015. Dose of jogging and long-term mortality: The Copenhagen City Heart Study. *Journal of the American College of Cardiology* 65(5): 411–419.

Swift, D. L., et al. 2018. The effects of exercise and physical activity on weight loss and maintenance. *Progress in Cardiovascular Diseases* 61(2): 206–213.

U.S. Department of Health and Human Services. 2018. *Physical Activity Guidelines for Americans,* 2nd ed. Washington, DC: U.S. Department of Health and Human Services.

Viana, R. B., et al. 2019. Is interval training the magic bullet for fat loss? A systematic review and meta-analysis comparing moderate-intensity continuous training with high-intensity interval training (HIIT). *British Journal Sports Medicine.* In press.

Watson, R. R. 2017. *Exercise and the Aging Brain: Effects of Exercise on Neurological Function.* London: Academic Press.

Wilson, M., et al. 2017. *IOC Manual of Sports Cardiology.* New York: Wiley.

Xiang, L., and R. L. Hester. 2017. *Cardiovascular Responses to Exercise,* 2nd ed. Williston, VT: Morgan & Claypool.

Name _____ Section _____ Date _____

LAB 3.1 Assessing Your Current Level of Cardiorespiratory Endurance

The conditions for exercise safety given in Chapter 2 apply to all fitness assessment tests. Talk to a physician if needed, and if you experience any unusual symptoms while taking a test, stop exercising and discuss your condition with your instructor. Additional cautions and prerequisites for the five test options presented in this lab are described below.

1-Mile Walk Test	Recommended for anyone who meets the criteria for safe exercise. This test can be used by people who cannot perform other tests because of low fitness level or injury.
3-Minute Step Test	If you suffer from joint problems in your ankles, knees, or hips or are significantly overweight, check with your physician before taking this test. People with balance problems or for whom a fall would be particularly dangerous, including older adults and pregnant women, should use special caution or avoid this test.
1.5-Mile Run-Walk Test	Recommended for people who are healthy and at least moderately active. If you have been sedentary, you should participate in a 4- to 8-week walk-run program before taking the test. Don't take this test in extremely hot or cold weather or if you aren't used to exercising under those conditions.
Beep Test	Recommended for fit individuals; the test is highly strenuous and requires the ability to jog, run, and sprint. Don't take this test unless you can complete at least 10 sets of 50-meter sprints.
12-Minute Swim Test	Recommended for relatively strong swimmers who are confident in the water; if needed, ask a qualified swimming instructor to evaluate your swimming ability before attempting this test.

Choose one of the tests based on your fitness level and available facilities. For best results, don't exercise strenuously or consume caffeine the day of the test, and don't smoke or eat a heavy meal within about three hours of the test.

The 1-Mile Walk Test

Equipment

1. A track or course that provides a measurement of 1 mile
2. A stopwatch, clock, or watch with a second hand
3. A weight scale

Preparation

Measure your body weight (in pounds) before taking the test.
Body weight: _____ lbs

Instructions

1. Warm up before taking the test. Do some walking, easy jogging, or calisthenics.
2. Cover the 1-mile course as quickly as possible. Walk at a pace that is brisk but comfortable. You must raise your heart rate above 120 beats per minute (bpm).
3. As soon as you complete the distance, note your time and take your pulse for 15 seconds.
   Walking time: _____ min _____ sec
   15-second pulse count: _____ beats
4. Cool down after the test by walking slowly for several minutes.

Determining Maximal Oxygen Consumption

1. Convert your 15-second pulse count into a value for exercise heart rate by multiplying it by 4.
   Exercise heart rate: _____ × 4 = _____ bpm
2. Convert your walking time from minutes and seconds to a decimal figure. For example, a time of 14 minutes and 45 seconds would be 14 + (45/60), or 14.75 minutes.
   Walking time: _____ min + (_____ sec ÷ 60 sec/min) = _____ min
3. Insert values for your age, gender, weight, walking time, and exercise heart rate in the following equation, where
   W = your weight (in pounds)
   A = your age (in years)

G = your gender (male = 1; female = 0)

T = your time to complete the 1-mile course (in minutes)

H = your exercise heart rate (in beats per minute)

$\dot{V}O_{2max} = 132.853 - (0.0769 \times W) - (0.3877 \times A) + (6.315 \times G) - (3.2649\ T) - (0.1565 \times H) =$ ml/kg/min (maximum oxygen consumption measured in milliliters of oxygen used per kilogram of body weight per minute)

For example, a 20-year-old, 190-pound male with a time of 14.75 minutes and an exercise heart rate of 152 bpm would calculate maximal oxygen consumption as follows:

$\dot{V}O_{2max} = 132.853 - (0.0769 \times 190) - (0.3877 \times 20) + (6.315 \times 1) - (3.2649 \times 14.75) - (0.1565 \times 152) = 45\ ml/kg/min$

$\dot{V}O_{2max} = \mathbf{132.853 - (0.0769 \times} \underline{\hspace{2cm}} \mathbf{) - (0.3877 \times} \underline{\hspace{2cm}} \mathbf{) + (6.315 \times} \underline{\hspace{2cm}} \mathbf{)}$
weight (lb)   age (years)   gender

$\mathbf{- (3.2649 \times} \underline{\hspace{2cm}} \mathbf{) - (0.1565 \times} \underline{\hspace{2cm}} \mathbf{) =} \underline{\hspace{2cm}}\mathbf{ml/kg/min}$
walking time (min)   exercise heart rate (bpm)

4. Copy this value for $\dot{V}O_{2max}$ into the appropriate place in the chart in the "Rating Your Cardiovascular Fitness" section.

The 3-Minute Step Test

Equipment

1. A step, bench, or bleacher step that is 16.25 inches from ground level

2. A stopwatch, clock, or watch with a second hand

3. A metronome

Preparation

Practice stepping up onto and down from the step before you begin the test. Each step has four beats: up-up-down-down. Males should perform the test with the metronome set for a rate of 96 beats per minute, or 24 steps per minute. Females should set the metronome at 88 beats per minute, or 22 steps per minute.

Instructions

1. Warm up before taking the test. Do some walking or easy jogging.

2. Set the metronome at the proper rate. Your instructor or a partner can call out starting and stopping times; otherwise, have a clock or watch within easy viewing during the test.

3. Begin the test and continue to step at the correct pace for three minutes.

4. Stop after three minutes. Remain standing and count your pulse for the 15-second period from 5 to 20 seconds into recovery.

    15-second pulse count: _____ beats

5. Cool down after the test by walking slowly for several minutes.

Determining Maximal Oxygen Consumption

1. Convert your 15-second pulse count to a value for recovery heart rate by multiplying by 4.

    Recovery heart rate: _____ × 4 = _____ bpm
    15-sec pulse count

2. Insert your recovery heart rate in the equation below, where

    H = recovery heart rate (in beats per minute)

    Males: $\dot{V}O_{2max} = 111.33 - (0.42 \times H)$

    Females: $\dot{V}O_{2max} = 65.81 - (0.18470 \times H)$

    For example, a man with a recovery heart rate of 162 bpm would calculate maximal oxygen consumption as follows:

    $\dot{V}O_{2max} = 111.33 - (0.42 \times 162) = 43\ ml/kg/min$

    Males: $\dot{V}O_{2max} = \mathbf{111.33 - (0.42 \times} \underline{\hspace{2cm}} \mathbf{) =} \underline{\hspace{2cm}}$ **ml/kg/min**
    recovery heart rate (bpm)

    Females: $\dot{V}O_{2max} = \mathbf{65.81 - (0.1847 \times} \underline{\hspace{2cm}} \mathbf{) =} \underline{\hspace{2cm}}$ **ml/kg/min**
    recovery heart rate (bpm)

3. Copy this value for $\dot{V}O_{2max}$ into the appropriate place in the chart in the "Rating Your Cardiovascular Fitness" section.

The 1.5-Mile Run-Walk Test

Equipment

1. A running track or course that is flat and provides exact measurements of up to 1.5 miles

2. A stopwatch, clock, or watch with a second hand

Preparation

You may want to practice pacing yourself prior to taking the test to avoid going too fast at the start and becoming prematurely fatigued. Allow yourself a day or two to recover from your practice run before taking the test.

Instructions

1. Warm up before taking the test. Do some walking or easy jogging.

2. Try to cover the distance as fast as possible without overexerting yourself. If possible, monitor your own time, or have someone call out your time at various intervals of the test to determine whether your pace is correct.

3. Record the amount of time, in minutes and seconds, it takes you to complete the 1.5-mile distance.

   Running-walking time: _____ min _____ sec

4. Cool down after the test by walking or jogging slowly for about five minutes.

Determining Maximal Oxygen Consumption

1. Convert your running time from minutes and seconds to a decimal figure. For example, a time of 14 minutes and 25 seconds would be 14 + (25/60), or 14.4 minutes.

   Running-walking time: _____ min + (_____ sec ÷ 60 sec/min) = _____ min

2. Insert your running time into the equation below, where

   T = running time (in minutes)

   $\dot{V}O_{2max} = (483 \div T) + 3.5$

   For example, a person who completes 1.5 miles in 14.4 minutes would calculate maximal oxygen consumption as follows:

   $\dot{V}O_{2max} = (483 \div 14.4) + 3.5 = 37$ *ml/kg/min*

   $\dot{V}O_{2max} = (483 \div$ _____) + 3.5 = _____ **ml/kg/min**
   run-walk time (min)

3. Copy this value for $\dot{V}O_{2max}$ into the appropriate place in the chart in the "Rating Your Cardiovascular Fitness" section.

The Beep Test

This is also called the Multi-Stage Fitness Test, Pacer Test, Yo Yo Test, or 20-Meter Shuttle Run Test.

Description

The Beep Test involves running a series of 20-meter shuttles at a specified pace. The pace gets faster each minute as you go to another level. For example, the series begins at a speed of 8.5 kilometers per hour and then increases by 0.5 kilometers per hour with each advancing level. The MP3 audio recording or phone app signals the end of a shuttle with a single beep and the start of the next level with three beeps. The object of the test is to keep up with the beeps as long as possible.

Facilities and Equipment

1. Running track, open field, or gymnasium

2. Two cones or field markers set 20 meters (21 yards, 32 inches) apart (use four cones if testing a large group)

3. Beep Test app or MP3 recording of beeps (widely available free on the Internet–e.g., http://www.beeptestacademy.com; free Beep Test apps are also available for the iPhone and Android smartphones)

4. Method of playing Beep Test: MP3 player with speaker, smartphone with speaker, iPad with speaker. You could run this test by yourself if you have an MP3 player with earphones.

Preparation

Don't take this test until you are prepared. A good technique is to run intervals on a track or playing field. For example, run 50 meters, rest 30 seconds, repeat. Gradually, increase the speed and number of repetitions until you can complete at least 10 sets of 50-meter sprints.

Instructions

The Beep Test is a popular assessment of cardiovascular endurance levels and maximal oxygen consumption.

1. Set up the audio alert system for the test (MP3 player with speaker, or personal MP3 player, or smartphone with headphones).

2. Run back and forth between two cones or field markers placed 20 meters apart, keeping pace with an audio beep that plays during the test. The test is arranged in levels. The beeps get faster with each increasing stage. A single beep will sound at the end of the time for each shuttle. A triple beep sounds at the end of each level. The triple beep is a signal that the pace will get faster. Do not stop when you hear the triple beat; continue running toward the other field marker or cone.

LABORATORY ACTIVITIES

3. The test ends when you can't keep pace with the beeps for two consecutive shuttles.

4. Note your level and the total number of shuttles you completed. Record your maximal oxygen consumption and enter it on the chart labeled "Rating Your Cardiovascular Fitness."

Videos of the test are widely available on the Internet.

Level	Speed (miles per hour)	Minutes per Mile	Total Shuttles	Predicted $\dot{V}O_{2max}$ (milliliters oxygen per kilogram body weight)
1	5.3	11.4	2	16.6
1	5.3	11.4	4	17.5
1	5.3	11.4	6	18.5
2	5.6	10.7	8	20.0
2	5.6	10.7	10	20.9
2	5.6	10.7	12	21.8
2	5.6	10.7	14	22.6
3	5.9	10.2	16	23.4
3	5.9	10.2	18	24.3
3	5.9	10.2	20	25.1
3	5.9	10.2	22	26.0
4	6.2	9.7	24	26.8
4	6.2	9.7	26	27.6
4	6.2	9.7	28	28.3
4	6.2	9.7	31	29.5
5	6.5	9.2	33	30.2
5	6.5	9.2	35	31.0
5	6.5	9.2	37	31.8
5	6.5	9.2	40	32.9
6	6.8	8.8	42	33.6
6	6.8	8.8	44	34.3
6	6.8	8.8	46	35.0
6	6.8	8.8	48	35.7
6	6.8	8.8	50	36.4
7	7.2	8.4	52	37.1
7	7.2	8.4	54	37.8
7	7.2	8.4	56	38.5
7	7.2	8.4	58	39.2
7	7.2	8.4	60	39.9
8	7.5	8.0	62	40.5
8	7.5	8.0	64	41.1
8	7.5	8.0	66	41.8
8	7.5	8.0	68	42.4
8	7.5	8.0	71	43.3
9	7.8	7.7	73	43.9
9	7.8	7.7	75	44.5
9	7.8	7.7	76	45.2
9	7.8	7.7	78	45.8
9	7.8	7.7	81	46.8
10	8.1	7.4	83	47.4
10	8.1	7.4	85	48.0
10	8.1	7.4	87	48.7
10	8.1	7.4	89	49.3
10	8.1	7.4	92	50.2

Level	Speed (miles per hour)	Minutes per Mile	Total Shuttles	Predicted $\dot{V}O_{2max}$ (milliliters oxygen per kilogram body weight)
11	8.4	7.2	94	50.8
11	8.4	7.2	96	51.4
11	8.4	7.2	98	51.9
11	8.4	7.2	100	52.5
11	8.4	7.2	102	53.1
11	8.4	7.2	104	53.7
12	8.7	6.9	106	54.3
12	8.7	6.9	108	54.8
12	8.7	6.9	110	55.4
12	8.7	6.9	112	56.0
12	8.7	6.9	114	56.5
12	8.7	6.9	116	57.1
13	9.0	6.7	118	57.6
13	9.0	6.7	120	58.2
13	9.0	6.7	122	58.7
13	9.0	6.7	124	59.3
13	9.0	6.7	126	59.8
13	9.0	6.7	129	60.6
14	9.3	6.4	131	61.1
14	9.3	6.4	133	61.7
14	9.3	6.4	135	62.2
14	9.3	6.4	137	62.7
14	9.3	6.4	139	63.2
14	9.3	6.4	142	64.0
15	9.6	6.2	144	64.6
15	9.6	6.2	146	65.1
15	9.6	6.2	148	65.6
15	9.6	6.2	150	66.2
15	9.6	6.2	152	66.7
15	9.6	6.2	154	67.5
16	9.9	6.0	156	68.0
16	9.9	6.0	158	68.5
16	9.9	6.0	160	69.0
16	9.9	6.0	162	69.5
16	9.9	6.0	164	69.9
16	9.9	6.0	166	70.5
16	9.9	6.0	168	70.9
17	10.3	5.9	170	71.4
17	10.3	5.9	172	71.9
17	10.3	5.9	174	72.4
17	10.3	5.9	176	72.9
17	10.3	5.9	178	73.4
17	10.3	5.9	180	73.9
17	10.3	5.9	182	74.4
18	10.6	5.7	184	74.8
18	10.6	5.7	186	75.3
18	10.6	5.7	188	75.8
18	10.6	5.7	190	76.2
18	10.6	5.7	192	76.7
18	10.6	5.7	194	77.2
18	10.6	5.7	197	77.9

LABORATORY ACTIVITIES

Level	Speed (miles per hour)	Minutes per Mile	Total Shuttles	Predicted $\dot{V}O_{2max}$ (milliliters oxygen per kilogram body weight)
19	10.9	5.5	199	78.3
19	10.9	5.5	201	78.8
19	10.9	5.5	203	79.2
19	10.9	5.5	205	79.7
19	10.9	5.5	207	80.2
19	10.9	5.5	209	80.6
19	10.9	5.5	212	81.3
20	11.2	5.4	214	81.8
20	11.2	5.4	216	82.2
20	11.2	5.4	218	82.6
20	11.2	5.4	220	83.0
20	11.2	5.4	222	83.5
20	11.2	5.4	224	83.9
20	11.2	5.4	226	84.8

SOURCE: Adapted from Ramsbottom, R., J. Brewer, and C. Williams. 1988. "A progressive shuttle run test to estimate maximal oxygen uptake." *British Journal of Sports Medicine* 22(4): 141–144.

Record your score. Copy this value for $\dot{V}O_{2max}$ into the appropriate place in the chart below:

Highest level: _____

Total shuttles run: _____

Predicted $\dot{V}O_{2max}$: _____

Rating Your Cardiovascular Fitness

Record your $\dot{V}O_{2max}$ score(s) and the corresponding fitness rating from the table below.

Women	Very Poor	Poor	Fair	Good	Excellent	Superior
Age: 18–29	Below 31.6	31.6–35.4	35.5–39.4	39.5–43.9	44.0–50.1	Above 50.1
30–39	Below 29.9	29.9–33.7	33.8–36.7	36.8–40.9	41.0–46.8	Above 46.8
40–49	Below 28.0	28.0–31.5	31.6–35.0	35.1–38.8	38.9–45.1	Above 45.1
50–59	Below 25.5	25.5–28.6	28.7–31.3	31.4–35.1	35.2–39.8	Above 39.8
60–69	Below 23.7	23.7–26.5	26.6–29.0	29.1–32.2	32.3–36.8	Above 36.8
Men						
Age: 18–29	Below 38.1	38.1–42.1	42.2–45.6	45.7–51.0	51.1–56.1	Above 56.1
30–39	Below 36.7	36.7–40.9	41.0–44.3	44.4–48.8	48.9–54.2	Above 54.2
40–49	Below 34.6	34.6–38.3	38.4–42.3	42.4–46.7	46.8–52.8	Above 52.8
50–59	Below 31.1	31.1–35.1	35.2–38.2	38.3–43.2	43.3–49.6	Above 49.6
60–69	Below 27.4	27.4–31.3	31.4–34.9	35.0–39.4	39.5–46.0	Above 46.0

SOURCE: Ratings based on norms from *The Physical Fitness Specialist Manual*, The Cooper Institute of Aerobic Research, Dallas, TX.; Revised 2002.

	$\dot{V}O_{2max}$	Cardiovascular Fitness Rating
1-Mile Walk Test		
3-Minute Step Test		
1.5-M Run-Walk Test		
Beep Test		

The 12-Minute Swim Test

If you enjoy swimming and prefer to build a cardiorespiratory training program around this type of exercise, you can assess your cardiorespiratory endurance by taking the 12-Minute Swim Test. You will receive a rating based on the distance you can swim in 12 minutes. A complete fitness program based on swimming is presented in Chapter 7.

Note, however, that this test is appropriate only for relatively strong swimmers who are confident in the water. If you are unsure about your swimming ability, this test may not be appropriate for you. If necessary, ask your school's swim coach or a qualified swimming instructor to evaluate your ability in the water before attempting this test.

Equipment

1. A swimming pool that provides measurements in yards
2. A wall clock that is clearly visible from the pool, or someone with a watch who can time you

Preparation

You may want to practice pacing yourself before taking the test to avoid going too fast at the start and becoming prematurely fatigued. Allow yourself a day or two to recover from your practice swim before taking the test.

Instructions

1. Warm up before taking the test. Do some walking or light jogging before getting in the pool. Once in the water, swim a lap or two at an easy pace to make sure your muscles are warm and you are comfortable.
2. Try to cover the distance as fast as possible without overexerting yourself. If possible, monitor your own time, or have someone call out your time at various intervals of the test to determine whether your pace is correct.
3. Record the distance, in yards, that you were able to cover during the 12-minute period.
4. Cool down after the test by swimming a lap or two at an easy pace.
5. Use the following chart to gauge your level of cardiorespiratory fitness.

DISTANCE IN YARDS

Men	Needs Work	Better	Fair	Good	Excellent
Age: 13–19	Below 500	500–599	600–699	700–799	Above 800
20–29	Below 400	400–499	500–599	600–699	Above 700
30–39	Below 350	350–449	450–549	550–649	Above 650
40–49	Below 300	300–399	400–499	500–599	Above 600
50–59	Below 250	250–349	350–449	450–549	Above 550
60 and over	Below 250	250–299	300–399	400–499	Above 500
Women					
Age: 13–19	Below 400	400–499	500–599	600–699	Above 700
20–29	Below 300	300–399	400–499	500–599	Above 600
30–39	Below 250	250–349	350–449	450–549	Above 550
40–49	Below 200	200–299	300–399	400–499	Above 500
50–59	Below 150	150–249	250–349	350–449	Above 450
60 and over	Below 150	150–199	200–299	300–399	Above 400

100 yards = 91 meters

SOURCE: Cooper, Kenneth H. 1982. *The Aerobics Program for Total Well-Being.* New York: Bantam Books.

Record your fitness rating:

	Cardiovascular Fitness Rating
12-Minute Swim Test	

LABORATORY ACTIVITIES

Using Your Results

How did you score? Does your rating for cardiovascular fitness surprise you? Are you satisfied with your current rating?

If you're not satisfied, set a realistic goal for improvement: _____

_____

Are you satisfied with your current level of cardiovascular fitness as evidenced in your daily life—your ability to walk, run, bicycle, climb stairs, do yard work, or engage in recreational activities?

If you're not satisfied, set some realistic goals for improvement, such as completing a 5K run or 25-mile bike ride: _____

_____

What should you do next? Enter the results of this lab in the Preprogram Assessment column in Appendix B. If you've set goals for improvement, begin planning your cardiorespiratory endurance exercise program by completing the plan in Lab 3.2. After several weeks of your program, complete this lab again, and enter the results in the Postprogram Assessment column of Appendix B. How do the results compare? (Remember, it's best to compare $\dot{V}O_{2max}$ scores for the same test.)

SOURCES: Brooks, G. A., T. D. Fahey, and K. Baldwin. 2005. *Exercise Physiology: Human Bioenergetics and its Applications*, 4th ed. New York: McGraw Hill; Kline, G. M., et al. 1987. "Estimation of $\dot{V}O_{2max}$ from a one-mile track walk, gender, age, and body weight," *Medicine and Science in Sports and Exercise* 19(3): 253–259; McArdle, W. D., F. I. Katch, and V. L. Katch. 2017. *Exercise Physiology: Nutrition, Energy, and Human Performance*, 8th ed. Philadelphia: Lea and Febiger.

Name _____ **Section** _____ **Date** _____

LAB 3.2 Developing an Exercise Program for Cardiorespiratory Endurance

1. *Goals.* List goals for your cardiorespiratory endurance exercise program. Your goals can be specific or general, short or long term. In the first section, include specific, measurable goals that you can use to track the progress of your fitness program. These goals might be things like raising your cardiorespiratory fitness rating from fair to good or swimming laps for 30 minutes without resting. In the second section, include long-term and more qualitative goals, such as improving self-confidence and reducing your risk for chronic disease.

   Specific Goals: Current Status   Final Goals

   _____   _____

   _____   _____

   _____   _____

   Other goals: _____
   _____

2. *Type of Activities.* Choose one or more endurance activities for your program. These can include any activity that uses large-muscle groups, can be maintained continuously, and is rhythmic and aerobic in nature. Examples include walking, jogging, cycling, ebike cycling, group exercise such as aerobic dance, rowing, rope-skipping, stair-climbing, cross-country skiing, swimming, skating, and endurance game activities such as soccer and tennis. Choose activities that are both convenient and enjoyable. Fill in the activity names on the program plan.

3. *Frequency.* On the program plan, fill in how often you plan to participate in each activity; the ACSM recommends participating in cardiorespiratory endurance exercise three to five days per week.

Program Plan

Type of Activity	Frequency (check ✓)							Intensity (bpm or RPE)	Time (min)
	M	T	W	TH	F	SA	SU		

4. *Intensity.* Determine your exercise intensity using one of the following methods, and enter it on the program plan. Begin your program at a lower intensity and slowly increase intensity as your fitness improves, so select a range of intensities for your program.

   a. *Target heart rate zone:* Calculate target heart rate zone in beats per minute and then calculate the corresponding 15-second exercise count by dividing the total count by 4. For example, the 15-second exercise counts corresponding to a target heart rate zone of 122–180 bpm would be 31–45 beats.

   Maximum heart rate: 220 − _____ = _____ bpm
                                                        age (years)

   #### Maximum Heart Rate Method

   65% training intensity = _____ bpm × 0.65 = _____ bpm
                                                   maximum heart rate

   90% training intensity = _____ bpm × 0.90 = _____ bpm
                                                   maximum heart rate

   Target heart rate zone = _____ to _____ bpm   15-second count = _____ to _____

LABORATORY ACTIVITIES

Heart Rate Reserve Method

Resting heart rate: _____ bpm (taken after 10 minutes of complete rest)

Heart rate reserve = _____ bpm − _____ bpm = _____ bpm
    maximum heart rate   resting heart rate

50% training intensity = (_____ bpm × 0.50) + _____ bpm = _____ bpm
    heart rate reserve   resting heart rate

85% training intensity = (_____ bpm × 0.85) + _____ bpm = _____ bpm
    heart rate reserve   resting heart rate

Target heart rate zone = _____ to _____ **bpm**   **15-second count** = _____ to _____

b. *Ratings of perceived exertion (RPE):* If you prefer, determine an RPE value that corresponds to your target heart rate range (see Figure 3.6).

5. *Time (Duration).* A total time of 20–60 minutes per exercise session is recommended; your duration of exercise will vary with intensity. For developing cardiorespiratory endurance, higher-intensity activities can be performed for a shorter duration; lower-intensity activities require a longer duration. Enter a duration (or a range of duration) on the program plan.

6. *Volume.* Volume is the product of frequency, intensity, and time. Vary each factor for variety. Sometimes use high-intensity interval training (HIIT) to boost fitness quickly. Other times, exercise longer but at a lower intensity.

7. *Monitoring Your Program.* Complete a log like the one below to monitor your program and track your progress. Note the date on top, and fill in the intensity and time (duration) for each workout. If you prefer, you can also track other variables such as distance. For example, if your cardiorespiratory endurance program includes walking and swimming, you may want to track miles walked and yards swum in addition to the duration of each exercise session.

Activity/Date														
1	Intensity													
	Time													
	Distance													
2	Intensity													
	Time													
	Distance													
3	Intensity													
	Time													
	Distance													
4	Intensity													
	Time													
	Distance													

8. *Progression and Making Progress.* Follow the guidelines in the chapter and in Table 3.5 and Figure 3.7 to slowly increase the amount of overload in your program. Continue keeping a log, and periodically evaluate your progress.

Progress Checkup: Week _____ of program

Goals: Original Status   Current Status

_____   _____

_____   _____

_____   _____

List each activity in your program and describe how satisfied you are with the activity and with your overall progress. List any problems you've encountered or any unexpected costs or benefits of your fitness program so far.

Muscular Strength and Endurance

LOOKING AHEAD...

After reading this chapter, you should be able to

- Describe the basic physiology of muscles and explain how strength training affects muscles.

- Define muscular strength and endurance, and describe how they relate to wellness.

- Assess muscular strength and endurance.

- Apply the FITT-VP principle to create a safe and successful strength-training program.

- Describe the effects of supplements and drugs that are marketed to active people and athletes.

- Explain how to safely perform common strength-training exercises using body weight, free weights, and weight machines.

TEST YOUR KNOWLEDGE

1. For women, weight training typically results in which of the following?
   a. bulky muscles
   b. significant increases in body weight
   c. improved body image

2. To maximize strength gains, it is a good idea to hold your breath as you lift a weight. True or false?

3. Regular strength training is associated with which of the following benefits?
   a. denser bones
   b. reduced risk of heart disease
   c. improved body composition
   d. fewer injuries
   e. improved metabolic health
   f. increased longevity
   g. all six

See answers on the next page.

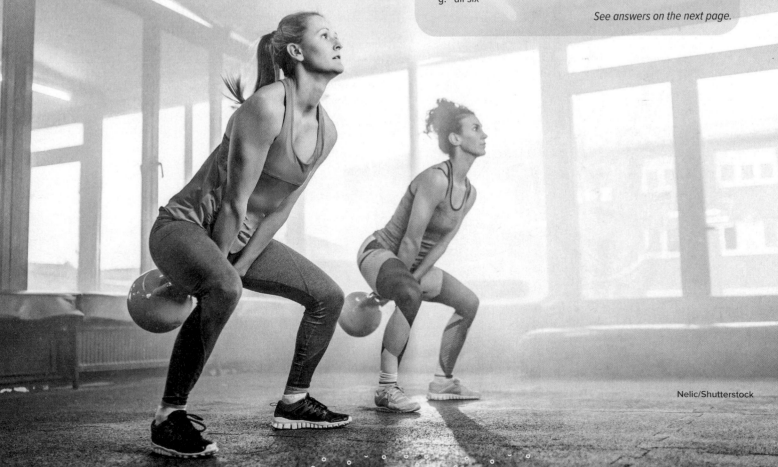

Nelic/Shutterstock

Muscles make up more than 40% of your body mass. You depend on them for movement, and, because of their mass, they are the sites of a large portion of the energy reactions (metabolism) that take place in your body. Strong, well-developed muscles help you perform daily activities with greater ease, protect you from injury, and enhance your well-being in other ways.

As described in Chapter 2, muscular strength is the force a muscle can produce with a single maximum effort, and muscular endurance is the ability to hold or repeat a muscular contraction for a long time. This chapter explains the benefits of *strength training* (also called *resistance training* or *weight training*) and describes methods of assessing muscular strength and endurance. It then explains the basics of strength training and provides guidelines for setting up your own training program.

BASIC MUSCLE PHYSIOLOGY AND THE EFFECTS OF STRENGTH TRAINING

Muscles move the body and enable it to exert force. When a muscle contracts (shortens), it moves a bone by pulling on the **tendon** that attaches the muscle to the bone.

Muscle Fibers

Muscles consist of individual muscle cells, or **muscle fibers**, connected in bundles called fascicles (Figure 4.1). A single muscle is made up of many bundles of muscle fibers and is covered by layers of connective tissue that hold the fibers together. Muscle fibers, in turn, are made up of smaller protein structures called **myofibrils**. Myofibrils consist of a series of contractile units called *sarcomeres,* which are composed largely of actin and myosin molecules. Muscle cells contract when the myosin molecules glide across the actin molecules in a ratchet-like movement. Each muscle cell has many **nuclei** containing genes that control cell function and direct the production of enzymes and structural proteins required for muscle contraction. Strength training activates structures called **satellite cells** that provide additional muscle cell nuclei, which in turn enhances muscle repair and muscle protein synthesis. These cells improve muscle function, and they persist even if you stop training intensely.

In response to strength training, myofibrils increase in size (thicken) and in number, resulting in larger individual muscle fibers. Larger muscle fibers mean a larger and stronger muscle. The development of large muscle fibers is called **hypertrophy** (Figure 4.2). The process of hypertrophy begins after about six to eight weeks of strength training. In some species, muscles can increase in size through a separate process called **hyperplasia**, which involves an increase in the *number* of muscle fibers rather than the *size* of muscle fibers. In humans, hyperplasia is not thought to play a significant role in determining muscle size. Consistent with the fitness principle of reversability, inactivity causes a decrease in muscle fiber size, known as **atrophy**, the reversal of this process.

Muscle fibers are classified as slow-twitch or fast-twitch fibers according to their strength, speed of contraction, and energy source. (See Chapter 3 for more on energy systems.)

- **Slow-twitch muscle fibers** are relatively fatigue resistant, but they don't contract as rapidly or strongly as fast-twitch

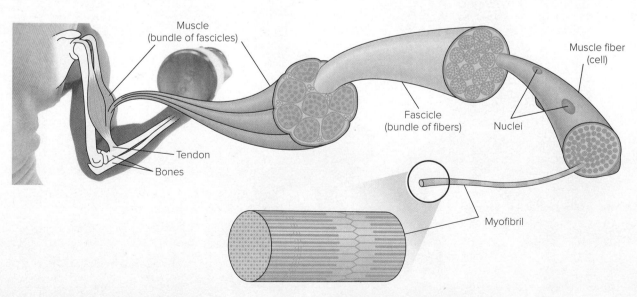

Figure 4.1 Components of skeletal muscle tissue.
Ryan McVay/Photodisc/Getty Images

Muscle (bundle of fascicles)

Muscle fiber (cell)

Tendon

Bones

Fascicle (bundle of fibers)

Nuclei

Myofibril

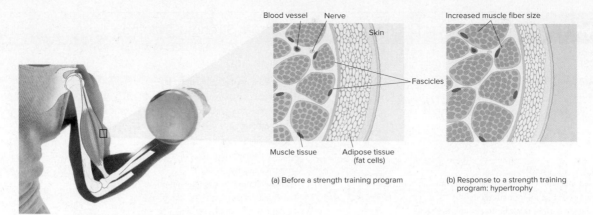

Figure 4.2   Process of muscle hypertrophy. Strength training leads to muscle hypertrophy, an increase in muscle mass and size. The increase occurs as a result of cellular enlargement—and increase in the size of individual muscle fibers—which in turn is due to an increase in the size and number of myofibrils. In this way, muscle fibers increase in size and in their capacity for generating force.

Ryan McVay/Photodisc/Getty Images

fibers. The principal energy system that fuels slow-twitch fibers is aerobic (oxidative). Slow-twitch muscle fibers are typically reddish in color.

- **Fast-twitch muscle fibers** contract more rapidly and forcefully than slow-twitch fibers but fatigue more quickly. Although oxygen is important in the energy system that fuels fast-twitch fibers, they rely more on anaerobic (nonoxidative) metabolism than do slow-twitch fibers. Fast-twitch muscle fibers are typically whitish in color (e.g., white meat versus dark meat in a turkey).

Most muscles contain both slow-twitch and fast-twitch fibers. The proportion of the types of fibers varies significantly among different muscles and different individuals, and that proportion is largely fixed at birth, although fibers can contract faster or slower following a period of training or a period of inactivity. The type of fiber that acts during a particular activity depends on the type of work required. Endurance activities like jogging tend to use slow-twitch fibers, whereas strength and **power** activities like sprinting, use fast-twitch fibers. Strength training can increase the size and strength of both fast-twitch and slow-twitch fibers, although fast-twitch fibers are preferentially increased.

Motor Units

To exert force, a muscle recruits one or more motor units to contract. A **motor unit** is made up of a nerve connected to a number of muscle fibers. The number of muscle fibers in a motor unit varies from two to hundreds. Small motor units contain slow-twitch fibers, whereas large motor units contain fast-twitch fibers. When a motor unit calls on its fibers to contract, all fibers contract to their full capacity. The number of motor units recruited depends on the amount of strength required: When you pick up a small weight, you use fewer and smaller motor units than when picking up a large weight.

The nervous system controls motor unit activation. Nerve cell components called **axons** are often covered in a special tissue called **myelin**, which speeds the rate of nerve conduction. Practicing a skill causes the nervous system to lay down more myelin, which increases the speed, efficiency, and coordination

TERMS

tendon   A tough band of fibrous tissue that connects a muscle to a bone or other body part and transmits the force exerted by the muscle.

muscle fiber   A single muscle cell, usually classified according to strength, speed of contraction, and energy source.

myofibrils   Protein structures that make up muscle fibers.

nucleus   A cell structure containing DNA and genes that direct the production of proteins; plural, *nuclei*.

satellite cells   Cells that provide additional cell nuclei in skeletal muscle, which enhances muscle protein synthesis and cell repair.

hypertrophy   An increase in the size of muscle fibers, usually stimulated by muscular overload, as occurs during strength training.

hyperplasia   An increase in the number of muscle fibers.

atrophy   A decrease in the size of muscle fibers, usually attributable to inactivity.

slow-twitch muscle fibers   Red muscle fibers that are fatigue resistant but have a slow contraction speed and a lower capacity for tension; usually recruited for endurance activities.

fast-twitch muscle fibers   White muscle fibers that contract rapidly and forcefully but fatigue quickly; usually recruited for actions requiring strength, power, or speed.

power   The ability to exert force rapidly.

motor unit   A motor nerve (one that initiates movement) connected to one or more muscle fibers.

axon   A long, slender part of the nerve cell that conducts the nerve impulse away from the nerve cell body.

myelin   A fatty material covering the nerve cell that insulates the axon. Practicing a motor skill lays down more myelin on the axon, which speeds neural conduction and improves skills such as hitting a tennis ball or baseball or skiing down a hill.

Table 4.1 — Physiological Changes and Benefits from Strength Training

CHANGE	BENEFITS
Increased muscle mass* and strength	Increased muscular strength
	Improved body composition
	Higher rate of metabolism
	Improved capacity to regulate fuel use with aging
	Toned, healthy-looking muscles
	Increased longevity
	Improved quality of life
Increased utilization of motor units during muscle contractions	Increased muscular strength and power
Improved coordination of motor units	Increased muscular strength and power
Increased strength of tendons, ligaments, and bones	Lower risk of injury to these tissues
Increased storage of fuel in muscles	Increased resistance to muscle fatigue
Increased size of fast-twitch muscle fibers (from a high-resistance program)	Increased muscular strength and power
Increased size of slow-twitch muscle fibers (from a high-repetition program)	Increased muscular endurance
Increased blood supply to muscles (from a high-repetition program) and improved blood vessel health	Increased delivery of oxygen and nutrients Faster elimination of wastes
Biochemical improvements (e.g., increased sensitivity to insulin)	Enhanced metabolic health and, possibly, increased life span
Improved blood fat levels	Reduced risk of heart disease
Increased muscle endurance	Enhanced ability to exercise for long periods and maintain good body posture

*Due to genetic and hormonal differences, men will build more muscle mass than women, but both men and women make about the same percentage gains in strength through a good program.

of the movement. In this way, basic movement skills become almost reflexive. The adage that practice makes perfect should be changed to "practice makes myelin." The nervous system contains more than one billion nerve cells, an indicator of how complex it is to control movement.

Strength training improves the body's ability to recruit motor units—a phenomenon called **muscle learning**—which increases strength even before muscle size increases. The physiological changes and benefits that result from strength training are summarized in Table 4.1; see the box "Gender Differences in Muscular Strength" for additional information on hormonal and nervous system influences on muscle tissue.

As a person ages, motor nerves can become disconnected from the portion of muscle they control. By age 70, 15% of the motor nerves in most people are no longer connected to muscle tissue. Aging and inactivity also cause muscles to become slower and therefore less able to perform quick, powerful movements. Strength training helps maintain motor nerve connections and the quickness of muscles, particularly when engaged in **purposeful strength training**.

---

muscle learning The improvement in the body's ability to recruit motor units, brought about through strength training.

purposeful strength training Activating muscle contractions explosively, regardless of weight used. Also called compensatory acceleration training.

TERMS

Osteoporosis (bone loss) is common in people over age 55, particularly postmenopausal women. Osteoporosis leads to fractures that can be life threatening. Hormonal changes from aging account for much of the bone loss that occurs, but lack of bone mass due to inactivity and a poor diet are contributing factors. Strength training can lessen bone loss even if it is taken up later in life; if practiced regularly, strength training may even build bone mass in postmenopausal women and older men. Strength training can also help prevent falls, which are a major cause of injury in people with osteoporosis (see the box "Benefits of Muscular Strength and Endurance").

Metabolic and Heart Health

Strength training helps prevent and manage both cardiovascular disease and diabetes by doing the following:

- Improving glucose metabolism
- Increasing maximal oxygen consumption
- Reducing blood pressure
- Increasing HDL cholesterol and reducing LDL cholesterol (in some people)
- Improving blood vessel health

Stronger muscles reduce the demand on the heart during ordinary daily activities such as lifting and carrying objects. The benefits of resistance exercise to the heart are so great that the American Heart Association recommends strength training two or three days per week for healthy adults and many low-risk cardiac patients. Resistance training may not be appropriate for people with some types of heart disease.

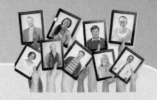
Men are generally stronger than women because they typically have larger bodies and a larger proportion of their total body mass is made up of muscle. But when strength is expressed per unit of cross-sectional area of muscle tissue (i.e., relative strength), men are only 1–2% stronger than women in the upper body and about equal to women in the lower body. However, because of the larger proportion of muscle tissue in the upper male body, men can more easily build upper-body strength than women can. Individual muscle fibers are larger in men, but the metabolism of cells within those fibers is the same in both sexes.

Two factors that help explain these disparities are **testosterone** levels and the speed of nervous control of muscle. Testosterone promotes the growth of muscle tissue in both males and females, but testosterone levels are 5–10 times higher in men than in women, allowing men to have larger muscles. Also, because the male nervous system can activate muscles faster, men have more power.

Women are often concerned that they will develop large muscles from strength training. Because of hormonal differences, however, most women do not develop big muscles unless they train intensely over many years or take anabolic steroids. Women do gain muscle and improve body composition through strength training, but they don't develop bulky muscles or gain significant weight. A study of average women who weight trained two or three days per week for eight weeks found they gained about 1.75 pounds of muscle and lost about 3.5 pounds of fat. Losing muscle over time is a much greater health concern for women than small gains in muscle weight, especially because any gains in muscle weight are typically more than offset by loss of fat weight. Both men and women lose muscle mass and power as they age, but because men start with more muscle and don't lose power as

quickly, older women generally have greater impairment of muscle function than older men. This may partially account for the higher incidence of life-threatening falls in older women.

The bottom line is that both men and women can increase strength through strength training. Women may not be able to lift as much weight as men, but pound for pound of muscle, they have nearly the same capacity to gain strength as men.

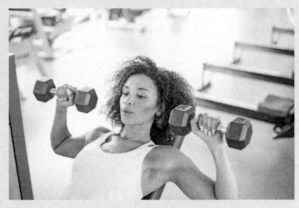

Vitapix/E+/Getty Images

ASSESSING MUSCULAR STRENGTH AND ENDURANCE

Muscular strength is usually assessed by measuring the maximum weight a person can lift in a single effort. This single maximum effort is called a **repetition maximum (RM)**. You can assess the strength of your major muscle groups by taking the one–repetition maximum (1-RM) test for the bench press and by taking functional leg strength tests. You can measure 1 RM directly or estimate it by doing multiple repetitions with a submaximal (lighter) weight. It is best to learn proper lifting techniques and to train for several weeks before attempting a direct 1-RM test; after you have a baseline value, you can retest after 6–12 weeks to check your progress. See Lab 4.1 for guidelines on taking these tests. For more accurate results, avoid strenuous weight training for 48 hours beforehand.

Muscular endurance is usually assessed by counting the maximum number of **repetitions** of an exercise a person can do (such as in push-ups or kettlebell snatches) or the maximum amount of time a person can hold a muscular contraction (such as in the flexed-arm hang). You can test the muscular endurance of major muscle groups in your body by taking the curl-up test, the push-up test, and the squat endurance test. See Lab 4.2 for complete instructions on

taking these assessment tests. Additional tests for low-back muscle endurance are found in Chapter 5.

CREATING A SUCCESSFUL STRENGTH TRAINING PROGRAM

When the muscles are stressed by a load greater than they are used to, they adapt and improve their function. The adaptation depends on the stress applied.

TERMS

testosterone The principal male hormone, responsible for the development of secondary sex characteristics and important in increasing muscle size.

repetition maximum (RM) The maximum resistance that can be moved a specified number of times. One RM is the maximum weight that can be lifted one time; 5 RM is the maximum weight that can be lifted five times.

repetitions The number of times an exercise is performed during one set.

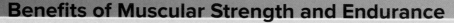
Enhanced muscular strength and endurance prevents injuries and improves exercise and sports performance, body composition, self-image, and muscle, bone, and metabolic health. Most important, greater muscular strength and endurance reduce the risk of premature death. Stronger people—particularly men—have a lower death rate due to all causes, including cardiovascular disease (CVD) and cancer. The link between strength and death rate is independent of age, physical activity, smoking, alcohol intake, body composition, and family history of CVD.

Improved Performance of Physical Activities

A person with a moderate to high level of muscular strength and endurance can perform everyday tasks—such as climbing stairs and carrying groceries—with ease. Increased strength can enhance enjoyment of recreational sports by making it possible to achieve high levels of performance and to handle advanced techniques. Strength training also results in modest improvements in maximal oxygen consumption. People with poor muscle strength tire more easily and are less effective in both everyday and recreational activities.

Injury Prevention

Increased muscular strength and endurance help protect you from injury in two key ways:

• By enabling you to maintain good posture. Good muscle strength and endurance help stabilize the spine and stiffen the **core**, which protects against back and neck injuries.

• By encouraging proper body mechanics during everyday activities such as walking and lifting.

Good muscle strength and endurance in the abdomen, hips, lower back, and legs maintain the spine in proper alignment and help prevent low-back pain, which afflicts over 85% of Americans at some time in their lives. (Prevention of low-back pain is discussed in Chapter 5.)

Training for muscular strength and endurance also makes the tendons, **ligaments**, and **cartilage** cells stronger and less susceptible to injury and improves bone marrow metabolism. Resistance exercise prevents injuries best when the training program is gradual and progressive and builds all the major muscle groups.

Improved Body Composition

Healthy body composition means that the body has a high proportion of fat-free mass and a relatively small proportion of fat. Strength training improves body composition by increasing muscle mass, tipping the body composition ratio toward fat-free mass and away from fat.

Building muscle mass through strength training also helps with losing fat because metabolic rate is related to muscle mass: The greater your muscle mass, the higher your metabolic rate. A high metabolic rate means that a nutritionally sound diet coupled with regular exercise will not lead to an increase in body fat. Strength training can boost resting metabolic rate by up to 15%, depending on how hard you train. Resistance exercise also increases muscle temperature, which slightly increases the rate at which you burn calories over the hours following a weight-training session.

Enhanced Self-Image and Quality of Life

Strength training leads to an enhanced self-image in both men and women by providing stronger, firmer muscles and a toned, healthy-looking body. Women lose inches, increase strength, and develop greater muscle definition. Men build larger, stronger muscles and improve muscle tone. The larger muscles in men combine with high levels of the hormone testosterone for a strong tissue-building effect; see the box "Gender Differences in Muscular Strength."

Because strength training involves measurable objectives (pounds lifted, repetitions accomplished), a person can easily recognize improved performance, leading to greater self-confidence and self-esteem. Strength training also improves quality of life by increasing energy, preventing injuries, and making daily activities easier and more enjoyable.

Improved Muscle and Bone Health with Aging

Research has shown that good muscular strength helps people live healthier lives. A lifelong program of regular strength training prevents muscle and nerve degeneration that can compromise the quality of life and increase the risk of hip fractures and other potentially life-threatening injuries.

In the general population, people lose muscle mass after age 30, a condition called *sarcopenia*. At first they may notice they cannot play sports as well as they could in high school. After more years of inactivity and strength loss, people may have trouble performing even the simple movements of daily life, such as walking up a flight of stairs or doing yard work. By age 75, strength decreases by 30% and power by 40%. Although aging contributes to decreased strength, inactivity causes most of the loss. Poor strength and power make it much more likely that a person will be injured during everyday activities.

Increased Longevity

Strength training helps you live longer. Greater muscular strength is linked to lower rates of death from all causes, including cancer and CVD. A study of over 9,000 men showed that compared to men with the lowest levels of muscular strength, stronger men were 1.5 times less likely to die from all causes; 1.6 times less likely to die from CVD; and 1.25 times less likely to die from cancer. The results were particularly striking in men age 60 and older with low levels of muscular strength, who were over four times more likely to die from cancer than similar-age men with greater muscular strength.

Static versus Dynamic Strength Training Exercises

Strength training exercises are generally classified as static or dynamic. Each involves a different way of using and strengthening muscles.

Static Exercise Also called **isometric** exercise, **static exercise** causes a muscle contraction without changing the length of the muscle or the angle in the joint on which the muscle acts (Figure 4.3A). In isometrics, the muscle contracts, but there is no movement. To perform an isometric exercise, a person can use an immovable object like a wall to provide resistance, or simply tighten a muscle while remaining still (e.g., tightening the abdominal muscles while sitting at a desk). The spine extension and the side bridge, shown in Exercises 5 and 6 (later in the chapter), are both isometric exercises.

Static exercises are important for developing stiff core or torso muscles that support the spine and provide a firm foundation for whole body motions. During most movements some muscles contract statically to support the skeleton so other muscles can contract dynamically. For example, when you throw something, hit a ball, or ski, the core muscles in the abdomen and back stabilize the spine. This stability allows more powerful contractions in the lower- and upper-body muscles. The core muscles also contract statically during dynamic exercises, such as squats, lunges, and overhead presses.

Static exercises are useful in strengthening muscles after an injury or surgery, when movement of the affected joint could delay healing. Isometrics are also used to overcome weak points in an individual's range of motion. Statically strengthening a muscle at its weakest point will allow more weight to be lifted with that muscle during dynamic exercise. Certain types of calisthenics and Pilates exercises (described in more detail later in the chapter) also involve static contractions. For maximum strength gains, hold the isometric contraction maximally for six seconds; do 2–10 repetitions.

Dynamic Exercise Also called **isotonic** exercise, **dynamic exercise** causes a muscle contraction and a change in the length of the muscle and the angle of the joint (Figure 4.3B and C). Dynamic exercises are the most popular for increasing muscle

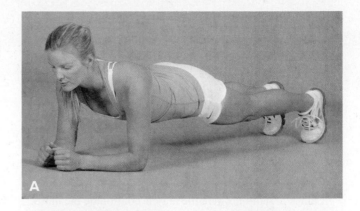

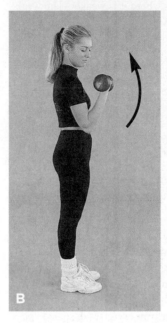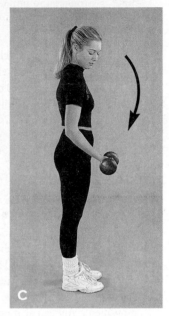

Figure 4.3 Static versus dynamic exercise. A static (isometric) exercise such as a plank (A) involves muscle contraction without movement; the position is held. A dynamic exercise such as a biceps curl involves muscle contraction with a change in the length of the muscle and angle of the joint. Dynamic muscle contractions can be concentric (B), in which the muscle shortens as it contracts, or eccentric (C), in which the muscle lengthens as it contracts.

(a): Photo taken by Taylor Robertson Photography: (b–c): Photo taken by Neil A. Tanner

---

> **TERMS**
>
> **core muscles** The trunk muscles extending from the hips to the upper back.
>
> **ligament** A tough band of tissue that connects the ends of bones to other bones or supports organs in place.
>
> **cartilage** Tough, resilient tissue that acts as a cushion between the bones in a joint.
>
> **isometric (static) exercise** Exercise causing a muscle contraction without a change in the muscle's length or a joint's angle.
>
> **isotonic (dynamic) exercise** Exercise causing a muscle contraction and a change in the muscle's length.
>
> **concentric muscle contraction** A dynamic contraction in which the muscle gets shorter as it contracts; also called a *miometric contraction*.
>
> **eccentric muscle contraction** A dynamic contraction in which the muscle lengthens as it contracts.

strength and seem to be most valuable for developing strength that can be transferred to other forms of physical activity. They can be performed with weight machines, free weights, or a person's own body weight (as in pull-ups or push-ups).

There are two kinds of dynamic muscle contractions:

- A **concentric muscle contraction** occurs when the muscle applies enough force to overcome resistance and shortens as it contracts.

- An **eccentric muscle contraction** (also called *a pliometric contraction*) occurs when the resistance is greater than the force applied by the muscle and the muscle lengthens as it contracts.

For example, in an arm curl, the biceps muscle works concentrically as the weight is raised toward the shoulder and eccentrically as the weight is lowered.

CONSTANT AND VARIABLE RESISTANCE Two of the most common dynamic exercise techniques are constant resistance exercise and variable resistance exercise. Both exercises are extremely effective for building muscular strength and endurance.

- **Constant resistance exercise** uses a constant load (weight) throughout a joint's full range of motion. Training with free weights is a form of constant resistance exercise; the amount of weight you move is the same during the entire exercise. A problem with this technique is that, because of differences in leverage, there are points in a joint's range of motion where the muscle controlling the movement is stronger and points where it is weaker. The weakest point in the range limits the amount of weight a person can lift.

- In **variable resistance exercise**, the load is changed to provide maximum load throughout the entire range of motion. This form of exercise uses machines that place more stress on muscles at the end of the range of motion, where a person has better leverage and can exert more force. Use elastic bands and chains with free weights to add variable resistance to the exercises.

OTHER DYNAMIC EXERCISE TECHNIQUES Athletes use four other kinds of isotonic techniques, primarily for training and rehabilitation.

- **Eccentric loading** places a load on a muscle as it lengthens. The muscle contracts eccentrically to control the weight. Eccentric loading is practiced during most types of resistance training, such as when you lower the weight to your chest during a bench press in preparation for the active movement. You can also perform exercises designed specifically to overload a muscle eccentrically, a technique called *negatives*.

- **Plyometrics** is the sudden eccentric loading and stretching of muscles followed by a forceful concentric contraction—a movement that scientists call the stretch-shortening cycle. An example would be the action of the lower-body muscles when jumping from a bench to the ground and then jumping back onto the bench. This type of exercise helps develop explosive strength; it also helps build and maintain bone density.

- In **speed loading** you move a weight as rapidly as possible in an attempt to approach the speeds used in movements like throwing a softball or sprinting. In the bench press, for example, speed loading might involve doing five repetitions as fast as possible using a weight that is half the maximum load you can lift. You can gauge your progress by timing how fast you can perform the repetitions. Purposeful strength training—performing exercises explosively, regardless of weight—is a type of speed loading that builds neuromuscular power and is useful in high-intensity power sports such as basketball, tennis, skiing, and volleyball.

    Training with a **kettlebell**—an iron ball with a handle—is another type of speed loading. Kettlebell training is highly ballistic, meaning that many exercises involve fast, pendulum-type motions, extreme decelerations, and high-speed eccentric muscle contractions. Kettlebell swings require dynamic concentric muscle contractions during the upward phase of the exercise followed by high-speed eccentric contractions to control the movement when returning to the starting position.

- **Isokinetic exercise** involves exerting force at a constant speed against an equal force exerted by a special strength-training machine. The isokinetic machine provides variable resistance at different points in the joint's range of motion, matching the effort applied by the individual while keeping the speed of the movement constant. Isokinetic exercises are excellent for building strength and endurance.

Comparing Static and Dynamic Exercise Static exercises require no equipment, so they can be done virtually anywhere. They build strength rapidly and are useful for rehabilitation of joints after injury or surgery and for stabilizing joints in the shoulder and spine. On the other hand, they have to be performed at several different angles for each joint to improve strength throughout its entire range of motion. Dynamic exercises can be performed without equipment (calisthenics) or with equipment (weight training). Not only are they excellent for building muscular strength and endurance, but they also tend to build strength through a joint's full range of motion. Most people develop muscular strength and endurance using dynamic exercises. Ultimately, however, the type of exercise a person chooses depends on individual goals, preferences, and access to equipment.

Weight Machines, Free Weights, and Body Weight Exercises

Muscles get stronger when made to work against resistance. Resistance can be provided by free weights, body weight, or exercise machines. Many people prefer machines because they are

---

constant resistance exercise A type of dynamic exercise that uses a constant load throughout a joint's full range of motion.

variable resistance exercise A type of dynamic exercise that uses a changing load, providing a maximum load at the strongest point in the affected joint's range of motion.

eccentric loading Loading the muscle while it is lengthening; sometimes called *negatives*.

plyometrics Rapid stretching of a muscle group that is undergoing eccentric stress (that is, the muscle is exerting force while it lengthens), followed by a rapid concentric contraction.

speed loading Moving a load as rapidly as possible.

kettlebell A large iron weight with a connected handle; used for ballistic weight-training exercises such as swings and one-arm snatches.

isokinetic exercise A type of dynamic exercise that provides variable resistance to a movement, so that the movement occurs at a constant speed no matter how much effort is exerted.

safe, convenient, and easy to use. You just set the resistance, sit down at the machine, and start working. Machines make it easy to isolate and work specific muscles. You don't need a **spotter**—someone who stands by to assist when free weights are used—and you don't have to worry about dropping a weight on yourself. Many machines provide support for the back.

Free weights, such as barbells and kettlebells, require more care, balance, and coordination to use than machines, but they strengthen your body in ways that are more adaptable to real life. They are also more popular with athletes for developing functional strength for sports, especially sports that require a great deal of strength. Free weights are widely available, inexpensive, and convenient for home use.

Exercises that use body weight, elastic bands, rocks, or soup cans as resistance enable you to do workouts at home. You can purchase elastic bands at sporting goods stores or any home improvement or hardware store. A basic principle of resistance exercise is to "train movements and not muscles." This means that you can overload the body in everyday movements like sitting and standing from a chair, climbing a fence, getting out of a swimming pool without a ladder, and standing after lying on the ground.

Other Training Methods and Types of Equipment

You don't need a fitness center or expensive equipment to strength train. If you prefer to train at home or like low-cost alternatives, consider the following options.

Resistance Bands Resistance or exercise bands are elastic strips or tubes of rubber material that are inexpensive, lightweight, and portable. They are available in a variety of styles and levels of resistance. Some are sold with instructional guides or online videos, and classes may be offered at fitness centers. Many free-weight exercises can be adapted for resistance bands. For example, you can do biceps curls by standing on the center of the band and holding one end of the band in each hand; the band provides resistance when you stretch it to perform the curl.

Exercise (Stability) Balls The exercise or stability ball is an extra-large inflatable ball. It was originally developed for use in physical therapy but has become a popular piece of exercise equipment for use in the home or gym. It can be used to work the entire body, but it is particularly effective for working the core stabilizing muscles in the abdomen, chest, and back—muscles that are important for preventing back problems. The ball's instability forces the exerciser to use the stability muscles to balance the body, even when just sitting on the ball. The "stir-the-pot" exercise—a plank position with elbows resting on the ball, which is then moved in small circles—is an example of a core-building exercise that uses the stability ball.

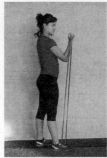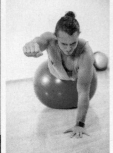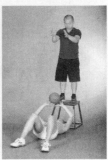

Fitness Tip Many options are available for resistance training, and many are low cost. Try different types of exercises to see what you enjoy and to add variety to your program. Shown here are exercises using an elastic band (left), stability ball (center), and medicine ball (right)

Dave Moyer/McGraw-Hill Education: Wavebreakmedia/iStock/Getty Images: Photo taken by Taylor Robertson Photography

You can incorporate a stability ball into a typical workout in many ways. For example, you can perform curl-ups while lying on a ball instead of on the floor. Lying facedown across a ball provides different leverage points for push-ups. A variety of resistance training exercises can be performed on a stability ball, but experts recommend using dumbbells rather than barbells when lifting weights on a ball.

When selecting a ball, make sure your thighs are parallel to the ground when you sit on it; if you are a beginner or have back problems, choose a larger ball so that your thighs are at an angle, with hips higher than knees. Beginners should use caution until they feel comfortable with the movements and take care to avoid poor form due to fatigue (Table 4.2).

Vibration Training Vibration training consists of doing basic exercises, such as squats, push-ups, lunges, and modified pull-ups, on a vibrating platform. Vibration is transferred to whichever part of the body is in contact with the vibrating plate or handlebars. Vibration activates stretch receptors in the muscles, which triggers thousands of small reflex muscle contractions. Most studies have found that vibration training caused little or no additional effects above weight training alone.

Pilates Pilates (*pil-LAH-teez*) was developed by German gymnast and boxer Joseph Pilates early in the 20th century. Pilates focuses on strengthening and stretching the core muscles in the back, abdomen, and buttocks to create a solid base of support for whole-body movement; the emphasis is on concentration, control, movement flow, and breathing. Pilates often makes use of specially designed resistance training devices, although some classes feature just mat or floor work. Mat exercises can be done at home, but because there are hundreds of Pilates exercises, some of them strenuous, it is best to begin with some qualified instruction.

Medicine Balls, Suspension Training, Stones, and Carrying Exercises Almost anything that provides resistance to movement will develop strength. Rubber medicine balls weighing up to 50 pounds can be used for a variety of functional

Table 4.2 — The Pros and Cons of Stability Balls

PROS	CONS
Stability balls activate muscle and nerve groups that might not otherwise get involved in a particular exercise.	Muscle activation when training on unstable surfaces is less effective than traditional training for building strength in muscle groups responsible for a movement or in trunk-stabilizing muscle groups.
Some exercises, such as the stir-the-pot exercise, can enhance the stability of supporting joints throughout the body.	Some exercises (such as curl-ups) can be more stressful to certain joints and muscles and promote back or shoulder pain in susceptible people.
Stability balls can be useful for some older adults because they require balance and can enhance overall stability.	Falling off an unstable surface, especially while holding weights, can cause serious injury.
Stability balls add variety and challenge to a workout.	

movements, such as squats and overhead throws. Suspension training (e.g., TRX system) uses body weight as the resistance in exercises using ropes or cords attached to a hook, bar, door jam, or sturdy tree branch. You can train with a stone found in your backyard or local riverbank in performing exercises such as squats, presses, and carries. Walking while carrying dumbbells, farmer's bars, or heavy stones is an easy and effective way to develop whole-body strength. Carrying exercises are particularly useful for building core muscle fitness.

Power-Based Conditioning Programs This type of training combines aerobics, weight training, gymnastics, and high-intensity interval training. Programs such as CrossFit and Gym Jones employ different exercises every day. More traditional circuit training methods often use the same exercises set up in series. (See the box "High-Intensity Conditioning Programs" in Chapter 3.)

Blood Flow Restriction Resistance Training **Blood flow restriction training** involves exercising with restricted blood flow to the working muscles. Blood flow restriction during low-intensity weight training promotes muscle hypertrophy because it creates severe metabolic stress that stimulates muscle protein synthesis and hypertrophy. Although blood flow restriction might be effective for injury rehabilitation, it is less effective than traditional training and may cause severe muscle injury in some people.

Applying the FITT-VP Principle: Selecting Exercises and Putting Together a Program

A complete weight training program works all the major muscle groups. It usually takes about 8–10 exercises to get a complete full-body workout. Use the FITT-VP principle—frequency, intensity, time, type, volume, and progression—to set the parameters of your program.

Frequency of Exercise For general fitness, the American College of Sports Medicine (ACSM) recommends a frequency of at least two nonconsecutive days per week for weight training. Allow your muscles at least one day of rest between workouts; if

you train too often, your muscles won't be able to work with enough intensity to improve their fitness, and soreness and injury are more likely to result. One technique, called split routines, works different muscle groups on alternate days. For example, work your arms and upper body one day, work your lower body the next day, and then return to upper-body exercises on the third day. Recent studies found, however, that training the same muscle groups three times a week was more effective than split routines.

Intensity of Exercise: Amount of Resistance The amount of weight (resistance) you lift in weight training exercises is equivalent to intensity in cardiorespiratory endurance training. It determines how your body will adapt to weight training and how quickly these adaptations will occur.

Choose weights based on your current level of muscular fitness and your fitness goals. The weight should be heavy enough to fatigue your muscles but light enough for you to complete the repetitions with good form. (For tips on perfecting your form, see the box "Improving Your Technique with Video.") To build strength rapidly, lift weights as heavy as 80% of your maximum capacity (1 RM). If you're more interested in building endurance, choose a lighter weight (perhaps 40–60% of 1 RM), and do more repetitions.

For example, if your maximum capacity for the leg press is 160 pounds, you might lift 130 pounds to build strength and 80 pounds with more repetitions to build endurance. For a general fitness program to develop both muscular strength and endurance, choose a weight in this range, perhaps 70% of 1 RM. Or you can create a program that includes both higher-intensity exercise (80% of 1 RM for 8–10 repetitions) and lower-intensity exercise (60% of 1 RM for 15–20 repetitions); this routine will develop both fast-twitch and slow-twitch muscle fibers.

Time of Exercise: Repetitions and Sets To improve fitness, you must repeat each exercise to fatigue your muscles. The number of repetitions needed to cause fatigue depends on

blood flow restriction training Exercising with restricted blood flow to working muscles. Also called Kaatsu training. **TERMS**

Want to get stronger? Then you need to focus on developing your skills at least as much as you focus on lifting more weight. Improving skill is the best way to increase strength during movements such as hitting a tennis ball or baseball, performing a bench press, driving a golf ball, skiing down a slope, or carrying a bag of groceries up a flight of stairs. In the world of weight training, skill means lifting weights with proper form; the better your form, the better your results.

The brain develops precise neural pathways as you learn a skill. As you improve, the pathways conduct nervous impulses faster and more precisely until the movement becomes almost reflexive. The best way to learn a skill is through focused practice that involves identifying mistakes, correcting them, and practicing the refined movement often. However, simply practicing the skill is not enough if you want to improve and perform more powerful movements. You must perform the movements correctly instead of practicing mistakes or poor form.

Here's where technology can help. Watch videos of people performing weight training movements correctly. You may be able to borrow videos from your instructor, purchase low-cost training videos through magazines and sporting goods stores, or find them on the Internet. If you watch training videos online, however, make sure they were produced by an authoritative source on weight training. Otherwise, you may be learning someone else's mistakes.

Film your movements using a phone camera or inexpensive video camera. Compare your movements with those of a more skilled person performing them correctly. Make a note of movement patterns that need work and try to change your technique to make it more mechanically correct. Share your videos with your instructor or a certified personal trainer, who can help you identify poor form and teach you ways to correct your form. Smartphone apps such as Coach's Eye, Hudl Technique, and Dartfish allow you to analyze movements in slow motion, compare movements side by side, and share your videos with others.

---

the amount of resistance: The heavier the weight, the fewer repetitions to reach fatigue. A heavy weight and a low number of repetitions (1-5) build strength and overload primarily fast-twitch fibers, whereas a light weight and a high number of repetitions (15-20) build endurance and overload primarily slow-twitch fibers.

For a general fitness program to build both strength and endurance, try to do about 8-12 repetitions of each exercise; a few exercises, such as abdominal crunches and calf raises, may require more. To avoid injury, older (approximately age 50-60 and above) and frailer people should perform more repetitions (10-15) using a lighter weight.

In weight training, a **set** refers to a group of repetitions of an exercise followed by a rest period. To develop strength and endurance for general fitness, you can make gains doing a single set of each exercise, provided you use enough resistance to fatigue your muscles. (You should just barely be able to complete the 8-12 repetitions—using good form—for each exercise.) Doing more than one set of each exercise will increase strength development; most serious weight trainers do at least three sets of each exercise (see the section "More Advanced Strength Training Programs" for guidelines).

If you perform more than one set of an exercise, you need to rest long enough between sets to allow your muscles to work with enough intensity to increase fitness. The length of the rest interval depends on the amount of resistance. In a program to develop a combination of strength and endurance for wellness, a rest

period of 1-3 minutes between sets is appropriate. If you are lifting heavier loads to build strength, rest 3-5 minutes between sets. You can save time in your workouts by alternating sets of different exercises. One muscle group can rest between sets while you work on another group.

Overtraining—doing more exercise than your body can recover from—can occur in response to heavy resistance training. Possible signs of overtraining include lack of progress or decreased performance, chronic fatigue, decreased coordination, and chronic muscle soreness. The best remedy for overtraining is rest; add more days of recovery between workouts. With extra rest, chances are you'll be refreshed and ready to train again. Adding variety to your program, as discussed later in the chapter, can also help you avoid overtraining with resistance exercise.

Type or Mode of Exercise For overall fitness, you need to include exercises for your neck, upper back, shoulders, arms, chest, abdomen, lower back, thighs, buttocks, and calves—about 8-10 exercises in all. If you are also training for a particular sport, include exercises to strengthen the muscles important for optimal performance *and* the muscles most likely to be injured. Weight training exercises for general fitness are presented later in this chapter.

BALANCE EXERCISES FOR OPPOSING MUSCLE GROUPS It is important to balance exercises between antagonistic muscle groups. When a muscle contracts, the opposing muscle must relax. Whenever you do an exercise that moves a joint in one direction, also select an exercise that works the joint in the opposite direction. For example, if you do knee extensions to develop the muscles on the front of your thighs, also do leg curls to develop the antagonistic muscles on the back of your thighs.

---

set A group of repetitions followed by a rest period.

TERMS

SETTING ORDER OF EXERCISES The order of exercises can also be important. Do exercises for large-muscle groups such as the chest and shoulders before you do exercises that use small-muscle groups such as the upper and lower arms. Alternate pushing and pulling exercises. This allows for more effective overload of the larger, more powerful muscle groups. Small-muscle groups fatigue more easily than larger ones, and small-muscle fatigue limits your capacity to overload large-muscle groups. For example, lateral raises, which work the shoulder muscles, should be performed after bench presses, which work the chest and arms in addition to the shoulders. If you fatigue your shoulder muscles by doing lateral raises first, you won't be able to lift as much weight and effectively fatigue all the key muscle groups used during the bench press.

Also, order exercises so that you work opposing muscle groups in sequence, one after the other. For example, follow biceps curls, which work the biceps, with triceps extensions, which exercise the triceps—the antagonistic muscle to the biceps.

Volume Volume is the product of frequency, intensity, and time. For weight training, the volume of a specific exercise during a workout would be the amount of weight lifted multiplied by the number of reps and sets. Choose a training volume that promotes progress and that you will do consistently. And change the components from time to time—that is, increase the weight on some days and the sets and reps on other days. Changing the training volume prevents the body from adapting to exercise stress and results in more consistent improvements in fitness.

Progression Training intensity is the most important factor promoting improvements in strength and power. You will progress rapidly when you begin training, but progress slows as you become more fit. Set fitness goals and progress systematically by adding weight or sets as you gain strength and power; see the section "Getting Started and Making Progress" for specific recommendations for adjusting training intensity in response to fitness improvements. After achieving your goal, maintain strength by training one to three times per week.

The Warm-Up and Cool-Down

As with cardiorespiratory endurance exercise, you should warm up before every weight training session and cool down afterward (Figure 4.4). You should do both a general warm-up—several minutes of walking or easy jogging and a warm-up for the weight training exercises you plan to perform. For example, if you plan to do one or more sets of 10 repetitions of bench presses with 125 pounds, you might do one set of 10 repetitions with 50 pounds as a warm-up. Do similar warm-up exercises for each exercise in your program.

To cool down, perform 5–10 minutes of increasingly less intense aerobic and muscular endurance activity so that your body transitions to a resting state. Although controversial, a few studies have suggested that including a period of post-exercise

Warm-up 5–10 minutes	Strength training exercises for major muscle groups (8–10 exercises)	Cool-down 5–10 minutes
	Sample program	
	Exercise — *Muscle group(s) developed*	
	Bench press — Chest, shoulders, triceps	
	Lat pulls — Lats, biceps	
	Shoulder press — Shoulders, trapezius, triceps	
	Upright rowing — Deltoids, trapezius	
	Biceps curls — Biceps	
	Lateral raises — Shoulders	
	Squats — Gluteals, quadriceps	
	Heel raises — Calves	
	McGill curl-ups — Abdominals	
	Spine extensions — Low- and mid-back spine extensors	
Start	Side bridges — Obliques, quadratus lumborum	***Stop***

Frequency: 2–3 nonconsecutive days per week

Intensity/resistance: Use weights heavy enough to cause muscle fatigue when exercises are performed with good form for the selected number of repetitions

Time: repetitions: 8–12 of each exercise (10–15 with a lower weight for people over age 50–60); **sets:** 1 (doing more than 1 set per exercise may result in faster and greater strength gains); rest 1–2 minutes between exercises.

Type of activity: 8–10 strength training exercises that focus on major muscle groups

Volume: An example might be 3 sets of 8-12 repetitions of each exercise with 1 minute rest between sets.

Progression: As you progress, add weight according to the "two-for-two" rule: When you can perform two additional repetitions with a given weight on two consecutive training sessions, increase the load. For example, if your target is to perform 8–10 repetitions per exercise, and you performed 12 repetitions in your previous two workouts, it would be appropriate to increase your load.

Figure 4.4   The FITT-VP principle for a strength training workout.

stretching may help prevent muscle soreness; warmed-up muscles and joints make the cool-down period a particularly good time to work on flexibility.

Getting Started and Making Progress

The first few sessions of weight training should be devoted to learning the movements and allowing your nervous system to practice communicating with your muscles so that you can develop strength effectively. To start, choose a weight that you can move easily through 8–12 repetitions, do only one set of each exercise, and rest 1-2 minutes between exercises. Gradually add weight and (if you want) sets to your program over the first few weeks until you are doing one to three sets of 8-12 repetitions of each exercise. If adding weight means you can do only 7 or 8 repetitions, stay with that weight until you can again complete 12 repetitions per set. If you can do only 4-6 repetitions after adding weight, or if you can't maintain good form, you've added too much and should take some off.

You can add more resistance in large-muscle exercises, such as squats and bench presses, than you can in small-muscle exercises, such as curls. For example, when you can complete 12 repetitions of squats with good form, you may be able to add 10-20 pounds of additional resistance; for curls, by contrast, you might add only 3-5 pounds. As a general guideline, try increases of approximately 5%, which is half a pound of additional weight for each 10 pounds you are currently lifting.

You can expect to improve rapidly during the first 6-10 weeks of training—a 10-30% increase in the amount of weight lifted. Gains will then come more slowly. Your rate of improvement will depend on how hard you work and how your body responds to resistance training. Factors such as age, gender, motivation, and heredity also will affect your progress.

After you achieve the level of strength and muscularity you want, you can maintain your gains by training two or three days per week. You can monitor the progress of your program by recording the amount of resistance and the number of repetitions and sets you perform on a workout card like the one shown in Figure 4.5.

More Advanced Strength Training Programs

The program just described is sufficient to develop and maintain muscular strength and endurance for general fitness. Performing more sets and fewer repetitions with a heavier load will cause greater increases in strength. Such a program might include three to five sets of 4-6 repetitions each; the load should be heavy enough to cause fatigue with the smaller number of repetitions. Rest long enough after a set (3-5 minutes) to allow your muscles to recover and work intensely during the next set. Train purposefully when lifting heavy weights—that is, make an effort to train explosively, no matter how much weight you are lifting. This increases the capacity of the nervous system to recruit motor units and maximize strength and power output.

Experienced weight trainers often practice some form of cycle training, also called *periodization,* in which the exercises, number of sets and repetitions, and intensity vary within a workout and/or between workouts. For example, you might do a particular exercise more intensely during some sets or on some days than others. You might also vary the exercises you perform for particular muscle groups. For more detailed information on these more advanced training techniques, consult a certified strength coach. If you decide to adopt a more advanced training regimen, start off slowly to give your body a chance to adjust and to minimize the risk of injury.

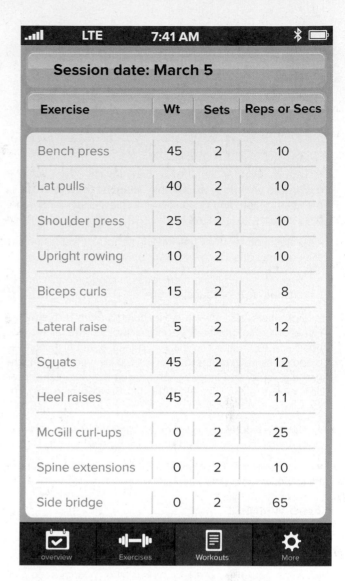

Session date: March 5			
Exercise	**Wt**	**Sets**	**Reps or Secs**
Bench press	45	2	10
Lat pulls	40	2	10
Shoulder press	25	2	10
Upright rowing	10	2	10
Biceps curls	15	2	8
Lateral raise	5	2	12
Squats	45	2	12
Heel raises	45	2	11
McGill curl-ups	0	2	25
Spine extensions	0	2	10
Side bridge	0	2	65

Figure 4.5 A sample workout log for a general fitness strength training program.

Weight Training Safety

Injuries happen in weight training. Maximum physical effort, elaborate machinery, rapid movements, and heavy weights can combine to make the weight room a dangerous place if proper precautions aren't taken. To help ensure that your workouts are safe and productive, follow the guidelines in the box "Safe Weight Training" and the suggestions that follow.

Use Proper Lifting Technique Every exercise has a proper technique that is important for obtaining maximum benefits and preventing injury. Your instructor or weight room attendant can help explain the specific techniques for different exercises and weight machines.

Perform exercises smoothly and with good form. Lift or push the weight forcefully during the active phase of the lift and then lower it with control. Perform all lifts through the full range of motion and strive to maintain a neutral spine position during each exercise.

General Guidelines

- When beginning a program or trying new exercises or equipment, ask a qualified trainer or instructor to show you how to do exercises safely and correctly.

- Lift weights from a stabilized body position; keep weights as close to your body as possible. **Hinge** at the hips, and use the large gluteal and quadriceps muscles, rather than fragile back muscles, to lift heavy loads.

- Protect your back by maintaining control of your spine and stiff core muscles. Don't twist your body while lifting.

- Observe proper lifting techniques and good form. Don't lift beyond the limits of your strength.

- Don't hold your breath while doing weight training exercises. Doing so causes a decrease in blood returning to the heart and can make you dizzy and faint. It can also increase blood pressure to dangerous levels. Exhale when exerting the greatest force, and inhale when moving the weight into position for the active phase of the lift. Breathe smoothly and steadily.

- Don't use defective equipment. Look for broken collars or bolts, frayed cables, broken chains, or loose cushions.

- Don't exercise if you are ill, injured, or overtrained. Do not try to work through the pain.

Free Weights

- Make sure the bar is loaded evenly on both sides and weights are secured with collars or spring clips.

- When you pick up a weight from the ground, keep your back straight and your head level. Don't bend at the waist with straight legs.

- Lift weights smoothly; don't jerk them. Control the weight through the entire range of motion.

- Maximize lifting strength by hinging at the hips rather than rounding the back. When doing standing lifts, maintain a good posture so that you protect your back. Feet should be shoulder-width apart, heels and balls of the feet in contact with the floor, and knees slightly bent.

- Don't bounce weights against your body during an exercise.

Spotting

- Use spotters for free-weight exercises in which the bar crosses the face or head (e.g., the bench press), is placed on the back (e.g., squats), or is racked in front of the chest (e.g., overhead press from the rack holding the weight).

- If one spotter is used, the spotter should stand behind the lifter; if two spotters are used, one spotter should stand at each end of the barbell.

- For squats with heavy resistance, use at least three spotters—one behind the lifter (hands near lifter's hips, waist, or torso) and one at each end of the bar. Squatting in a power rack will increase safety during this exercise. A power rack consists of four vertical posts with two movable horizontal bar catchers on each side.

- Spot dumbbell exercises at the forearms, as close to the weights as possible.

- For over-the-face and over-the-head lifts, the spotter should hold the bar with an alternate grip (one palm up and one palm down) inside the lifter's grip.

- Spotter and lifter should ensure good communication by agreeing on verbal signals before the exercise.

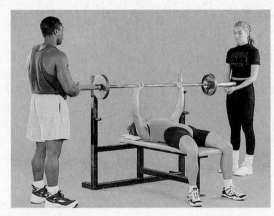

Photo taken by Neil A. Tanner

Use Spotters and Collars with Free Weights Spotters are necessary when an exercise has potential for danger; a weight that is out of control or falls can cause a serious injury. A spotter can assist you if you cannot complete a lift or if the weight tilts. A spotter can also help you move a weight into position before a lift and provide help or additional resistance during a lift. Spotting requires practice and coordination between the lifter and the spotter(s).

Collars are devices that secure weight disks or plates to a barbell or dumbbell; they may have a coiled spring mechanism or a clamp or bolt. Although people lift weights without collars, doing so is dangerous. It is easy to lose your balance or to raise one side of the weight faster than the other. Without collars, the

> **hinge** A powerful movement in the lower body involving first hip flexion and then hip extension; the hip hinge maximizes the use of the gluteal and quadriceps muscles while maintaining a stiff core to keep the spine in a neutral position.
>
> **TERMS**

weights can slip off and crash to the floor. If you use spring clip collars, make sure they fit the bar tightly. Worn spring collars can slide off the bar easily.

Be Alert for Injuries Report any obvious muscle or joint injuries to your instructor or physician, and stop exercising the affected area. Training with an injured joint or muscle can lead to a more serious injury. Get the necessary first aid. Even minor injuries heal faster if you use the R-I-C-E principle of treating injuries described in Chapter 3.

Consult a physician if you have any unusual symptoms during exercise or if you're uncertain whether weight training is a proper activity for you. Weight training can aggravate conditions such as heart disease and high blood pressure. Immediately report symptoms such as headaches; dizziness; labored breathing; numbness; vision disturbances; and chest, neck, or arm pain. Pushing muscles to failure can sometimes result in **rhabdomyolysis** (destruction of muscle cells), which can cause serious illness or even death.

Supplements and Drugs

Active people may use nutritional supplements and drugs—called **ergogenic aids**—in the quest to improve performance and appearance, and more specifically, for these reasons:

- To enhance muscle hypertrophy, strength, power, and endurance
- To speed recovery and prevent the effects of overtraining
- To increase training intensity and aggressiveness
- To control fat, body water, and appetite

This section discusses a selection of "performance aids" along with their potential side effects. Although some of these substances improve performance, most are ineffective and expensive, and some are dangerous. Also remember that dietary supplements are not regulated in the same way that drugs are. A balanced diet should be your primary nutritional strategy.

Drug scandals involving Olympic or professional athletes may lead people to believe that only elite athletes use performance-enhancing drugs. In fact, recreationally active young adults (18–35 years old) are the principle users of sports supplements such as protein and creatine monohydrate and muscle-building drugs such as anabolic steroids and growth hormone. Nonathletes also use performance aids to improve physical appearance and improve fitness.

Anabolic-Androgenic Steroids People take anabolic steroids (AS) for much the same reasons they take other ergogenic aids, but AS have many undesirable and dangerous side effects, including the following:

- Liver toxicity and tumors
- Decreased high-density lipoproteins (good cholesterol)
- Cardiac **arrhythmia**
- Reduced sperm count

- Lowered testosterone production
- High blood pressure
- Increased risk of HIV infection (from shared needles)
- Depressed immune function
- **Glucose intolerance**
- Psychological disturbances
- Masculinization in women and children
- Premature closure of the bone growth centers
- Increased cancer risk

Creatine Monohydrate Creatine monohydrate (i.e., creatine) is among the most popular and widely used supplements taken by athletes to build strength and muscle mass, enhance recovery, and improve exercise capacity. Taking creatine increases the creatine phosphate content of the muscles by about 20%. Creatine phosphate is an important high-energy chemical that maintains ATP levels. Recall from the discussion of exercise physiology in Chapter 3 that ATP supplies the energy for most of the body's hundreds of physiological functions.

Research shows that creatine supplementation improves performance in short-term, high-intensity, repetitive exercise, which might make it a valuable supplement for some physically active people. It may improve performance by augmenting creatine phosphate availability and possibly by regulating the rate of muscle sugar breakdown. It may also increase muscle-building capacity during resistance exercise by allowing athletes to train more intensely.

The long-term safety or effectiveness is currently unknown, however. Over 100 studies on this supplement have failed to report any significant side effects. Creatine monohydrate should be used with caution, especially in youth.

Protein, Amino Acid, and Polypeptide Supplements Athletes may take amino acids and polypeptide supplements to promote muscle hypertrophy, decrease body fat, and stimulate growth hormone release. Little scientific proof exists to support a benefit to taking amino acid or polypeptide supplementation. The protein requirement for active athletes is not much greater than for the average person—0.8–1.5 grams of protein per kilogram body weight per day. However, the timing of protein and amino acid ingestion may be important for stimulating muscle

---

rhabdomyolysis   Destruction of muscle tissue   **TERMS** resulting in the release of enzymes and electrolytes from the cell contents, which can cause kidney damage and even death. This usually occurs during traumatic injuries such as automobile accidents. Overzealous training programs can also cause "rhabdo."

ergogenic aids   Substances consumed to improve athletic performance.

arrhythmia   A change in the normal pattern of the heartbeat.

glucose intolerance   Elevated blood glucose (blood sugar) levels caused by metabolic problems.

growth. Radioactive tracer studies that precisely chronicle the metabolism of various fuels reported that taking a protein supplement either 30 minutes before weight training or immediately after speeds the movement of amino acids into muscle and stimulates protein synthesis.

Other Supplements Carbohydrate beverages consumed during and immediately following physical activity enhance recovery from intense training, speeding the replenishment of liver and muscle glycogen. Benefits of other substances used to

> **caffeine** A central nervous system stimulant found in coffee, tea, chocolate, and energy drinks; it increases energy level and alertness.
>
> **TERMS**

speed recovery—N-acetyl-L-cysteine (NAC), inosine, and beta-hydroxy beta-methylbutyrate (HMB)—are not consistently supported by research.

Caffeine is found in coffee, cola, tea, energy drinks, plants, beans and seeds, some over-the-counter medicines, and chocolate. It is a favorite stimulant of physically active people and is the principle ingredient in energy drinks. It stimulates the central nervous system to release adrenaline (epinephrine). In athletics, caffeine is used as a stimulant and to mobilize fatty acids. Caffeine may improve endurance, strength, and power, and promote recovery from intense exercise. However, caffeine increases the risk of heart arrhythmias and insomnia. It is a controlled substance in the National Collegiate Athletic Association but is not controlled in Olympic or professional sports.

Popular ergogenic aids appear in Table 4.3.

Table 4.3	Performance Aids Marketed to Weight Trainers		
SUBSTANCE	**SUPPOSED EFFECTS**	**ACTUAL EFFECTS**	**SELECTED POTENTIAL SIDE EFFECTS**
Adrenal androgens, such as dehydroepiandrosterone (DHEA), androstenedione	Increased testosterone, muscle mass, and strength; decreased body fat	Increased testosterone, strength, and fat-free mass; decreased fat in older subjects (more studies needed in younger people)	Gonadal suppression, prostate hypertrophy, breast development in males, masculinization in women and children; long-term effects unknown
Amphetamines	Prevention of fatigue; increased confidence and training intensity	Increased arousal, wakefulness, and confidence; feeling of enhanced decision-making ability	Depression and fatigue, extreme confusion; aggressiveness, paranoia, hallucinations, restlessness, irritability, heart arrhythmia, high blood pressure, and chest pain
Anabolic steroids (steroids are controlled substances*)	Increased muscle mass, strength, power, psychological aggressiveness, and endurance	Increased strength, power, fat-free mass, and aggression; no effects on endurance	Liver damage and tumors, abnormal blood lipids, impaired reproductive health, hypertension, depressed immunity, insulin resistance, psychological disturbances, acne, breast development in males, masculinization in women and children, heart disease, thicker blood, and increased risk of cancer
Caffeine	Weight loss; improved endurance, strength, and power output; stimulant effect	Improves sports performance in low to moderate doses (2–6 mg/kg body weight); improves endurance and high-intensity exercise capacity	Abnormal heart rhythm and insomnia in some people; caffeine is addictive
Creatine monohydrate	Increased creatine phosphate levels in muscles, muscle mass, and capacity for high-intensity exercise	Increased muscle mass and performance in some types of high-intensity exercise	Minimal side effects; long-term effects unknown
Diuretics	Promote loss of body fluid	Promote loss of body fluid to accentuate muscle definition; often taken with potassium supplements and very low-calorie diets	Muscle cell destruction, low blood pressure, blood chemistry abnormalities, and heart problems
Energy drinks	Increased energy, strength, power	Increased training volume; caffeine and carbohydrates are main ingredients; products are overpriced	Insomnia, increased blood pressure, heart palpitations
Erythropoietin	Enhanced performance during endurance events	Stimulated growth of red blood cells; enhanced oxygen uptake and endurance	Increased blood viscosity (thickness), can cause potentially fatal blood clots
Ginseng	Decreased effects of physical and emotional stress; increased oxygen consumption	Most well-controlled studies show no effect on performance	No serious side effects; high doses can cause high blood pressure, nervousness, and insomnia

(Continued)

SUBSTANCE	SUPPOSED EFFECTS	ACTUAL EFFECTS	SELECTED POTENTIAL SIDE EFFECTS
Growth hormone (extremely expensive controlled substance*)	Increased muscle mass, strength, and power; decreased body fat	Increased muscle mass and strength; decreased fat mass; little effect on exercise performance	Elevated blood sugar, high insulin levels, and carpal tunnel and tarsal syndrome; enlargement of the heart and other organs
Insulin	Increased muscle mass	Effectiveness in stimulating muscle growth unknown	Insulin shock (characterized by extremely low blood sugar), which can lead to unconsciousness and death
"Metabolic-optimizing" meals for athletes	Increased muscle mass and energy supply; decreased body fat	No proven effects beyond those of balanced meals	No reported side effects, extremely expensive
Nitric oxide boosters (arginine, beet root)	Increased blood flow by stimulating nitric oxide production in blood vessels	Might increase endurance (beet root); little evidence that they promote muscle hypertrophy	Generally safe; could lower blood pressure in some people and make herpes infections worse
Protein, amino acids such as leucine and their metabolites (beta-hydroxy beta-methylbutyrate (HMB)	Increased muscle mass and growth hormone release; accelerated muscle development and protein synthesis; decreased body fat	No effects if dietary protein intake is adequate; may promote protein synthesis if taken immediately before or after weight training	Can be dangerous for people with liver or kidney disease; substituting amino acid or polypeptide supplements for protein-rich food can cause nutrient deficiencies; protein supplements and sports foods such as bars and gels are more expensive than whole foods

*Possession of a controlled substance is illegal without a prescription, and physicians are not allowed to prescribe controlled substances for the improvement of athletic performance. In addition, the use of anabolic steroids, growth hormone, or any of several other substances listed in this table is banned for athletic competition. Some apparently safe supplements may contain substances banned for use in sports.

SOURCES: Office of Dietary Supplements, National Institutes of Health. 2017. *Dietary Supplements for Exercise and Athletic Performance: Fact Sheet for Health Professionals,* 2017 (https://ods.od.nih.gov/factsheets/ExerciseAndAthleticPerformance-HealthProfessional); Fahey, T., et al. 2015. "Sport and exercise physiology: Performance-enhancing substances—anabolic steroids, in Sports Science and Physical Education," ed., L. Georgescu, *Encyclopedia of Life Support Systems (EOLSS)*; Brooks, G. A., et al. 2005. *Exercise Physiology: Human Bioenergetics and Its Applications,* 4th ed. New York: McGraw-Hill; Pasiakos, S. M., et al. 2015. "The effects of protein supplements on muscle mass, strength, and aerobic and anaerobic power in healthy adults: A systematic review," *Sports Medicine*, vol. 45, no. 1: 111–131; Thomas, D.T., et al. 2016. "American College of Sports Medicine joint position statement. Nutrition and athletic performance," *Medicine and Science in Sports and Exercise* 48(3): 543–568.

TIPS FOR TODAY AND THE FUTURE

To improve and maintain your muscle fitness, perform strength training exercise for major muscle groups at least twice a week.

RIGHT NOW YOU CAN

- Stand up and do some body weight exercises—air squats, lunges, side bridges, and planks.
- Identify your current options for equipment and facilities for strength training. If you are interested in a machine weight-training program, research low-cost facility options on your campus or in your community.

IN THE FUTURE YOU CAN

- Add variety to your strength training workouts by trying different equipment and types of exercises; for example, if you normally use machines, try free weights. Also make changes in the specific exercises you do for major muscle groups.
- Reassess your muscular strength and endurance by repeating tests from the lab activities. Evaluate the progress of your program to date, and make changes to your FITT-VP factors. For example, you might start training less frequently but with heavier weights and/or more sets.

WEIGHT TRAINING EXERCISES

A general book on fitness and wellness cannot include a detailed description of all weight training exercises. The following pages present a basic program for developing muscular strength and endurance for general fitness using body weight (no equipment), free weights, and weight machines. Photographs and a list of the muscles being trained accompany instructions for each exercise; Table 4.4 lists exercises and major muscles and functions for the major muscle groups that you should train in your program. See Figure 4.6 for a clear illustration of the deep and superficial muscles referenced in the exercises.

Labs 4.2 and 4.3 will help you assess your current level of muscular endurance and design your own weight training program. If you want to develop strength for a particular activity, your program should contain exercises for general fitness, exercises for the muscle groups most important for the activity, and exercises for muscle groups most often injured. Regardless of the goals of your program or the type of equipment you use, your program should be structured so that you obtain maximum results without risking injury.

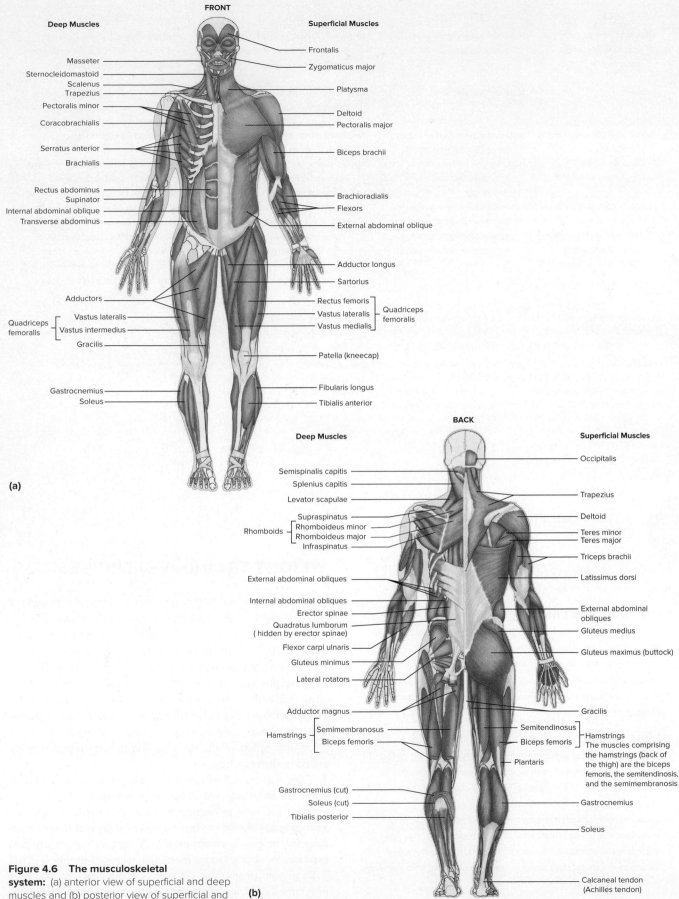

FRONT

Deep Muscles — Superficial Muscles

- Frontalis
- Masseter
- Sternocleidomastoid
- Scalenus
- Trapezius
- Zygomaticus major
- Platysma
- Pectoralis minor
- Coracobrachialis
- Deltoid
- Pectoralis major
- Serratus anterior
- Brachialis
- Biceps brachii
- Rectus abdominus
- Supinator
- Internal abdominal oblique
- Transverse abdominus
- Brachioradialis
- Flexors
- External abdominal oblique
- Adductor longus
- Sartorius
- Adductors
- Rectus femoris
- Vastus lateralis — Quadriceps femoralis
- Vastus lateralis
- Quadriceps femoralis — Vastus intermedius
- Vastus medialis
- Gracilis
- Patella (kneecap)
- Gastrocnemius
- Soleus
- Fibularis longus
- Tibialis anterior

(a)

BACK

Deep Muscles — Superficial Muscles

- Occipitalis
- Semispinalis capitis
- Splenius capitis
- Levator scapulae
- Trapezius
- Supraspinatus
- Deltoid
- Rhomboids — Rhomboideus minor
- Rhomboideus major
- Infraspinatus
- Teres minor
- Teres major
- Triceps brachii
- External abdominal obliques
- Latissimus dorsi
- Internal abdominal obliques
- Erector spinae
- Quadratus lumborum (hidden by erector spinae)
- Flexor carpi ulnaris
- Gluteus minimus
- Lateral rotators
- External abdominal obliques
- Gluteus medius
- Gluteus maximus (buttock)
- Adductor magnus
- Gracilis
- Hamstrings — Semimembranosus
- Biceps femoris
- Semitendinosus
- Biceps femoris
- Hamstrings The muscles comprising the hamstrings (back of the thigh) are the biceps femoris, the semitendinosis, and the semimembranosis
- Plantaris
- Gastrocnemius (cut)
- Soleus (cut)
- Tibialis posterior
- Gastrocnemius
- Soleus
- Calcaneal tendon (Achilles tendon)

(b)

Figure 4.6 The musculoskeletal system: (a) anterior view of superficial and deep muscles and (b) posterior view of superficial and deep muscles

Table 4.4

Muscle Groups, Major Muscles and Functions, and Strength Training Exercises

MUSCLE GROUP	MAJOR MUSCLES AND FUNCTIONS	STRENGTH TRAINING EXERCISES
Neck and upper back	Trapezius: A large muscle in the upper back and neck that moves the shoulder blades. Latissimus dorsi: A large muscle in the back that extends, adducts (lowers) the shoulder down and to the side, and helps stabilize the shoulder. Rhomboids: Moves (retracts and elevate) the shoulder blades.	Front plank, pull-up, shoulder press, upright rowing, kettlebell swing, horizontal rowing, kettlebell one-arm snatch, kettlebell carry, lat pull, assisted pull-up, overhead press, pullover, lateral raise
Shoulders	Deltoids: Large round shoulder muscles that lift the arm to the front (flexion) and to the side (abduction). Rhomboids: Moves and stabilizes the shoulder blades; assists during rowing motions. Rotator cuff: Internally and externally rotates the shoulder; consists of the supraspinatus, infraspinatus, teres minor, and subscapularis.	Burpees with a push-up, spine extension, thrusters, front plank, push-ups, bench press, shoulder press, upright rowing, lateral raise, kettlebell one-arm snatch, overhead press, lateral raise, assisted dip
Arms	Biceps: Muscle on the front of the upper arm that bends the elbow (elbow flexion) and lifts the shoulder (shoulder flexion). Triceps: A muscle on the back of the arm that extends (straightens) the elbow. Brachialis: Muscle in the upper arm that bends (flexes) the elbows.	Thrusters, push-ups, bench press, pull-up, shoulder press, upright rowing , biceps curl, lat pull, assisted pull-up, overhead press, pullover, triceps extension, assisted dip
Chest	Pectoralis major and minor: Large chest muscles that move the shoulder (flexion, adduction, and rotation).	Burpees with a push-up, thrusters, front plank, push-ups, bench press, pullover, assisted dip
Abdomen	Rectus abdominis: A large muscle on the front part of the abdomen that flexes the spine and stabilizes the core. Sometimes called the "six-pack" muscle. Obliques: Muscles on the side of the abdomen that stabilize the core and bend the trunk to the side (lateral flexion). Transversus abdominis: A muscle that stabilizes the core.	Curl-up, isometric side bridge, front plank, kettlebell carry, pullover
Lower back	Erector spinae: Muscles running along the spinal column that straighten and rotate the back and stabilize the core. Quadratus lumborum: A deep core muscle connecting the spine, hip, and ribs. It stabilizes the core, bends the trunk to the side, and rotates the hip.	Spine extension, isometric side bridge, front plank, kettlebell carry
Thighs	Quadriceps: Muscle group on the front of the thighs consisting of the vastus lateralis, vastus intermedius, vastus medialis, and rectus femoris. Hamstrings: Muscle group on the back of the thigh consisting of the semimembranosis, semitendinosis, biceps femoris.	Squats (all types), lunges, burpees with a push-up, spine extension, thrusters, kettlebell swing, kettlebell one-arm snatch, kettlebell carry, leg press, leg extension, seated leg curl
Buttocks	Gluteals: Muscles of the buttocks, consisting of the gluteus maximus, gluteus minimus, and gluteus medius.	Squats (all types), lunges, burpees with a push-up, spine extension, thrusters, front plank, kettlebell swing, kettlebell one-arm snatch, leg press
Calves	Calf muscles: Muscles on the back of the lower leg consisting of the gastrocnemius, soleus, and plantaris.	Squats, lunges, burpees with a push-up, thrusters, heel raise, seated leg curl, heel raise

EXERCISE 1

Air Squats

Instructions: (a) Keep your back straight and head level; stand with feet slightly more than shoulder-width apart and toes pointed slightly outward. Hold your hands out in front of you. **(b)** Squat down until your thighs are below parallel with the floor. Let your thighs move laterally (outward) so that you "squat between your legs." Hinge at your hips and don't let your back sag. This will help keep your back straight and your heels on the floor. Drive upward toward the starting position, hinging at the hips and keeping your back in a fixed position throughout the exercise.

Muscles developed: Quadriceps, gluteals, hamstrings, calf

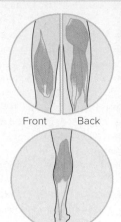

Front   Back

Back

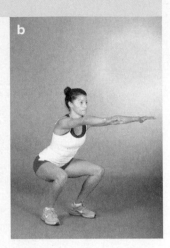

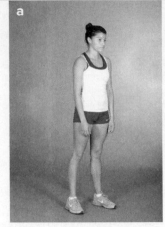

(a–b): Photo taken by Taylor Robertson Photography

EXERCISE 2

Lunges

Instructions: (a) Stand with one foot about two feet in front of the other. **(b)** Lunge forward with the front leg, bending it until the thigh is parallel to the floor. The heel of the lead leg should stay on the ground. Do not shift your weight so far forward that the knee moves out past the toes. Repeat the exercise using the other leg. Keep your back and head as straight as possible and maintain control while performing the exercise.

Muscles developed: Quadriceps, gluteals, hamstrings, calf

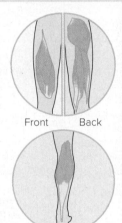

Front   Back

Back

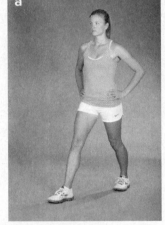

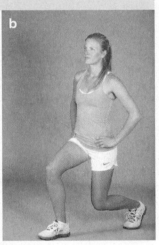

(a–b): Photo taken by Taylor Robertson Photography

EXERCISE 3

Burpees with a Push-Up

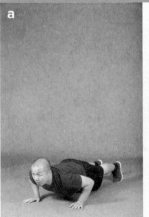

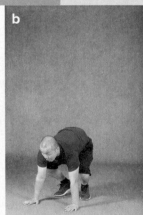

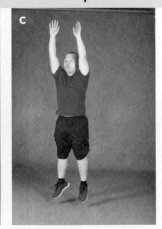

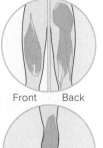

Front   Back

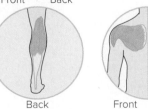

Back

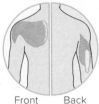

Front   Back

(a–c): Photo taken by Taylor Robertson Photography

Instructions: From a standing position, squat down and place your hands on the floor; and then **(a)** kick your legs behind you and land in the "up" push-up position. Do a push-up. **(b)** Then move your knees forward returning to the squat position; **(c)** spring up as high as you can into a full jump. Repeat.

Muscles developed: Quadriceps, gluteals, hamstrings, calf, deltoids, pectoralis major, triceps

McGill Curl-Up

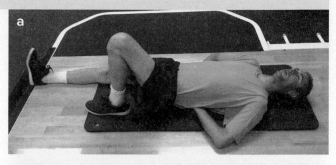

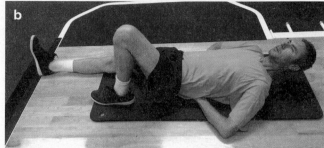

Instructions: (a) Lie on your back on the floor with one leg bent, foot placed flat on the floor, and the other leg straight. Place your hands under the small of your back or fold your arms across your chest. **(b)** Slowly raise the chest, shoulders, and head as a unit while maintaining a neutral spine. Try to isolate the rectus abdominis. Do not grasp your hands around your head when doing crunches because you might injure your neck.

Muscles developed: Rectus abdominis, obliques

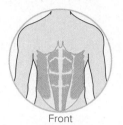

Front

(a–b): Photo taken by Tom Fahey

Spine Extension ("Bird Dog") (Isometric Exercise)

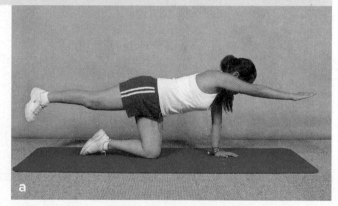

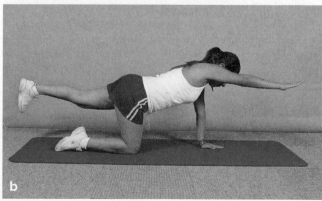

Instructions: Begin on all fours with your knees below your hips and your hands below your shoulders.

Unilateral spine extension: (a) Extend your right leg to the rear and reach forward with your right arm. Keep your spine neutral and your raised arm and leg in line with your torso. Don't arch your back or let your hip or shoulder sag. Hold this position for 10–30 seconds. Repeat with your left leg and left arm.

Bilateral spine extension: (b) Extend your left leg to the rear and reach forward with your right arm. Keep your spine neutral and your raised arm and leg in line with your torso. Don't arch your back or let your hip or shoulder sag. Hold this position for 10–30 seconds. Repeat with your right leg and left arm.

You can make this exercise more difficult by making box patterns with your arms and legs.

Muscles developed: Erector spinae, gluteus maximus, hamstrings, deltoids

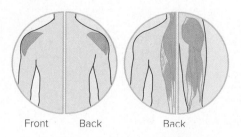

Front   Back   Back

(a–b): Photo taken by Wayne Glusker

Isometric Side Bridge

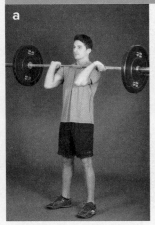

Photo taken by Joseph Quever

Instructions: Lie on the floor on your side with your knees bent and your top arm lying alongside your body. Lift and drive your hips forward so that your weight is supported by your forearm and knee. Hold this position for 3–10 seconds, breathing normally. Repeat on the other side. Perform 3–10 repetitions on each side.

Variation: You can make the exercise more difficult by keeping your legs straight and supporting yourself with your feet and forearm (see Lab 5.3) or with your feet and hand (with elbow straight). An advanced version of this exercise that builds the core and shoulder muscles is to do a side bridge on the right side, rotate to a front plank, and then rotate to a side bridge on the left side. Hold each position for 3 seconds.

Muscles developed: Obliques, quadratus lumborum

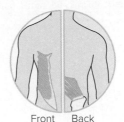

Front   Back

Thrusters

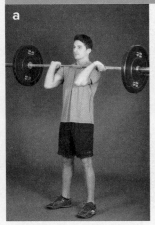
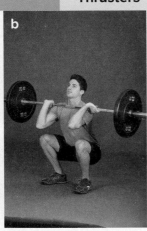
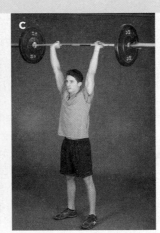

(a–c): Photo taken by Taylor Robertson Photography

Muscles developed: Quadriceps, gluteus maximus, hamstrings, gastrocnemius, deltoids, pectoralis major, triceps

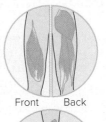

Front   Back

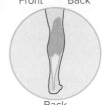

Back

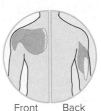

Front   Back

Instructions: **(a)** From a standing position, hold stones, soup cans, dumbbells, or barbells (or a single rock with both hands) at chest level with palms facing outward. **(b)** Squat down until your thighs are parallel with the floor. **(c)** Immediately stand and press the objects overhead in one continuous motion. Lower the objects to the starting position and immediately repeat the exercise.

EXERCISE 8

Overhead Squats

Instructions: (a) Stand holding a broom handle, stones, barbell, or soup cans overhead with straight arms, feet placed slightly more than shoulder-width apart, toes pointed out slightly, head neutral, and back straight. Center your weight over your arches or slightly behind. **(b)** Squat down, keeping your weight centered over your arches, and actively flex the hips (hinge at the hips with buttocks back) until your legs break parallel (hips below knees). During the movement, keep your spine neutral, shoulders back, and chest out, and let your thighs part to the side so that you are "squatting between your legs." Try to "spread the floor" with your feet. Push up to the starting position, maximizing the use of the posterior hip and thigh muscles, and maintaining a straight back and neutral head position.

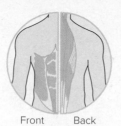

Front   Back

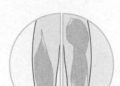

Front   Back

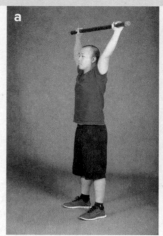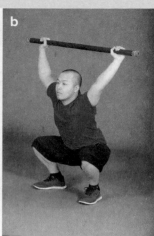

(a–b): Photo taken by Taylor Robertson Photography

Muscles developed: Quadriceps, hamstrings, gluteal muscles, core muscles

EXERCISE 9

Front Plank

Instructions: Lying on your front with body straight, raise your body upward, supporting your weight on forearms and toes. Hold the position. Begin with 10-second holds and progress until you can hold the plank for at least two minutes. Breathe normally. Tighten your abs, glutes, and quads as you do this exercise.

Muscles developed: Rectus abdominis, erector spinae, trapezius, rhomboids, deltoids, pectorals, gluteal muscles

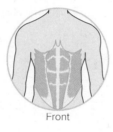

Front

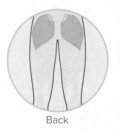

Back

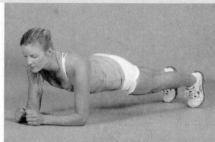

Photo taken by Taylor Robertson Photography

EXERCISE 10

Push-Ups

Instructions: (a) Start in the push-up position with your body weight supported by your hands and feet. Your arms and back should be straight and your fingers pointed forward. Lower your chest to the floor with your back straight, and then return to the starting position.

Variation: (b) Do modified push-ups if you can't do at least 10 regular push-ups. Start with your body weight supported by your hands and knees. Your arms and back should be straight and your fingers pointed forward. Lower your chest to the floor with your back straight, and then return to the starting position.

Muscles developed: Pectorals, triceps, deltoids

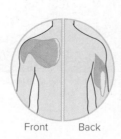

Front   Back

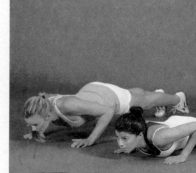

Photo taken by Taylor Robertson Photography

EXERCISE 1	Bench Press

Instructions: (a) Lying on a bench on your back with your feet on the floor, grasp the bar with palms upward and hands shoulder-width apart. If the weight is on a rack, move the bar carefully from the supports to a point over the middle of your chest or slightly above it (at the lower part of the sternum). **(b)** Lower the bar to your chest. Then press it in a straight line to the starting position. Don't arch your back or bounce the bar off your chest. You can also do this exercise with dumbbells or one arm at a time (unilateral training).

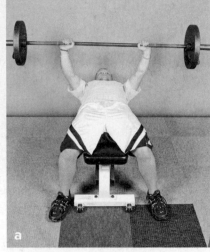
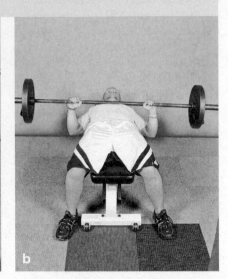

(a–b): Photo taken by Wayne Glusker

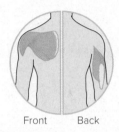

Front   Back

Muscles developed: Pectoralis major, triceps, deltoids

Note: *To allow an optimal view of exercise technique, a spotter does not appear in these demonstration photographs; however, spotters should be used for this exercise.*

EXERCISE 2	Pull-Up

Instructions: (a) Begin by grasping the pull-up bar with both hands, palms facing forward and elbows extended fully. **(b)** Pull yourself upward until your chin goes above the bar. Then return to the starting position.

Assisted pull-up: (c) This is done as described for a pull-up, except that a spotter assists the person by pushing upward at the waist, hips, or legs during the exercise.

Muscles developed: Latissimus dorsi, biceps

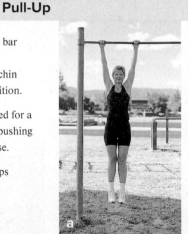
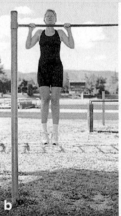
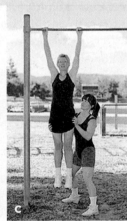

(a–c): Photo taken by Neil A. Tanner

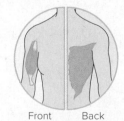

Front   Back

<table>
<tr><td>**EXERCISE 3**</td><td>**Shoulder Press (Overhead or Military Press)**</td></tr>
</table>

Instructions: This exercise can be done standing or seated, with dumbbells or a barbell. The shoulder press begins with the weight at your chest, preferably on a rack. **(a)** Grasp the weight with your palms facing away from you. **(b)** Push the weight overhead until your arms are extended. Then return to the starting position (weight at chest). Be careful not to arch your back excessively.

If you are a more advanced weight trainer, you can "clean" the weight (lift it from the floor to your chest). The clean should be attempted only after instruction from a knowledgeable coach; otherwise, it can lead to injury.

Muscles developed:
Deltoids, triceps, trapezius

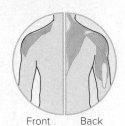

Front   Back

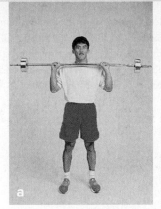

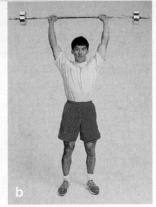

(a–b): Photo taken by Joseph Quever

<table>
<tr><td>**EXERCISE 4**</td><td>**Upright Rowing**</td></tr>
</table>

Instructions: (a) From a standing position with arms extended fully, grasp a barbell with a close grip (hands about 6–12 inches apart) and palms facing the body. **(b)** Raise the bar to about the level of your collarbone, keeping your elbows above bar level at all times. Return to the starting position.

This exercise can be done using dumbbells, a weighted bar (shown), or a barbell.

Muscles developed:
Trapezius, deltoids, biceps

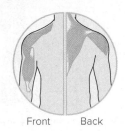

Front   Back

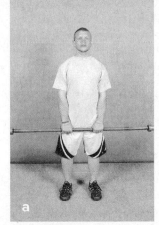

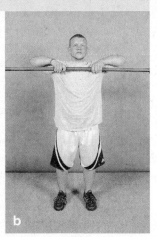

(a–b): Photo taken by Wayne Glusker

<table>
<tr><td>**EXERCISE 5**</td><td>**Biceps Curl**</td></tr>
</table>

Instructions: (a) From a standing position, grasp the bar with your palms facing away from you and your hands shoulder-width apart. **(b)** Keeping your upper body rigid, flex (bend) your elbows until the bar reaches a level slightly below the collarbone. Return the bar to the starting position.

This exercise can be done using dumbbells, a curl bar (shown), or a barbell; some people find that using a curl bar places less stress on the wrists.

Muscles developed:
Biceps, brachialis

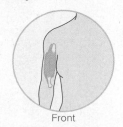

Front

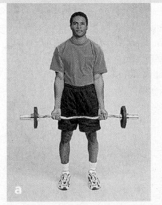

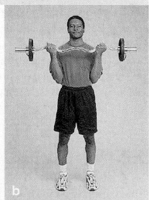

(a–b): Photo taken by Joseph Quever

EXERCISE 6   Lateral Raise

Instructions: (a) Stand with feet shoulder-width apart and a dumbbell in each hand. Hold the dumbbells in front of you and parallel to each other. **(b)** With elbows slightly bent, slowly lift both weights to the side until they reach shoulder level. Keep your wrists in a neutral position, in line with your forearms. Return to the starting position.

Muscles developed: Deltoids

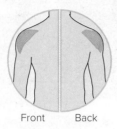

Front   Back

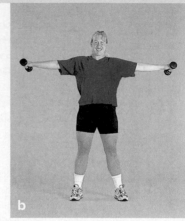

(a–b): Photo taken by Neil A. Tanner

EXERCISE 7   Squat

Instructions: (a) If the bar is racked, place the bar on the fleshy part of your upper back and grasp the bar at shoulder width. Keeping your back straight and head level, remove the bar from the rack and take a step back. Stand with feet slightly more than shoulder-width apart and toes pointed slightly outward. Rest the bar on the back of your shoulders, holding it there with palms facing forward. **(b)** Keeping your head level and lower back straight and pelvis back, squat down until your thighs are below parallel with the floor. Let your thighs move laterally (outward) so that you "squat between your legs." This will help keep your back straight and keep your heels on the floor. Drive upward toward the starting position, hinging at the hips and keeping your back in a fixed position throughout the exercise.

Muscles developed:
Quadriceps, gluteals, hamstrings, calf

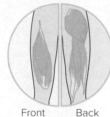

Front   Back

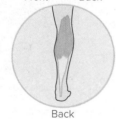

Back

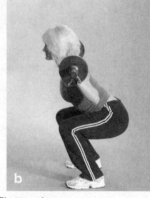

(a–b): Photo taken by Taylor Robertson Photography

EXERCISE 8   Heel Raise

Instructions: Stand with feet shoulder-width apart and toes pointed straight ahead. **(a)** Rest the bar on the back of your shoulders, holding it there with palms facing forward. **(b)** Press down with your toes while lifting your heels. Return to the starting position.

Muscle developed:
Calf

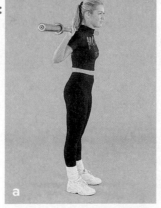

Back

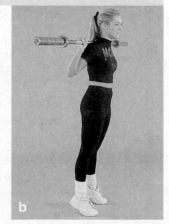

(a–b): Photo taken by Neil A. Tanner

EXERCISE 9

Kettlebell Swing

Instructions: (a) Begin by holding the kettlebell in both hands with palms facing toward you, in a standing position with knees bent, feet placed slightly more than shoulder-width apart, hips flexed, back straight, chest out, and head in a neutral position. **(b)** Holding the kettlebell at knee level, swing the weight to a horizontal position by initiating the motion with the hips, thighs, and abs (tighten the quads, glutes, and ab muscles as hard as you can), keeping your arm straight and relaxed during the movement. Let the weight swing back between your legs in a "football hiking motion" and then repeat the exercise. During the movement, hinge at the hips and not at the spine.

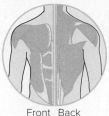
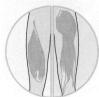

Front Back

Front Back

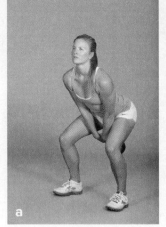

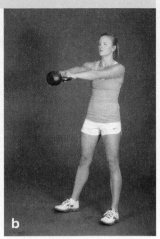

(a–b): Photo taken by Taylor Robertson Photography

Muscles developed: Quadriceps, hamstrings, latisimus dorsi, erector spinae, gluteals, core

EXERCISE 10

Kettlebell One-Arm Snatch

Instructions: (a) Begin by holding the kettlebell in one hand with your palm facing toward you, in a standing position with knees bent, feet placed slightly more than shoulder-width apart, hips flexed, back straight, chest out, and head in a neutral position.

Hold the kettlebell at knee level. **(b)** Swing the weight to a horizontal position by initiating the motion with the hips, thighs, and abs (tighten the quads, glutes, and ab muscles as hard as you can), bending your arm as it approaches the chest and continuing the motion until straightening it overhead.

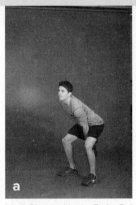
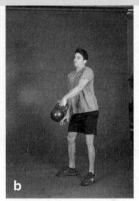
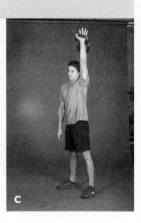

(a–c): Photo taken by Taylor Robertson Photography

The kettlebell should rotate from the front of your hand to the back during the motion. Use an upward punching motion at the top of the movement to prevent injuring your forearm. **(c)** Let the weight swing back between your legs in a "football hiking motion" and then repeat the exercise. During the movement, hinge at the hips and not at the spine.

Muscles developed: Quadriceps, gluteals, hamstrings, core, deltoids, trapezius, erector spinae, latissimus dorsi, pectoralis major

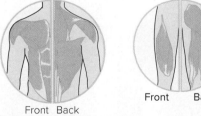

Front Back

Front Back

EXERCISE 11

Kettlebell or Dumbbell Carry ("Suitcase Carry")

Instructions: This is an excellent exercise for building the core muscles. Pick up a dumbbell or kettlebell in one or both hands. Maintaining good posture, walk 20 to 100 yards carrying the weight. Carry 10 to several hundred pounds, depending on your fitness.

Muscles developed: Core, trapezius, quadriceps, gluteals

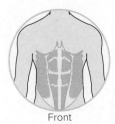

Front

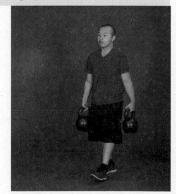

Photo taken by Taylor Robertson Photography

EXERCISE 1

Bench Press (Chest or Vertical Press) Weight Machines

Instructions: Sit or lie on the seat or bench, depending on the type of machine and the manufacturer's instructions. Your back, hips, and buttocks should be pressed against the machine pads. Place your feet on the floor or the foot supports.

(a) Grasp the handles with your palms facing away from you; the handles should be aligned with your armpits.

(b) Push the bars until your arms are fully extended, but don't lock your elbows. Return to the starting position.

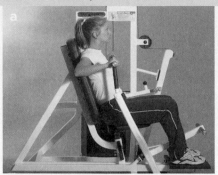
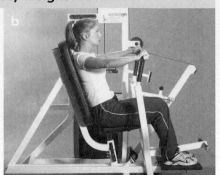

(a–b): Photo taken by Taylor Robertson Photography

Muscles developed: Pectoralis major, anterior deltoids, triceps

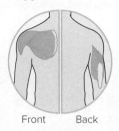

Front   Back

EXERCISE 2

Lat Pull

Instructions: Begin in a seated or kneeling position, depending on the type of lat machine and the manufacturer's instructions.

(a) Grasp the bar of the machine with arms fully extended.

(b) Slowly pull the weight down until it reaches the top of your chest. Slowly return to the starting position.

Muscles developed: Latissimus dorsi, biceps

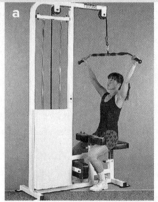
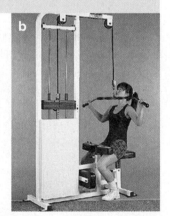

(a–b): Photo taken by Neil A. Tanner

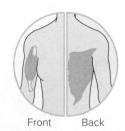

Front   Back

Note: *This exercise focuses on the same major muscles as the assisted pull-up (Exercise 3); choose an appropriate exercise for your program based on your preferences and equipment availability.*

EXERCISE 3 — Assisted Pull-Up

Instructions: Set the weight according to the amount of assistance you need to complete a set of pull-ups—the heavier the weight, the more assistance provided.

(a) Stand or kneel on the assist platform, and grasp the pull-up bar with your elbows fully extended and your palms facing away.

(b) Pull up until your chin goes above the bar, and then return to the starting position.

Muscles developed: Latissimus dorsi, biceps

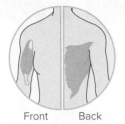

Front   Back

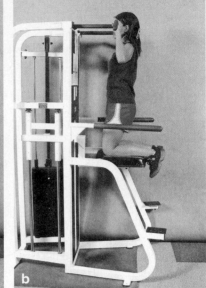
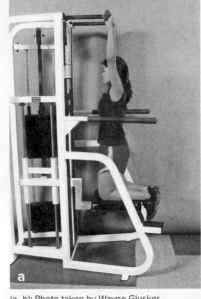

a   b

(a–b): Photo taken by Wayne Glusker

EXERCISE 4 — Overhead Press (Shoulder Press)

Instructions: Adjust the seat so that your feet are flat on the ground and the hand grips are slightly above your shoulders. **(a)** Sit down, facing away from the machine, and grasp the hand grips with your palms facing forward. **(b)** Press the weight upward until your arms are extended. Return to the starting position.

Muscles developed: Trapezius, triceps, deltoids, pectoralis major, rotator cuff

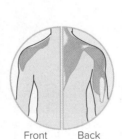

Front   Back

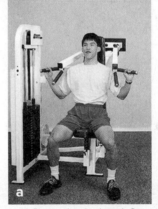
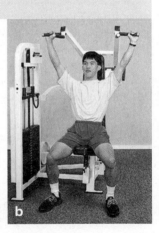

a   b

(a–b): Photo taken by Joseph Quever

EXERCISE 5 — Biceps Curl

Instructions: **(a)** Adjust the seat so that your back is straight and your arms rest comfortably against the top and side pads. Place your arms on the support cushions and grasp the hand grips with your palms facing up. **(b)** Keeping your upper body still, flex (bend) your elbows until the hand grips almost reach your collarbone. Return to the starting position.

Muscles developed: Biceps, brachialis

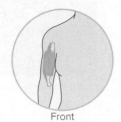

Front

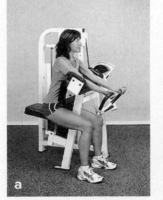
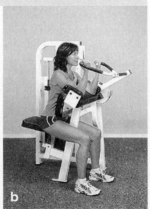

a   b

(a–b): Photo taken by Joseph Quever

EXERCISE 6 — Pullover

Instructions: Adjust the seat so that your shoulders are aligned with the cams. Push down on the foot pads with your feet to bring the bar forward until you can place your elbows on the pads. Rest your hands lightly on the bar. If possible, place your feet flat on the floor. **(a)** To get into the starting position, let your arms go backward as far as possible. **(b)** Pull your elbows forward until the bar almost touches your abdomen. Return to the starting position.

Muscles developed: Latissimus dorsi, pectorals, triceps, rectus abdominis

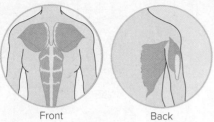

Front   Back

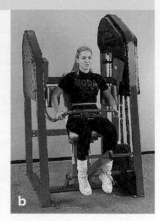

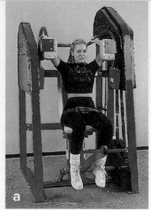

(a–b): Photo taken by Neil A. Tanner

EXERCISE 7 — Lateral Raise

Instructions: **(a)** Adjust the seat so that the pads rest just above your elbows when your upper arms are at your sides, your elbows are bent, and your forearms are parallel to the floor. Lightly grasp the handles. **(b)** Push outward and up with your arms until the pads are at shoulder height. Lead with your elbows rather than trying to lift the bars with your hands. Return to the starting position.

Muscles developed: Deltoids, trapezius

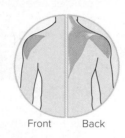

Front   Back

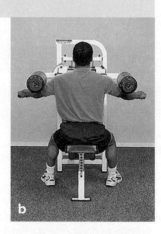

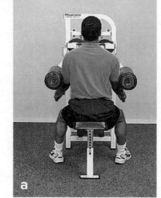

(a–b): Photo taken by Joseph Quever

EXERCISE 8 — Triceps Extension

Instructions: **(a)** Adjust the seat so that your back is straight and your arms rest comfortably against the top and side pads. Place your arms on the support cushions and grasp the hand grips with palms facing inward. **(b)** Keeping your upper body still, extend your elbows as much as possible. Return to the starting position.

Muscles developed: Triceps

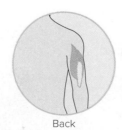

Back

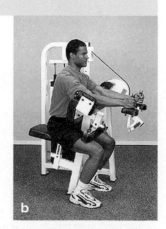

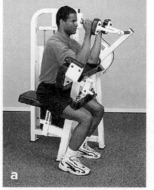

(a–b): Photo taken by Joseph Quever

Note: *This exercise focuses on some of the same muscles as the Assisted Dip (Exercise 9); choose an appropriate exercise for your program based on your preferences and equipment availability.*

EXERCISE 9 — Assisted Dip

Instructions: Set the weight according to the amount of assistance you need to complete a set of dips—the heavier the weight, the more assistance provided. **(a)** Stand or kneel on the assist platform with your body between the dip bars. With your elbows fully extended and palms facing your body, support your weight on your hands. **(b)** Lower your body until your upper arms are almost parallel with the bars. Then push up until you reach the starting position.

Muscles developed: Triceps, deltoids, pectoralis major

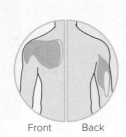

Front   Back

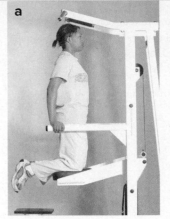

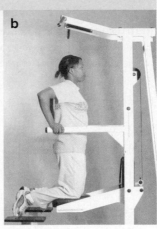

(a–b): Photo taken by Taylor Robertson Photography

EXERCISE 10 — Leg Press

Instructions: Sit or lie on the seat or bench, depending on the type of machine and the manufacturer's instructions. Your head, back, hips, and buttocks should be pressed against the machine pads. Loosely grasp the handles at the side of the machine. **(a)** Begin with your feet flat on the foot platform about shoulder-width apart. Extend your legs, but do not forcefully lock your knees. **(b)** Slowly lower the weight by bending your knees and flexing your hips until your knees are bent at about a 90-degree angle or your heels start to lift off the foot platform. Keep your lower back flat against the support pad. Then extend your knees and return to the starting position.

Muscles developed: Gluteals, quadriceps, hamstrings

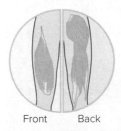

Front   Back

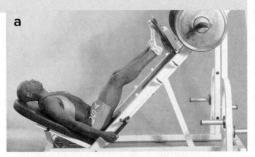

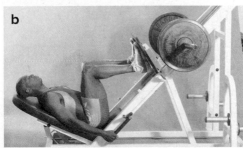

(a–b): Photo taken by Taylor Robertson Photography

EXERCISE 11 — Leg Extension (Knee Extension)

Instructions: **(a)** Adjust the seat so that the pads rest comfortably on top of your lower shins. Loosely grasp the handles. **(b)** Extend your knees until they are almost straight. Return to the starting position.

Knee extensions cause kneecap pain in some people. If you have kneecap pain during this exercise, check with an orthopedic specialist before repeating it.

Muscles developed: Quadriceps

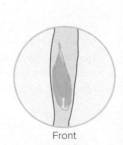

Front

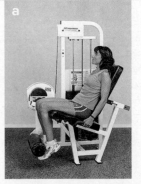

(a–b): Photo taken by Joseph Quever

Instructions: (a) Sit on the seat with your back against the back pad and the leg pad below your calf muscles. **(b)** Flex your knees until your lower and upper legs form a 90-degree angle. Return to the starting position.

Muscles developed: Hamstrings, calf

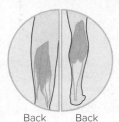

Back   Back

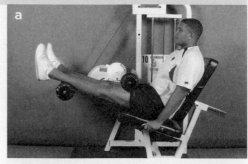

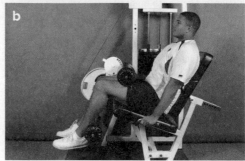

(a–b): Photo taken by Wayne Glusker

Instructions: (a) Stand with your head between the pads and one pad on each shoulder. The balls of your feet should be on the platform. Lightly grasp the handles. **(b)** Press down with your toes while lifting your heels. Return to the starting position. Changing the direction your feet are pointing (straight ahead, inward, and outward) will work different portions of your calf muscles.

Muscle developed: Calf

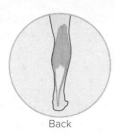

Back

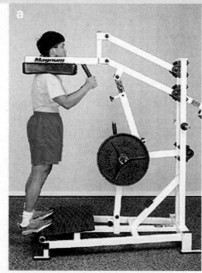

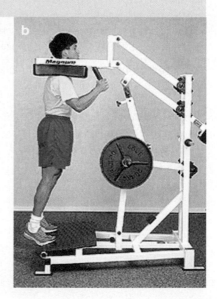

(a–b): Photo taken by Joseph Quever

Note: *Abdominal machines, low-back machines, and trunk rotation machines are not recommended because of injury risk. Refer to the "Body Weight" and "Free Weights" exercise sections for appropriate exercises to strengthen the abdominal and low-back muscles. For the rectus abdominis, obliques, and transverse abdominis,* *perform curl-ups (Exercise 4 in the "Body Weight" section) and the stir-the-pot exercise (Exercise 11 in the "Flexibility and Low-Back Health" chapter), and for the erector spinae and quadratus lumborum, perform the spine extension and the isometric side bridge (Exercises 5 and 6 in the "Body Weight" section).*

COMMON QUESTIONS ANSWERED

Q Will I gain weight if I do resistance exercises?

A Your weight probably will not change significantly as a result of a general fitness program: one set of 8–12 repetitions of 8–10 exercises, performed on at least two nonconsecutive days per week. You will lose body fat but also increase muscle mass, so your weight will stay about the same. You may notice a change in how your clothes fit, however, because muscle is denser than fat. Increased muscle mass will help you control body fat. Muscle increases your metabolism, which means you burn more calories every day. If you combine resistance exercises with endurance exercises, you will be on your way to developing a healthier body composition. Concentrate on fat loss rather than weight loss.

Q Do I need more protein in my diet when I train with weights?

A No. Although some evidence indicates that power athletes involved in heavy training have a higher-than-normal protein requirement, there is no reason for most people to consume extra protein. Most Americans take in more protein than they need, so even if there is an increased protein need during heavy training, the average diet probably supplies it. However, recent studies from Canada showed that the combination of high-intensity training (high-intensity interval training and weight training), caloric restriction, and high protein intake (2.4 grams per kilogram body weight per day) resulted in substantial increases in lean mass and decreases in body fat. Consuming a protein-rich snack before or after training may promote muscle hypertrophy. You may find protein bars and shakes to be convenient, but keep in mind that they are more expensive than whole foods and do not contain all the nutrients found in a well-rounded diet.

Q What causes muscle soreness the day or two following a weight training workout?

A The muscle pain you feel a day or two after a heavy weight training workout is caused by injury to the muscle fibers and surrounding connective tissue. Contrary to popular belief, delayed-onset muscle soreness is not caused by lactic acid buildup. Scientists believe that injury to muscle fibers causes inflammation, which in turn causes the release of chemicals that break down part of the muscle tissue and cause pain. After a bout of intense exercise that causes muscle injury and delayed-onset muscle soreness, the muscles produce protective proteins that prevent soreness during future workouts. If you don't work out regularly, you lose these protective proteins and become susceptible to soreness again.

Q Will strength training improve my sports performance?

A Strength developed in the weight room does not automatically increase your power in sports such as skiing, tennis, or cycling. Hitting a forehand in tennis and making a turn on skis are precise skills that require coordination between your nervous system and muscles. For skilled people, movements become reflex; you don't think about them when you do them. Increasing strength can disturb this coordination. Only by simultaneously practicing a sport and improving fitness can you expect to become more powerful in the skill. Practice helps you integrate your new strength with your skills, which makes you more powerful. Consequently, you can hit the ball harder in tennis or make more forceful turns on the ski slopes. (Refer to Chapter 2 for more on the concept of specificity in physical training.)

Q Will I improve faster if I train every day?

A No. Your muscles need time to recover between training sessions. Doing resistance exercises every day will cause you to become overtrained, which will increase your chance of injury and impede your progress. If your strength training program reaches a plateau, try one of these strategies:

- Vary the number of sets. If you have been performing one set of each exercise, add sets.

- Train less frequently. If you are currently training the same muscle groups three or more times per week, you may not be allowing your muscles to fully recover from intense workouts.

- Change exercises. Using different exercises for the same muscle group may stimulate further strength development.

- Vary the load and number of repetitions. Try increasing or decreasing the loads you are using and changing the number of repetitions accordingly.

- If you are training alone, find a motivated training partner. A partner can encourage you and assist you with difficult lifts, forcing you to work harder.

- Train explosively (purposefully). This trains the nervous system and the muscles, which results in greater improvements in strength and power than training more slowly.

Q If I stop training, will my muscles turn to fat?

A No. Fat and muscle are two different kinds of tissue, and one cannot turn into the other. Muscles that aren't used become smaller (atrophy), and body fat may increase if caloric intake exceeds calories burned. Although the result of inactivity may be smaller muscles and more fat, the change is caused by two separate processes.

Q Should I wear a weight belt when I lift?

A Until recently, most experts advised people to wear weight belts. However, several studies have shown that weight belts do not prevent back injuries and may, in fact, increase the risk of injury by encouraging people to lift more weight than they are capable of lifting with good form. Although wearing a belt may allow you to lift more weight in some lifts, you may not get the full benefit of your program because use of a weight belt reduces the effectiveness of the workout on the muscles that help support your spine.

Q I don't live near a convenient gym; what exercises can I do at home in a small space?

A Purchase a kettlebell and do whole body exercises such as kettlebell swings, squats, and clean and press. Do body weight exercises such as push-ups, pull-ups, and isometric core exercises. Simulate weight exercises with elastic bands available in sports stores and the Internet.

Q How do I tell the differences between regular muscle soreness and an injury?

A Muscle soreness is caused by small injuries to muscles and tendons. The pain is transient and goes away in a day or so. More serious injuries result in prolonged pain and disability and might require medical attention and RICE (rest, ice, compression, elevation).

SUMMARY

• Hypertrophy (increased muscle fiber size) occurs when weight training causes the size and number of myofibrils to increase, thereby increasing total muscle size. Strength also increases through muscle learning. Most women do not develop large muscles from weight training.

• Improvements in muscular strength and endurance lead to enhanced physical performance, protection against injury, improved body composition, better self-image, improved muscle and bone health with aging, reduced risk of chronic disease, and decreased risk of premature death.

• Muscular strength can be assessed by determining the amount of weight that can be lifted in one repetition of an exercise. Muscular endurance can be assessed by determining the number of repetitions of a particular exercise that can be performed.

• Static (isometric) exercises involve contraction without movement. They are most useful when a person is recovering from an injury or surgery or needs to overcome weak points in a range of motion.

• Dynamic (isotonic) exercises involve contraction that results in movement. The two most common types are constant resistance (free weights and body weight) and variable resistance (many weight machines).

• Free weights and weight machines have pluses and minuses for developing fitness, although machines tend to be safer.

• Lifting heavy weights for only a few repetitions helps develop strength. Lifting lighter weights for more repetitions helps develop muscular endurance.

• A strength training program for general fitness includes at least one set of 8–12 repetitions (enough to cause fatigue) of 8–10 exercises, along with warm-up and cool-down periods. The program should be carried out at least two nonconsecutive days per week.

• Safety guidelines for strength training include using proper technique, using spotters and collars when necessary, and taking care of injuries.

• Supplements or drugs that are promoted as instant or quick "cures" usually don't work and are either dangerous, expensive, or both. Although some elite athletes take performance-enhancing drugs, the largest consumers are physically active young adults (18–35 years old) who want to improve appearance and physical performance.

FOR FURTHER EXPLORATION

American College of Sports Medicine Position Stand: Progression Models in Resistance Training for Healthy Adults. Provides an in-depth look at strategies for setting up a strength training program and making progress based on individual program goals.

http://journals.lww.com/acsm-msse/Fulltext/2009/03000/Progression_Models_in_Resistance_Training_for.26.aspx

Crossfit. Extensive written and video resources for people interested in cross-training and resistive exercise.

https://www.crossfit.com/

Dan John. An excellent website for people serious about improving strength and fitness, written by a world-class athlete and coach in track and field and Highland games.

http://danjohn.net

InnerBody. Provides text, illustrations, and animations about the muscular system, nerve-muscle connections, muscular contraction, and other topics.

http://www.innerbody.com/htm/body.html

Mayo Clinic: Weight Training: Improve Your Muscular Fitness. Provides a basic overview of weight training essentials along with links to many other articles on specific weight-training-related topics.

https://www.mayoclinic.org/healthy-lifestyle/fitness/in-depth/weight-training/art-20047116

National Strength and Conditioning Association. A professional organization that focuses on strength development for fitness and athletic performance.

http://www.nsca.com

Pilates Method Alliance. Provides information about Pilates and about instructor certification; includes a directory of instructors.

http://www.pilatesmethodalliance.org

Strong First: A website hosted by kettlebell master Pavel Tsatsouline that presents excellent information on strength training.

http://www.strongfirst.com/

University of California, San Diego: Muscle Physiology Home Page. Provides an introduction to muscle physiology, including information about types of muscle fibers and energy cycles.

http://muscle.ucsd.edu/musintro/jump.shtml

University of Michigan: Muscles in Action. Interactive descriptions of muscle movements.

http://www.med.umich.edu/lrc/Hypermuscle/Hyper.html

Yoga Alliance. A resource site for yoga instructors and people interested in yoga.

http://www.yogaalliance.org

See also the listings in Chapter 2.

SELECTED BIBLIOGRAPHY

American College of Sports Medicine. 2011. American College of Sports Medicine position stand: Progression models in resistance training for healthy adults. *Medicine and Science in Sports and Exercise* 43(7): 1334–1359.

American College of Sports Medicine. 2013. *ACSM's Resource Manual for Guidelines for Exercise Testing and Prescription,* 7th ed. Philadelphia: Lippincott Williams and Wilkins.

American College of Sports Medicine. 2018. *ACSM's Guidelines for Exercise Testing and Prescription,* 10th ed. Philadelphia: Wolters Kluwer.

Andersen, V., et al. 2016. Core muscle activation in one-armed and two-armed kettlebell swing. *Journal of Strength and Conditioning Research* 30: 1196–1204.

Andrews, M. A., et al. 2018. Physical effects of anabolic-androgenic steroids in healthy exercising adults: A systematic review and meta-analysis. *Current Sports Medicine Reports* 17(7): 232–241.

Antonio, J. 2019. High-protein diets in trained individuals. *Research in Sports Medicine* 27(2): 195–203.

Awan, R., and E. R. Laskowski. 2019. Yoga: Safe for all? *Mayo Clinic Proceedings* 94(3): 385–387.

Baechle, T., and R. W. Earl. 2016. *National Strength and Conditioning Association's Essentials of Strength and Conditioning,* 4th ed. Champaign, Ill.: Human Kinetics.

Batrakoulis, A., et al. 2018. High intensity, circuit-type integrated neuromuscular training alters energy balance and reduces body mass and fat in obese women: A 10-month training-detraining randomized controlled trial. *PLoS One* 13(8): e0202390.

Beck, B. R., et al. 2016. Exercise and Sports Science Australia (ESSA) position statement on exercise prescription for the prevention and management of osteoporosis. *Journal of Science and Medicine in Sport* S1440-2440(16)30217-1.

Beckham, G. K., et al. 2019. Influence of sex and maximum strength on reactive strength index-modified. *Journal Sports Science Medicine* 18(1): 65–72.

Behm, D. G., et al. 2010. Canadian Society for Exercise Physiology position stand: The use of instability to train the core in athletic and nonathletic conditioning. *Applied Physiology, Nutrition and Metabolism* 35(1): 109–112.

Brennan, R., et al. 2016. The injecting use of image and performance-enhancing drugs (IPED) in the general population: A systematic review. *Health and Social Care in the Community.* doi:10.1111/hsc.12326

Brooks, G. A., et al. 2005. *Exercise Physiology: Human Bioenergetics and Its Applications,* 4th ed. New York: McGraw-Hill.

Chen, H. T., et al. 2018. Effects of 8-week kettlebell training on body composition, muscle strength, pulmonary function, and chronic low-grade inflammation in elderly women with sarcopenia. *Experimental Gerontology* 112: 112–118.

De Souza, E. O., et al. 2018. Different patterns in muscular strength and hypertrophy adaptations in untrained individuals undergoing non-periodized and periodized strength regimens. *Journal Strength Conditioning Research* 32(5): 1238–1244.

Fahey, T. D. 2011. *Basic Weight Training for Men and Women,* 8th ed. New York: McGraw-Hill.

Figueroa, A., et al. 2019. Impact of high- and low-intensity resistance training on arterial stiffness and blood pressure in adults across the lifespan: A review. *Pflugers Archives* 471(3): 467–478.

Garcia-Hermoso, A., et al. 2018. Muscular strength as a predictor of all-cause mortality in an apparently healthy population: A systematic review and meta-analysis of data from approximately 2 million men and women. *Archives Physical Medicine Rehabilitation* 99(10): 2100–2113, e2105.

Hackett, D., et al. 2016. Olympic weightlifting training improves vertical jump height in sportspeople: A systematic review with meta-analysis. *British Journal Sports Medicine* 50: 865–872.

Ihalainen, J. K., et al. 2019. Strength training improves metabolic health markers in older individual regardless of training frequency. *Frontiers Physiology* 10: 32.

Jimenez-Garcia, J. D., et al. 2019. Suspension training HIIT improves gait speed, strength and quality of life in older adults. *International Journal Sports Medicine* 40(2): 116–124.

Kang, D. Y., et al. 2015. The effects of bodyweight-based exercise with blood flow restriction on isokinetic knee muscular function and thigh circumference in college students. *Journal of Physical Therapy Science* 27: 2709–2712.

Kerksick, C. M., et al. 2018. ISSN exercise & sports nutrition review update: research & recommendations. *Journal International Society of Sports Nutrition* 15(1): 38.

Laine, M. K., et al. 2016. Former male elite athletes have better metabolic health in late life than their controls. *Scandinavian Journal of Medicine Science in Sports* 26: 284–290.

Landi, F., et al. 2017. Age-related variations of muscle mass, strength, and physical performance in community-dwellers: Results from the Milan EXPO Survey. *Journal of the American Medical Directors Association* 88(1): e17–88.

Lee, B., and S. McGill. 2015. The effect of long-term isometric training on core/torso stiffness. *Journal of Strength and Conditioning Research* 29(6): 1515–1526.

Lippi, G., et al. 2018. Diagnostic biomarkers of muscle injury and exertional rhabdomyolysis. *Clinical Chemistry Laboratory Medicine* 57(2): 175–182.

Longland, T. M., et al. 2016. Higher compared with lower dietary protein during an energy deficit combined with intense exercise promotes greater lean mass gain and fat mass loss: A randomized trial. *American Journal Clinical Nutrition* 2103(3): 738–746.

Lorenzetti, S., et al. 2018. How to squat? Effects of various stance widths, foot placement angles and level of experience on knee, hip and trunk motion and loading. *BMC Sports Science Medicine Rehabilitation* 10: 14.

Maughan, R. J., et al. 2018. IOC consensus statement: dietary supplements and the high-performance athlete. *British Journal Sports Medicine* 52(7): 439–455.

McKendry, J., et al. 2016. Short inter-set rest blunts resistance exercise-induced increases in myofibrillar protein synthesis and intracellular signaling in young males. *Experimental Physiology* 101(7): 866–882.

Metter, E. J. 1997. Age-associated loss of power and strength in the upper extremities in women and men. *Journal of Gerontology: Biological Sciences.* 52A(5): 8267–8276.

Nakahara, H., et al. 2015. Low-frequency severe-intensity interval training improves cardiorespiratory functions. *Medicine and Science in Sports and Exercise* 47(4): 789–798.

Ostry, D. J., et al. 2016. Sensory plasticity in human motor learning. *Trends in Neuroscience* 39: 114–123.

Outram, S., and B. Stewart. 2015. Doping through supplement use: A review of the available empirical data. *International Journal of Sports Nutrition and Exercise Metabolism* 25(1): 54–59.

Paoli, A., et al. 2017. Resistance training with single vs. multi-joint exercises at equal total load volume: effects on body composition, cardiorespiratory fitness, and muscle strength. *Frontiers Physiology* 8: 1105.

Pedersen, B. K. 2019. Which type of exercise keeps you young? *Current Opinion Clinical Nutrition Metabolic Care* 22(2): 167–173.

Roshanravan, B., et al. 2017. Association of muscle endurance, fatigability, and strength with functional limitation and mortality in the Health Aging and Body Composition Study. *Journal of Gerontology Series A: Biological Sciences and Medical Sciences* 72(2): 284–291.

Saeterbakken, A. H., and M. S. Fimland. 2013. Electromyographic activity and 6RM strength in bench press on stable and unstable surfaces. *Journal of Strength and Conditioning Research* 27(4): 1101–1107.

Sanchis-Gomar, F., et al. 2014. 'Olympic' centenarians: Are they just biologically exceptional? *International Journal of Cardiology* 175(1): 216–217.

Schmidt, D., et al. 2016. The effect of high-intensity circuit training on physical fitness. *Journal of Sports Medicine and Physical Fitness* 56: 534–540.

Slimani, M., et al. 2018. A meta-analysis to determine strength training related dose-response relationships for lower-limb muscle power development in young athletes. *Frontiers of Physiology* 9: 1155.

Suchomel, T. J., et al. 2018. The importance of muscular strength: Training considerations. *Sports Medicine* 48(4): 765–785.

Sung, D. J., et al. 2018. Rhabdomyolysis from resistance exercise and caffeine intake. *Iranian Journal Public Health* 47(1): 138–139.

Tibana, R. A., and N. M. F. de Sousa. 2018. Are extreme conditioning programmes effective and safe? A narrative review of high-intensity functional training methods research paradigms and findings. *British Medical Journal Open Sports Exercise Medicine* 4(1): e000435.

Van de Vijver, P. L., et al. 2016. Early and extraordinary peaks in physical performance come with a longevity cost. *Aging* 8: 1822–1829.

Vechin, F. C., et al. 2015. Comparisons between low-intensity resistance training with blood flow restriction and high-intensity resistance training on quadriceps muscle mass and strength in elderly. *Journal of Strength and Conditioning Research* 29(4): 1071–1076.

Viana, R. B., et al. 2019. Is interval training the magic bullet for fat loss? A systematic review and meta-analysis comparing moderate-intensity continuous training with high-intensity interval training (HIIT). *British Journal Sports Medicine.* In press.

Vikmoen, O., et al. 2016. Effects of heavy strength training on running performance and determinants of running performance in female endurance athletes. *PLoS One* 11: e0150799.

Villanueva, M. G., et al. 2015. Short rest interval lengths between sets optimally enhance body composition and performance with 8 weeks of strength resistance training in older men. *European Journal Applied Physiology* 115(2): 295–308.

Zhou, M., et al. 2018. Tai chi improves brain metabolism and muscle energetics in older adults. *Journal Neuroimaging* 28(4): 359–364.

Name _____ Section _____ Date _____

LAB 4.1 Assessing Your Current Level of Muscular Strength

Assess your muscular strength using one or more of the tests in this lab. Bench press 1 RM can be assessed directly or by performing multiple repetitions to predict 1 RM. The functional lower body movement test assesses lower body strength. For best results, don't do any strenuous weight training within 48 hours of any test. Use great caution when completing 1-RM tests; do not take the maximum bench press test if you have any injuries to your shoulders, elbows, back, hips, or knees. In addition, do not take these tests until you have had at least one month of weight training experience and competent instruction in the techniques.

The Maximum Bench Press Test

Equipment
The free weights bench press test uses the following equipment

1. Flat bench (with or without racks)
2. Barbell
3. Assorted weight plates with collars to hold them in place
4. One or two spotters
5. Weight scale

If a weight machine is preferred, use the following equipment:

1. Bench press machine
2. Weight scale

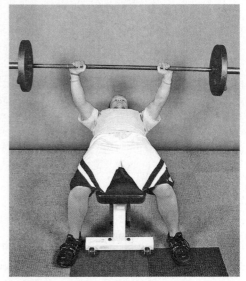

Photo taken by Wayne Glusker

Preparation
Try a few bench presses with a small amount of weight so that you can practice your technique, warm up your muscles, and, if you use free weights, coordinate your movements with those of your spotters. Weigh yourself and record the results.

Body weight: _____ lb.

Instructions

1. Use a weight that is lower than the amount you believe you can lift. For free weights, men should begin with a weight about two-thirds of their body weight; women should begin with the weight of just the bar (45 lb).

2. Lie on the bench with your feet firmly on the floor. If you are using a weight machine, grasp the handles with palms away from you; the tops of the handles should be aligned with the tops of your armpits.

    If you are using free weights, grasp the bar slightly wider than shoulder width with your palms away from you. If you have one spotter, she or he should stand directly behind the bench; if you have two spotters, they should stand to the side, one at each end of the barbell. Signal to the spotter when you are ready to begin the test by saying, "1, 2, 3." On "3," the spotter should help you lift the weight to a point over your mid-chest (nipple line).

3. Push the handles or barbell until your arms are fully extended. Exhale as you lift. If you are using free weights, the weight moves from a low point at the chest straight up. Keep your feet firmly on the floor, don't arch your back, and push the weight evenly with your right and left arms. Don't bounce the weight on your chest.

4. Rest for several minutes, then repeat the lift with a heavier weight. It will probably take several attempts to determine the maximum amount of weight you can lift (1 RM).

    1 RM: _____ lb

    Check one: _____ Free weights _____ Universal _____ Other

5. If you used free weights, convert your free weights bench press score to an estimated value for 1 RM on the Universal bench press or other bench press machine using the appropriate formula:

    Males: Estimated Universal 1 RM = (1.016 × free weights 1 RM _____ lb) + 18.41 = _____ lb

    Females: Estimated Universal 1 RM = (0.848 × free weights 1 RM _____ lb) + 21.37 = _____ lb

(Note: this formula might not be accurate on other bench press machines.)

LABORATORY ACTIVITIES

Rating Your Bench Press Result

1. Divide your 1-RM value by your body weight.

   1 RM _____ lb ÷ body weight _____ lb = _____

2. Find this ratio in the table to determine your bench press strength rating. Record the rating here and in the chart at the end of this lab.

   Bench press strength rating: _____

Strength Ratings for the Maximum Bench Press Test

	Pounds Lifted/Body Weight (lb)					
Men	*Very Poor*	*Poor*	*Fair*	*Good*	*Excellent*	*Superior*
Age: Under 20	Below 0.89	0.89–1.05	1.06–1.18	1.19–1.33	1.34–1.75	Above 1.75
20–29	Below 0.88	0.88–0.98	0.99–1.13	1.14–1.31	1.32–1.62	Above 1.62
30–39	Below 0.78	0.78–0.87	0.88–0.97	0.98–1.11	1.12–1.34	Above 1.34
40–49	Below 0.72	0.72–0.79	0.80–0.87	0.88–0.99	1.00–1.19	Above 1.19
50–59	Below 0.63	0.63–0.70	0.71–0.78	0.79–0.89	0.90–1.04	Above 1.04
60 and over	Below 0.57	0.57–0.65	0.66–0.71	0.72–0.81	0.82–0.93	Above 0.93
Women						
Age: Under 20	Below 0.53	0.53–0.57	0.58–0.64	0.65–0.76	0.77–0.87	Above 0.87
20–29	Below 0.51	0.51–0.58	0.59–0.69	0.70–0.79	0.80–1.00	Above 1.00
30–39	Below 0.47	0.47–0.52	0.53–0.59	0.60–0.69	0.70–0.81	Above 0.81
40–49	Below 0.43	0.43–0.49	0.50–0.53	0.54–0.61	0.62–0.76	Above 0.76
50–59	Below 0.39	0.39–0.43	0.44–0.47	0.48–0.54	0.55–0.67	Above 0.67
60 and over	Below 0.38	0.38–0.42	0.43–0.46	0.47–0.53	0.54–0.71	Above 0.71

SOURCE: The Cooper Institute of Aerobic Research, Dallas, TX; from *The Physical Fitness Specialist Manual*, revised 2005.

Predicting 1 RM from Multiple-Repetition Lifts Using Free Weights

Instead of doing the 1-RM maximum strength bench press test, you can predict your 1 RM from multiple-repetition lifts.

Instructions

1. Choose a weight you think you can bench press five times.

2. Follow the instructions for lifting the weight given in the maximum bench press test.

3. Do as many repetitions of the bench press as you can. A repetition counts only if done correctly

4. Refer to the chart below, or calculate predicted 1 RM using the Brzycki equation:

   1 RM = *weight* ÷ (1.0278 – [0.0278 × *number of repetitions*])

   1 RM = _____ lb ÷ (1.0278 – [0.0278 × _____ repetitions]) = _____

5. Divide your predicted 1-RM value by your body weight.

   1 RM _____ lb ÷ body weight _____ lb = _____

6. Find this ratio in the table above to determine your bench press strength rating. Record the rating here and in the chart at the end of the lab.

   Bench press strength rating: _____

Weight Lifted (lb.)	Repetitions											
	1	*2*	*3*	*4*	*5*	*6*	*7*	*8*	*9*	*10*	*11*	*12*
66	66	68	70	72	74	77	79	82	85	88	91	95
77	77	79	82	84	87	89	92	96	99	103	107	111
88	88	91	93	96	99	102	106	109	113	117	122	127
99	99	102	105	108	111	115	119	123	127	132	137	143
110	110	113	116	120	124	128	132	137	141	147	152	158
121	121	124	128	132	136	141	145	150	156	161	168	174
132	132	136	140	144	149	153	158	164	170	176	183	190
143	143	147	151	156	161	166	172	178	184	191	198	206
154	154	158	163	168	173	179	185	191	198	205	213	222
165	165	170	175	180	186	192	198	205	212	220	229	238
176	176	181	186	192	198	204	211	219	226	235	244	254
187	187	192	198	204	210	217	224	232	240	249	259	269
198	198	204	210	216	223	230	238	246	255	264	274	285
209	209	215	221	228	235	243	251	259	269	279	289	301
220	220	226	233	240	248	256	264	273	283	293	305	317
231	231	238	245	252	260	268	277	287	297	308	320	333
242	242	249	256	264	272	281	290	300	311	323	335	349
253	253	260	268	276	285	294	304	314	325	337	350	364
264	264	272	280	288	297	307	317	328	340	352	366	380
275	275	283	291	300	309	319	330	341	354	367	381	396
286	286	294	303	312	322	332	343	355	368	381	396	412
297	297	305	314	324	334	345	356	369	382	396	411	428
308	308	317	326	336	347	358	370	382	396	411	427	444

SOURCE: Brzycki, M. 1993. "Strength testing—predicting a one-rep max from reps to fatigue," *The Journal of Physical Education, Recreation and Dance* 64: 88–90.

Functional Lower Body Movement Tests

The following tests assess functional leg movement skills using squats. Most people do squats improperly, increasing their risk of knee and back pain. Before you add weight-bearing squats to your weight training program, you should determine your functional leg movement skills, check your ability to squat properly, and give yourself a chance to master squatting movements. The following leg strength tests will help you in each of these areas.

These tests are progressively more difficult, so do not move to the next test until you have scored at least a 3 on the current test. On each test, give yourself a rating of 0, 1, 3, or 5, as described in the instructions that follow the last test.

1. Chair Squat

Instructions

1. Sit up straight in a chair with your back resting against the backrest and your arms at your sides. Your feet should be placed more than shoulder-width apart so that you can get them under the body.

2. Begin the motion of rising out of the chair by flexing (bending) at the hips—not the back. Then squat up using a hip hinge movement (no spine movement). Stand without rocking forward, bending your back, or using external support, and keep your head in a neutral position.

3. Return to the sitting position while maintaining a straight back and keeping your weight centered over your feet. Your thighs should abduct (spread) as you sit back in the chair. Use your rear hip and thigh muscles as much as possible as you sit.

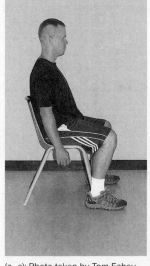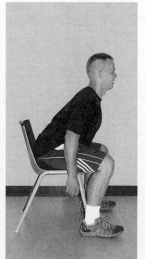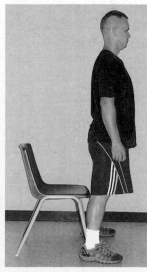

(a–c): Photo taken by Tom Fahey

Do five repetitions.

Your rating: _____

(See rating instructions that follow.)

2. Single-Leg Step-Up

Instructions

1. Stand facing a bench, with your right foot placed on the middle of the bench, right knee bent at 90 degrees, and arms at your sides.

2. Step up on the bench until your right leg is straight, maximizing the use of the hip muscles.

3. Return to the starting position. Keep your hips stable, back straight, chest up, shoulders back, and head neutral during the entire movement.

Do five repetitions for each leg.

Your rating: _____

(See rating instructions that follow.)

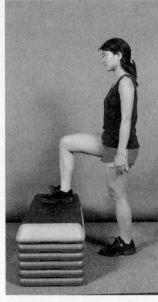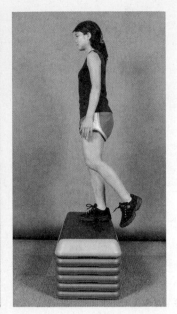

(a–b): Photo taken by Wayne Glusker

3. Unweighted Squat

Instructions

1. Stand with your feet placed slightly more than shoulder-width apart, toes pointed out slightly, hands on hips or across your chest, head neutral, and back straight. Center your weight over your arches or slightly behind.

2. Squat down, keeping your weight centered over your arches and actively flexing (bending) your hips until your legs break parallel. During the movement, keep your back straight, shoulders back, and chest out, and let your thighs part to the side so that you are "squatting between your legs."

3. Push back up to the starting position, hinging at the hips and not with the spine, maximizing the use of the rear hip and thigh muscles, and maintaining a straight back and neutral head position.

Do five repetitions.

Your rating: _____

(See rating instructions that follow.)

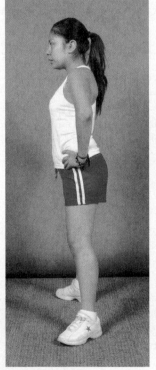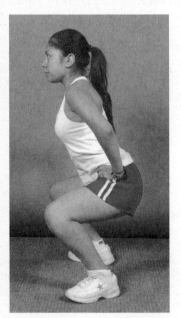

(a–b): Photo taken by Wayne Glusker

4. Single-Leg Lunge-Squat with Rear-Foot Support

Instructions

1. Stand about three feet in front of a bench (with your back to the bench).
2. Place the top of your left foot on the bench, and put most of your weight on your right leg (your left leg should be bent), with your hands at your sides.
3. Squat on your right leg until your thigh is parallel with the floor. Keep your back straight, chest up, shoulders back, and head neutral.
4. Return to the starting position.

   Do three repetitions for each leg.
   Your rating: _____
   (See rating instructions that follow.)

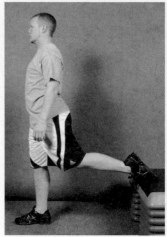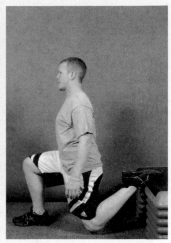

(a–b): Photo taken by Wayne Glusker

Rating Your Functional Leg Strength Test Results

5 points: Performed the exercise properly with good back and thigh position, weight centered over the middle or rear of the foot, chest out, and shoulders back; good use of hip muscles on the way down and on the way up, with head in a neutral position throughout the movement; maintained good form during all repetitions; abducted (spread) the thighs on the way down during chair squats and double-leg squats; for single-leg exercises, showed good strength on both sides; for single-leg lunge-squat with rear-foot support, maintained straight back, and knees stayed behind toes.

3 points: Weight was forward on the toes, with some rounding of the back; used thigh muscles excessively, with little use of hip muscles; head and chest were too far forward; showed little abduction of the thighs during double-leg squats; when going down for single-leg exercises, one side was stronger than the other; form deteriorated with repetitions; for single-leg lunge-squat with rear-foot support, could not reach parallel (thigh parallel with floor).

1 point: Had difficulty performing the movement, rocking forward and rounding back badly; used thigh muscles excessively, with little use of hip muscles on the way up or on the way down; chest and head were forward; on unweighted squats, had difficulty reaching parallel and showed little abduction of the thighs; on single-leg exercises, one leg was markedly stronger than the other; could not perform multiple repetitions.

0 points: Could not perform the exercise.

Summary of Results

Maximum bench press test from either the 1-RM test or the multiple-repetition test: Weight pressed: _____ lb   Rating: _____
Functional leg strength tests (0–5):
Chair squat: _____
Single-leg step-up: _____
Unweighted squat: _____
Single-leg lunge-squat with rear-foot support: _____

Remember that muscular strength is specific: Your ratings may vary considerably for different parts of your body.

LABORATORY ACTIVITIES

Using Your Results

How did you score? Are you surprised by your ratings for muscular strength? Are you satisfied with your current ratings?

If you're not satisfied, set realistic goals for improvement:

Are you satisfied with your current level of muscular strength as evidenced in your daily life—for example, your ability to lift objects, climb stairs, and engage in sports and recreational activities?

If you're not satisfied, set realistic goals for improvement:

What should you do next? Enter the results of this lab in the Preprogram Assessment column in Appendix B. If you've set goals for improvement, begin planning your strength training program by completing the plan in Lab 4.3. After several weeks of your program, complete this lab again and enter the results in the Postprogram Assessment column of Appendix B. How do the results compare?

Name_____ Section _____ Date _____

LAB 4.2 Assessing Your Current Level of Muscular Endurance

For best results, don't do any strenuous weight training within 48 hours of any test. To assess endurance of the abdominal muscles, perform the curl-up test. To assess endurance of muscles in the upper body, perform the push-up test. To assess endurance of the muscles in the lower body, perform the squat endurance test.

The Curl-Up Test

Equipment

1. Two six-inch strips of self-stick Velcro or heavy tape
2. Ruler
3. Partner
4. Mat (optional)

Preparation

Affix the strips of Velcro or long strips of tape on the mat or testing surface. Place the strips 3 inches apart.

Instructions

1. Start by lying on your back on the floor or mat, arms straight and by your sides, shoulders relaxed, palms down and on the floor, and fingers straight. Adjust your position so that the longest fingertip of each hand touches the end of the near strip of Velcro or tape. Your knees should be bent about 90 degrees, with your feet about 12–18 inches from your buttocks.

2. To perform a curl-up, flex your spine while sliding your fingers across the floor until the fingertips of each hand reach the second strip of Velcro or tape. Then return to the starting position; the shoulders must be returned to touch the mat between curl-ups, but the head need not touch. Shoulders must remain relaxed throughout the curl-up, and feet and buttocks must stay on the floor. Breathe easily, exhaling during the lift phase of the curl-up; do not hold your breath.

3. Once your partner says "go," perform as many curl-ups as you can at a steady pace with correct form. Your partner counts the curl-ups you perform and calls a stop to the test if she or he notices any incorrect form or drop in your pace.

Number of curl-ups: _____

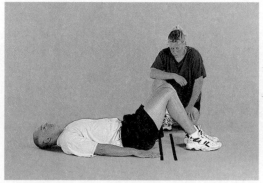 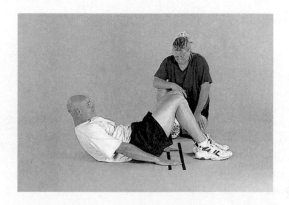

(a–b): Photo taken by Neil A. Tanner

LABORATORY ACTIVITIES

Rating Your Curl-Up Test Result

Your score is the number of completed curl-ups. Refer to the appropriate portion of the table for a rating of your abdominal muscular endurance. Record your rating below and in the summary at the end of this lab.

Rating: _____

Ratings for the Curl-Up Test

			Number of Curl-Ups			
Men	*Very Poor*	*Poor*	*Average*	*Good*	*Excellent*	*Superior*
Age: 16–19	Below 48	48–57	58–64	65–74	75–93	Above 93
20–29	Below 46	46–54	55–63	64–74	75–93	Above 93
30–39	Below 40	40–47	48–55	56–64	65–81	Above 81
40–49	Below 38	38–45	46–53	54–62	63–79	Above 79
50–59	Below 36	36–43	44–51	52–60	61–77	Above 77
60–69	Below 33	33–40	41–48	49–57	58–74	Above 74
Women						
Age: 16–19	Below 42	42–50	51–58	59–67	68–84	Above 84
20–29	Below 41	41–51	52–57	58–66	67–83	Above 83
30–39	Below 38	38–47	48–56	57–66	67–83	Above 83
40–49	Below 36	36–45	46–54	55–64	65–83	Above 83
50–59	Below 34	34–43	44–52	53–62	63–81	Above 81
60–69	Below 31	31–40	41–49	50–59	60–78	Above 78

SOURCE: Ratings based on norms calculated from data collected by Robert Lualhati on 4545 college students, 16–80 years of age, at Skyline College, San Bruno, CA.

The Push-Up Test

Equipment:

Mat or towel (optional)

Preparation

In this test, you will perform either standard push-ups or modified push-ups, in which you support yourself with your knees. The Cooper Institute developed the ratings for this test with men performing push-ups and women performing modified push-ups. Biologically, males tend to be stronger than females; the modified technique reduces the need for upper-body strength in a test of muscular endurance. Therefore, for an accurate assessment of upper-body endurance, men should perform standard push-ups and women should perform modified push-ups. However, in using push-ups as part of a strength training program, individuals should choose the technique most appropriate for increasing their level of strength and endurance—regardless of gender.

Instructions

1. *For push-ups:* Start in the push-up position with your body supported by your hands and feet. *For modified push-ups:* Start in the modified push-up position with your body supported by your hands and knees. *For both positions,* keep your arms and your back straight and your fingers pointed forward.

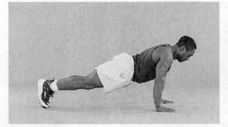 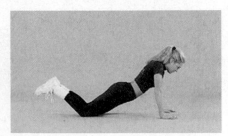

(a–b): Photo taken by Neil A. Tanner

2. Lower your chest to the floor with your back straight, and then return to the starting position.

3. Perform as many push-ups or modified push-ups as you can without stopping.

   Number of push-ups: _____ Number of modified push-ups: _____

Rating Your Push-Up Test Result

Your score is the number of completed push-ups or modified push-ups. Refer to the appropriate portion of the table for a rating of your upper-body endurance. Record your rating below and in the summary at the end of this lab.

Rating: _____

Ratings for the Push-Up and Modified Push-Up Tests

	Number of Push-Ups					
Men	*Very Poor*	*Poor*	*Fair*	*Good*	*Excellent*	*Superior*
Age: 18–29	Below 22	22–28	29–36	37–46	47–61	Above 61
30–39	Below 17	17–23	24–29	30–38	39–51	Above 51
40–49	Below 11	11–17	18–23	24–29	30–39	Above 39
50–59	Below 9	9–12	13–18	19–24	25–38	Above 38
60 and over	Below 6	6–9	10–17	18–22	23–27	Above 27
	Number of Modified Push-Ups					
Women	*Very Poor*	*Poor*	*Fair*	*Good*	*Excellent*	*Superior*
Age: 18–29	Below 17	17–22	23–29	30–35	36–44	Above 44
30–39	Below 11	11–18	19–23	24–30	31–38	Above 38
40–49	Below 6	6–12	13–17	18–23	24–32	Above 32
50–59	Below 6	6–11	12–16	17–20	21–27	Above 27
60 and over	Below 2	2–4	5–11	12–14	15–19	Above 19

SOURCE: The Cooper Institute of Aerobic Research, Dallas, TX; from *The Physical Fitness Specialist Manual*, revised 2002.

The Squat Endurance Test

Instructions

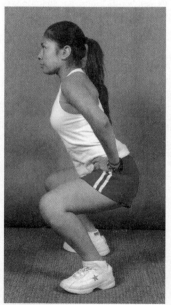

1. Stand with your feet placed slightly more than shoulder-width apart, toes pointed out slightly hands on hips or across your chest, head neutral, and back straight. Center your weight over your arches or slightly behind.

2. Squat down, keeping your weight centered over your arches, until your thighs are parallel with the floor. Push back up to the starting position, maintaining a straight back and neutral head position.

3. Perform as many squats as you can without stopping.

   Number of squats: _____

Rating Your Squat Endurance Test Result

Your score is the number of completed squats. Refer to the appropriate portion of the table for a rating of your leg muscular endurance. Record your rating below and in the summary at the end of this lab.

Rating: _____

Photo taken by Wayne Glusker

LABORATORY ACTIVITIES

Ratings for the Squat Endurance Test

Number of Squats Performed

Men	Very Poor	Poor	Below Average	Average	Above Average	Good	Excellent
Age: 18–25	<25	25–30	31–34	35–38	39–43	44–49	>49
26–35	<22	22–28	29–30	31–34	35–39	40–45	>45
36–45	<17	17–22	23–26	27–29	30–34	35–41	>41
46–55	<13	13–17	18–21	22–24	25–28	29–35	>35
56–65	<9	9–12	13–16	17–20	21–24	25–31	>31
65+	<7	7–10	11–14	15–18	19–21	22–28	>28
Women	*Very Poor*	*Poor*	*Below Average*	*Average*	*Above Average*	*Good*	*Excellent*
Age: 18–25	<18	18–24	25–28	29–32	33–36	37–43	>43
26–35	<13	13–20	21–24	25–28	29–32	33–39	>39
36–45	<7	7–14	15–18	19–22	23–26	27–33	>33
46–55	<5	5–9	10–13	14–17	18–21	22–27	>27
56–65	<3	3–6	7–9	10–12	13–17	18–24	>24
65+	<2	2–4	5–10	11–13	14–16	17–23	>23

SOURCE: Squat Test at Home, Topend Sports Network, www.topendsports.com/testing/tests/home-squat.htm.

Summary of Results

Curl-up test: Number of curl-ups: _____ Rating: _____

Push-up test: Number of push-ups: _____ Rating: _____

Squat endurance test: Number of squats: _____ Rating: _____

Remember that muscular endurance is specific: Your ratings may vary considerably for different parts of your body.

Using Your Results

How did you score? Are you surprised by your ratings for muscular endurance? Are you satisfied with your current ratings?

If you're not satisfied, set realistic goals for improvement:

Are you satisfied with your current level of muscular endurance as evidenced in your daily life—for example, your ability to carry groceries or your books, hike, and do yard work?

If you're not satisfied, set realistic goals for improvement:

What should you do next? Enter the results of this lab in the Preprogram Assessment column in Appendix B. If you've set goals for improvement, begin planning your strength training program by completing the plan in Lab 4.3. After several weeks of your program, complete this lab again and enter the results in the Postprogram Assessment column of Appendix B. How do the results compare?

Name _____ Section _____ Date _____

LAB 4.3   Designing and Monitoring a Strength Training Program

1. *Set goals.* List goals for your strength training program. Your goals can be specific or general, short or long term. In the first section, include specific, measurable goals that you can use to track the progress of your fitness program—for example, raising your upper-body muscular strength rating from fair to good or being able to complete 10 repetitions of a lat pull with 125 pounds of resistance. In the second section, include long-term and more qualitative goals, such as improving self-confidence and reducing your risk for back pain.

Specific Goals: Current Status   Final Goals

_____   _____

_____   _____

_____   _____

Other goals: _____

_____

2. *Choose exercises.* Based on your goals, choose 8–10 exercises to perform during each weight training session. If your goal is general training for wellness, use the sample program in Figure 4.4. List your exercises and the muscles they develop in your program plan.

3. *Frequency: Choose the number of training sessions per week.* Work out at least two nonconsecutive days per week. Indicate the days you will train in your program plan; be sure to include days of rest to allow your body to recover.

4. *Intensity: Choose starting weights.* Experiment with different amounts of weight until you settle on a good starting weight, one that you can lift easily for 10–12 repetitions. As you progress in your program, add more weight. Fill in the starting weight for each exercise in your program plan.

5. *Time: Choose a starting number of sets and repetitions.* Include at least one set of 8–12 repetitions of each exercise. (When you add weight, you may have to decrease the number of repetitions slightly until your muscles adapt to the heavier load.) If your program is focusing on strength alone, your sets can contain fewer repetitions using a heavier load. If you are over approximately age 50–60, your sets should contain more repetitions (10–15) using a lighter load. Fill in the starting number of sets and repetitions of each exercise in your program plan.

6. *Volume.* Choose a training volume (weight lifted multiplied by number of reps and sets) that promotes progress and that you will do consistently. Vary the components from time to time—for example, increase the weight on some days and the sets and reps on other days.

7. *Monitor your progress.* Use a phone app or the workout card here to monitor your progress and keep track of exercises, weights, sets, and repetitions.

Many excellent weight training program apps, such as the Beast Sensor, Strong, and Stronger are available for smartphones. The Beast Sensor includes a wearable accelerometer that tracks power and strength and stores workout data on the cloud. Though sophisticated and motivating, it is fairly expensive. Strong and Stronger are low-cost apps that serve as online workout cards and can also store data on the cloud.

Program Plan for Weight Training											
Exercise	Muscle(s) Developed	Frequency (✓)							Intensity: Weight (lb.)	Time	
		M	T	W	Th	F	Sa	Su		Repetitions	Sets

LABORATORY ACTIVITIES

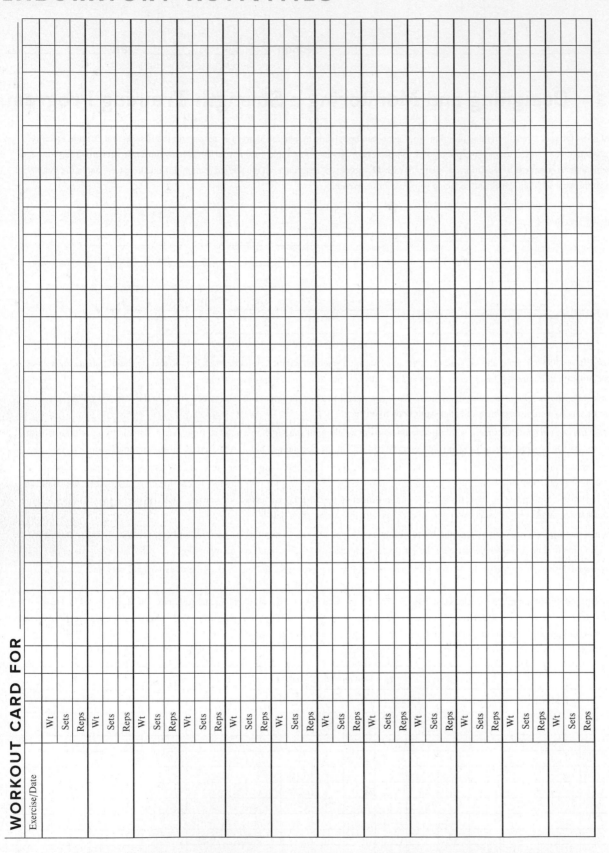

WORKOUT CARD FOR _____

Design elements: Evidence for Exercise box (shoes and stethoscope): Vstock LLC/Tetra Images/Getty Images; Take Charge box (lady walking): VisualCommunications/E+/Getty Images; Critical Consumer box (man): Sam74100/iStock/Getty Images; Diversity Matters box (holding devices): Robert Churchill/iStockphoto/Rawpixel Ltd/Getty Images; Wellness in the Digital Age box (Smart Watch): Hong Li/DigitalVision/Getty Images

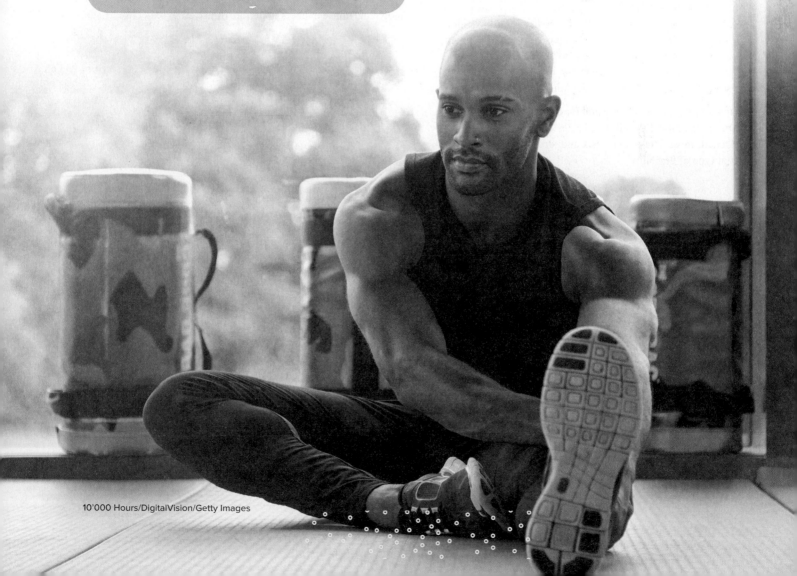

CHAPTER 5

Flexibility and Low-Back Health

LOOKING AHEAD...

After reading this chapter, you should be able to

- Identify the potential benefits of flexibility and stretching exercises.

- List the factors that affect a joint's flexibility.

- Describe the types of stretching exercises and how they affect muscles.

- Describe the frequency, intensity, duration, volume, and progression for a successful flexibility program.

- List safe stretching exercises for major joints.

- Explain how low-back pain can be prevented and managed.

TEST YOUR KNOWLEDGE

1. Static stretching exercises should be performed
   a. at the start of a warm-up.
   b. first thing in the morning.
   c. after endurance exercise or strength training.

2. If you injure your back, it's usually best to rest in bed until the pain is completely gone. True or false?

3. It is better to hold a stretch for a short time than to "bounce" while stretching. True or false?

See answers on the next page.

10'000 Hours/DigitalVision/Getty Images

Flexibility—the ability of a joint to move through its normal, full **range of motion**—is important for general fitness and wellness. Flexibility is a highly adaptable physical fitness component: It increases in response to a regular program of stretching exercises and decreases with inactivity. Flexibility is also specific: Good flexibility in one joint doesn't necessarily mean good flexibility in another. You can increase your overall flexibility by doing regular stretching exercises for all your major joints.

This chapter describes the factors that affect flexibility and the benefits of maintaining good flexibility. It provides guidelines for assessing your current level of flexibility and putting together a successful stretching program. It also examines the common problem of low-back pain.

TYPES OF FLEXIBILITY

There are two types of flexibility:

- *Static flexibility* is the ability to hold an extended position at one end or point in a joint's range of motion. For example, static flexibility determines how far you can extend your arm across the front of your body or out to the side. Static flexibility depends on your ability to tolerate stretched muscles, the structure of your joints, and the elasticity of muscles.

- *Dynamic flexibility* is the ability to move a joint through its range of motion with little resistance. It would affect your ability to pitch a ball or swing a golf club. Dynamic flexibility depends on static flexibility, but it also involves strength, coordination, and resistance to movement.

Dynamic flexibility is important for daily activities and sports. But because static flexibility is easier to measure and better researched, most assessment tests and stretching programs target that type of flexibility.

WHAT DETERMINES FLEXIBILITY?

The flexibility of a joint is affected by its structure, by muscle elasticity and length, and by nervous system regulation. Joint structure can't be changed, but other factors, such as the length of resting muscle fibers, can be changed through exercise; these factors should be the focus of a program to develop flexibility.

Joint Structure

How flexible a joint is depends partly on the nature and structure of the joint (Figure 5.1). Hinge joints such as those in your fingers and knees allow only limited forward and backward movement; they lock when fully extended. Ball-and-socket joints like the hip enable movement in many directions and provide for a greater range of motion. **Joint capsules**, semielastic structures that give joints strength and stability but limit movement, surround the major joints. The bone surfaces within the joint are lined with cartilage and separated by a joint cavity containing *synovial fluid,* which cushions the bones and reduces friction as the joint moves. Breakdown in joint cartilage from injury or aging leads to **arthritis**, which severely limits joint flexibility. Ligaments, both inside and outside the joint capsule, strengthen and reinforce the joint.

Heredity plays a part in joint structure and flexibility. For example, although everyone has a broad range of motion in the hip joint, not everyone can do a split. Gender may also play a role. Some studies have found that women have greater flexibility in certain joints.

Muscle Elasticity and Length

Soft tissues—including skin, muscles, tendons, and ligaments—also affect the flexibility of a joint. Muscle tissue is the key to developing flexibility because regular stretching can lengthen it. The most important component of muscle tissue related to flexibility is the connective tissue that envelops every part of muscle tissue, from individual muscle fibers to entire muscles. Connective tissue

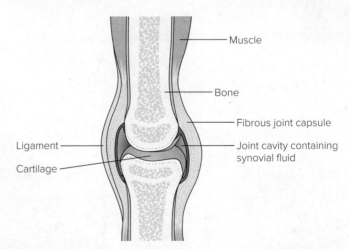

Figure 5.1   Basic joint structures.

---

range of motion   The full motion possible in a joint.

joint capsules   Semielastic structures, composed primarily of connective tissue, that surround major joints.

arthritis   A disorder of the joints characterized by joint pain, stiffness, and inflammation. Osteoarthritis, the most common form, is a degenerative joint disease. Rheumatoid arthritis is an autoimmune disease that typically affects the hands and feet.

soft tissues   Tissues of the human body that include skin, fat, linings of internal organs and blood vessels, connective tissues, tendons, ligaments, muscles, and nerves.

TERMS

provides structure, elasticity, and bulk and makes up about 30% of muscle mass. Two principal types of connective tissue are **collagen**—white fibers that provide structure and support—and **elastin**—yellow fibers that are elastic and flexible. The collagen and elastin are closely intertwined, so muscle tissue exhibits the properties of both types of fibers. A structural protein in muscles called *titin* also has elastic properties and contributes to flexibility.

When a muscle is stretched, the wavelike elastin fibers straighten; when the stretch is relieved, they rapidly snap back to their resting position. This temporary lengthening is called **elastic elongation**. If stretched gently and regularly, connective tissues may lengthen and flexibility may improve. This long-term lengthening is called **plastic elongation**. Without regular stretching, the process reverses: These tissues shorten, resulting in decreased flexibility. Regular stretching may contribute to flexibility by lengthening muscle fibers through the addition of contractile units called *sarcomeres*.

A muscle can tolerate a limited amount of stretch. As the limits of its flexibility are reached, connective tissue becomes more brittle and may rupture if overstretched. A safe and effective program stretches muscles enough to slightly elongate the tissues but not so much that they are damaged. Research has shown that flexibility is improved best by stretching when muscles are warm (following exercise or the application of heat) and the stretch is applied gradually and conservatively. Sudden, high-stress stretching is less effective and can lead to muscle damage.

Nervous System Regulation

Proprioceptors are nerves that send information about changes in the muscular and skeletal systems to the nervous system, which responds with signals to help control the speed, strength, and coordination of muscle contractions. When a muscle is stretched (lengthened), proprioceptors detect the amount and rate of the change in muscle length. The nerves send a signal to the spinal cord, which then sends a signal back to the muscle, triggering a muscle contraction that resists the change in muscle length. Another signal is sent to the opposing muscle (**antagonist**), causing it to relax and facilitate contraction of the stretched (agonist) muscle. These reflexes occur frequently in active muscles and allow for fine control of muscle length and movement. Muscle flexibility is linked to strength. Practicing lower-body eccentric exercise (lengthening contractions) increases strength and flexibility and might decrease the risk of lower-body muscle injury.

Small movements that only slightly stimulate the nerves cause small reflex actions. Rapid, powerful, and sudden changes in muscle length strongly stimulate the nerve receptors and can cause large and powerful reflex muscle contractions. Thus, stretches that involve rapid, bouncy movements can be dangerous and cause injury. Each bounce causes a reflex contraction, which means a muscle might be stretching at the same time it is contracting. Performing a gradual stretch and then holding it allows the proprioceptors to adjust to the new muscle length and to reduce the signals sent to the spine, thereby allowing muscles to lengthen and, over time, improving flexibility.

The stretching technique called *proprioceptive neuromuscular facilitation (PNF)*, described later, takes advantage of nerve activity to improve flexibility. For example, contracting a muscle prior to stretching it can help allow the muscle to stretch farther. The advanced strength training technique called plyometrics (Chapter 4) also takes advantage of the nervous system action in stretching and contracting muscles.

Modifying nervous control through movement and specific exercises is the best way to improve the functional range of motion. Regular stretching trains the proprioceptors to allow the muscles to lengthen. Proprioceptors adapt quickly to stretching (or lack of stretching), so frequent stretching helps develop flexibility. Stretching before exercising, however, can disturb proprioceptors and interfere with motor control during exercise. This is another good reason to stretch *after* exercising.

BENEFITS OF FLEXIBILITY

Good flexibility provides benefits for the entire musculoskeletal system. Flexibility training increases range of motion, and it may prevent muscle strains. As long as you don't overstretch, flexibility training will increase strength and the quality of movement, which might decrease the risk of some sports injuries. Most studies, however, show that stretching does not prevent overuse injuries.

Joint Health

Good flexibility is essential to good joint health. When the muscles and other tissues that support a joint are tight, the joint is subject to abnormal stresses that can cause joint deterioration. For example, tight thigh muscles cause excessive pressure on the kneecap, leading to pain in the knee joint. Poor joint flexibility can also cause abnormalities in joint lubrication, leading to deterioration of the sensitive cartilage cells lining the joint; pain and further joint injury can result.

Improved flexibility can greatly improve your quality of life, particularly as you get older. People tend to exercise less as they age, leading to loss of joint mobility and increased incidence of joint pain. Aging also decreases the natural elasticity of muscles, tendons, and joints, resulting in stiffness. The problem is often compounded by arthritis (see the box "Does Physical Activity Increase or Decrease the Risk of Bone and Joint Disease?").

TERMS

collagen   White fibers that provide structure and support in connective tissue.

elastin   Yellow fibers that make connective tissue flexible.

elastic elongation   Temporary change in the length of muscles, tendons, and supporting connective tissues.

plastic elongation   Long-term change in the length of muscles, tendons, and supporting connective tissues.

proprioceptor   A nerve that sends information about the muscular and skeletal systems to the nervous system.

antagonist muscle   A muscle that opposes the action of another. For example, the biceps brachius muscle (agonist) flexes the elbow, while the triceps brachius (antagonist) extends the elbow.

THE EVIDENCE FOR EXERCISE
Does Physical Activity Increase or Decrease the Risk of Bone and Joint Disease?

Most college students don't worry much about fall-related fractures or chronic bone-related illnesses, such as **osteoporosis** (loss of bone mass) or osteoarthritis (degeneration of the cartilage inside joints). But bone health should be a concern throughout life. This is because girls amass 85% of their adult bone mass by age 18, and boys build the same amount by age 20, but most people lose bone mass beginning around age 30. For many people, poor diet and lack of exercise accelerate bone loss. According to the National Osteoporosis Foundation, 10 million Americans have osteoporosis. Meanwhile, 44 million Americans are at risk of the disease because of low bone mass. Overall, osteoporosis is a health threat for about 55% of Americans age 50 and older.

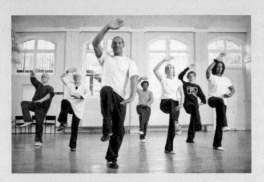

Tim Platt/DigitalVision/Getty Images

Getting enough nutrients is important for bone health (see Chapter 8), but mounting evidence shows that exercise can also help preserve or improve bone health. For example, several studies have shown an inverse relationship between physical activity and the risk for bone fractures: The more you exercise, the less likely you are to suffer fractures, especially of the upper leg and hip. Research has not determined conclusively how much exercise is required to reduce fracture risk, but people who walk at least four hours per week and devote at least one hour per week to other forms of physical activity appear to reduce that risk. These findings seem consistent for women and men, but because some studies disagree on this point, further research is needed.

One way that exercise helps both men and women is by increasing the mineral density of bones, or at least by decreasing the loss of mineral density over time. Several one-year-long studies found that exercise can increase bone mineral density by 1–2% per year, which is significant—especially considering that the same bone mineral density can be lost every one to four years in older persons. The American College of Sports Medicine recommends that adults perform weight-bearing physical activities (such as walking) three to five days per week and strength training exercises two or three days per week to increase bone mass or avoid loss of mineral density. They also recommend that adults practice neuromotor exercise training exercises, such as yoga or tai chi, to prevent falls and bone fractures. Exercise is particularly important in lactating (breastfeeding) women for preventing bone loss.

The evidence is less conclusive for the effect of exercise on osteoarthritis but still fairly positive. All experts agree that regular, moderate-intensity exercise is necessary for joint health. However, they also warn that vigorous or too-frequent exercise may contribute to joint damage and encourage the onset of osteoarthritis. Experts try to strike a balance in their exercise recommendations, especially for those with a family history of osteoarthritis. Research seems to support this cautious approach. Some studies have found that regular physical activity (as recommended for general health) at least does not increase osteoarthritis risk. Other studies show that moderate activity may provide some protection against the disease, but this evidence is limited.

A few studies also reveal that the type of exercise you do may increase your risk. For example, competitive or strenuous sports such as ballet, orienteering, football, basketball, soccer, and tennis have been associated with the disease, whereas sports such as cross-country skiing, running, swimming, biking, and walking have not.

The bottom line is that the earlier in life you become physically active, the greater your protection against bone loss and bone-related diseases. However, if you have a family history of osteoporosis or osteoarthritis, or if you have already developed symptoms of one of these ailments, talk to your physician before beginning an exercise program.

SOURCE: American College of Sports Medicine. 2018. *ACSM's Guidelines for Exercise Testing and Prescription,* 10th ed. Philadelphia: Wolters Kluwer; Giangregorio, L. M., et al. 2015. "Too fit to fracture: Outcomes of a Delphi consensus process on physical activity and exercise recommendations for adults with osteoporosis with or without vertebral fractures," *Osteoporosis International* 26(3): 891–910; American College of Sports Medicine. 2004. "ACSM position stand: Physical activity and bone health," *Medicine and Science in Sports and Exercise* 36(11): 1985–1996.

Good joint flexibility may help prevent arthritis, and stretching may lessen pain in people with the condition. Another benefit of good joint flexibility for older adults is that it increases balance and stability.

osteoporosis A condition in which the bones become extremely thin and brittle and break easily.

TERMS

Prevention of Low-Back Pain and Injuries

Poor spinal stability puts pressure on the nerves leading out from the spinal column and can lead to low-back pain. Strength and flexibility in the back, pelvis, and thighs may help prevent back pain but may or may not improve back health or reduce the risk of injury. Good hip and knee flexibility protects the spine from excessive motion during the tasks of daily living.

Although scientific evidence is limited, people with either high or low flexibility seem to have an increased risk of injury. Extreme flexibility reduces joint stability, and poor flexibility limits a joint's range of motion. Persons of average fitness should try to attain normal flexibility in joints throughout the body, meaning each joint can move through its normal range of motion with no difficulty. Stretching programs are particularly important for older adults, people engaged in high-power sports that require rapid changes in direction (such as football and tennis), workers involved in brief bouts of intense exertion (such as police officers and firefighters), and people who sit for prolonged periods (such as office workers and students).

However, as we have seen, static stretching *before* a high-intensity activity (such as sprinting or basketball) may increase the risk of injury by interfering with neuromuscular control and reducing muscles' natural ability to stretch and contract. When injuries occur, flexibility exercises can reduce symptoms and help restore normal range of motion in affected joints.

Additional Potential Benefits of Flexibility

• *Relief of aches and pains.* Studying or working in one place for a long time can make your muscles tense. Stretching helps relieve tension and joint stiffness, so you can go back to work refreshed and effective. Stretching reduces the symptoms of exercise-induced muscle damage, and flexible muscles are less susceptible to the damage.

• *Relief of muscle cramps.* Recent research suggests that exercise-related muscle cramps are caused by increased electrical activity within the affected muscle. The best treatment for muscle cramps is gentle stretching, which reduces the electrical activity and allows the muscle to relax.

• *Improved body position and strength for sports (and life).* Good flexibility lets you assume more efficient body positions and exert force through a greater range of motion. For example, swimmers with more flexible shoulders have stronger strokes because they can pull their arms through the water in the optimal position. Some studies also suggest that flexibility training enhances strength development.

• *Maintenance of good posture and balance.* Good flexibility also contributes to body symmetry and good posture. Bad posture can gradually change your body structures. Sitting in a slumped position, for example, can lead to tightness in the muscles in the front of your chest and overstretching and looseness in the upper spine, causing a rounding of the upper back. This condition, called *kyphosis,* is common in older people. Stretching regularly may prevent it.

• *Relaxation.* Flexibility exercises, particularly when combined with yoga or tai chi, reduce mental tension, slow your breathing rate, and reduce blood pressure.

• *Improving impaired mobility.* Stretching often decreases pain and improves functional capacity in people with arthritis, stroke, or muscle and nerve diseases and in people who are recovering from surgery or injury.

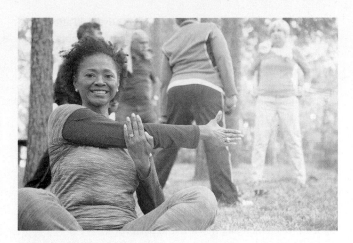

Wellness Tip Flexibility training helps maintain pain-free joints as you age. You don't have to be at the gym to stretch. There are lots of simple, small-movement stretches you can do anywhere—whether at your desk or on the go. For some examples, visit a good health website such as http://www.MayoClinic.com and search for "stretching exercises."

Fstop123/E+/Getty Images

ASSESSING FLEXIBILITY

Because flexibility is specific to each joint, there are no tests of general flexibility. The most commonly used flexibility test is the sit-and-reach test, which rates the flexibility of the muscles in the lower back and hamstrings. To assess your flexibility and identify inflexible joints, complete Lab 5.1.

CREATING A SUCCESSFUL PROGRAM TO DEVELOP FLEXIBILITY

A successful program for developing flexibility includes safe exercises executed with the most effective techniques. Your goal should be to attain normal flexibility in the major joints. Balanced flexibility (not too much or too little) provides joint stability and facilitates smooth, economical movement patterns. You can achieve balanced flexibility by performing stretching exercises regularly and by using a variety of stretches and stretching techniques.

Applying the FITT-VP Principle

As with other programs, the acronym FITT-VP can help you remember key components of a stretching program: Frequency, Intensity, Time, Type, Volume, and Progression of exercise.

Frequency The American College of Sports Medicine (ACSM) recommends that stretching exercises be performed at least two or three days per week, but more often is even better. To prevent injury and improve flexibility, it's best to stretch when your muscles are warm, either after a warm-up or after cardio-respiratory endurance exercise or weight training.

As described earlier, static stretching can adversely affect muscle performance in the short term. So, if you are planning a workout for which high performance is important, it is best to perform static stretches after your workout but while your muscles are still warm and your joints are lubricated. Stretching isn't the same thing as a cool-down, so be sure to do the cardiorespiratory cool-down first, so that you can transition to a lower level of intensity before stretching. If the plan for your workout includes a moderate activity like walking, then static stretching prior to your workout isn't likely to impact performance in a significant way.

Dynamic stretching, described in the next section, may have less of an impact on muscle performance and so is sometimes included as part of an active warm-up. However, dynamic stretching is more challenging to learn and perform.

Intensity and Time (Duration) For each exercise, slowly stretch your muscles to the point of slight tension or mild discomfort—but not to the point of pain. Hold the stretch for 10–30 seconds. As you hold the stretch, the feeling of slight tension should subside slowly; at that point, try to stretch a bit farther. Throughout the stretch, try to relax and breathe easily. Rest for about 30–60 seconds between each stretch, and do 2–4 repetitions of each stretch for a total of 60 seconds per exercise. A complete flexibility workout usually takes about 10–30 minutes (Figure 5.2).

Types of Stretching Techniques Stretching techniques vary from simply stretching the muscles during the course of normal activities to sophisticated methods based on patterns of muscle reflexes. Improper stretching can do more harm than good, so it's important to understand the different types of stretching exercises and how they affect the muscles. Four common techniques are static stretches, ballistic stretches, dynamic stretches, and proprioceptive neuromuscular facilitation (PNF).

STATIC STRETCHING In **static stretching**, each muscle is gradually stretched, and the stretch is held for 10–30 seconds. A slow stretch prompts less reaction from proprioceptors, and the muscles can safely stretch farther than usual. Static stretching is the type most often recommended by fitness experts because it is safe and effective.

The key to this technique is to stretch the muscles and joints to the point where a pull is felt, but not to the point of pain. (One

---

Warm-up 5–10 minutes or following an endurance or strength training workout	Stretching exercises for major joints **Sample program**	
	Exercise	*Areas stretched*
	Head turns and tilts	Neck
	Towel stretch	Triceps, shoulders, chest
	Across-the-body and overhead stretches	Shoulders, upper back, back of arm
	Upper-back stretch	Upper back
	Lateral stretch	Trunk muscles
	Step stretch	Hip, front of thigh
	Side lunge	Inner thigh, hip, calf
	Inner-thigh stretch	Inner thigh, hip
	Hip and trunk stretch	Trunk, outer thigh, hip, buttocks, lower back
	Modified hurdler stretch	Back of thigh, lower back
	Alternate leg stretcher	Back of thigh, hip, knee, ankle, buttocks
	Lower-leg stretch	Calf, soleus, Achilles tendon

Frequency: 2 or 3 days per week (minimum); 5–7 days per week (ideal).

Intensity: Stretch to the point of mild discomfort, not pain.

Time (duration): Hold static stretches for 10–30 seconds.

Type of activity: Stretching exercises that focus on major joints.

Volume: Perform 2–4 repetitions for a total stretching time of 60 seconds for each exercise.

Progression: Progressively build flexibility, striving for a normal range of motion; avoid excessive flexibility.

Figure 5.2   The FITT-VP principle for a flexibility program.

note of caution: Excess static stretching can decrease joint stability and increase the risk of injury. This may be a particular concern for women, whose joints are less stable and more flexible than are men's.) The sample stretching program presented later in this chapter features static stretching exercises.

BALLISTIC STRETCHING In **ballistic stretching**, the muscles are stretched suddenly in a forceful bouncing movement. For example, touching the toes repeatedly in rapid succession is a ballistic stretch for the hamstrings. A problem with this technique is that the heightened activity of proprioceptors caused by the rapid stretches can continue for some time, possibly causing injuries during any physical activities that follow. Another concern is that triggering strong responses from the nerves can cause a reflex muscle contraction that makes it harder to stretch. For these reasons, ballistic stretching is usually not recommended, especially for people of average fitness.

Ballistic stretching trains the muscle dynamically, so it can be an appropriate stretching technique for some well-trained athletes. For example, tennis players stretch their hamstrings and quadriceps ballistically when they lunge for a ball during a tennis match. Because this movement is part of their sport, they might benefit from ballistic training of these muscle groups.

DYNAMIC (FUNCTIONAL) STRETCHING The emphasis in **dynamic stretching** is on functional movements. Dynamic

---

TERMS

static stretching   A technique in which a muscle is slowly and gently stretched and then held in the stretched position.

ballistic stretching   A technique in which muscles are stretched by the force generated as a body part is repeatedly bounced, swung, or jerked.

dynamic stretching   A technique in which muscles are stretched by moving joints slowly and fluidly through their range of motion in a controlled manner; also called *functional stretching*.

passive stretching   A technique in which muscles are stretched by force applied by an outside source.

active stretching   A technique in which muscles are stretched by the contraction of the opposing muscles.

stretching is similar to ballistic stretching in that it includes movement, but it differs in that it does not involve rapid bouncing. Instead, dynamic stretching moves the joints in an exaggerated but controlled manner through the range of motion used in a specific exercise or sport; movements are fluid rather than jerky. An example of a dynamic stretch is the lunge walk, in which a person takes slow steps with an exaggerated stride length and reaches a lunge stretch position with each step.

Slow dynamic stretches can lengthen the muscles in many directions without developing high tension in the tissues. These stretches elongate the tissues and train the neuromuscular system. Because dynamic stretches are based on sports movements or movements used in daily life, they develop functional flexibility that translates well into activities.

Dynamic stretches are more challenging than static stretches because they require balance and coordination and may carry a greater risk of muscle soreness and injury. People just beginning a flexibility program might want to start off with static stretches and try dynamic stretches only after they are comfortable with static stretching and have improved their flexibility. It is also a good idea to seek expert advice on dynamic stretching technique and program development.

Functional flexibility training can be combined with functional strength training. For example, lunge curls, which combine dynamic lunges with free weights biceps curls, stretch the hip, thigh, and calf muscles; stabilize the core muscles in the trunk; and build strength in the arm muscles. Many activities build functional flexibility and strength at the same time, including yoga, Pilates, tai chi, Olympic weight lifting, plyometrics, stability training (including Swiss and Bosu ball exercises), medicine ball exercises, and functional training machines (for example, Life Fitness and Cybex).

PROPRIOCEPTIVE NEUROMUSCULAR FACILITATION (PNF)

PNF techniques use reflexes initiated by both muscle and joint nerves to cause greater training effects. The most popular PNF stretching technique is the contract-relax stretching method, in which a muscle is contracted before it is stretched. The contraction activates proprioceptors, causing relaxation in the muscle about to be stretched. For example, in a seated stretch of calf muscles, the first step in PNF is to contract the calf muscles. The individual or a partner can provide resistance for an isometric contraction. Following a brief period of relaxation, the next step is to stretch the calf muscles by pulling the tops of the feet toward the body. A duration of 3–6 seconds for the contraction at 20–75% of maximum effort and 10–30 seconds for the stretch is recommended. PNF appears to be most effective if the individual pushes hard during the isometric contraction.

Another example of a PNF stretch is the contract-relax-contract pattern. In this technique, begin by contracting the muscle to be stretched and then relaxing it. Next, contract the opposing muscle (the antagonist). Finally, stretch the first muscle. For example, using this technique to stretch the hamstrings (the muscles in the back of the thigh) would require the following steps: Contract the hamstrings, relax the hamstrings, contract the quadriceps (the muscles in the front of the thigh), and then stretch the hamstrings.

PNF appears to allow more effective stretching and greater increases in flexibility than static stretching, but it tends to cause more muscle stiffness and soreness. It also usually requires a partner and takes more time.

PASSIVE VERSUS ACTIVE STRETCHING Stretches can be done either passively or actively. In **passive stretching**, an outside force or resistance provided by yourself, a partner, gravity, or a weight helps your joints move through their range of motion. For example, a seated stretch of the hamstring and back muscles can be done by reaching the hands toward the feet until a pull is felt in those muscles. You can achieve a greater range of motion (a more intense stretch) using passive stretching. However, because the stretch is not controlled by the muscles themselves, there is a greater risk of injury. Communication between partners in passive stretching is important to ensure that joints aren't forced outside their normal functional range of motion.

In **active stretching**, a muscle is stretched by a contraction of the opposing muscle (the muscle on the opposite side of the limb). For example, an active seated stretch of the calf muscles occurs when a person actively contracts the muscles on the top of the shin. The contraction of this opposing muscle produces a reflex that relaxes the muscles to be stretched. The muscle can be stretched farther with a low risk of injury. The only disadvantage of active stretching is that a person may not be able to produce enough stress (enough stretch) to increase flexibility using only the contraction of opposing muscle groups.

The safest and most convenient technique is *active static stretching,* with an occasional passive assist. For example, you might stretch your calves both by contracting the muscles on the top of your shin and by pulling your feet toward you.

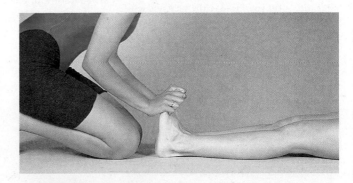

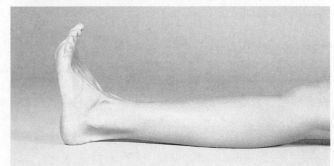

Fitness Tip In passive stretching (top), an outside force—such as pressure exerted by another person—helps move the joint and stretch the muscles. In active stretching (bottom), the force to move the joint and stretch the muscles is provided by a contraction of the opposing muscles.

(top and bottom): Photo taken by Shirlee Stevens

This way you combine the advantages of active stretching—safety and the relaxation reflex—with those of passive stretching—greater range of motion. People who are just beginning flexibility training may be better off doing active rather than passive stretches. For PNF techniques, it is particularly important to have a knowledgeable partner.

Making Progress

As with any type of training, you will make progress and improve your flexibility if you stick with your program. Judge your progress by noting your body position while stretching. For example, note how far you can lean forward during a modified hurdler stretch. Repeat the assessment tests that appear in Lab 5.1 periodically and be sure to take the test at the same time of day each time. You will likely notice some improvement after only two to three weeks of stretching, but you may need at least two months to attain significant improvements. By then, you can expect flexibility increases of about 10–20% in many joints. Don't continue

to try to increase flexibility once you have achieved a normal range of motion in your joints; excessive flexibility can cause joint instability.

EXERCISES TO IMPROVE FLEXIBILITY: A SAMPLE PROGRAM

There are hundreds of exercises that can improve flexibility. Your program should include exercises that work all the major joints of the body by stretching their associated muscle groups (refer back to Figure 5.2). The exercises on the following pages are simple to do and pose a minimum risk of injury. Use these exercises to create a well-rounded program for developing flexibility. Be sure to perform each stretch using the proper technique. Hold each position for 10–30 seconds and perform 2–4 repetitions of each exercise. Complete Lab 5.2 when you're ready to start your program.

FLEXIBILITY EXERCISES

EXERCISE 1   Head Turns and Tilts

Instructions:

Head turns: Turn your head to the right and hold the stretch. Repeat to the left.

Head tilts: Tilt your head to the right and left side. Hold the stretch. Repeat to the left. Do not hyperextend the neck (bend it backward) because this can cause injury.

Area stretched: Neck

Variation: Place your right palm on your right cheek; try to turn your head to the right as you resist with your hand. Repeat on the left side.

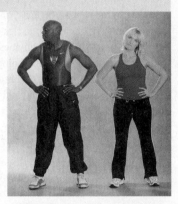

Photo taken by Taylor Robertson Photography

EXERCISE 2   Towel Stretch

Instructions: Roll up a towel and grasp it with both hands, palms down. With your arms straight, slowly lift the towel back over your head as far as possible. The closer together your hands are, the greater the stretch.

Areas stretched: Triceps, shoulders, chest (pectorals)

Variation: Repeat the stretch with your arms down and the towel behind your back. Grasp the towel with your palms forward and thumbs pointing out. Gently raise your arms behind your back. This exercise can also be done without a towel.

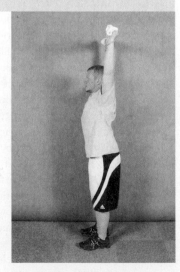

Photo taken by Wayne Glusker

EXERCISE 3

Across-the-Body and Overhead Stretches

Instructions: (**a**) Keeping your back straight, cross your right arm in front of your body and grasp it with your left hand. Stretch your arm, shoulders, and back by gently pulling your arm as close to your body as possible. Hold. (**b**) Bend your right arm over your head, placing your right elbow as close to your right ear as possible. Grasp your right elbow with your left hand over your head. Stretch the back of your arm by gently pulling your right elbow back and toward your head. Hold. Repeat both stretches on your left side.

Areas stretched: Shoulders, upper back, back of the arm (triceps)

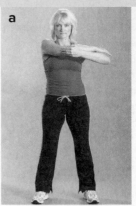
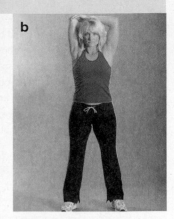

(a–b): Photo taken by Taylor Robertson Photography

EXERCISE 4

Upper-Back Stretch

Instructions: Stand with your feet shoulder-width apart, knees slightly bent, and pelvis tucked under. Lace your fingers in front of your body and press your palms forward.

Area stretched: Upper back

Variation: In the same position, wrap your arms around your body as if you were giving yourself a hug.

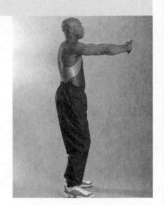

Photo taken by Taylor Robertson Photography

EXERCISE 5

Lateral Stretch

Instructions: Stand with your feet shoulder-width apart, knees slightly bent, and pelvis tucked under. Raise one arm over your head and bend sideways from the waist. Support your trunk by placing the hand or forearm of your other arm on your thigh or hip for support. Be sure you bend directly sideways and don't move your body below the waist. Repeat on the other side.

Areas stretched: Core muscles

Variation: Perform the same exercise in a seated position.

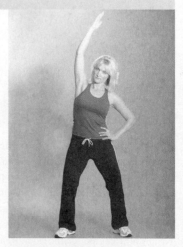

Photo taken by Taylor Robertson Photography

EXERCISE 6 — Step Stretch

Instructions: Step forward and bend your forward knee, keeping it directly above your ankle. Stretch your other leg back so that your shin is parallel to the floor. Press your hips forward and down to stretch. Your arms can be at your sides, on top of your knee, or on the ground for balance. Repeat on the other side.

Areas stretched: Hip flexors and quadriceps

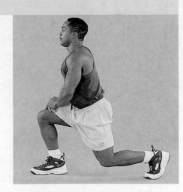

Photo taken by Neil A. Tanner

EXERCISE 7 — Side Lunge

Instructions: Stand in a wide straddle with your legs turned out from your hip joints and your hands on your thighs. Lunge to one side by bending one knee and keeping the other leg straight. Keep your bent knee directly over your ankle; do not bend it more than 90 degrees. Repeat on the other side.

Areas stretched: Inner thigh, hip, calf

Variation: In the same position, lift the heel of the bent knee to provide additional stretch. The exercise may also be performed with your hands on the floor for balance.

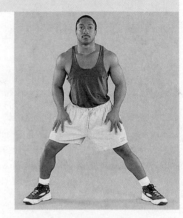

Photo taken by Neil A. Tanner

EXERCISE 8 — Inner-Thigh Stretch

Instructions: Sit on the floor with the soles of your feet together. Push your knees toward the floor using your hands or forearms.

Areas stretched: Inner thigh, hip

Variation: When you first begin to push your knees toward the floor, use your legs to resist the movement. Then relax and press your knees down as far as they will go.

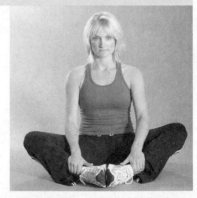

Photo taken by Taylor Robertson Photography

EXERCISE 9 — Hip and Trunk Stretch

Instructions: Sit on the floor with your left leg straight, right leg bent and crossed over the left knee, and right hand on the floor next to your right hip. Turn your trunk as far as possible to the right by pushing against your right leg with your left forearm or elbow. Keep your right foot on the floor. Repeat on the other side.

Areas stretched: Core, outer thigh, gluteal muscles, lower back

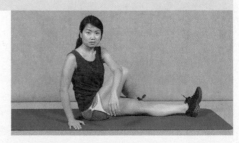

Photo taken by Wayne Glusker

EXERCISE 10 — Modified Hurdler Stretch (Seated Single-Leg Hamstring)

Instructions: Sit on the floor with your left leg straight and your right leg tucked close to your body. Reach toward your left ankle as far as possible. Repeat for the other leg.

Areas stretched: Hamstrings, lower back

Variation: As you stretch forward, point your toe as much as possible. Repeat for the other leg. Alternately flex and point the foot of your extended leg.

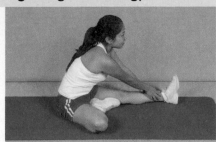

Photo taken by Wayne Glusker

EXERCISE 11 — Leg Stretcher

Instructions: Lie flat on your back with both legs straight. **(a)** Grasp your left leg behind the thigh, and pull it in to your chest. **(b)** Hold this position, and then extend your left leg toward the ceiling. **(c)** Hold this position, and then bring your left knee back to your chest and pull your toes toward your shin (hamstring), hip, knee, ankle, and buttocks with your left hand. Stretch the back of the leg by attempting to straighten your knee. Repeat for the other leg.

Areas stretched: Hamstrings, gluteal muscles, calf

Variation: Perform the stretch on both legs at the same time.

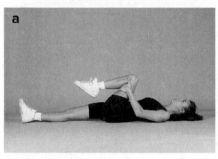
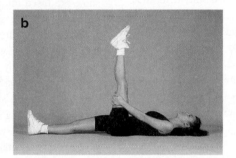
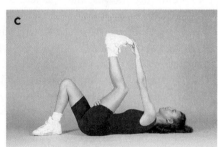

(a–c): Photo taken by Shirlee Stevens

EXERCISE 12 — Lower-Leg Stretch

Instructions: Stand with one foot about 1–2 feet in front of the other, with both feet pointing forward. **(a)** Keeping your back leg straight, lunge forward by bending your front knee and pushing your rear heel backward. Hold. **(b)** Then pull your back foot in slightly and bend your back knee. Shift your weight to your back leg. Hold. Repeat on the other side.

Areas stretched: Hamstrings, calf

Variation: Place your hands on a wall and extend one foot back, pressing your heel down to stretch, or stand with the balls of your feet on a step or bench and allow your heels to drop below the level of your toes.

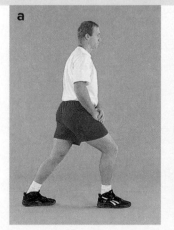
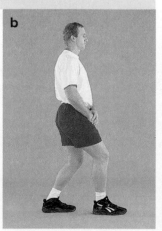

(a–b): Photo taken by Neil A. Tanner

Instructions: Start with a dumbbell or kettlebell placed slightly outside the foot of one leg. Bend down to the weight by hinging at the hips and bending at the knee. Your other leg should be bent and relaxed. Pick up the weight and tighten your body and extend the hip and knee as you stand straight, locking out your hip and contracting your glute. Repeat with the other leg.

Areas stretched: This exercise stretches and loads the hamstrings and gluteal muscles both eccentrically and concentrically (lengthening and shortening contractions).

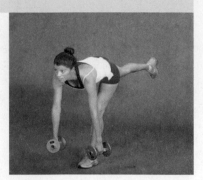

Photo taken by Taylor Robertson Photography

PREVENTING AND MANAGING LOW-BACK PAIN

More than 85% of Americans experience back pain by age 50. Low-back pain is the second most common ailment in the United States—headache tops the list—and the second most common reason for absences from work and visits to a physician. Low-back pain is estimated to cost as much as $50 billion a year in lost productivity, medical and legal fees, and disability insurance and compensation.

Back pain can result from sudden traumatic injuries, but it is more often the long-term result of weak and inflexible muscles, poor posture, or poor body mechanics during activities like lifting and carrying. Any abnormal strain on the back can result in pain. Most cases of low-back pain clear up within a few weeks or months, but some people have recurrences or suffer from chronic pain.

Function and Structure of the Spine

The spinal column performs many important functions in the body:

- It provides structural support for the body, especially the thorax (upper-body cavity).
- It surrounds and protects the spinal cord.
- It supports much of the body's weight.

- It serves as an attachment site for a large number of muscles, tendons, and ligaments.
- It allows movement of the neck and back in all directions.

The spinal column is made up of bones called **vertebrae** that provide structural support to the body and protect the spinal cord (Figure 5.3). The spine consists of 7 cervical vertebrae in the neck, 12 thoracic vertebrae in the upper back, and 5 lumbar vertebrae in the lower back. The 9 vertebrae at the base of the spine are fused into two sections and form the sacrum and the coccyx (tailbone). The spine has four curves: the cervical, thoracic, lumbar, and sacral curves (see Figure 5.3). These curves help bring the body weight supported by the spine in line with the axis of the body.

Although the structure of vertebrae depends on their location on the spine, all vertebrae share common characteristics. Each consists of a body, an arch, and several bony processes (Figure 5.4). The vertebral body is cylindrical, with flattened surfaces where **intervertebral disks** are attached. The vertebral body carries the stress of body weight and physical activity. The vertebral arch surrounds and protects the spinal cord. Irregularly shaped bony outgrowths serve as joints for adjacent vertebrae and attachment sites for muscles and ligaments. **Nerve roots** from the spinal cord pass through notches in the vertebral arch.

Intervertebral disks are shock absorbers that disperse the stresses placed on the spine and separate vertebrae from one another. Disks consist of a gel- and water-filled nucleus surrounded by a series of fibrous rings. The liquid nucleus can change shape when compressed, allowing the disk to absorb shock. The intervertebral disks also help maintain the spaces between vertebrae where the spinal nerve roots are located.

Core Muscle Fitness

The **core muscles** are the trunk muscles in the middle of the body extending from the hips to the upper back, including those in the abdomen, pelvic floor, sides of the trunk, back, buttocks, hip, and pelvis (Figure 5.5). These muscles are attached to the ribs, hips, spinal column, and other bones in the trunk of the body. The core muscles stabilize the spine and help transfer force

TERMS

vertebrae Bony segments composing the spinal column that provide structural support for the body and protect the spinal cord.

intervertebral disk An elastic disk located between adjoining vertebrae, consisting of a gel- and water-filled nucleus surrounded by fibrous rings; serves as a shock absorber for the spinal column.

nerve roots The bases of the 31 pairs of spinal nerves that branch off the spinal cord through spaces between vertebrae.

core muscles The trunk muscles extending from the hips to the upper back.

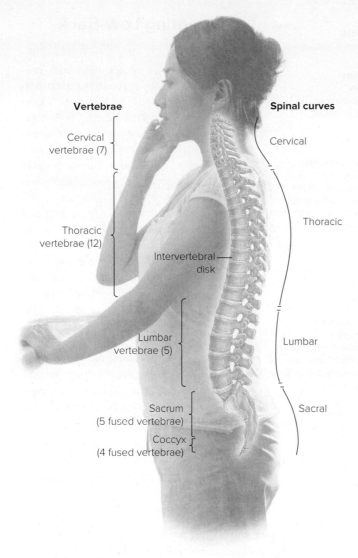

Vertebrae

Cervical vertebrae (7)

Thoracic vertebrae (12)

Intervertebral disk

Lumbar vertebrae (5)

Sacrum (5 fused vertebrae)

Coccyx (4 fused vertebrae)

Spinal curves

Cervical

Thoracic

Lumbar

Sacral

Figure 5.3 The spinal column. The spine is made up of five separate regions and has four distinct curves. An intervertebral disk is located between adjoining vertebrae.

Image Source/Photodisc/Getty Images

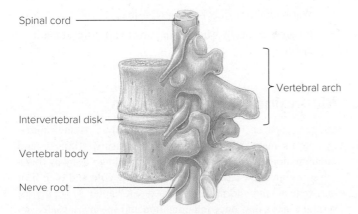

Spinal cord

Intervertebral disk

Vertebral body

Nerve root

Vertebral arch

Figure 5.4 Vertebrae and an intervertebral disk.

between the upper body and lower body. They stabilize the midsection when you sit, stand, reach, walk, jump, twist, squat, throw, or bend. The muscles on the front, back, and sides of your trunk support your spine when you sit in a chair and fix your midsection as you use your legs to stand up. When hitting a forehand in tennis or batting a softball, most of the force is transferred from the legs and hips, across the core muscles, to the arms. Strong stiff core muscles make movements more forceful and help prevent back pain.

During any dynamic movement, the core muscles work together. Some shorten to cause movement, while others contract and hold to provide stability, lengthen to brake the movement, or send signals to the brain about the movements and positions of the muscles and bones (proprioception). When specific core muscles are weak or tired, the nervous system steps in and uses other muscles. This substitution causes abnormal stresses on the joints, decreases power, and increases the risk of injury.

The best exercises for low-back health are whole-body exercises that force the core muscles to stabilize and support the spine in many directions. The low-back exercises presented later in this chapter include several exercises that focus on the core muscles, including the step stretch (lunge), side bridges, and spine extensions. These exercises are generally safe for beginning exercisers and, with physician approval, people who have some back pain. More challenging core exercises utilize stability balls or free weights. Stability ball exercises require the core muscles to stabilize the ball (and the body) while performing nearly any type of exercise. Many traditional exercises with free weights can strengthen the core muscles if you do them in a standing position. Weight machines train muscles in isolation, while exercises with free weights done while standing help train the body for real-world movements—an essential principle of core training.

Causes of Back Pain

Back pain can occur at any point along your spine. The lumbar area, because it bears the majority of your weight, is the most common site. Any movement that puts excessive stress on the spinal column can cause injury and pain. The spine is well equipped to bear body weight and the force or stress of body movements along its long axis. However, it is less capable of bearing loads at an angle to its long axis or when the trunk is flexed (bent). You do not have to carry a heavy load or participate in a vigorous contact sport to injure your back. Picking up a pencil from the floor while using poor body mechanics—reaching too far out in front of you or bending over with your knees straight, for example—can also result in back pain.

Risk factors associated with low-back pain include age greater than 34 years, degenerative diseases such as arthritis or osteoporosis, a family or personal history of back pain or trauma, a sedentary lifestyle, low job satisfaction, low socioeconomic status, excess body weight, smoking (which appears to hasten degenerative changes in the spine), and psychological stress or depression (which can cause muscle tension and back pain). Occupations and activities associated with low-back pain are those requiring physically hard work, such as frequent lifting, twisting, bending, standing up, or straining in forced positions; those requiring

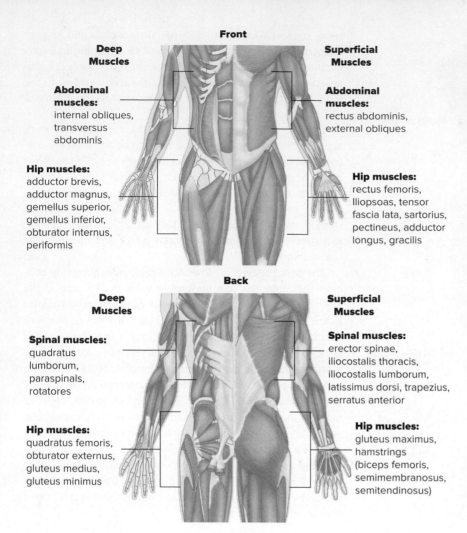

Front

Deep
Muscles

Abdominal muscles:
internal obliques, transversus abdominis

Hip muscles:
adductor brevis, adductor magnus, gemellus superior, gemellus inferior, obturator internus, periformis

Superficial
Muscles

Abdominal muscles:
rectus abdominis, external obliques

Hip muscles:
rectus femoris, Iliopsoas, tensor fascia lata, sartorius, pectineus, adductor longus, gracilis

Back

Deep
Muscles

Spinal muscles:
quadratus lumborum, paraspinals, rotatores

Hip muscles:
quadratus femoris, obturator externus, gluteus medius, gluteus minimus

Superficial
Muscles

Spinal muscles:
erector spinae, iliocostalis thoracis, iliocostalis lumborum, latissimus dorsi, trapezius, serratus anterior

Hip muscles:
gluteus maximus, hamstrings (biceps femoris, semimembranosus, semitendinosus)

Figure 5.5   Major core muscles.

high concentration demands while seated (such as computer programming); and those involving vibrations affecting the entire body (such as truck driving).

Underlying causes of back pain include poor muscle endurance and strength in the core muscles; excess body weight; poor posture or body position when standing, sitting, or sleeping; and poor body mechanics when performing actions like lifting and carrying or sports movements. Strained muscles, tendons, or ligaments can cause pain and, over time, lead to injuries to vertebrae, intervertebral disks, and surrounding muscles and ligaments.

Physical stress can cause disks to break down and lose some of their ability to absorb shock. A damaged disk may bulge out between vertebrae and pressure a nerve root, which causes pain. Painful pressure on nerves can also occur if damage to a disk narrows the space between two vertebrae. With age, you lose fluid from the disks, making them more likely to bulge and pressure nerve roots. Depending on the pressure on a nerve, symptoms may include numbness in the back, hip, leg, or foot; radiating pain; loss of muscle function; depressed reflexes; and muscle spasm. If the pressure is severe enough, loss of function can be permanent.

Preventing Low-Back Pain

Incorrect posture causes many back injuries. Strategies for maintaining good posture are presented in the box "Good Posture and Low-Back Health." Follow the same guidelines when you engage in sports or recreational activities. Control your movements, and warm up thoroughly before you exercise. Take special care when lifting weights.

The role of exercise in preventing and treating back pain is still being investigated. However, many experts recommend exercise, especially for people who have experienced an episode of low-back pain. The exercise can be a workout aimed at increasing muscle endurance and strength in the back and abdomen or just regular lifestyle physical activity such as walking. Movement helps lubricate your spinal joints and increases muscle fitness in your trunk and legs. Other lifestyle recommendations for preventing back pain include the following:

- Maintain a healthy weight. Excess fat contributes to poor posture, which can place harmful stresses on the spine.
- Stop smoking and reduce stress.
- Avoid sitting, standing, or working in the same position for too long. Stand up every hour or half-hour and move around.
- Use a supportive seat and a medium-firm mattress.
- Use lumbar support when driving, particularly for long distances, to prevent muscle fatigue and pain.
- Warm up thoroughly before exercising.
- Progress gradually when attempting to improve strength or fitness.

Managing Acute Back Pain

Sudden (acute) back pain usually involves tissue injury. Symptoms may include pain, muscle spasms, stiffness, and inflammation. Many cases of acute back pain go away by themselves within a few days or weeks. Applying cold and then heat may reduce pain and inflammation (see Chapter 3). Apply ice several times a day; once inflammation and spasms subside, you can apply heat using a heating pad or a warm bath. If the pain is bothersome, an over-the-counter nonsteroidal anti-inflammatory medication such as ibuprofen or naproxen may be helpful. Stronger pain medications and muscle relaxants are available by prescription.

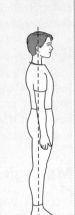

Changes in everyday posture and behavior can help prevent and alleviate low-back pain.

- **Lying down.** When resting or sleeping, lie on your side with your knees and hips bent. If you lie on your back, place a pillow under your knees. However, do not elevate your knees so much that the curve in your lower spine is flattened. Don't lie on your stomach. Use a medium-firm mattress.

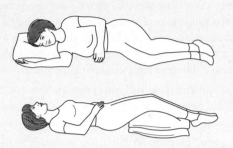

- **Sitting at a computer.** Sit in a slightly reclined position of 100–110 degrees, not an upright 90-degree position. Adjust your chair so your knees are slightly lower than your hips. If your back flattens as you sit, try using a lumbar roll to maintain your back's natural curvature. Place your feet flat on the floor or on a footrest. Place the monitor directly in front of you and adjust it so your eyes are level with the top of the screen; you should be looking slightly downward at the middle of the screen. Adjust the keyboard and mouse so your forearms and wrists are in a neutral position, parallel with the floor. Stand up and walk a short distance at least once every hour.

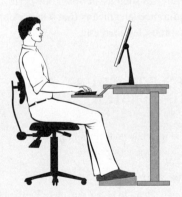

- **Lifting.** If you need to bend down to grasp an object, hinge at the hips and bend at the knees rather than at the waist. Your feet should be about shoulder-width apart. Lift gradually, keeping your arms straight, by standing up or by pushing with your hip muscles. Keep the object close to your body. Don't twist; if you have to turn with the object, change the position of your feet so you pivot your entire body rather than twisting at your waist or shoulders. Maintain a stiff core and neutral spine (natural spinal curves).

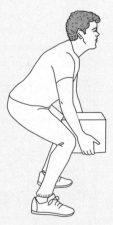

- **Standing.** When standing, a straight line should run from the top of your ear through the center of your shoulder, the center of your hip, the back of your kneecap, and the front of your ankle bone. Support your weight mainly on your heels, with one or both knees slightly bent. Don't let your pelvis tip forward or your back arch. Shift your weight back and forth from foot to foot. Avoid prolonged standing.

To check your posture, stand normally with your back to a wall. Your upper back and buttocks should touch the wall; your heels may be a few inches away. Slide one hand into the space between your lower back and the wall. It should slide in easily but should almost touch both your back and the wall. Adjust your posture as needed, and try to hold this position as you walk away from the wall.

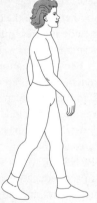

- **Walking.** Walk with your toes pointed straight ahead. Keep your back flat, head up and centered over your body, and chin in. Swing your arms freely. Don't wear tight or high-heeled shoes. Walking briskly is better for back health than walking slowly.

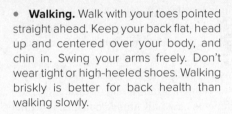

Bed rest immediately following the onset of back pain may make you feel better, but it should be of short duration. Prolonged bed rest—five days or more—was once thought to be an effective treatment for back pain, but most physicians now advise against it because it may weaken muscles and actually worsen pain. Limit bed rest to one day and begin moderate physical activity soon. Exercise can increase muscular endurance and flexibility and protect disks from loss of fluid. Three of the back exercises discussed later in the chapter may be especially helpful following an episode of acute back pain: McGill curl-ups, side bridges, and spine extensions ("bird dogs").

See your physician if acute back pain doesn't resolve within a short time. Other warning signals of a more severe problem that requires a professional evaluation include severe pain, numbness, pain that radiates down one or both legs, problems with bladder or bowel control, fever, and rapid weight loss.

Managing Chronic Back Pain

Low-back pain is considered chronic if it persists over three months. Symptoms vary—some people experience stabbing or shooting pain, and others a steady ache accompanied by stiffness. Sometimes pain is localized; in other cases, it radiates to another part of the body. Underlying causes of chronic back pain include injuries, infection, muscle or ligament strains, and disk herniations.

Because symptoms and causes are so varied, different people benefit from different treatment strategies, and researchers have found that many treatments have only limited benefits. Potential treatments include over-the-counter or prescription medications; exercise; physical therapy, massage, yoga, or chiropractic care; acupuncture; percutaneous electrical nerve stimulation (PENS), in which acupuncture-like needles deliver an electrical current; education and advice about posture, exercise, and body mechanics; and surgery (see the box "Yoga for Relaxation and Pain Relief").

Psychological therapy may also be beneficial in some cases. Reducing emotional stress that causes muscle tension can provide direct benefits, and other therapies can help people deal better with chronic pain and its effects on their daily lives. Support groups and expressive writing are beneficial for people with chronic pain and other conditions.

EXERCISES FOR THE PREVENTION AND MANAGEMENT OF LOW-BACK PAIN

The tests in Lab 5.3 can help you assess low-back muscular endurance. The exercises that follow can help you maintain a healthy back by stretching and strengthening the major muscle groups that affect the back—the abdominal muscles, the muscles along your spine and sides, and the muscles of your hips and thighs. If you have back problems, check with your physician before beginning any exercise program. Perform the exercises slowly and progress gradually. Stop and consult your physician if

any exercise causes back pain. General guidelines for back exercise programs include the following:

- Do low-back exercises at least three days per week. Most experts recommend daily back exercises.

- Emphasize muscular endurance rather than muscular strength—endurance is more protective.

- Don't do spine exercises involving a full range of motion early in the morning. Because your disks have a high fluid content early in the day, injuries may result.

- Engage in regular endurance exercise such as cycling or walking in addition to performing exercises that specifically build muscular endurance and flexibility. Brisk walking with a natural arm swing may help relieve back pain. Start with fast walking if your core muscles are weak or you have back pain.

- Be patient and stick with your program. Increased back fitness and pain relief may require as long as three months of regular exercise.

- The adage "no pain, no gain" does not apply to back exercises. Always use good form and stop if you feel pain.

- Build core stiffness through stabilization exercises because they strengthen muscles, improve muscular endurance, reduce low back pain, and boost sports performance. Greater core stiffness transfers strength and speed to the limbs, increases the load-bearing capacity of the spine, and protects the internal organs during sports movements. When working on abdominal muscles, emphasize stabilization exercises, such as side bridges, carry exercises, planks, bird dogs, and the stir-the-pot exercise rather than spinal flexion exercises such as sit-ups. Poor performance on the spinal endurance labs means that you are not training your abdominal muscles correctly.

TIPS FOR TODAY AND THE FUTURE

To improve and maintain your flexibility, perform stretches that work the major joints at least twice a week.

RIGHT NOW YOU CAN
- Stand up and stretch—do either the upper-back stretch or the across-the-body stretch shown in the chapter.
- Practice the recommended sitting and standing postures described in the chapter. If needed, adjust your chair or find something to use as a footrest.

IN THE FUTURE YOU CAN
- Build up your flexibility by incorporating more sophisticated stretching exercises into your routine. Increase the frequency of your flexibility workouts to five or more days per week.
- Increase the efficiency of your workouts by adding stretching exercises to the cool-down period of your endurance or strength workouts.
- Incorporate low-back exercises into your daily routine.

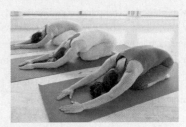

Exercise, such as yoga and tai chi, can provide relief from back pain, depending on the pain's underlying cause. Effective exercises stretch the muscles and connective tissue in the hips, stabilize the spine, and strengthen and build endurance in the core muscles of the back and abdomen.

Yoga may be an option for many back pain sufferers because it offers a variety of exercises that target the spine and the core muscles. Yoga is an ancient practice involving slow, gentle movements performed with controlled breathing and focused attention. Yoga practitioners slowly move into a specific posture (called an *asana*) and hold the posture for up to 60 seconds. There are hundreds of asanas, many of which are easy to do and provide good stretches.

Yoga also involves simple breathing exercises that gently stretch the muscles of the upper back while helping the practitioner focus. Yoga experts say that breathing exercises not only encourage relaxation but also clear the mind and can

help relieve mild to moderate pain. Yoga enthusiasts end their workouts energized and refreshed but calm and relaxed.

Many medical professionals now recommend yoga for patients with back pain, particularly asanas that arch and gently stretch the back, such as the cat pose (similar to the cat stretch shown in the "Low-Back Exercises" section) and the child pose (see photo). These are basic asanas that most people can perform repeatedly and hold for a relatively long time.

Because asanas must be performed correctly to be beneficial, qualified instruction is recommended. For those with back pain, physicians advise choosing an instructor not only accomplished in yoga but also knowledgeable about back pain and its causes. Such instructors can steer students away from exercises that do more harm than good. It is especially important to choose postures that will benefit the back without worsening the underlying problem. Some asanas can aggravate an injured or painful back if they are performed incorrectly or

too aggressively. People with back pain should avoid a few yoga postures, such as a standing forward bend.

Wavebreakmedia Ltd/Getty Images

If you have back pain, see your physician to determine its cause before beginning an exercise program. Even gentle exercise or stretching can be bad for an already injured back, especially if the spinal disks or nerves are involved. For some back conditions, rest or therapy may be a better option than exercise, at least in the short term.

SUMMARY

• Flexibility, the ability of a joint to move through its full range of motion, is highly adaptable and specific to each joint.

• Range of motion can be limited by joint structure, muscle inelasticity, and proprioceptor activity.

• Developing flexibility depends on stretching the elastic tissues within muscles regularly and gently until they lengthen. Overstretching can make connective tissue brittle and lead to rupture.

• Signals sent between muscle and tendon nerves and the spinal cord can enhance flexibility.

• The benefits of flexibility include preventing abnormal stresses that lead to joint deterioration and possibly reducing the risk of injuries.

• Static stretches should be held for 10–30 seconds and performed with 2–4 repetitions for a total stretching time of 60 seconds per exercise. Flexibility training should be done at least two or three days per week, preferably following activity, when muscles are warm.

• Static stretching is slow and held to the point of mild tension; ballistic stretching, consisting of bouncing stretches, can lead to injury. Dynamic stretching moves joints slowly and fluidly through their range of motions. Proprioceptive neuromuscular facilitation uses muscle receptors in contracting and relaxing a muscle.

• Passive stretching, using an outside force to move muscles and joints, achieves a greater range of motion (and has a higher injury risk) than active stretching, which uses opposing muscles to initiate a stretch.

• The spinal column consists of vertebrae separated by intervertebral disks. It provides structure and support for the body and protects the spinal cord. The core muscles stabilize the spine and transfer force between the upper and lower body.

• Acute back pain can be treated as a soft tissue injury, with cold treatment followed by application of heat (once swelling subsides); prolonged bed rest is not recommended. A variety of treatments have been suggested for chronic back pain, including regular exercise, physical therapy, acupuncture, education, and psychological therapy.

• Besides good posture, proper body mechanics, and regular physical activity, a program for preventing low-back pain includes exercises that develop flexibility, strength, and endurance in the muscle groups that affect the lower back.

• Build core stiffness through stabilization exercises because they strengthen muscles, improve muscular endurance, reduce low-back pain, and boost sports performance. Greater core stiffness transfers strength and speed to the limbs, increases the load-bearing capacity of the spine, and protects the internal organs during sports movements.

EXERCISE 1 — Cat Stretch

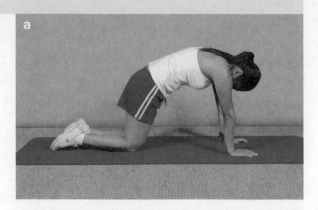

Instructions: Begin on all fours with your knees below your hips and your hands below your shoulders. Slowly and deliberately move through a cycle of extension and flexion of your spine. **(a)** Begin by slowly pushing your back up and dropping your head slightly until your spine is extended (rounded). **(b)** Then slowly lower your back and lift your chin slightly until your spine is flexed (relaxed and slightly arched). *Do not press at the ends of the range of motion.* Stop if you feel pain. Do 10 slow, continuous cycles of the movement.

Target: Improved strength and flexibility in the erector spinae, relaxation, and reduced stiffness in the spine.

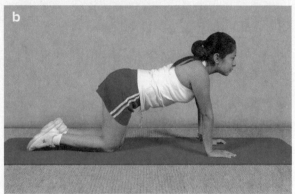

(a–b): Photo taken by Wayne Glusker

EXERCISE 2 — Step Stretch (see Exercise 6 in the flexibility program)

Instructions: Hold each stretch for 10–30 seconds and do 2–4 repetitions on each side.

Target: Improved flexibility, strength, and endurance in the hip flexors and hip extensors and stiffens the core.

EXERCISE 3 — Leg Stretcher (see Exercise 11 in the flexibility program)

Instructions: Hold each stretch for 10–30 seconds and do 2–4 repetitions on each side.

Target: Improved flexibility in the hip extensors and hamstrings.

EXERCISE 4 — Trunk Twist

Instructions: Lie on your side with top knee bent, lower leg straight, lower arm extended in front of you on the floor, and upper arm at your side. Push down with your upper knee while you twist your trunk to the opposite side. Try to get your shoulders and upper body flat on the floor, turning your head as well. Return to the starting position, and then repeat on the other side. Hold the stretch for 10–30 seconds and do 2–4 repetitions on each side.

Target: Improved flexibility in the lower back and core muscles.

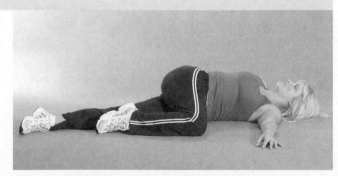

Photo taken by Taylor Robertson Photography

| EXERCISE 5 | McGill Curl-Up (see Exercise 4 in the body weight program in Chapter 4) |

Instructions: Lie on your back with one knee bent and arms crossed on your chest or hands under your lower back. Maintain a neutral spine. Tuck your chin in and slowly curl up, one vertebra at a time, as you use your abdominal muscles to lift your head first and then your shoulders. Stop when you can see your knees and hold for 5–10 seconds before returning to the starting position. Do 10 or more repetitions.

Target: Improved strength, endurance, and stiffness in the abdomen.

| EXERCISE 6 | Isometric Side Bridge (see Exercise 6 in the body weight program in Chapter 4) |

Instructions: Hold the bridge position for 10 seconds, breathing normally. Build up to five or more repetitions on each side.

Target: Increased strength and endurance in the muscles along the sides of the abdomen and deep lateral muscles that support the spine.

Variation: You can make the exercise more difficult by keeping your legs straight and supporting yourself with your feet and forearm (see Lab 5.3) or with your feet and hand (with elbow straight).

| EXERCISE 7 | Spine Extensions ("Bird Dogs"; see Exercise 5 in the body weight program in Chapter 4) |

Instructions: Hold each position for 5–15 seconds. Begin with one repetition on each side, and work up to five or more repetitions.

Target: Increased strength and endurance in the back, gluteal muscles, and hamstrings.

Variation: If you have experienced back pain in the past or if this exercise is difficult for you, do the exercise with both hands on the ground rather than with one arm lifted. You can make this exercise more difficult by doing it balancing on an exercise ball. Find a balance point on your chest while lying face down on the ball with one arm and the opposite leg on the ground. Tense your abdominal muscles while reaching and extending with one arm and reaching and extending with the opposite leg. Repeat this exercise using the other arm and leg.

| EXERCISE 8 | Wall Squat (Phantom Chair) |

Instructions: Lean against a wall and bend your knees as though you are sitting in a chair. Support your weight with your legs. Begin by holding the position for 5–10 seconds. Squeeze your gluteal muscles together as you do the exercise. Build up to one minute or more. Perform one or more repetitions.

Target: Increased strength and endurance in the lower back, quadriceps, gluteal muscles, and core muscles.

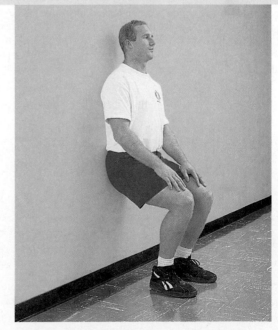

Photo taken by Neil A. Tanner

EXERCISE 9 — Pelvic Tilt

Instructions: Lie on your back with knees bent and arms extended to the side. Tilt your pelvis under and try to flatten your lower back against the floor. Tighten your buttock and abdominal muscles while you hold this position for 5–10 seconds. Don't hold your breath. Work up to 10 repetitions of the exercise. Pelvic tilts can also be done standing or leaning against a wall. *Note:* Although this is a popular exercise with many therapists, some experts question the safety of pelvic tilts. Stop if you feel pain in your back at any time during the exercise.

Target: Increased strength and endurance in the gluteal muscles and core muscles.

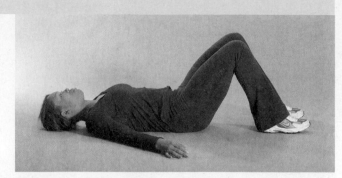

Photo taken by Taylor Robertson Photography

EXERCISE 10 — Back Bridge

Instructions: Lie on your back with knees bent and arms extended to the side. Tuck your pelvis under; contract your gluteal muscles; then lift your tailbone, buttocks, and lower back from the floor. Hold this position for 5–10 seconds with your weight resting on your feet, arms, and shoulders, and then return to the starting position. Work up to 10 repetitions of the exercise.

Target: Increased strength and endurance in quadriceps, gluteal muscles, and core muscles.

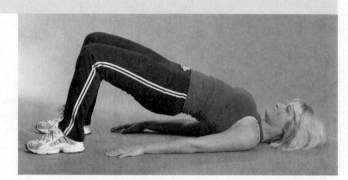

Photo taken by Taylor Robertson Photography

EXERCISE 11 — Stir the Pot

Instructions: Assume a plank position on an exercise ball, with forearms on the ball and legs extended to the rear. Maintaining a stiff torso and neutral spine, rotate on the ball in a clockwise direction for 10 repetitions and then repeat in a counterclockwise direction for 10 repetitions.

Target: Increased strength and endurance in the core muscles and shoulders.

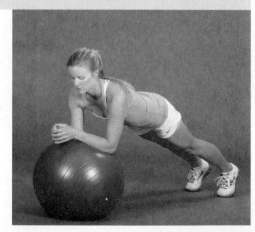

Photo taken by Taylor Robertson Photography

EXERCISE 12 — Kettlebell or Dumbbell Carry ("Suitcase Carry"; see Exercise 11 in the free weights program in Chapter 4)

Instructions: This is an excellent exercise for building the core muscles. Pick up a dumbbell or kettlebell in one or both hands. Maintaining good posture, walk 20 to 100 yards carrying the weights. Carry 10 to several hundred pounds, depending on your fitness.

Target: Core muscles, trapezius, quadriceps and gluteal muscles.

COMMON QUESTIONS ANSWERED

Q **Is stretching the same as warming up?**

A No. They are two distinct activities. A warm-up is light exercise that involves moving the joints through the same motions used during a more intense activity; it increases body temperature so that your metabolism works better when you're exercising at high intensity. Stretching increases the movement capability of your joints, so that you can move more easily with less risk of injury. It is best to stretch when your muscles are warm. Warmed muscles stretch better than cold ones and are less prone to injury.

Q **How much flexibility do I need?**

A This question is not always easy to answer. If you're involved in a sport such as gymnastics, figure skating, or ballet, you are often required to reach extreme joint motions to achieve success. However, non-athletes do not need to reach these extreme joint positions. In fact, too much flexibility may, in some cases, create joint instability and increase your risk of injury. As with other types of fitness, moderation is the key. You should regularly stretch your major joints and muscle groups but not aspire to reach extreme flexibility.

Q **Can I stretch too far?**

A Yes. As muscle tissue is progressively stretched, it reaches a point where it becomes damaged and may rupture. The greatest danger occurs during passive stretching when a partner is doing the stretching for you. It is critical that your stretching partner not force your joint outside its normal functional range of motion.

Q **Can physical training limit flexibility?**

A When done properly, weight training increases flexibility. However, because of the limited range of motion used during the running stride, jogging tends to compromise flexibility. It is important for runners to do flexibility exercises for the hamstrings and quadriceps regularly.

Q **Does static stretching affect muscular strength?**

A Flexibility training increases muscle strength over time, but many recent studies have found that stretching causes short-term decreases in strength, power, and motor control. This is one reason some experts suggest that people not stretch as part of their exercise warm-up, particularly if they plan to engage in a high-performance activity. It is important to warm up before any workout by engaging in 5–10 minutes of light exercise such as walking or slow jogging.

FOR FURTHER EXPLORATION

American Academy of Orthopaedic Surgeons. Provides information about a variety of joint problems.

http://orthoinfo.aaos.org

American Heart Association: Stretching and Flexibility Exercises. Describes a basic program of stretching exercises.

https://www.heart.org/en/health-topics/cardiac-rehab/getting-physically-active/stretching-and-flexibility-exercises

Back Fit Pro. A website maintained by Dr. Stuart McGill, a professor of spine biomechanics at the University of Waterloo, which provides evidence-based information on preventing and treating back pain.

http://www.backfitpro.com

Georgia State University: Flexibility. Provides information about the benefits of stretching and ways to develop a safe and effective program; includes illustrations of stretches.

http://www2.gsu.edu/~wwwfit/flexibility.html

International Fitness Association: Stretching and Flexibility. Provides information on the physiology of stretching and different types of stretching exercises.

http://www.ifafitness.com/stretch/stretch5.htm

International Yoga Alliance. A good resource for yoga organizations around the world.

https://www.yogaalliance.org/

Mayo Clinic: Focus on Flexibility. Presents basic information on flexibility and stretching exercises for a beginning program and for an office setting.

https://www.mayoclinic.org/healthy-lifestyle/fitness/in-depth/stretching/art-20047931

NIH Back Pain. Provides basic information on the prevention and treatment of back pain.

https://www.niams.nih.gov/health-topics/back-pain

See also the listings for Chapters 2 and 4.

SELECTED BIBLIOGRAPHY

American College of Sports Medicine. 2018. *ACSM's Guidelines for Exercise Testing and Prescription,* 10th ed. Philadelphia: Wolters Kluwer.

Avloniti, A., et al. 2016. The effects of static stretching on speed and agility: One or multiple repetition protocols? *European Journal of Sport Science* 16(4): 402–408.

Awan, R., and E. R. Laskowski. 2019. Yoga: safe for all? *Mayo Clinic Proceedings* 94(3): 385–387.

Ayala, C.A., et al. 2017. Acute effects of three neuromuscular warm-up strategies on several physical performance measures in football players. *PlosOne* 12(1): e0169660.

Barengo, N. C., et al. 2014. The impact of the FIFA 11+ training program on injury prevention in football players: A systematic review. *International Journal of Environmental Research and Public Health* 11(11): 1198-2000.

Baxter, C., et al. 2017. Impact of stretching on the performance and injury risk of long-distance runners. *Research in Sports Medicine* 25(1): 78-90.

Blazevich, A. J., et al. 2018. No effect of muscle stretching within a full, dynamic warm-up on athletic performance. *Medicine Science Sports and Exercise* 50(6): 1258-1266.

Cayco, C. S., et al. 2019. Hold-relax and contract-relax stretching for hamstrings flexibility: A systematic review with meta-analysis. *Physical Therapy in Sport* 35: 42-55.

Chang, D. G., et al. 2016. Yoga as a treatment for chronic low back pain: A systematic review of the literature. *Journal of Orthopedics and Rheumatology* 3(1): 1-8.

Chatzopoulos, D., et al. 2014. Acute effects of static and dynamic stretching on balance, agility, reaction time and movement time. *Journal of Sports Science and Medicine* 13(2): 403-409.

Evangelista, A. L., et al. 2019. Interset stretching vs. traditional strength training: Effects on muscle strength and size in untrained individuals. *Journal Strength and Conditioning Research.* In press.

Haddad, M., et al. 2014. Static stretching can impair explosive performance for at least 24 hours. *Journal of Strength and Conditioning Research* 28(1): 140-146.

Haladay, D. E., et al. 2013. Quality of systematic reviews on specific spinal stabilization exercise for chronic low back pain. *Journal of Orthopedic Sports Physical Therapy* 43(4): 242-250.

Howley, E., and D. Thompson. 2017. *Fitness Professional's Handbook,* 7th ed. Champaign, Ill.: Human Kinetics.

Ikeda, N., and T. Ryushi. 2018. Effects of 6-week static stretching of knee extensors on flexibility, muscle strength, jump performance, and muscle endurance. *Journal Strength and Conditioning Research.* In press.

Inami, T., et al. 2015. Acute changes in peripheral vascular tonus and systemic circulation during static stretching. *Research in Sports Medicine* 23(2): 167-178.

Iversen, V. M., et al. 2018. Resistance band training or general exercise in multidisciplinary rehabilitation of low back pain? A randomized trial. *Scandinavian Journal Medicine Science in Sports* 28(9): 2074-2083.

Kawada, T. 2018. Exercise therapy for low back pain: a systematic review. *American Journal Physical Medicine Rehabilitation* 97(10): e96.

Keilman, B. M., et al. 2017. The short-term effect of kettlebell swings on lumbopelvic pressure pain thresholds: A randomized controlled trial. *Journal Strength and Conditioning Research* 31(11): 3001-3009.

Kirmizigil, B., et al. 2014. Effects of three different stretching techniques on vertical jumping performance. *Journal of Strength and Conditioning Research* 28(5): 1263-1271.

Konrad, A., and M. Tilp. 2014. Increased range of motion after static stretching is not due to changes in muscle and tendon structures. *Clinical Biomechanics* 29(6): 636-642.

Konrad A., et al. 2016. The effects of acute static, ballistic, and PNF stretching exercise on the muscle and tendon tissue properties. *Scandinavian Journal of Medicine and Science in Sports.* doi:10.1111/sms.12725

Lee, B. C. Y., and S. M. McGill. 2015. Effect of long-term isometric training on core/torso stiffness. *Journal of Strength and Conditioning Research* 29(6): 1515-1526.

Lima, C. D., et al. 2016. Acute effects of static vs. ballistic stretching on strength and muscular fatigue between ballet dancers and resistance-trained women. *Journal of Strength and Conditioning Research* 30(11): 3220-3227.

Lima, C. D., et al. 2018. Effects of static versus ballistic stretching on hamstring: Quadriceps strength ratio and jump performance in ballet dancers and resistance trained women. *Journal Dance Medicine and Science* 22(3): 160-167.

Lopes, T. J. A., et al. 2018. Physical performance measures of flexibility, hip strength, lower limb power and trunk endurance in healthy navy cadets: Normative data and differences between sex and limb dominance. *Journal Strength and Conditioning Research.* In press

Matsuo, S., et al. 2015. Changes in force and stiffness after static stretching of eccentrically damaged hamstrings. *European Journal of Applied Physiology* 115(5): 981-991.

McGill, S. 2007. *Low Back Disorders: Evidence-Based Prevention and Rehabilitation,* 2nd ed. Champaign, Ill.: Human Kinetics.

McGill, S. 2014. *Ultimate Back Fitness and Performance,* 5th ed. Waterloo, Canada: Backfit Pro.

McGill, S. 2015. *Back Mechanics.* Waterloo, Canada: Backfit Pro.

McGill, S., et al. 2013. Movement quality and links to measures of fitness in firefighters. *Work* 45(3): 357-366.

McGill, S. M., and L. W. Marshall. 2012. Kettlebell swing, snatch, and bottoms-up carry: back and hip muscle activation, motion, and low back loads. *Journal of Strength and Conditioning Research* 26(1): 16-27.

McGill, S. M., et al. 2013. Low back loads while walking and carrying: Comparing the load carried in one hand or in both hands. *Ergonomics* 56(2): 293-302.

McGill, S. M., et al. 2014. Analysis of pushing exercises: Muscle activity and spine load while contrasting techniques on stable surfaces with a labile suspension strap training system. *Journal of Strength and Conditioning Research* 28(1): 105-116.

Miller, K. C., and J. A. Burne. 2014. Golgi tendon organ reflex inhibition following manually applied acute static stretching. *Journal of Sports Science* 32(15): 1491-1497.

Nakao, S., et al. 2019. Chronic effects of a static stretching program on hamstring strength. *Journal Strength and Conditioning Research.* In press.

Plouvier, S., et al. 2015. Occupational biomechanical exposure predicts low back pain in older age among men in the Gazel Cohort. *International Archives of Occupational and Environmental Health* 88: 501-510.

Ribeiro, A. S., et al. 2014. Static stretching and performance in multiple sets in the bench press exercise. *Journal of Strength and Conditioning Research* 28(4): 1158-1163.

Ryan, E. D., et al. 2014. Acute effects of different volumes of dynamic stretching on vertical jump performance, flexibility and muscular endurance. *Clinical Physiology and Functional Imaging* 34(6): 485-492.

Smith, J. C., et al. 2018. Acute effect of foam rolling and dynamic stretching on flexibility and jump height. *Journal Strength and Conditioning Research* 32(8): 2209-2215.

Swain, C. T. V., et al. 2019. The epidemiology of low back pain and injury in dance: A systematic review. *Journal Orthopedic Sports Physical Therapy,* 1-41.

Taniguchi, K., et al. 2015. Acute decrease in the stiffness of resting muscle belly due to static stretching. *Scandinavian Journal of Medicine and Science in Sports* 25(1): 32-40.

Thomas, E., et al. 2018. The relation between stretching typology and stretching duration: The effects on range of motion. *International Journal Sports Medicine* 39(4): 243-254.

Trajano, G., et al. 2015. Static stretching increases muscle fatigue during submaximal sustained isometric contractions. *Journal of Sports Medicine and Physical Fitness* 55(1-2): 43-50.

Wewege, M. A., et al. 2018. Aerobic vs. resistance exercise for chronic non-specific low back pain: A systematic review and meta-analysis. *Journal Back Musculoskeletal Rehabilitation* 31(5): 889-899.

Wieland, L. S., et al. 2017. Yoga treatment for chronic non-specific low back pain. *Cochrane Database System Review.* Published online January 12.

Yamaguchi, T., et al. 2015. Acute effect of dynamic stretching on endurance running performance in well-trained male runners. *Journal of Strength and Conditioning Research* 29 (11): 3045-3052.

Yu, A. P., et al. 2018. Revealing the neural mechanisms underlying the beneficial effects of tai chi: A neuroimaging perspective. *American Journal Chinese Medicine* 46(2): 231-259.

Name _____ Section _____ Date _____

LAB 5.1 Assessing Your Current Level of Flexibility

Part I Sit-and-Reach Test

Equipment

Use a modified Wells and Dillon flexometer or construct your own measuring device using a firm box or two pieces of wood about 30 centimeters (12 inches) high attached at right angles to each other. Attach a metric ruler to measure the extent of reach. With the low numbers of the ruler toward the person being tested, set the 26-centimeter mark of the ruler at the footline of the box. Individuals who cannot reach as far as the footline will have scores below 26 centimeters; those who can reach past their feet will have scores above 26 centimeters. Most studies show no relationship between performance on the sit-and-reach test and the incidence of back pain.

Preparation

Warm up your muscles with a low-intensity activity such as walking or easy jogging. Then perform slow stretching movements.

Instructions

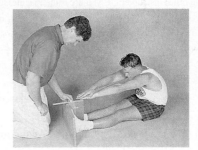

Photo taken by Shirlee Stevens

1. Remove your shoes and sit facing the flexibility measuring device with your knees fully extended and your feet flat against the device about 10 centimeters (4 inches) apart.

2. Reach as far forward as you can, with palms down, arms evenly stretched, and knees fully extended; hold the position of maximum reach for about two seconds.

3. Perform the stretch 2 times, recording the distance of maximum reach to the nearest 0.5 centimeters:

   _____ cm

Rating Your Flexibility

Find the score in the following table to determine your flexibility rating. Record it here and on the final page of this lab.
Rating: _____

Ratings for Sit-and-Reach Test

	Rating/Score (cm)*				
Men	*Needs Improvement*	*Fair*	*Good*	*Very Good*	*Excellent*
Age: 15–19	Below 24	24–28	29–33	34–38	Above 38
20–29	Below 25	25–29	30–33	34–39	Above 39
30–39	Below 23	23–27	28–32	33–37	Above 37
40–49	Below 18	18–23	24–28	29–34	Above 34
50–59	Below 16	16–23	24–27	28–34	Above 34
60–69	Below 15	15–19	20–24	25–32	Above 32
Women					
Age: 15–19	Below 29	29–33	34–37	38–42	Above 42
20–29	Below 28	28–32	33–36	37–40	Above 40
30–39	Below 27	27–31	32–35	36–40	Above 40
40–49	Below 25	25–29	30–33	34–37	Above 37
50–59	Below 25	25–29	30–32	34–38	Above 38
60–69	Below 23	23–26	27–30	31–34	Above 34

*Footline is set at 26 cm.

SOURCE: Canadian Society for Exercise Physiology. 2003. *The Canadian Physical Activity, Fitness & Lifestyle Approach: CSEP-Health & Fitness Program's Health-Related Appraisal and Counseling Strategy*, 3rd ed.

LABORATORY ACTIVITIES

Part II Range-of-Motion Assessment

This portion of the lab can be completed by doing visual comparisons or by measuring joint range of motion with a goniometer or other instrument.

Equipment

1. A partner to do visual comparisons or to measure the range of motion of your joints. (You can also use a mirror to perform your own visual comparisons.)

2. For the measurement method, you need a goniometer, flexometer, or other instrument to measure range of motion.

Preparation

Warm up your muscles with some low-intensity activity such as walking or easy jogging.

Instructions

On the following pages, the average range of motion is illustrated and listed quantitatively for some of the major joints. Visually assess the range of motion in your joints, and compare it to that shown in the illustrations. For each joint, note (with a check mark) whether your range of motion is above average, average, or below average and in need of improvement. Average values for range of motion are given in degrees for each joint in the assessment. You can also complete the assessment by measuring your range of motion with a goniometer, flexometer, or other instrument. If you are using this measurement method, identify your rating (above average, average, or below average) and record your range of motion in degrees next to the appropriate category. Although the measurement method is more time consuming, it allows you to track the progress of your stretching program more precisely and to note changes within the broader ratings categories (below average, above average).

Record your ratings on the following pages and on the chart on the final page of this lab. (Ratings were derived from several published sources.)

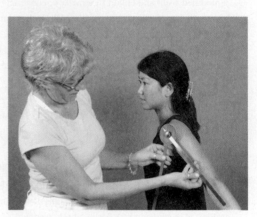

Photo taken by Wayne Glusker

1. Shoulder Abduction and Adduction

For each position and arm, check one of the following; fill in degrees if using the measurement method.

Shoulder abduction—raise arm up to the side.

Right	Left	
_____	_____	Below average/needs improvement
_____	_____	Average (92-95°)
_____	_____	Above average

Shoulder adduction—move arm down and in front of body.

Right	Left	
_____	_____	Below average/needs improvement
_____	_____	Average (124-127°)
_____	_____	Above average

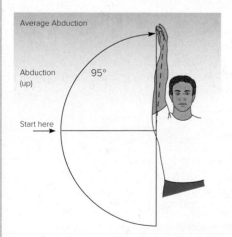

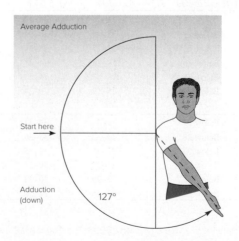

2. Shoulder Flexion and Extension

For each position and arm, check one of the following; fill in degrees if using the measurement method.

Shoulder flexion—raise arm up in front of the body.

Right *Left*

_____ _____ Below average/needs improvement

_____ _____ Average (92–95°)

_____ _____ Above average

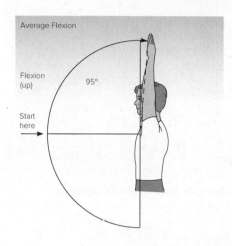

Shoulder extension—move arm down and behind the body.

Right *Left*

_____ _____ Below average/needs improvement

_____ _____ Average (145–150°)

_____ _____ Above average

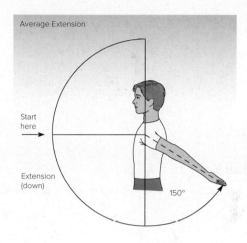

3. Trunk/Low-Back Lateral Flexion

Bend directly sideways at your waist. To prevent injury, keep your knees slightly bent, and support your trunk by placing your hand or forearm on your thigh. Check one of the following for each side; fill in degrees if using the measurement method.

Right *Left*

_____ _____ Below average/needs improvement

_____ _____ Average (36–40°)

_____ _____ Above average

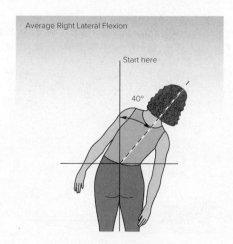

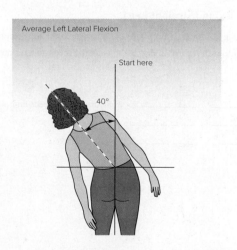

LABORATORY ACTIVITIES

4. Hip Abduction

Raise your leg to the side at the hip. Check one of the following for each leg; fill in degrees if using the measurement method.

Right　　　*Left*

_____　　_____　　Below average/needs improvement

_____　　_____　　Average (40–45°)

_____　　_____　　Above average

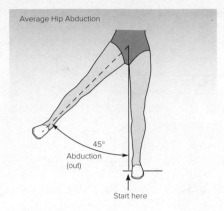

Average Hip Abduction

45°
Abduction (out)

Start here

5. Hip Flexion (Bent Knee)

With one leg flat on the floor, bend the other knee and lift the leg up at the hip. Check one of the following for each leg; fill in degrees if using the measurement method.

Right　　　*Left*

_____　　_____　　Below average/needs improvement

_____　　_____　　Average (121–125°)

_____　　_____　　Above average

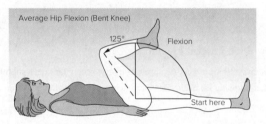

Average Hip Flexion (Bent Knee)

125°　　Flexion

Start here

6. Hip Flexion (Straight Leg)

With one leg flat on the floor, raise the other leg at the hip, keeping both legs straight. Take care not to put excess strain on your back. Check one of the following for each leg; fill in degrees if using the measurement method.

Right　　　*Left*

_____　　_____　　Below average/needs improvement

_____　　_____　　Average (79–81°)

_____　　_____　　Above average

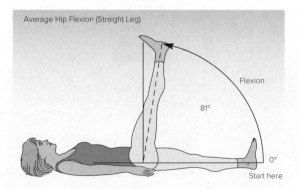

Average Hip Flexion (Straight Leg)

Flexion

81°

0°

Start here

7. Ankle Dorsiflexion and Plantar Flexion

For each position and foot, check one of the following; fill in degrees if using the measurement method.

Ankle dorsiflexion–pull your toes toward your shin.

Right   Left

_____   _____   Below average/needs improvement

_____   _____   Average (9–13°)

_____   _____   Above average

Right   Left

_____   _____   Below average/needs improvement

_____   _____   Average (50–55°)

_____   _____   Above average

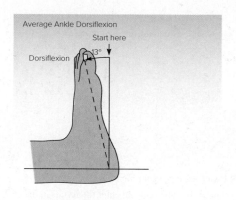

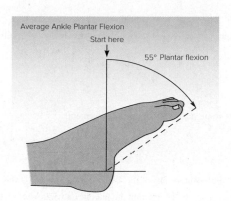

Plantar flexion–point your toes.

Rating Your Flexibility

Sit-and-reach test: Score: _____ cm Rating: _____

Range-of-Motion Assessment

Identify your rating for each joint on each side of the body. If you used the comparison method, put check marks in the appropriate categories; if you measured range of motion, enter the degrees for each joint in the appropriate category.

Joint/Assessment		Right Below Average	Right Average	Right Above Average	Left Below Average	Left Average	Left Above Average
1. Shoulder abduction and adduction	Abduction						
	Adduction						
2. Shoulder flexion and extension	Flexion						
	Extension						
3. Trunk/low-back lateral flexion	Flexion						
4. Hip abduction	Abduction						
5. Hip flexion (bent knee)	Flexion						
6. Hip flexion (straight leg)	Flexion						
7. Ankle dorsiflexion and plantar flexion	Dorsiflexion						
	Plantar flexion						

LABORATORY ACTIVITIES

Using Your Results

How did you score? Do your scores for the flexibility tests surprise you? Are you satisfied with your current ratings?

If you're not satisfied, set a realistic goal for improvement:

Are you satisfied with your current level of flexibility as expressed in your daily life—for example, your ability to maintain good posture and move easily and without pain?

If you're not satisfied, set some realistic goals for improvement:

What should you do next? Enter the results of this lab in the Preprogram Assessment column in Appendix B. If you've set goals for improvement, begin planning your flexibility program by completing the plan in Lab 5.2. After several weeks of your program, complete this lab again and enter the results in the Postprogram Assessment column of Appendix B. How do the results compare?

Name _____ **Section** _____ **Date** _____

LAB 5.2   Creating a Personalized Program for Developing Flexibility

1. *Goals.* List goals for your flexibility program. On the left, include specific, measurable goals that you can use to track the progress of your fitness program. These goals might be things like raising your sit-and-reach score from fair to good or your bent-leg hip flexion rating from below average to average. On the right, include long-term and more qualitative goals, such as reducing your risk for back pain.

Specific Goals: Current Status   Final Goals

_____   _____

_____   _____

_____   _____

Other Goals: _____

_____

2. *Exercises.* The exercises in the following program plan are from the general stretching program presented in Chapter 5. You can add or delete exercises depending on your needs, goals, and preferences. For any exercises you add, fill in the areas of the body affected.

3. *Frequency.* A minimum frequency of two or three days per week is recommended; five to seven days per week is ideal. You may want to do your stretching exercises the same days you plan to do cardiorespiratory endurance exercise or weight training because muscles stretch better following exercise, when they are warm.

4. *Intensity.* All stretches should be done to the point of mild discomfort, not pain.

5. *Time/duration.* All stretches should be held for 10–30 seconds. (PNF techniques should include a 6-second contraction followed by a 10- to 30-second assisted stretch.) All stretches should be performed 2–4 times, for a total volume of 60 seconds per exercise.

Program Plan for Flexibility

Exercise	Areas Stretched	Frequency (check ✓)						
		M	T	W	Th	F	Sa	Su
Head turns and tilts	Neck							
Towel stretch	Triceps, shoulders, chest							
Across-the-body and overhead stretches	Shoulders, upper back, back of the arm							
Upper-back stretch	Upper back							
Lateral stretch	Trunk muscles							
Step stretch	Hip, front of thigh							
Side lunge	Inner thigh, hip, calf							
Inner-thigh stretch	Inner thigh, hip							
Hip and trunk stretch	Trunk, outer thigh and hip, lower back							
Modified hurdler stretch	Back of the thigh, lower back							
Leg stretcher	Back of the thigh, hip, knee, ankle, buttocks							
Lower-leg stretch	Back of the lower leg							
Single-leg deadlift	Hamstrings and gluteal muscles							

LABORATORY ACTIVITIES

You can monitor your program using a chart like the one here.

Flexibility Program Chart

Fill in the dates you perform each stretch, the number of seconds you hold each stretch (should be 10–30), and the number of repetitions of each (should be 2–4). For an easy check on the duration of your stretches, count "one thousand one, one thousand two," and so on. You will probably find that over time you'll be able to hold each stretch longer (in addition to being able to stretch farther).

Exercise/Date																					
	Duration																				
	Reps																				
	Duration																				
	Reps																				
	Duration																				
	Reps																				
	Duration																				
	Reps																				
	Duration																				
	Reps																				
	Duration																				
	Reps																				
	Duration																				
	Reps																				
	Duration																				
	Reps																				
	Duration																				
	Reps																				
	Duration																				
	Reps																				
	Duration																				
	Reps																				
	Duration																				
	Reps																				
	Duration																				
	Reps																				
	Duration																				
	Reps																				
	Duration																				
	Reps																				
	Duration																				
	Reps																				
	Duration																				
	Reps																				
	Duration																				
	Reps																				

Name _____ Section _____ Date _____

LAB 5.3 Assessing Muscular Endurance for Low-Back Health

The four tests in this lab evaluate the muscular endurance of major spine-stabilizing muscles. These tests are the trunk flexor endurance test, back extensor endurance test, side bridge endurance test, and front plank endurance test.

Trunk Flexor Endurance Test (also called the V-Sit Flexor Endurance Test)

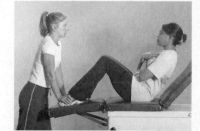

Photo taken by Taylor Robertson Photography

Equipment

1. Stopwatch or clock with a second hand
2. Exercise mat or padded exercise table
3. Two helpers
4. A wedge angled at 55 degrees from the floor or padded bench (optional)

Preparation
Warm up with some low-intensity activity such as walking or easy jogging.

Instructions

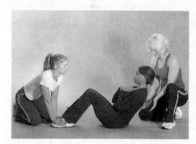

Photo taken by Taylor Robertson Photography

1. To start, assume a sit-up posture with your back supported at an angle of 55 degrees from the floor; support can be provided by a wedge, a padded bench, or a spotter (see photos). Your knees and hips should both be flexed at 90 degrees, and your arms should be folded across your chest with your hands placed on the opposite shoulders. Your toes should be secured under a toe strap or held by a partner.

2. Your goal is to hold the starting position (isometric contraction) as long as possible after the support is pulled away. To begin the test, a helper should pull the wedge or other support back about 10 centimeters (4 inches). The helper should keep track of the time; if a spotter is acting as your support, she or he should be ready to support your weight as soon as your torso begins to move back. Your final score is the total time you are able to hold the contraction—from the time the support is removed until any part of your back touches the support or you request to discontinue the test. Remember to breathe normally throughout the test.

3. Record your time here and on the chart at the end of the lab. Trunk flexors endurance time: _____ sec

Back Extensor Endurance Test (also called the Biering-Sorensen extension test)

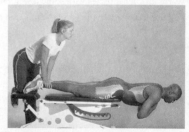

Photo taken by Taylor Robertson Photography

Equipment

1. Stopwatch or clock with a second hand
2. Extension bench with padded ankle and hip support or any padded bench
3. Partner

Preparation
Warm up with some low-intensity activity such as walking or easy jogging.

Instructions

1. Lie face down on the test bench with your upper body extending out over the end of the bench and your pelvis, hips, and knees flat on the bench. Your arms should be folded across your chest with your hands placed on the opposite shoulders. Your legs and hips should be secured under padded straps or held by a partner.

LABORATORY ACTIVITIES

2. Your goal is to hold your upper body in a straight horizontal line with your lower body as long as possible. Keep your neck straight and neutral; don't raise your head and don't arch your back. Breathe normally. Your partner should keep track of the time and watch your form. Your final score is the total time you are able to hold the horizontal position—from the time you assume the position until your upper body drops from the horizontal position.

3. Record your time here and on the chart at the end of the lab. Back extensor endurance time: _____ sec

Side Bridge Endurance Test

Equipment

1. Stopwatch or clock with a second hand
2. Exercise mat
3. Partner

Preparation

Warm up your muscles with some low-intensity activity such as walking or easy jogging. Practice assuming the side bridge position described next.

Photo taken by Joseph Quever

Instructions

1. Lie on the mat on your side with your legs extended. Place your top foot in front of your lower foot for support. Lift your hips off the mat so that you are supporting yourself on one elbow and your feet (see photo). Your body should maintain a straight line. Breathe normally; don't hold your breath.

2. Hold the position as long as possible. Your partner should keep track of the time and make sure that you maintain the correct position. Your final score is the total time you are able to hold the side bridge with correct form—from the time you lift your hips until your hips return to the mat.

3. Rest for five minutes and then repeat the test on the other side. Record your times here and on the chart at the end of the lab.

Right side bridge time: _____ sec

Left side bridge time: _____ sec

Front Plank Test

Equipment

1. Stopwatch or clock with a second hand
2. Exercise mat
3. Partner

Preparation

Warm up your muscles with some low-intensity activity such as walking or easy jogging. Practice assuming the front plank position described next.

Instructions

1. Assume a front plank position by lying on your front and then lifting your hips, supporting your weight on your forearms and toes and keeping the torso rigid (see photo). Your body should maintain a straight line; keep your hands together and elbows directly under your shoulders. Breathe normally and don't hold your breath.

2. Hold the position as long as possible. Your partner should keep track of the time and make sure that you maintain the correct position. Your final score is the total time you are able to hold the front plank with correct form—from the time you lift your hips until your hips return to the mat.

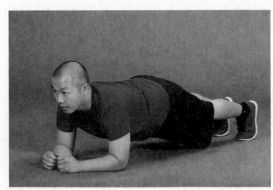
Photo taken by Taylor Robertson Photography

3. Record your time here and on the chart at the end of the lab.

Front plank time: _____ sec

Rating Your Test Results for Muscular Endurance for Low-Back Health

The following table shows percentiles for torso endurance tests for healthy young college students, ages 17–25, based on a study of 181 university students. Compare your scores with the times shown in the table. Your percentile on each test tells you the percentage of the students in the study who scored at or below your score.

Percentiles Ranks for Torso Muscle Endurance Tests for College-Age Men and Women (age 17–25)

Percentiles	Trunk flexor test (sec)		Back extensor test (sec)		Side bridge test, right (sec)		Side bridge test, left (sec)		Front plank test (sec)	
	Men	Women	Men	Women	Men	Women	Men	Women	Men	Women
99%	276	246	246	265	193	130	187	133	400	213
95%	234	208	215	232	164	112	160	114	336	181
90%	211	188	199	215	149	102	146	104	302	165
85%	196	174	188	204	140	96	137	97	280	154
80%	184	163	179	194	131	91	129	92	261	145
75%	174	154	171	186	124	86	122	87	245	137
70%	164	145	164	179	118	83	116	83	231	130
65%	156	138	159	173	113	79	111	79	219	124
60%	148	130	152	167	107	76	106	75	206	118
55%	140	123	147	161	102	72	101	72	195	112
50%	132	116	141	155	97	69	96	68	183	106
45%	124	109	135	149	92	66	91	64	171	100
40%	117	102	130	143	87	63	86	61	160	95
35%	108	94	123	137	81	59	81	57	147	88
30%	100	87	118	131	76	55	76	53	135	82
25%	90	78	111	124	70	52	70	49	121	75
20%	80	69	103	116	63	47	63	44	105	67
15%	68	58	94	106	54	42	55	39	86	58
10%	53	44	83	95	45	36	46	32	64	47
5%	30	24	67	78	30	26	32	22	30	31
1%	0	0	36	45	1	8	5	3	0	0

NOTE: The percentiles were based on data collected on 181 university kinesiology students ages 17–25. The results might not be representative of other populations.

Source: Percentile charts calculated from the data of McGill, S., M. Belore, I. Crosby, and C. Russell. "Clinical tools to quantify torso flexion endurance: normative data from student and firefighter populations," *Occupational Ergonomics* 9, no. 1 (2010): 55–61.

Record Your Scores

Test	Time	Percentile
Trunk Flexor Endurance Test		
Back Extensor Endurance Test		
Side Bridge Endurance Test, right side		
Side Bridge Endurance Test, left side		
Front Plank Test		

LABORATORY ACTIVITIES

Using Your Results

How did you score? Are you surprised by your scores for the low-back tests? Are you satisfied with your current ratings?

If you're not satisfied, set a realistic goal for improvement. The norms in this lab are based on healthy young adults, so a score above the mean may or may not be realistic for you. Instead, you may want to set a specific goal based on time rather than rating; for example, set a goal of improving your time by 10%. Imbalances in muscular endurance have been linked with back problems, so if your rating is significantly lower for one of the three tests, you should focus particular attention on that area of your body.

Goal:

What should you do next? Enter the results of this lab in the Preprogram Assessment column in Appendix B. If you've set a goal for improvement, begin a program of low-back exercises such as that suggested in this chapter. After several weeks of your program, complete this lab again and enter the results in the Postprogram Assessment column of Appendix B. How do the results compare?

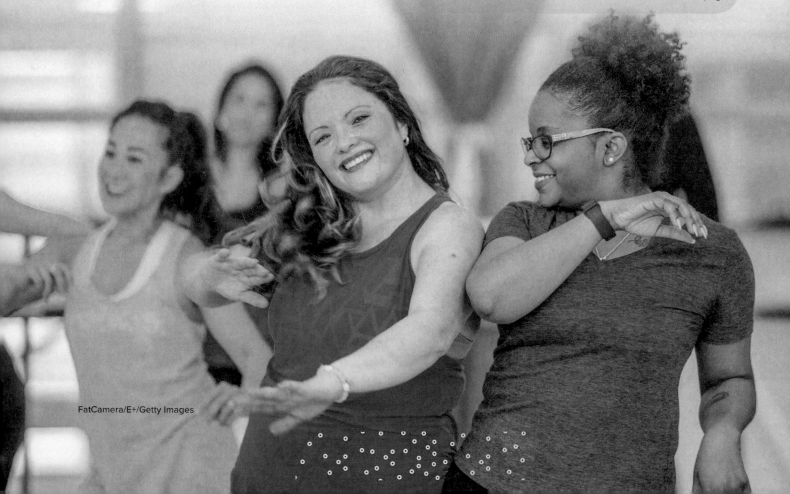

CHAPTER 6

Body Composition

LOOKING AHEAD...

After reading this chapter, you should be able to

- Define fat-free mass and body fat, and describe their functions in the body.
- Explain how body composition affects overall health and wellness.
- Describe how body mass index, body composition, and body fat distribution are measured and assessed.
- Explain how to determine recommended body weight and body fat distribution.

TEST YOUR KNOWLEDGE

1. Exercise helps reduce the risks associated with overweight and obesity even if it doesn't result in improvements in body composition. True or false?

2. Which of the following is the most significant controllable risk factor for the most common type of diabetes (type 2 diabetes)?
   a. smoking
   b. low-fiber diet
   c. overweight or obesity
   d. inactivity

3. In women, excessive exercise and low energy (calorie) intake can cause which of the following?
   a. unhealthy reduction in body fat levels
   b. amenorrhea (absent menstruation)
   c. bone density loss and osteoporosis
   d. muscle wasting and fatigue
   e. all of these

See answers on the next page.

FatCamera/E+/Getty Images

Body composition, the body's relative amounts of fat and fat-free mass, is an important component of fitness for health and wellness. People with an optimal body composition tend to be healthier, to move more efficiently, and to feel better about themselves. They also have a lower risk of many chronic diseases.

Many people, however, don't succeed in their efforts to obtain a fit and healthy body because they set unrealistic goals and emphasize short-term weight loss rather than permanent lifestyle changes that lead to fat loss and a healthy body composition. Successful management of body composition requires the long-term, consistent coordination of many aspects of a wellness program, particularly dietary choices and physical activity. Even in the absence of changes in body composition, an active lifestyle improves wellness and decreases the risk of disease and premature death (later in the chapter, see the box "Why Is Physical Activity Important Even If Body Composition Doesn't Change?").

This chapter focuses on defining and measuring body composition. The aspects of lifestyle that affect body composition—physical activity and exercise, nutrition, weight management, and stress management—are discussed in detail in other chapters.

WHAT IS BODY COMPOSITION, AND WHY IS IT IMPORTANT?

The human body can be divided into fat-free mass and body fat. As defined in Chapter 2, fat-free mass comprises all the body's nonfat tissues: bone, water, muscle, connective tissue, organ tissues, and teeth.

Body fat is incorporated into the nerves, brain, heart, lungs, liver, mammary glands, and other body organs and tissues. A certain amount of body fat is necessary for the body to function. It is the main source of stored energy in the body; it also cushions body organs and helps regulate body temperature. This **essential fat** makes up about 3–5% of total body weight in men and about 8–12% in women (Figure 6.1). The percentage is higher in women due to fat deposits in the breasts, uterus, and other gender-specific sites.

Most of the fat in the body is stored in fat cells, or **adipose tissue**, located under the skin (**subcutaneous fat**) and around major organs (**visceral fat** or *intra-abdominal fat*). People have a genetically determined number of fat cells, but these cells can

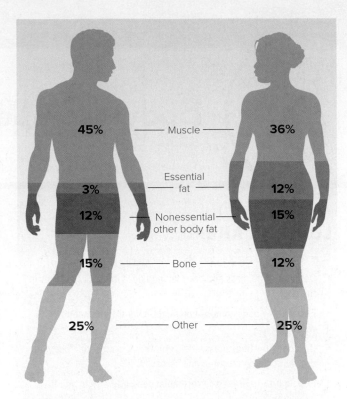

Figure 6.1   Body composition of a typical man and woman, 20–24 years old. Each number represents each component's contribution to total body mass.

SOURCES: Brooks, G. A., et al. 2005. *Exercise Physiology: Human Bioenergetics and Its Applications*, 4th ed. New York: McGraw-Hill; Santos, D.A., et al. 2014. "Reference Values for body composition and anthropometric measurements in athletes," *PLoS ONE*, vol. 9, no. 5: e97846; Santos, D., et al. 2014. "Reference Values for Body Composition and Anthropometric Measurements in Athletes." *PLoS ONE* 9, no. 5: 1–11. https://DOI:10.1371/journal.pone.0097846.

become larger or smaller depending on how much fat is being stored. The amount of stored fat depends on several factors, including age, gender, metabolism, diet, and activity level. The primary source of excess body fat is excess calories consumed in the diet—that is, calories consumed beyond what are expended in metabolism, physical activity, and exercise. A pound of body fat is equivalent to 3,500 calories. Over the short term, consuming 3,500 more or fewer calories would result in a gain or loss of about one pound. Over the long term, the relationship between changes in calorie intake and body weight is more complex, as metabolism and calorie needs change as body weight changes; see Chapter 9 for more on strategies for making changes in body composition. Excess stored body fat is associated with increased risk of chronic diseases like diabetes and cardiovascular disease, as described later in this chapter.

Overweight and Obesity Defined

When looking at body composition, the most important consideration is the proportion of the body's total weight that is fat—the **percent body fat**. For example, two women may be 5 feet 5 inches tall and weigh 130 pounds. But one woman may have only 15% of her body weight as fat, whereas the other woman could have 34% body fat. Although neither woman is overweight by most standards, the second woman is considered overfat. Too much body fat (not just total weight) has a negative effect on health and well-being. Just as the proportion of body fat is important, so is its location on your body. Visceral fat is more harmful to health than subcutaneous fat.

Overweight is usually defined as total body weight above the recommended range for good health as determined by large-scale population surveys. **Obesity** is defined as a more serious degree of overweight that carries multiple major health risks. The cutoff point for obesity may be set in terms of percent body fat or in terms of some measure of total body weight.

Prevalence of Overweight and Obesity among Americans

Americans are getting fatter. Since 1960, the average American man's weight has increased from 166 to 198 pounds, and the average American woman's weight has increased from 140 to 171 pounds. The prevalence of obesity has increased from about 13% in 1960 to 39.8% in 2016. Today, 62–69% of Americans are obese or overweight (Figure 6.2). In 2016, according to the National Center for Health Statistics, about 35–41% of adult men and 37–45% of adult women were obese. Since 1960, overweight and obesity rates have increased in both men and women, in every age and socioeconomic group, and in people living in every part of the country. Obesity rates are particularly high in blacks, in low-income Americans, and in the South and Midwest; between 2008 and 2019, obesity rates increased most among middle-aged and older adults.

Possible explanations for this increase include increased calorie intake, more time spent in sedentary work and leisure activities, fewer short trips on foot and more by automobile, fewer daily gym classes for students, more meals eaten outside the home, greater consumption of fast food, increased portion sizes, and increased consumption of soft drinks and convenience foods. According to National Health and Nutrition Examination Survey (NHANES), energy intake increased from 1,955 calories per day in 1971 to 2,105 in 2016. People are gaining weight because they are consuming too many calories and not doing enough physical activity. Chapter 9 reviews individual and environmental factors that contribute to overweight and obesity.

Excess Body Fat and Wellness

As rates of overweight and obesity increase, so do the problems associated with them. Obesity doubles mortality rates and can reduce life expectancy by 10–20 years. In fact, if the current trends in overweight and obesity (and their related health problems) continue, scientists believe the average American's life expectancy may soon decline by as much as several years.

Diabetes *Diabetes* is a disease that disrupts normal metabolism. The pancreas normally secretes the hormone insulin, which stimulates cells to take up glucose (blood sugar) to produce energy. Diabetes interferes with this process, causing a buildup of glucose in the bloodstream. Diabetes is associated

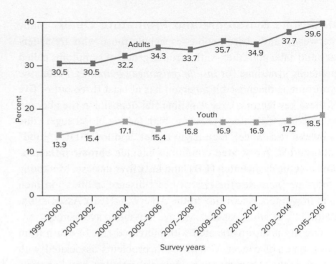

Figure 6.2   Obesity trends for U.S. adults age 20 and over and youth ages 2–19, 1999–2016. Since 1999, the proportion of American adults who are obese (body mass index ≥ 30) has increased substantially.

SOURCE: Hales, C., et al. 2017. "Prevalence of obesity among adults and youth: United States, 2015–2016," *National Center Health Statistics Data Brief*, No. 288, Hyattsville, MD: National Center for Health Statistics.

with kidney failure; nerve damage; erectile dysfunction; circulation problems; retinal damage and blindness; and increased rates of heart attack, stroke, and hypertension. Diabetes is currently the seventh leading cause of death in the United States.

Even mild to moderate overweight is associated with a substantial increase in the risk of type 2 diabetes, the most common form, and excess body fat is the key controllable risk factor for diabetes. Obese people are more than three times as likely as nonobese people to develop type 2 diabetes. The incidence of this disease among Americans has increased dramatically as the rate of obesity has climbed, more than doubling between 1995 and 2016.

See Chapter 11 for more on types, diagnosis, treatment, and prevention of diabetes.

TERMS

essential fat   Fat incorporated in various tissues of the body that is critical for normal body functioning.

adipose tissue   Tissue in which fat is stored; fat cells.

subcutaneous fat   Fat located under the skin.

visceral fat   Fat located around major organs; also called *intra-abdominal fat.*

percent body fat   The percentage of total body weight that is composed of fat.

overweight   Body weight above the recommended range for good health; sometimes defined as a body mass index between 25 and 29.9, a measure of the proportion of weight to height.

obesity   Severely overweight, characterized by an excessive accumulation of body fat; may also be defined in terms of some measure of total body weight or a body mass index of 30 or more.

Metabolic Syndrome and Premature Death Many overweight and obese people—especially those who are sedentary and eat a poor diet—suffer from a group of symptoms called **metabolic syndrome** (or *insulin resistance syndrome*). Metabolic syndrome is diagnosed if a person has at least three out of five of these key factors: large waistline (fat deposits in the abdominal region), high blood pressure, high fasting blood sugar (due to **insulin resistance**), high triglycerides, and low HDL ("good" cholesterol). Associated conditions include **chronic inflammation**, **erectile dysfunction (ED)**, and **fatty liver** disease. Metabolic syndrome increases the risk of heart disease, more so in men than in women. According to the American Heart Association, about 34% of adult Americans have metabolic syndrome.

Obesity is also associated with increased risk of death from many types of cancer. Other health problems associated with obesity include hypertension, impaired immune function, gallbladder and kidney diseases, skin problems, sleep and breathing disorders, erectile dysfunction, pregnancy complications, back pain, arthritis, and other bone and joint disorders.

Body Fat Distribution and Health The distribution of body fat (the locations of fat on the body) is also an important indicator of health. Men and postmenopausal women usually store fat in the upper regions of their bodies, particularly in the abdominal area (the "apple shape"). Premenopausal women usually store fat in the hips, buttocks, and thighs (the "pear shape"). Excess fat in the abdominal area increases risk of high blood pressure, diabetes, early-onset heart disease, stroke, certain cancers, and mortality. The reason for this increase in risk is not entirely clear, but abdominal fat is more easily mobilized and sent into the bloodstream, increasing disease-related blood fat levels.

> **TERMS**
>
> **metabolic syndrome** A cluster of symptoms present in many overweight and obese people that greatly increases their risk of heart disease, diabetes, and other chronic illnesses; symptoms include insulin resistance, abnormal blood fats, abdominal fat deposition, type 2 diabetes, high blood pressure, and high blood glucose.
>
> **insulin resistance** A condition in which body cells do not respond normally to insulin and cannot easily absorb glucose from the bloodstream; excess glucose can build up in the blood.
>
> **chronic inflammation** A response of blood vessels to harmful substances, such as germs, damaged cells, or irritants; can lead to heart disease, cancer, allergies, and muscle degeneration.
>
> **erectile dysfunction (ED)** Inability of a man to develop an erection firm enough for sex. ED is a risk factor of coronary artery disease.
>
> **fatty liver** Increased fat storage in the liver that can lead to liver inflammation and failure.
>
> **amenorrhea** Absent or infrequent menstruation, sometimes related to unhealthily low levels of body fat and excessive quantity or intensity of exercise.

A measure of waist circumference helps assess the risks of unhealthy body fat distribution. A total waist measurement of over 40 inches (102 cm) for men and over 35 inches (88 cm) for women is associated with a significantly increased risk of disease. Waist circumference is usually higher in taller people, so waist-to-height ratio can be a more accurate measure than waist circumference alone. Your waist measurement should be less than half your height. Using this index, a person 5 feet 8 inches (68 inches) tall should have a waist circumference of less than 34 inches. A person 6 feet 4 inches (76 inches) tall should have a waist circumference of less than 38 inches.

Performance of Physical Activities Too much body fat makes physical activity difficult because moving the body through everyday activities entails working harder and using more energy. In general, overfat people are less fit than others and don't have the muscular strength, endurance, and flexibility that make normal activity easy. Because exercise is more difficult, they do less of it, depriving themselves of an effective way to improve body composition.

Emotional Wellness and Self-Image Obesity can affect psychological and physical wellness. Being perceived as fat can be a source of judgment, ostracism, and sometimes discrimination by others; it can contribute to psychological problems such as depression, anxiety, and low self-esteem.

The popular image of the "ideal" body has changed greatly in the past 50 years, evolving from slightly plump to unhealthily thin. The ideal body—as presented by the media—is an unrealistic goal for most Americans. This is because one's ability to change body composition depends on heredity as well as diet and exercise. Body image, problems with body image, and unhealthy ways of dealing with a negative body image are discussed in Chapter 9. We need to change popular perceptions so active obese people are regarded as more fit, and normal-weight sedentary people as less fit.

Problems Associated with Very Low Levels of Body Fat

Though not as prevalent a problem as overweight or obesity, having too little body fat is also dangerous. Essential fat is necessary for the functioning of the body, and health experts generally view too little body fat—less than 8-12% for women and 3-5% for men—as a threat to health. Extreme leanness is linked with reproductive, respiratory, circulatory, and immune system disorders and with premature death in both men and women. Extremely lean people may experience muscle wasting and fatigue. They are also more likely to have eating disorders (described in more detail in Chapter 9). For women, an extremely low percentage of body fat is associated with loss of bone mass and **amenorrhea**—absent or infrequent menstruation (see the box "The Female Athlete Triad"). In older adults, having a low level of lean body mass and muscle strength are better predictors of premature death than body mass index.

ASSESSING BODY MASS INDEX, BODY COMPOSITION, AND BODY FAT DISTRIBUTION

Although a scale can tell your total weight, it can't reveal whether a fluctuation in weight is due to a change in muscle, body water, or fat. Most important, a scale can't differentiate between overweight and overfat. Some methods of assessing and classifying body composition are based on body fat and others on total body weight. Methods based on total body weight are less accurate, but they are commonly used because body weight is easier to measure than body fat. (Various methods of assessing body composition are described later in the chapter.)

In the past, many people relied on height-weight tables (which were based on insurance company mortality statistics) to determine whether they were at a healthy weight. Such tables, however, can be highly inaccurate for some people. Because muscle tissue is denser and heavier than fat, a fit person can easily weigh more than the recommended weight on a height-weight table. For the same reason, an unfit person may weigh less than the table's recommended weight.

There are several simple, inexpensive ways to estimate healthy body weight and healthy body composition more accurately than height-weight tables. These assessments can provide you with information about the health risks associated with your body weight and body composition. They can also help you establish reasonable goals and set a starting point for current and future decisions about weight loss and weight gain.

Calculating Body Mass Index

Body mass index (BMI) is useful for classifying the health risks of body weight if you don't have access to more sophisticated methods. Though more accurate than height-weight tables, body mass index is also based on the concept that weight should be proportional to height. BMI is easy to calculate and rate. Researchers frequently use BMI with waist circumference in studies that examine the health risks associated with body weight.

BMI is calculated by dividing your body weight (expressed in kilograms) by the square of your height (expressed in meters). The following example is for a person 5 feet 3 inches tall (63 inches), weighing 130 pounds:

1. Divide body weight in pounds by 2.2 to convert weight to kilograms: $130 \div 2.2 = 59.1$

2. Multiply height in inches by 0.0254 to convert height to meters: $63 \times 0.0254 = 1.6$

3. Multiply the result of step 2 by itself to get the square of the height measurement: $1.6 \times 1.6 = 2.56$

4. Divide the result of step 1 by the result of step 3 to determine BMI: $59.1 \div 2.56 = 23$

An alternative equation, based on pounds and inches, is

$$BMI = [weight/(height \times height)] \times 703$$

Space for your own calculations can be found in Lab 6.1, and a complete BMI chart appears in Lab 6.2. The online CDC Adult BMI calculator (https://www.cdc.gov/healthyweight/assessing/bmi/adult_bmi/english_bmi_calculator/bmi_calculator.html) and many apps can also calculate BMI.

A BMI between 18.5 and 24.9 is considered normal and desirable under separate standards from the National Institutes of Health (NIH) and the World Health Organization (WHO). A person with a BMI of 25 or above is classified as overweight, and someone with a BMI of 30 or above is classified as obese (Table 6.1). A person with a BMI below 18.5 is classified as underweight, although low BMI values may be healthy in some cases if they are not the result of smoking, an eating disorder, or an underlying disease. A BMI of 17.5 or less is sometimes used as a diagnostic criterion for the eating disorder anorexia nervosa.

A meta-analysis from the National Center for Health Statistics, pooling data from studies of nearly 3 million people, found those with severe obesity (BMI greater than 34.9) had a higher death rate from all causes than did people with normal weight (BMI = 18.5–24.9). However, overweight people (BMI = 25–29.9) had a *lower* all-cause death rate than normal weight people, and moderately obese people (BMI = 30–34.9) had

Table 6.1	Classifications from the World Health Organization

BODY MASS INDEX (BMI) CLASSIFICATIONS

WEIGHT STATUS CLASSIFICATION	BODY MASS INDEX
Underweight	<18.5
Severe thinness	<16.0
Moderate thinness	16.0–16.9
Mild thinness	17.0–18.4
Normal	18.5–24.9
Overweight	25.0–29.9
Obese, Class I	30.0–34.9
Obese, Class II	35.0–39.9
Obese, Class III	≥40.0

WAIST CIRCUMFERENCE CLASSIFICATIONS

RISK CLASSIFICATION	WAIST CIRCUMFERENCE IN INCHES (CENTIMETERS) WOMEN	MEN
Normal	<32 in. (80 cm)	<37 in. (94 cm)
Increased	≥32 in. (80 cm)	≥37 in. (94 cm)
Substantially increased	≥35 in. (88 cm)	≥40 in. (102 cm)

SOURCE: World Health Organization. 2008. *Waist Circumference and Waist-to-Hip Ratio. Report of a WHO Expert Consultation.* Geneva: WHO.

body mass index (BMI) A measure of relative body weight correlating highly with more direct measures of body fat, calculated by dividing total body weight (in kilograms) by the square of body height (in meters). **TERMS**

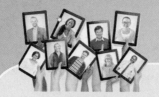

DIVERSITY MATTERS
The Female Athlete Triad

Even though obesity is at epidemic levels in the United States, many girls and women strive for unrealistic thinness in response to pressure from peers and a society obsessed with appearance. This quest for thinness has led to an increasingly common, under-reported condition called the **female athlete triad**.

The triad consists of three interrelated disorders: abnormal eating patterns (and excessive exercising), followed by lack of menstrual periods (amenorrhea), followed by decreased bone density (premature osteoporosis). Left untreated, the triad can lead to decreased physical performance, reproductive problems, increased incidence of bone fractures, disturbances of heart rhythm and metabolism, and even death.

Abnormal eating ranges from moderately restricting food intake, to binge eating and purging (bulimia), to severely restricting food intake (anorexia nervosa). Whether serious or relatively mild, disordered eating prevents women from getting enough calories to meet their bodies' needs. Low energy intake can lead to unhealthy changes in both body composition and many body functions.

Disordered eating, combined with intense exercise and emotional stress, can suppress the hormones that control the menstrual cycle. Energy availability and, especially, menstrual status directly influence bone health. If the menstrual cycle stops for three consecutive months, the condition is called amenorrhea. Chronic

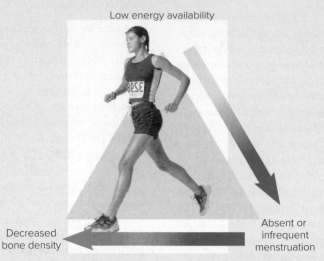

Low energy availability

Decreased bone density

Absent or infrequent menstruation

Alan Bailey/Rubberball/Getty Images

disruption of the menstrual cycle can lead to osteoporosis. Bone density may erode to the point that a woman in her 20s has the bone density of a woman in her 60s. Women with osteoporosis have fragile, easily fractured bones. Even a few missed menstrual periods can decrease bone density.

All physically active women and girls have the potential to develop one or more components of the female athlete triad. For example, it is estimated that 5–20% of women who exercise regularly and vigorously may develop amenorrhea. But the triad is most prevalent among athletes who participate in certain sports: those in which appearance is highly important, those that emphasize a prepubertal body shape, those that require contour-revealing clothing for competition, those that require endurance, and those that use weight categories for participation. Such sports include

gymnastics, figure skating, swimming, distance running, cycling, cross-country skiing, track, volleyball, rowing, horse racing, and cheerleading.

The female athlete triad can be life threatening. Typical signs of the eating disorders that trigger the condition are extreme weight loss, dry skin, loss of hair, brittle fingernails, cold hands and feet, low blood pressure and heart rate, swelling around the ankles and hands, and weakening of the bones. Female athletes who have repeated stress fractures may be suffering from the condition.

Early intervention is the key to stopping this series of interrelated conditions. Unfortunately, once the condition has progressed, long-term consequences, especially bone loss, are unavoidable. Teenagers may need only to learn about good eating habits; college-age women with a long-standing problem may require psychological counseling.

SOURCES: Tenforde, A. S., et al. 2017. "Association of the female athlete triad risk assessment stratification to the development of bone stress injuries in collegiate athletes," *American Journal of Sports Medicine* 45(2): 302–310; Mountjoy, M., et al. 2014. "The IOC consensus statement: Beyond the female athlete triad—relative energy deficiency in sport," *British Journal Sports Medicine* 48(7): 491–497; Joy, E., et al. 2014. "2014 Female Athlete Triad Coalition consensus statement on treatment and return to play of the female athlete triad." *Current Sports Medicine Reports* 13(4): 219–232.

---

similar death rates to normal-weight people. These controversial results showed that there are problems associated with using a one-time measure of BMI to predict health and longevity. Other

> **female athlete triad** A condition consisting of three interrelated disorders: abnormal eating patterns (and excessive exercising) followed by lack of menstrual periods (amenorrhea) and decreased bone density (premature osteoporosis).
>
> **TERMS**

factors, such as amount of physical activity, lean body mass, body fat changes over time, level of stress, dietary composition, and social factors, might account for the results.

Fat percentage varies for people with a given BMI. In the NHANES, for example, people with BMIs less than 25 had fat percentages ranging from 10% to nearly 32%. Factors influencing fat percentage at a given BMI included age, race, gender, and physical activity.

In classifying the health risks associated with overweight and obesity, the NIH and WHO guidelines also consider body fat distribution and other disease risk factors. As described earlier, excess fat in the abdomen is of greater concern than excess fat in other areas. Measurement of waist circumference (see Table 6.1) is one method of assessing body fat distribution. At a given level of overweight, people with a large waist circumference and/or additional disease risk factors are at risk for health problems. For example, a man with a BMI of 27, a waist circumference over 40 inches, and high blood pressure is at greater risk for health problems than another man with a BMI of 27 but a smaller waist circumference and no other risk factors.

Thus, optimal BMI for good health depends on many factors; if your BMI is 25 or above, consult a physician for help in determining a healthy BMI for you. While BMI and waist circumference are important measures of health, they must be considered with other factors such as high blood pressure, diabetes, blood fats, and insulin resistance.

Because BMI doesn't distinguish between fat weight and fat-free weight, it is only an indirect indicator of body fatness and so will not accurately classify all individuals. Factors including muscle mass, age, sex, and race/ethnicity, and height influence the relationship between BMI and actual percent body fat:

- *Muscle mass:* An athlete who weight trains will have more muscle mass than a less trained person of the same height and weight. Although both might be classified as overweight by the BMI scale, that classification would be inaccurate for the athlete because her or his "excess" weight is in the form of muscle, and it is healthy.

- *Age:* Older adults tend to have more body fat than younger adults for an equivalent BMI.

- *Sex:* Women are likely to have more body fat at a given BMI than men, although among healthy adults, women naturally have a higher percent body fat than men.

- *Race/ethnicity:* BMI measurements have over- and underestimated the prevalence of obesity in several groups, such as Hispanics and blacks, because of racial and ethnic differences in muscle mass and muscle density.

- *Height:* BMI is a poor predictor of health in people of **short stature**, whose gene function may have been altered by environmental factors early in life.

If you are an athlete, a serious weight trainer, or a person of short stature, do not use BMI as your primary means of assessing whether your current weight is healthy. Instead, try one of the methods described in the next section for estimating percent body fat. Further, BMI is not particularly useful for tracking changes in body composition over time—gains in muscle mass and losses of fat.

Estimating Percent Body Fat

Assessing body composition involves estimating percent body fat. The dissection and chemical analysis of the body is the only method for directly measuring the percentage of body weight that is fat. However, there are indirect techniques that can provide an *estimate* of percent body fat. One of the most accurate is underwater weighing. Other techniques include the Bod Pod, skinfold measurements, bioelectrical impedance analysis, and dual-energy X-ray absorptiometry.

All of these methods have a margin of error, so it is important not to focus too much on precise values. For example, underwater weighing has a margin of error of about ±3%, meaning that if a person's percent body fat is actually 17%, the test result could range from 14% to 20%. The results of different methods may also vary. If you plan to track changes in body composition over time, perform the assessment using the same method each time. See Table 6.2 for body composition ratings based on percent

Table 6.2	Percent Body Fat Classification						
	PERCENT BODY FAT (%)				PERCENT BODY FAT (%)		
	20–39 YEARS	*40–59* YEARS	*60–79* YEARS		*20–39* YEARS	*40–59* YEARS	*60–79* YEARS
Women				**Men**			
Essential*	8–12	8–12	8–12	Essential*	3–5	3–5	3–5
Low/athletic**	13–20	13–22	13–23	Low/athletic**	6–7	6–10	6–12
Recommended	21–32	23–33	24–35	Recommended	8–19	11–21	13–24
Overfat†	33–38	34–39	36–41	Overfat†	20–24	22–27	25–29
Obese†	≥39	≥40	≥42	Obese†	≥25	≥28	≥30

NOTE: The cutoffs for recommended, overfat, and obese ranges in this table are based on a study that linked BMI classifications from the NIH with predicted percent body fat (measured using dual-energy X-ray absorptiometry).

*Essential body fat is necessary for the basic functioning of the body.

**Percent body fat in the low/athletic range may be appropriate for some people as long as it is not the result of illness or disordered eating habits.

†Health risks increase as percent body fat exceeds the recommended range.

SOURCES: American College of Sports Medicine. 2018. *ACSM's Guidelines for Exercise Testing and Prescription*, 10th ed. Philadelphia: Wolters Kluwer; Borrud, L.G., et al. 2010. "Body composition data for individuals 8 years of age and older: U.S. population, 1999–2004," *Vital Health Stat*, vol. 11, no. 250: 1–87; Gallagher, D., et al. 2009. "Healthy percentage body fat ranges: An approach for developing guidelines based on body mass index," *American Journal of Clinical Nutrition*, vol. 72: 694–701. https://doi.org/10.1093/ajcn/72.3.694.

body fat as a criterion for obesity. It should be noted, however, that the NIH has not developed an official standard linking body fat percentage with obesity.

Underwater Weighing In hydrostatic (underwater) weighing, an individual is submerged and weighed under water. The percentages of fat and fat-free weight are calculated from body density. Muscle has a higher density and fat a lower density than water. Therefore, people with more body fat float and weigh less under water, and lean people sink and weigh more under water. Many university exercise physiology departments or sports medicine laboratories have an underwater weighing facility. For an accurate assessment of your body composition, find a place that does underwater weighing or has a Bod Pod (described in the next section).

The Bod Pod The Bod Pod, a small chamber containing computerized sensors, measures body composition by air displacement. The technique's technical name is *plethysmography*. It determines the percentage of fat by calculating body density from how much air is displaced by the person sitting inside the chamber. The Bod Pod has an error rate of about ±2–4% in determining percent body fat.

Skinfold Measurements Skinfold measurement is a simple, inexpensive, and practical way to assess body composition. Equations can link the thickness of skinfolds at various sites to percent body fat calculations from more precise laboratory techniques.

Skinfold assessment typically involves measuring the thickness of skinfolds at several places on the body. You can sum the skinfold values as an indirect measure of body fatness. For example, if you plan to create a fitness (and dietary change) program to improve body composition, you can compare the sum of skinfold values over time as an indicator of your program's progress and of improvements in body composition. You can also plug your skinfold values into equations like those in Lab 6.1 that predict percent body fat. When using these equations, however, remember that they have a fairly substantial margin of error (±4% if performed by a skilled technician), so don't focus too much on specific values. The sum represents only a relative measure of body fatness.

Skinfolds are measured with a device called a **caliper**, which is a pair of spring-loaded, calibrated jaws. High-quality calipers are made of metal and have parallel jaw surfaces and constant spring tension. Inexpensive plastic calipers are also available, but you need to make sure they are spring-loaded and have metal jaws to ensure accuracy. Refer to Lab 6.1 for instructions on how to take skinfold measurements.

> **short stature** Women less than 5 ft 0 in (153 centimeters) tall and men less than 5 ft 5 in (166 centimeters) tall.
>
> **caliper** A pressure-sensitive measuring instrument with two jaws that can be adjusted to determine thickness of the skinfold.
>
> **TERMS**

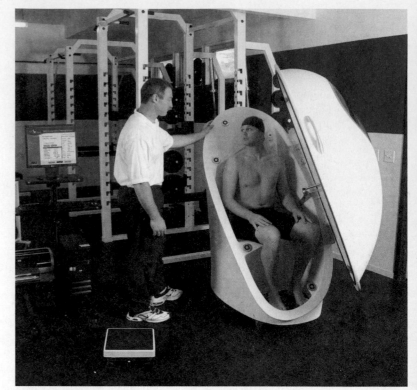

BOD POD® Body Composition Tracking System photo provided courtesy of COSMED USA, Inc.

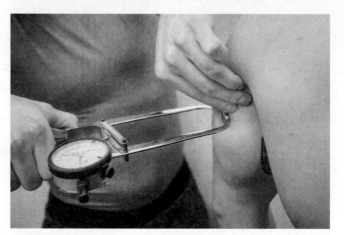

Fitness Tip If you plan to track body composition, be sure to use the same assessment method each time. In addition, don't become overly focused on precise values, because even the most accurate methods have a margin of error. The Bod Pod estimates body composition by air displacement and has a margin of error of about ±2–4%. Skinfold assessment is based on measurement of the thickness of several skinfolds, including the back of the arm, as shown here; equations translate these measurements into a percent body fat estimate, with about a ±4% margin of error.

Zefrog/Alamy Stock Photo

Taking accurate measurements with calipers requires patience, experience, and considerable practice. It's best to take several measurements at each site (or have several people take each measurement). Take the measurements in the exact location called for in the procedure. Because the amount of water in your body changes during the day, skinfold measurements taken

Scientists can use several techniques to accurately measure body composition. As described in the chapter, these techniques include underwater weighing, air displacement, and more advanced methods such as dual-energy X-ray absorptiometry (DEXA) and total body electrical conductivity (TOBEC). These methods, however, are costly and require technical expertise.

You can estimate your body fat and fat-free weight simply and accurately, at home, without the help of a technician. All you need is a digital home scale with a built-in bioelectrical impedance analyzer or a hand-held BIA unit. BIA works by measuring the resistance in the body to a small electric current. Electricity flows more slowly through fat tissue than through muscle, so the more fat you have, the more slowly such a current will flow through your body. Conversely, a current will pass through your body more quickly if you have more fat-free (muscle) weight.

To use a BIA scale or hand-held unit, just stand on the scale with bare feet or grasp the handles with each hand. As it checks your weight, the BIA unit sends a low-voltage electrical current through your body and analyzes the speed at which the current travels. Checking your weight and body composition takes no longer than checking your weight alone. Most BIA units can remember your last weight and body composition measurement, making it easy to compare the measurements from day to day or week to week. Some scales can remember measurements for multiple people.

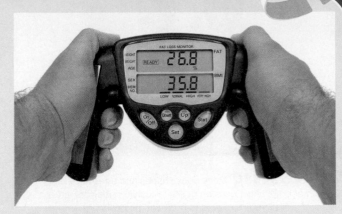

Lebazele/E+/Getty Images

A study of 22 weight-trained men showed that BIA compared favorably to underwater weighing for measuring body composition. Measurements of fat and lean mass are most valuable for measuring changes in body composition during diet and exercise programs.

Popular BIA scales and hand-held BIA devices are manufactured by Taylor, Whynter, Omron, Remedy, and Tanita. These scales and devices are available in most department stores and online, and cost between $30 and $200, depending on features.

in the morning and evening often differ. If you repeat the measurements to track changes in your body composition, measure skinfolds at approximately the same time of day.

Bioelectrical Impedance Analysis (BIA) The BIA technique works by sending a small electrical current through the body and measuring the body's resistance to it. Fat-free tissues, where most body water is located, are good conductors of electrical current, whereas fat is not (see the box "Using BIA at Home"). Thus, the resistance to electrical current is related to the amount of fat-free tissue in the body (the lower the resistance, the greater the fat-free mass) and can be used to estimate percent body fat.

Bioelectrical impedance analysis has an error rate of about ±4–5%. To reduce error, follow the manufacturer's instructions carefully and avoid overhydration or underhydration (having more or less body water than normal). Because measurement varies with the analyzer, use the same instrument to compare measurements over time.

Advanced Techniques: DEXA and TOBEC Dual-energy X-ray absorptiometry (DEXA) works by measuring the tissue absorption of high- and low-energy X-ray beams. The procedure has an error rate of about ±2%. Total body electrical conductivity (TOBEC) estimates lean body mass by passing a body through a magnetic field. These methods are often used in sophisticated research projects but are seldom available to the average person. We mention them because they are often used for comparison with some of the field tests described in this chapter.

Assessing Body Fat Distribution

Researchers have studied many methods for measuring body fat distribution. Two of the simplest to perform are waist circumference measurement and waist-to-hip ratio calculation. In the first method, you measure your waist circumference; in the second, you divide your waist circumference by your hip circumference. Waist circumference is a better indicator of abdominal fat than waist-to-hip ratio. More research is needed to determine the risk associated with specific values for these two assessments of body fat distribution. However, a total waist measurement over 40 inches (102 cm) for men and 35 inches (88 cm) for women and a waist-to-hip ratio above 0.94 for young men and 0.82 for young women are associated with an increased risk of heart disease and diabetes. Lab 6.1 shows you how to measure your body fat distribution.

Somatotype

Somatotype describes your basic body build. The three somatotypes are endomorph, mesomorph, and ectomorph:

- *Endomorphs* are round and pear shaped, with wide hips and shoulders. They gain weight easily and will typically regain weight rapidly if they resume their normal lifestyle after losing weight. Endomorphs often excel at weight lifting and might enjoy weight-supported aerobic exercises such as swimming or cycling. Conversely, they might find distance running difficult and painful.

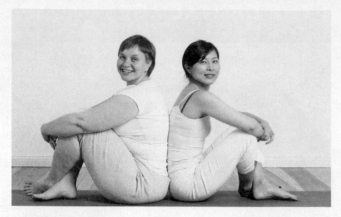

Wellness Tip Many body shapes and sizes are associated with good health. Focus on positive lifestyle behaviors rather than on unrealistic goals related to body weight or shape.

FredFroese/E+/Getty Images

- *Mesomorphs* are lean and muscular and respond well to exercise. They have wedged-shaped bodies, broad shoulders, narrow hips, and little body fat. They gain fitness easily and usually excel at almost any physical activity or sport.
- *Ectomorphs* are thin and linear, with narrow hips and shoulders. They typically have little muscle or fat. Their light frame helps make them successful in activities such as distance running and gymnastics.

Few people have extreme body types—most of us are a mixture of all three. People with every body type can benefit from physical activity.

SETTING BODY COMPOSITION GOALS

If assessment tests indicate that fat loss would be beneficial for your health, your first step is to establish a goal. You can use the ratings in Table 6.1 or Table 6.2 to choose a target value for BMI or percent body fat (depending on which assessment you completed).

Set a realistic goal that will ensure good health. Heredity limits your capacity to change your body composition, and few people can expect to develop the body of a fashion model or competitive bodybuilder. However, you can improve your body composition through a program of regular exercise and a healthy diet. If your body composition is in or close to the recommended range, set a lifestyle goal rather than a specific percent body fat or BMI goal. For example, you might set a goal of increasing your daily physical activity from 20 to 60 minutes or beginning a program of weight training, and then let any improvements in body composition occur as a secondary result of your primary target (physical activity). Remember, a lifestyle that includes regular exercise may be more important for health than trying to reach any ideal weight.

If you are significantly overfat or if you have known risk factors for disease (such as high blood pressure or high cholesterol), consult your physician to determine a body composition goal for your individual risk profile. For people who are obese, even small losses of body weight (5–15%) over a 6- to 12-month period can cause significant health improvements.

After you've established a body composition goal, you can then set a target range for body weight. Although body weight is not an accurate method of assessing body composition, it's a useful method for tracking progress in a program to change body composition. If you're losing a small or moderate amount of weight and exercising, you're probably losing fat while building muscle mass. Lab 6.2 will help you determine a range for recommended body weight.

Using percent body fat or BMI will generate a fairly accurate target body weight for most people. However, it's best not to stick rigidly to a recommended body weight calculated from any formula; individual genetic, cultural, and lifestyle factors are also important. Decide whether the body weight that the formulas generate for you is realistic, meets all your goals, is healthy, *and* is reasonable for you to maintain.

MAKING CHANGES IN BODY COMPOSITION

Chapter 9 includes specific strategies for losing or gaining weight and improving body composition. Lifestyle should be your focus—moderate energy intake, regular physical activity, endurance exercise, and strength training. For most people who lose weight and body fat, cutting calories is central during the weight loss phase, with physical activity playing a critical role for weight loss maintenance. In studies of people who have lost weight and maintained the loss, reduced calorie intake and increased physical activity are the keys to long-term success. In many studies, a combination approach—including dietary changes, endurance exercise, and resistance training—yields the best results for weight loss and improved body composition. But even absent significant changes in body composition, an active lifestyle improves wellness and decreases the risk of disease and premature death; see the box "Why Is Physical Activity Important Even If Body Composition Doesn't Change?"

You can track your progress toward your target body composition by checking your body weight regularly. Also, focus on how much energy you have and how your clothes fit. If feasible, you can also track risk factors such as waist measurement and blood glucose or cholesterol levels. To get a more accurate idea of your progress, reassess your body composition occasionally during your program: Body composition changes as weight changes, although body composition can change even if your weight remains the same. If you lose a significant amount of weight, you will usually lose both body fat and some muscle weight because muscles need not work as hard to move a lighter body. However, the decline in weight will favor fat loss, and the proportion of body fat will decline, meaning an improvement in body composition.

Many studies have found that engaging in exercise preserves muscle mass during weight loss; consuming adequate protein is also important. A short-term study by researchers in Canada had otherwise healthy overweight young men engage in a "boot camp" style program combining significant calorie restriction, high-intensity interval and weight training, and relatively high dietary protein intake; participants on average lost more than 10 pounds of fat and gained 2.4 pounds of lean tissue in four weeks. None of the participants wished to continue the regimen after the study period, but the researchers hope to develop a more sustainable program in the future; the results did point to the power of lifestyle changes to impact body composition. A 2017 review of studies on preserving healthy muscle during weight loss recommended a reduced-calorie diet with adequate protein in combination with increased physical activity; the review concluded that both endurance and resistance exercise help preserve muscle mass and that resistance exercise also builds strength. A complete exercise program is best for overall health as well as for developing and maintaining a healthy body composition.

TIPS FOR TODAY AND THE FUTURE

A wellness lifestyle can lead naturally to a body composition that is healthy and appropriate for you.

RIGHT NOW YOU CAN

- Find out what types of body composition assessment techniques are available at facilities on your campus or in your community.
- Do 30 minutes of physical activity five days per week—walk, jog, bike, swim, or climb stairs.
- Drink a glass of water instead of a soda, and include a high-fiber food such as whole-grain bread or cereal, popcorn, apples, berries, or beans in your next snack or meal.

IN THE FUTURE YOU CAN

- Think about your image of the ideal body type for your sex. Consider where your idea comes from, whether you use this image to judge your own body, and whether it is a realistic goal for you.
- Recognize media messages (especially visual images) that make you feel embarrassed or insecure about your body. Remind yourself that these messages are usually designed to sell a product; they should not form the basis of your body image.

SUMMARY

- The human body is composed of fat-free mass (which includes bone, muscle, organ tissues, and connective tissues) and body fat.

- Having too much body fat has negative health consequences, especially in terms of cardiovascular disease and diabetes. Distribution of fat is also a significant factor in health.

- A fit and healthy looking body, with the right body composition for a particular person, develops from habits of proper nutrition and exercise.

- Measuring body weight alone is not an accurate way to assess body composition because this measure does not differentiate between muscle weight and fat weight.

- Body mass index (calculated from weight and height measurements) and waist circumference can help classify the health risks associated with being overweight. BMI is sometimes inaccurate, however, particularly in muscular people.

- Techniques for estimating percent body fat include underwater weighing, the Bod Pod, skinfold measurements, bioelectrical impedance analysis (BIA), dual-energy X-ray absorptiometry (DEXA), and total body electrical conductivity (TOBEC).

- Body fat distribution can be assessed through waist measurement or the waist-to-hip ratio.

- Somatotype—endomorph (round), mesomorph (muscular), ectomorph (linear)—is a useful tool for describing basic body characteristics.

- You can determine a recommended body composition and weight by choosing a target BMI or target body fat percentage. Keep heredity in mind when setting a goal, and focus on positive changes in lifestyle.

FOR FURTHER EXPLORATION

Consumer Reports: Body Fat Scale Review: An Evaluation of Home Body-Fat Scales. The full report requires a membership with the Consumer Union.

https://www.consumerreports.org/body-fat-scales/body-fat-scale-review/

Georgia State University: The Exercise and Physical Fitness Page. Provides an excellent discussion of body composition assessment methods.

http://www2.gsu.edu/~wwwfit/bodycomp.html

National Health and Nutrition Examination Survey (NHANES). Ongoing survey and assessment of health status and practices in the United States.

http://www.cdc.gov/nchs/nhanes/new_nhanes.htm

National Heart, Lung, and Blood Institute: Obesity Education Initiative. Provides information on the latest federal obesity standards and a BMI calculator.

http://www.nhlbi.nih.gov/about/oei/index.htm

National Institute of Diabetes and Digestive and Kidney Diseases: Weight-control Information Network. Provides information about adult obesity: how it is defined and assessed, the risk factors associated with it, and its causes.

http://win.niddk.nih.gov

Robert Wood Johnson Foundation. Promotes the health and health care of Americans through research and distribution of information on healthy lifestyles. The foundation publishes an annual report on the status of the national obesity problem.

http://www.rwjf.org

USDA Food and Nutrition Information Center: Weight and Obesity. Provides links to recent reports and studies on the issue of obesity among Americans.

http://fnic.nal.usda.gov/weight-and-obesity

See also the listings for Chapters 2, 8, and 9.

THE EVIDENCE FOR EXERCISE
Why Is Physical Activity Important Even If Body Composition Doesn't Change?

Physical fitness and physical activity are important for health even if they produce little or no change in body composition—that is, even if a person remains overweight or obese. Physical activity and fitness confer benefits no matter how much you weigh; conversely, physical inactivity operates as a risk factor for health problems independently of body composition.

High fitness levels block many of the destructive effects of obesity. For example, cardiorespiratory fitness is linked to lower blood pressure, lower blood glucose and cholesterol levels, and improved body fat distribution. It also lowers the risk of cardiovascular disease, diabetes, and premature death. Although physical activity and fitness produce these improvements quickly in some people and slowly in others, due to genetic differences, the improvements do occur. Physical activity is important for the many people with *metabolic syndrome* or *prediabetes,* both of which are characterized by *insulin resistance.* Exercise improves blood sugar control. Exercise makes fat cells fit by improving the function of their mitochondria (powerhouses of the cell) and decreasing inflammation.

Although being physically active and not being sedentary may sound identical, experts describe them as different dimensions of the same health issue. Data suggest that it is important not only to be physically active but also to avoid prolonged sitting. In one study, people who watched TV or used a computer four or more hours a day had twice the risk of having metabolic syndrome as those who spent less than one hour a day in these activities; other studies reported similar results. Increasing physical activity and avoiding or reducing sedentary behavior are both important and challenging health goals.

Physical activity, then, is important even if it doesn't change body composition. Large population studies show that moderate to high levels of cardiorespiratory fitness reduce the risk of heart disease, diabetes, and premature death in obese people. Fit but fat people are largely spared from the health risks of a high body mass index.

The question is sometimes asked: Which is more important in combating the adverse health effects of obesity—physical activity or physical fitness? Many studies suggest that both are important; the more active and fit you are, the lower your risk of having health problems and dying prematurely. Of the two, however, physical fitness is most critical for long-term health and longevity. You can build fitness by meeting the recommended exercise goal of the equivalent of 150 minutes per week of moderate-intensity exercise or 75 minutes per week or high-intensity exercise.

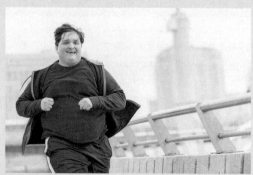

Kali9/E+/Getty Images

SOURCES: Blair-Kennedy, A., et al. 2018. "Fitness or fatness. Which is more important?" *Journal American Medical Association* 319(3): 231–232; Gaesser, G., and S. Blair. 2019. "The health risks of obesity have been exaggerated." *Medicine & Science in Sport & Exercise* 51(1): 218–221; Ortega, F. B., et al. 2018. "Role of physical activity and fitness and in the characterization and prognosis of the metabolically healthy obesity phenotype: A systematic review and meta-analysis." *Progress in Cardiovascular Disease* 61: 190–205.

SELECTED BIBLIOGRAPHY

Aatashak, S., et al. 2016. Cardiovascular risk factors adaptation to concurrent training in overweight sedentary middle-aged men. *Journal of Sports Medicine and Physical Fitness* 56(5): 624–630.

American College of Sports Medicine. 2018. *ACSM's Guidelines for Exercise Testing and Prescription,* 10th ed. Philadelphia: Wolters Kluwer.

Ashwell, M., and S. Gibson. 2014. A proposal for a primary screening tool: "Keep your waist circumference to less than half your height." *BMC Medicine* 12: 207.

Aune, D., et al. 2016. BMI and all cause mortality: Systematic review and non-linear dose-response meta-analysis of 230 cohort studies with 3.74 million deaths among 30.3 million participants. *BMJ* 353:i2156. doi:10.1136/bmj.i2156

Becroft, L., et al. 2018. Validity of multi-frequency bioelectric impedance methods to measure body composition in obese patients: A systematic review. *International Journal of Obesity.* Published online.

Blair-Kennedy, A., et al. 2018. Fitness or fatness. Which is more important? *Journal American Medical Association* 319(3): 231–232.

Cava, E., N. C. Yeat, and B. Mittendorfer. 2017. Preserving healthy muscle during weight loss. *Advances in Nutrition* 8(3): 511–519.

Cavedon, V., et al. 2018. Anthropometric prediction of DXA-measured body composition in female team handball players. *PeerJ* 6: e5913.

Ceniccola, G. D., et al. 2018. Current technologies in body composition assessment: Advantages and disadvantages. *Nutrition* 62: 25–31.

Deiseroth, A., et al. 2018. Influence of body composition and physical fitness on arterial stiffness after marathon running. *Scandinavian Journal Medicine Science in Sports* 28(12): 2651–2658.

Estrella, M. L., et al. 2019. Correlates of and body composition measures associated with metabolically healthy obesity phenotype in Hispanic/Latino women and men: The Hispanic Community Health Study/Study of Latinos (HCHS/SOL). *Journal of Obesity* 2019: 1251456.

Fahey, T., and M. Fahey. 2014. Nutrition, physical activity, and the obesity epidemic: Issues, policies, and solutions (1960s–present). In T. Oliver, ed., *The Guide to U.S. Health and Health Care Policy,* pp. 363–374. New York: DWJ Books.

Fothergill, E., et al. 2016. Persistent metabolic adaptation 6 years after "The Biggest Loser" competition. *Obesity* 24(8): 1612–1619.

Fryar, C. D., D. Kruszon-Moran, Q. Gu, and C. L. Ogden. 2018. Mean body weight, height, waist circumference, and body mass index among adults: United States, 1999–2000 through 2015–2016. *National Health Statistics Reports,* No 122. Hyattsville, MD: National Center for Health Statistics.

COMMON QUESTIONS ANSWERED

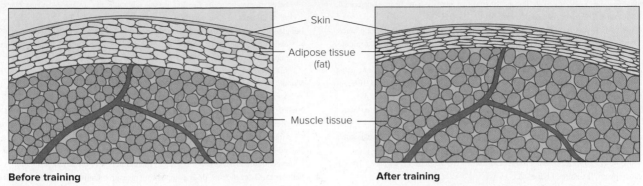

Before training | After training

Effects of Exercise on Body Composition. Endurance exercise and strength training both reduce body fat and increase muscle mass.

Q **Is spot reducing effective?**

A *Spot reducing* refers to attempts to lose body fat in specific parts of the body by doing exercises for those parts. Danish researchers have shown that fat use increases in adipose tissue surrounding active muscle, but it is not known if short-term fat use helps reduce fat in specific sites. Most studies show that spot-reducing exercises contribute to fat loss only to the extent that they burn calories. The best way to reduce fat in any specific area is to create an overall negative energy balance: Take in less energy (food) than you use through exercise and metabolism.

Q **How does exercise affect body composition?**

A Cardiorespiratory endurance exercise burns calories, thereby helping create a negative energy balance. Weight training does not use many calories and therefore is of little use in creating a negative energy balance. However, weight training increases muscle mass, which maintains a higher metabolic rate (the body's rate of energy use) and helps improve body composition. To minimize body fat and increase muscle mass, thereby improving body composition, combine cardiorespiratory endurance exercise and weight training (see figure).

Q **Are people who have a desirable body composition physically fit?**

A Having a healthy body composition is not necessarily associated with overall fitness. For example, many bodybuilders have very little body fat but have poor cardiorespiratory capacity and flexibility. Some athletes, such as NFL linemen, weigh 300 pounds or more; they have to lose the weight when they retire if they don't want to jeopardize their health. To be fit, you must rate high on all the components of fitness.

Q **What is liposuction, and will it help me lose body fat?**

A Suction lipectomy, popularly known as *liposuction,* has become the most popular type of elective surgery in the world. The procedure involves removing limited amounts of fat from specific areas. Typically, no more than 2.5 kilograms (5.5 pounds) of adipose tissue are removed at a time. The procedure is usually successful if the amount of excess fat is limited and skin elasticity is good. The procedure is most effective if integrated into a program of dietary restriction and exercise. Side effects include infection, dimpling, and wavy skin contours. Liposuction has a death rate of 1 in 5,000 patients, primarily from pulmonary thromboembolism (a blood clot in the lungs) or fat embolism (circulatory blockage caused by a dislodged piece of fat). In contrast, the death rate for all other surgeries performed in the United States is 1 in 100,000. Other serious complications include shock, bleeding, and impaired blood flow to vital organs.

Q **What is cellulite, and how do I get rid of it?**

A *Cellulite* is the name commonly given to rippling, wavy fat deposits that collect just under the skin. The "cottage cheese" appearance stems from the breakdown of tissues supporting the fat. These rippling fat deposits are really the same as fat deposited anywhere else in the body. The only way to control them is to create a negative energy balance—that is, burn more calories than you take in. There are no creams or lotions that will rub away surface (subcutaneous) fat deposits, and spot reducing is also ineffective. The solution is sensible eating habits and exercise.

Funk, L. M., et al. 2017. Electronic health record data versus the National Health and Nutrition Examination Survey (NHANES); a comparison of overweight and obesity rates. *Medical Care* 55(6): 598-605.

Gaesser, G., and S. Blair. 2019. The health risks of obesity have been exaggerated. *Medicine & Science in Sport & Exercise* 51(1): 218-221.

Gonzalez, M. C., et al. 2018. Body composition using bioelectrical impedance: Development and validation of a predictive equation for fat-free mass in a middle-income country. *Clinical Nutrition.* Published online.

Goto, K., et al. 2018. Longitudinal changes and body composition assessment using bioelectrical impedance in elderly patients with mild disequilibrium and different care needs. *Journal of Physical Therapy Science* 30(12): 1473-1476.

Griffith, J. R., et al. 2018. Comparison of body composition metrics for United States Air Force Airmen. *Military Medicine* 183(3-4): e201-e207.

Hales, C. M., et al. 2017. Prevalence of obesity among adults and youth: United States 2015-2016. *National Center Health Statistics Data Brief,* No. 288.

Heyward, V. H. 2014. *Advanced Fitness Assessment and Exercise Prescription,* 7th ed. Champaign, IL: Human Kinetics.

Hong, H. O., and B. A. Lee. 2016. The effects of the academic performance of college students whose major is sports on body composition and abdominal fat rates. *Journal of Exercise Rehabilitation* 12(4): 328-332.

Hopkins, M., and J. E. Blundell. 2016. Energy balance, body composition, sedentariness and appetite regulation: Pathways to obesity. *Clinical Science* 130(18): 1615-1628.

Joy, E., et al. 2014. 2014 Female Athlete Triad Coalition consensus statement on treatment and return to play of the female athlete triad. *Current Sports Medicine Reports* 13(4): 219-232.

Kee, C. C., et al. 2017. Association of BMI with risk of CVD mortality and all-cause mortality. *Public Health Nutrition* 12: 1-9.

Kim, S., et al. 2016. Reappraisal of waist circumference cutoff value according to general obesity. *Nutrition & Metabolism* 13: 26.

Kiviruusu, O., et al. 2016. Self-esteem and body mass index from adolescence to mid-adulthood. A 26-year follow-up. *International Journal of Behavioral Medicine* 23(3): 355-363.

Lang, P. O., et al. 2015. Markers of metabolic and cardiovascular health in adults: Comparative analysis of DEXA-based body composition components and BMI categories. *Journal of Cardiology* 65(1): 42-49.

Lee, K., et al. 2019. Recent issues on body composition imaging for sarcopenia evaluation. *Korean Journal of Radiology* 20(2): 205-217.

Lee, S., and S. Arslanian. 2019. Body composition and cardiorespiratory fitness between metabolically healthy versus metabolically unhealthy obese black and white adolescents. *Journal Adolescent Health* 64(3): 327-332.

Longland, T. M., et al. 2016. Higher compared to lower dietary protein during an energy deficit combined with intense exercise promotes greater lean mass gain and fat mass loss: A randomized trial. *American Journal of Clinical Nutrition* 103: 738-746.

Mundi, M. S., et al. 2019. Body composition technology: Implications for the ICU. *Nutrition in Clinical Practice* 34(1): 48-58.

Nichols, G. A., et al. 2017. Cardiometabolic risk factors among 1.3 million adults with overweight or obesity, but not diabetes, in 10 geographically diverse regions of the United States, 2012-2013. *Preventing Chronic Diseases* 14: E22.

Ostendorf, D. M., et al. 2019. Physical activity energy expenditure and total daily energy expenditure in successful weight loss maintainers. *Obesity* 27(3): 496-504.

Pellonpera, O., et al. 2019. Body composition measurement by air displacement plethysmography in pregnancy: Comparison of predicted versus measured thoracic gas volume. *Nutrition* 60: 227-229.

Porto, L. G., et al. 2016. Agreement between BMI and body fat obesity definitions in a physically active population. *Archives of Endocrinology and Metabolism* 60(6): 515-525.

Reynolds, G. 2016. A diet and exercise plan to lose weight and gain muscle. *New York Times* (https://well.blogs.nytimes.com/2016/02/03/a-diet-and-exercise-plan-to-lose-weight-and-gain-muscle).

Tian, S., et al. 2016: Age-related changes in segmental body composition by ethnicity and history of weight change across the lifespan. *International Journal of Environmental Research and Public Health* 13: 821-838.

U.S. Department of Agriculture, Agricultural Research Service. 2018. Nutrient intakes from food and beverages: Mean amounts consumed per individual, by gender and age. *What We Eat in America,* National Health and Nutrition Examination Survey (NHANES) 2015-2016.

Weiss, E. P., et al. 2017. Effects of weight loss on lean mass, strength, bone, and aerobic capacity. *Medicine and Science in Sports and Exercise* 49(1): 206-217.

Xu, H., L. A. Cupples, A. Stokes, and C.-T. Liu. 2018. Association of obesity with mortality over 24 years of weight history: Findings from the Framingham Heart Study. *JAMA Network Open* 1(7): e184587.

Name _____ Section _____ Date _____

LAB 6.1 Assessing Body Mass Index and Body Composition

Body Mass Index

Equipment

1. Weight scale

2. Tape measure or other means of measuring height

Instructions

Measure your height and weight, and record the results. Be sure to record the unit of measurement.

Height: _____ Weight: _____

Calculating BMI (see also the shortcut chart of BMI values in Lab 6.2)

1. Convert your body weight to kilograms by dividing your weight in pounds by 2.2.

   Body weight _____ lb ÷ 2.2 lb/kg = body weight _____ kg

2. Convert your height measurement to meters by multiplying your height in inches by 0.0254.

   Height _____ in. × 0.0254 m/in. = height _____ m

3. Square your height measurement.

   Height _____ m × height _____ m = height m^2

4. BMI equals body weight in kilograms divided by height in meters squared (kg/m^2).

   Body weight _____ kg ÷ height _____ m^2 = BMI _____ kg/m^2
              (from step 1)   (from step 3)

Rating Your BMI

Refer to the table for a rating of your BMI. Record the results here and on the final page of this lab.

Classification	BMI (kg/m^2)
Underweight	<18.5
Normal	18.5–24.9
Overweight	25.0–29.9
Obesity (I)	30.0–34.9
Obesity (II)	35.0–39.9
Extreme obesity (III)	≥40.0

BMI _____ kg/m^2

Classification _____

Skinfold Measurements

Equipment

1. Skinfold caliper

2. Partner to take measurements

3. Marking pen (optional)

LABORATORY ACTIVITIES

Instructions

1. *Select and locate the correct sites for measurement.* All measurements should be taken on the right side of the body with the subject standing. Skinfolds are normally measured on the natural fold line of the skin, either vertically or at a slight angle. The skinfold measurement sites for males are chest, abdomen, and thigh; for females, triceps, suprailium, and thigh. If the person taking skinfold measurements is inexperienced, it may be helpful to mark the correct sites with a marking pen.

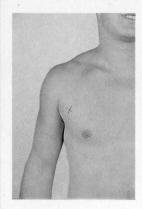 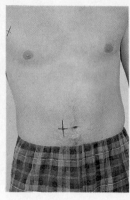 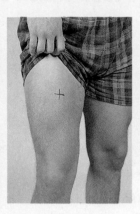 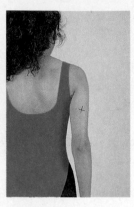 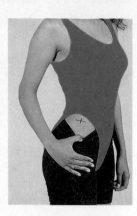

(a) Chest   (b) Abdomen   (c) Thigh   (d) Triceps   (e) Suprailium

(all): Photo taken by Shirlee Stevens

(a) *Chest.* Pinch a diagonal fold halfway between the nipple and the shoulder crease. (b) *Abdomen.* Pinch a vertical fold about 1 inch to the right of the umbilicus (navel). (c) *Thigh.* Pinch a vertical fold midway between the top of the hipbone and the kneecap. (d) *Triceps.* Pinch a vertical skinfold on the back of the right arm midway between the shoulder and elbow. The arm should be straight and should hang naturally. (e) *Suprailium.* Pinch a fold at the top front of the right hipbone. The skinfold here is taken slightly diagonally according to the natural fold tendency of the skin.

2. *Measure the appropriate skinfolds.* Pinch a fold of skin between your thumb and forefinger. Pull the fold up so that no muscular tissue is included; don't pinch the skinfold too hard. Hold the calipers perpendicular to the fold and measure the skinfold about 0.25 inch away from your fingers. Allow the tips of the calipers to close on the skinfold and let the reading settle before marking it down. Take readings to the nearest half-millimeter. Continue to repeat the measurements until two consecutive measurements match, releasing and repinching the skinfold between each measurement. Make a note of the final measurement for each site.

Time of day of measurements: _____

Men	*Women*
Chest: _____ mm	Triceps: _____ mm
Abdomen: _____ mm	Suprailium: _____ mm
Thigh: _____ mm	Thigh: _____ mm

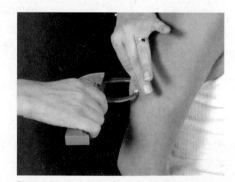

Photo taken by Wayne Glusker

Determining Percent Body Fat

Add the measurements of your three skinfolds. Use this sum as a point of comparison for future assessments and/or to find the percent body fat that corresponds to your total in the appropriate table. For example, a 20-year-old female with measurements of 17 mm, 21 mm, and 22 mm would have a skinfold sum of 60 mm; according to the following table, her percent body fat is 23.5. The table lists ages in increments of five. If your age is not listed on the table, use the column for the age closest to your own.

Sum of three skinfolds: _____ mm   Percent body fat: _____ %

Prediction of Fat Percentage in Females from the Sum of Three Skinfolds

Sum of Skinfolds (mm)	Age (Years)								
	20	*25*	*30*	*35*	*40*	*45*	*50*	*55*	*60 and over*
20	9.3	9.6	9.9	10.2	10.5	10.8	11.1	11.4	11.7
25	11.2	11.5	11.8	12.1	12.4	12.7	13.0	13.3	13.6
30	13.1	13.4	13.7	14.0	14.3	14.6	14.9	15.2	15.5
35	14.9	15.2	15.5	15.8	16.1	16.4	16.7	17.0	17.3
40	16.7	17.0	17.3	17.6	17.9	18.2	18.5	18.8	19.1
45	18.4	18.8	19.1	19.4	19.7	20.0	20.3	20.6	20.9
50	20.2	20.5	20.8	21.1	21.4	21.7	22.0	22.4	22.7
55	21.9	22.2	22.5	22.8	23.1	23.4	23.7	24.1	24.4
60	23.5	23.8	24.1	24.4	24.8	25.1	25.4	25.7	26.0
65	25.1	25.4	25.7	26.1	26.4	26.7	27.0	27.3	27.7
70	26.7	27.0	27.3	27.6	27.9	28.3	28.6	28.9	29.2
75	28.2	28.5	28.8	29.1	29.5	29.8	30.1	30.4	30.8
80	29.7	30.0	30.3	30.6	31.0	31.3	31.6	31.9	32.3
85	31.1	31.4	31.7	32.1	32.4	32.7	33.0	33.4	33.7
90	32.5	32.8	33.1	33.5	33.8	34.1	34.4	34.8	35.1
95	33.8	34.1	34.5	34.8	35.1	35.5	35.8	36.1	36.5
100	35.1	35.4	35.8	36.1	36.4	36.8	37.1	37.4	37.8
105	36.3	36.7	37.0	37.3	37.7	38.0	38.3	38.7	39.0
110	37.5	37.9	38.2	38.5	38.9	39.2	39.5	39.9	40.2
115	38.7	39.0	39.3	39.7	40.0	40.4	40.7	41.0	41.4
120	39.8	40.1	40.4	40.8	41.1	41.5	41.8	42.1	42.5
125	40.8	41.2	41.5	41.8	42.2	42.5	42.9	43.2	43.5
130	41.8	42.1	42.5	42.8	43.2	43.5	43.9	44.2	44.5
135	42.7	43.1	43.4	43.8	44.1	44.5	44.8	45.1	45.5

NOTE: Find the value on the chart that most closely corresponds to your age and the sum of measurement skinfolds. To calculate the value more precisely, plug your age and sum of skinfolds into the appropriate formula:

% Body Fat = ([4.95 ÷ [1.0994921 − (.0009929 × sum of skinfolds) + (.0000023 × the square of sum of skinfolds) − (.0001392 × age)] − 4.5} × 100), where the skinfold sites (measured in mm) are triceps, suprailium, and thigh

SOURCES: Jackson, A. S., M. L. Pollock, and A. Ward. 1980. "Generalized equations for predicting body density in women," *Medicine and Science in Sports and Exercise*, vol. 12: 175–182; Seri, W. E. 1956. "Gross composition of the body," *Advances in Biological and Medical Physics*, 4ed, ed. J. H. Lawrence and C. A. Tobias. New York: Academic Press; Seri, W. E. 1956. "The gross composition of the body," *Advances in Biological and Medical Physics* 4: 239–280. (https://doi.org/10.1016/B978-1-4832-3110-5.50011-X).

LABORATORY ACTIVITIES

Prediction of Fat Percentage in Males from the Sum of Three Skinfolds

Sum of Skinfolds (mm)	Age (Years)								
	20	25	30	35	40	45	50	55	60 and over
10	1.6	2.1	2.7	3.2	3.7	4.3	4.8	5.3	5.9
15	3.2	3.8	4.3	4.8	5.4	5.9	6.4	7.0	7.5
20	4.8	5.4	5.9	6.4	7.0	7.5	8.1	8.6	9.2
25	6.4	6.9	7.5	8.0	8.6	9.1	9.7	10.2	10.8
30	8.0	8.5	9.1	9.6	10.2	10.7	11.3	11.8	12.4
35	9.5	10.0	10.6	11.2	11.7	12.3	12.8	13.4	13.9
40	11.0	11.6	12.1	12.7	13.2	13.8	14.4	14.9	15.5
45	12.5	13.1	13.6	14.2	14.7	15.3	15.9	16.4	17.0
50	14.0	14.5	15.1	15.6	16.2	16.8	17.3	17.9	18.5
55	15.4	16.0	16.5	17.1	17.7	18.2	18.8	19.4	19.9
60	16.8	17.4	17.9	18.5	19.1	19.7	20.2	20.8	21.4
65	18.2	18.8	19.3	19.9	20.5	21.1	21.6	22.2	22.8
70	19.5	20.1	20.7	21.3	21.9	22.4	23.0	23.6	24.2
75	20.9	21.5	22.0	22.6	23.2	23.8	24.4	24.9	25.5
80	22.2	22.8	23.3	23.9	24.5	25.1	25.7	26.3	26.9
85	23.4	24.0	24.6	25.2	25.8	26.4	27.0	27.6	28.2
90	24.7	25.3	25.9	26.5	27.0	27.6	28.2	28.8	29.4
95	25.9	26.5	27.1	27.7	28.3	28.9	29.5	30.1	30.7
100	27.1	27.7	28.3	28.9	29.5	30.1	30.7	31.3	31.9
105	28.2	28.8	29.4	30.0	30.6	31.2	31.8	32.4	33.0
110	29.3	29.9	30.5	31.1	31.7	32.4	33.0	33.6	34.2
115	30.4	31.0	31.6	32.2	32.8	33.5	34.1	34.7	35.3
120	31.5	32.1	32.7	33.3	33.9	34.5	35.1	35.7	36.4
125	32.5	33.1	33.7	34.3	34.9	35.6	36.2	36.8	37.4

NOTE: Find the value on the chart that most closely corresponds to your age and the sum of measurement skinfolds. To calculate the value more precisely, plug your age and sum of skinfolds into the appropriate formula:

% Body Fat = ([4.95 ÷ [1.109380 − (.0008267 × sum of skinfolds) + (.0000016 × square of the sum of skinfolds) − (.0002574 × age)] − 4.5] × 100), where the skinfold sites (measured in mm) are chest, abdomen, and thigh

SOURCES: Jackson, A. S., and M. L. Pollock. 1978. "Generalized equations for predicting body density in men," *British Journal of Nutrition*, vol. 40, no. 3: 497–504; Jackson, A. S., M. L. Pollock, and A. Ward. 1980. "Generalized equations for predicting body density in women," *Medicine and Science in Sports and Exercise*, vol. 12, no. 3: 175–182; Seri, W. E. 1956. "Gross composition of the body," *Advances in Biological and Medical Physics*, 4ed, ed. J. H. Lawrence and C. A. Tobias. New York: Academic Press: 239–280. https://doi.org/10.1016/B978-1-4832-3110-5.50011-X.

Bioelectrical Impedance Analysis (BIA)

Equipment

A bioelectrical impedance analyzer such as Omron Body Fat Analyzer: The BIA device sends an extremely weak electrical current through your body to determine the amount of total body water. You will not feel the current during the test. The body fat percentage is calculated from a formula that uses body water, electric resistance, height, weight, age, and gender.

Instructions

1. Enter your height, weight, gender, and age into the BIA device.

2. Grasp the left and right handles and wrap your middle finger around the groove in the handle. With your thumbs facing up and resting on the unit, place the palms of your hands on the top and bottom electrodes.

3. Hold your arms straight out at a 90-degree angle to your body.

4. Confirm the ready to measure display and the **READY** indicator turns on. Push the start button and the display **START** turns on. The unit automatically detects that it is held and starts measurement. Do not move during measurement.

5. Record your fat, percent fat, and fat-free weight.

   Fat: _____

   Percent fat: _____

   Fat-free weight: _____

6. Compare the BIA measurements with other techniques of assessing body composition.

U.S. Navy Circumference Method of Measuring Percent Fat

This method measures fat percentage from abdominal circumference, neck circumference, and height in men, and from abdominal circumference, hip circumference, neck circumference, and height in women.

Equipment

1. Measuring tape

2. Stadiometer or tape on wall to measure height

Instructions

1. Measure height without shoes using a stadiometer or tape measure. A stadiometer is a height-measuring device that is often part of a scale found in a gym or physician's office.

   Height (inches): _____

2. Measure neck circumference below the larynx (Adam's apple), with the tape sloping slightly downward at the front.

   Neck circumference (inches): _____

3. Measure waist circumference at navel level for men and at the smallest point for women.

   Waist circumference (inches): _____

4. Measure hip circumference (women only) at the largest point.

   Hip circumference (inches): _____

Calculating percent fat using charts developed by the U.S. Navy

Men:

Calculate circumference value: Abdominal circumference − neck circumference: _____

Read percent fat from the chart from where the circumference value intersects with height. Enter fat percentage: _____

Women:

Calculate circumference value: Abdominal circumference + hip circumference − neck circumference (in inches): _____

Read percent fat from the chart from where the circumference value intersects with height. Enter fat percentage: _____

LABORATORY ACTIVITIES

U.S. Navy Circumference Chart for Predicting Percent Fat in Men

Circumference	Height (inches)																				
	60	61	62	63	64	65	66	67	68	69	70	71	72	73	74	75	76	77	78	79	80
13	8	8	7	7	6	6	5	5	4	4	3	3									
14	11	10	10	9	9	8	8	7	7	7	6	6	5	5	4	4	4	3	3		
15	13	13	12	12	11	11	10	10	10	9	9	8	8	7	7	7	6	6	5	5	5
16	16	15	15	14	14	13	13	12	12	12	11	11	10	10	9	9	9	8	8	7	7
17	18	18	17	17	16	16	15	15	14	14	13	13	13	12	12	11	11	10	10	10	9
18	20	20	19	19	18	18	17	17	16	16	15	15	15	14	14	13	13	13	12	12	11
19	22	22	21	21	20	20	19	19	18	18	18	17	17	16	16	15	15	15	14	14	13
20	24	24	23	23	22	22	21	21	20	20	19	19	19	18	18	17	17	17	16	16	15
21	26	25	25	24	24	24	23	23	22	22	21	21	20	20	20	19	19	18	18	18	17
22	28	27	27	26	26	25	25	24	24	23	23	23	22	22	21	21	20	20	20	19	19
23	29	29	28	28	27	27	26	26	26	25	25	24	24	23	23	23	22	22	21	21	21
24	31	30	30	29	29	28	28	28	27	27	26	26	25	25	25	24	24	23	23	23	22
25	32	32	31	31	30	30	30	29	29	28	28	27	27	26	26	26	25	25	24	24	24
26	34	33	33	32	32	31	31	31	30	30	29	29	28	28	28	27	27	26	26	26	25
27	35	35	34	34	33	33	32	32	32	31	31	30	30	29	29	29	28	28	27	27	27
28	37	36	36	35	35	34	34	33	33	32	32	32	31	31	30	30	29	29	29	28	28
29	38	37	37	37	36	36	35	35	34	34	33	33	32	32	32	31	31	30	30	30	29
30	39	39	38	38	37	37	36	36	35	35	35	34	34	33	33	32	32	32	31	31	31
31	40	40	39	39	39	38	38	37	37	36	36	35	35	35	34	34	33	33	33	32	32
32	42	41	41	40	40	39	39	38	38	37	37	37	36	36	35	35	34	34	34	33	33
33	43	42	42	41	41	40	40	39	39	39	38	38	37	37	36	36	36	35	35	34	34
34	44	43	43	42	42	42	41	41	40	40	39	39	38	38	38	37	37	36	36	36	35
35	45	45	44	44	43	43	42	42	41	41	40	40	39	39	39	38	38	37	37	37	36

U.S. Navy Circumference Chart for Predicting Percent Fat in Women

Circumference	Height (inches)																				
	58	59	60	61	62	63	64	65	66	67	68	69	70	71	72	73	74	75	76	77	78
45	19	18	18	17	16	16	15	14	14	13	12	12	11	11	10	9	9	8	8		
46	21	20	19	19	18	17	17	16	15	15	14	13	13	12	12	11	10	10	9	9	8
47	22	22	21	20	19	19	18	17	17	16	16	15	14	14	13	12	12	11	11	10	10
48	24	23	22	22	21	20	20	19	18	18	17	16	16	15	15	14	13	13	12	12	11
49	25	24	24	23	22	22	21	20	20	19	18	18	17	17	16	15	15	14	14	13	13
50	27	26	25	24	24	23	22	22	21	21	20	19	19	18	17	17	16	16	15	15	14
51	28	27	27	26	25	25	24	23	23	22	21	21	20	19	19	18	18	17	17	16	15
52	29	29	28	27	27	26	25	25	24	23	23	22	21	21	20	20	19	19	18	17	17
53	31	30	29	29	28	27	27	26	25	25	24	23	23	22	22	21	20	20	19	19	18
54	32	31	31	30	29	29	28	27	27	26	25	25	24	24	23	22	22	21	21	20	20
55	33	33	32	31	31	30	29	29	28	27	27	26	25	25	24	24	23	22	22	21	21
56	35	34	33	33	32	31	30	30	29	29	28	27	27	26	25	25	24	24	23	23	22
57	36	35	34	34	33	32	32	31	30	30	29	29	28	27	27	26	26	25	24	24	23
58	37	36	36	35	34	34	33	32	32	31	30	30	29	29	28	27	27	26	26	25	25
59	38	38	37	36	36	35	34	34	33	32	32	31	30	30	29	29	28	27	27	26	26
60	40	39	38	37	37	36	35	35	34	33	33	32	32	31	30	30	29	29	28	28	27
61	41	40	39	39	38	37	37	36	35	35	34	33	33	32	32	31	30	30	29	29	28
62	42	41	40	40	39	38	38	37	36	36	35	35	34	33	33	32	32	31	30	30	29
63	43	42	42	41	40	40	39	38	38	37	36	36	35	34	34	33	33	32	32	31	30
64	44	43	43	42	41	41	40	39	39	38	37	37	36	36	35	34	34	33	33	32	32
65	45	45	44	43	42	42	41	40	40	39	38	38	37	37	36	35	35	34	34	33	33
66	46	46	45	44	43	43	42	41	41	40	40	39	38	38	37	37	36	35	35	34	34
67	47	47	46	45	45	44	43	43	42	41	41	40	39	39	38	38	37	36	36	35	35
68	48	48	47	46	46	45	44	44	43	42	42	41	40	40	39	39	38	38	37	36	36
69	49	49	48	47	47	46	45	45	44	43	43	42	41	41	40	40	39	39	38	37	37
70	50	50	49	48	48	47	46	46	45	44	44	43	43	42	41	41	40	40	39	38	38
71	51	51	50	49	49	48	47	47	46	45	45	44	44	43	42	42	41	41	40	39	39
72	52	52	51	50	50	49	48	48	47	46	46	45	45	44	43	43	42	42	41	40	40
73	53	53	52	51	51	50	49	49	48	47	47	46	45	45	44	44	43	43	42	41	41
74	54	54	53	52	52	51	50	50	49	48	48	47	46	46	45	45	44	44	43	42	42
75	55	55	54	53	53	52	51	51	50	49	49	48	47	47	46	46	45	44	44	43	43

SOURCE: Hodgdon, J. A., and K. Friedl. 1998. *Development of the DoD Body Composition Estimation Equations.* Washington, D.C.: Bureau of Medicine and Surgery, Naval Health Research Center. Technical Document 99–2B.

Rating Your Body Composition

Refer to the following chart to rate your percent body fat. Record it here and in the chart at the end of this lab.

Rating: _____

Percent Body Fat Classification

	Percent Body Fat (%)				Percent Body Fat (%)		
	20–39 Years	*40–59 Years*	*60–79 Years*		*20–39 Years*	*40–59 Years*	*60–79 Years*
Women				**Men**			
Essential*	8–12	8–12	8–12	Essential*	3–5	3–5	3–5
Low/athletic**	13–20	13–22	13–23	Low/athletic**	6–7	6–10	6–12
Recommended	21–32	23–33	24–35	Recommended	8–19	11–21	13–24
Overfat†	33–38	34–39	36–41	Overfat†	20–24	22–27	25–29
Obese†	≥39	≥40	≥42	Obese†	≥25	≥28	≥30

NOTE: The cutoffs for recommended, overfat, and obese ranges in this table are based on a study that linked BMI classifications from the NIH with predicted percent body fat (measured using dual-energy X-ray absorptiometry).

*Essential body fat is necessary for the basic functioning of the body.

**Percent body fat in the low/athletic range may be appropriate for some people as long as it is not the result of illness or disordered eating habits.

†Health risks increase as percent body fat exceeds the recommended range.

SOURCES: Gallagher, D., et al. 2013. "Healthy percentage body fat ranges: An approach for developing guidelines based on body mass index," *American Journal of Clinical Nutrition*, vol 72, no. 3: 694–701; Swain, D. P. 2013. *ACSM's Resource Manual for Guidelines for Exercise Testing and Prescription*, 7th ed. Philadelphia: Lippincott Williams & Wilkins.

Other Methods of Assessing Percent Body Fat

If you use a different method, record the name of the method and the result here and in the chart at the end of this lab. Find your body composition rating on the previous chart.

Method used: _____ Percent body fat: _____

% Rating (from previous chart): _____

Body Fat Distribution

Waist Circumference and Waist-to-Hip Ratio

Equipment

1. Tape measure
2. Partner to take measurements

Preparation

Wear clothes that will not add significantly to your measurements.

Instructions

Stand with your feet together and your arms at your sides. Raise your arms only high enough to allow for taking the measurements. Your partner should make sure the tape is horizontal around the entire circumference and pulled snugly against your skin. The tape shouldn't be pulled so tight that it causes indentations in your skin. Record measurements to the nearest millimeter or one-sixteenth of an inch.

Waist. Measure at the smallest waist circumference. If you don't have a natural waist, measure at the level of your navel.

Waist measurement: _____

Hip. Measure at the largest hip circumference. Hip measurement: _____

Waist-to-Hip Ratio: You can use any unit of measurement (e.g., inches or centimeters) as long as you are consistent. Waist-to-hip ratio equals waist measurement divided by hip measurement.

Waist-to-hip ratio: ÷ _____ = _____ _____

            (hip measurement)   **(waist measurement)**

LABORATORY ACTIVITIES

Determining Your Risk

The following table indicates values for waist circumference and waist-to-hip ratio above which the risk of health problems increases significantly. If your measurement or ratio is above either cutoff point, put a check on the appropriate line here and in the chart at the end of this lab.

Waist circumference: _____ (✓ high risk) Waist-to-hip ratio: _____ (✓ high risk)

Body Fat Distribution

Cutoff Points for High Risk

	Waist Circumference	Waist-to-Hip Ratio
Men	More than 40 in. (102 cm)	More than 0.94
Women	More than 35 in. (88 cm)	More than 0.82

SOURCE: National Heart, Lung, and Blood Institute. 1998. *Clinical Guidelines on the Identification, Evaluation, and Treatment of Overweight and Obesity in Adults: The Evidence Report.* Bethesda, MD: National Institutes of Health; Heyward, V. H., and D. R. Wagner. 2004. *Applied Body Composition Assessment,* 2nd ed. Champaign, IL.: Human Kinetics.

Rating Your Body Mass Index, Body Composition, and Body Fat Distribution

Assessment	Value	Classification
BMI	_____ kg/m^2	_____
Skinfold measurements or alternative method of determining percent body fat. Specify method: _____	_____ % body fat	_____
Bioelectrical Impedance Analysis (BIA)	_____ % body fat	_____
U.S. Navy Circumference Method	_____ % body fat	_____
Waist circumference	_____ in. or cm	_____ (✓ high risk)
Waist-to-hip ratio	_____ (ratio)	_____ (✓ high risk)

Using Your Results

How did you score? Are you surprised by your ratings for body composition and body fat distribution? Are your current ratings in the range for good health? Are you satisfied with your current body composition? Why or why not?

If you're not satisfied, set a realistic goal for improvement:

What should you do next? Enter the results of this lab in the Preprogram Assessment column in Appendix B. If you've determined that you need to improve your body composition, set a specific goal by completing Lab 6.2, and then plan your program using the labs in Chapters 8 and 9. After several weeks or months of an exercise and/or dietary change program, complete this lab again and enter the results in the Postprogram Assessment column of Appendix B. How do the results compare?

Name _____ **Section** _____ **Date** _____

LAB 6.2 Setting Goals for Target Body Weight

This lab is designed to help you set body weight goals based on a target BMI or percent body fat. If the results of Lab 6.1 indicate that a change in body composition would be beneficial for your health, you may want to complete this lab to help you set goals.

Remember, though, that a wellness lifestyle—including a balanced diet and regular exercise—is more important for your health than achieving any specific body weight, BMI, or percent body fat. You may want to set goals for improving your diet and increasing physical activity and let your body composition change as a result. If so, use the labs in Chapters 3, 4, 8, and 9 as your guides.

Equipment

Calculator (or pencil and paper for calculations)

Preparation

Determine percent body fat and/or calculate BMI as described in Lab 6.1. Keep track of height and weight as measured for these calculations.

Height: _____ Weight: _____

Instructions: Target Body Weight from Target BMI

Use the following chart to find the target body weight that corresponds to your target BMI. Find your height in the left column, and then move across the appropriate row until you find the weight that corresponds to your target BMI. Remember, BMI is only an indirect measurement of body composition. It is possible to improve body composition without any significant change in weight. For example, a weight training program may result in increased muscle mass and decreased fat mass without any change in overall weight. For this reason, you may want to set alternative or additional goals, such as improving the fit of your clothes or decreasing your waist measurement.

	<18.5 Underweight		18.5–24.9 Normal						25–29.9 Overweight					30–34.9 Obesity (Class I)					35–39.9 Obesity (Class II)				>40 Extreme Obesity
BMI	17	18	19	20	21	22	23	24	25	26	27	28	29	30	31	32	33	34	35	36	37	38	39	40
Height												Body Weight (pounds)												
4' 10"	81	86	91	96	101	105	110	115	120	124	129	134	139	144	148	153	158	163	168	172	177	182	187	192
4' 11"	84	89	94	99	104	109	114	119	124	129	134	139	144	149	154	159	163	168	173	178	183	188	193	198
5'	87	92	97	102	108	113	118	123	128	133	138	143	149	154	159	164	169	174	179	184	190	195	200	205
5' 1"	90	95	101	106	111	117	122	127	132	138	143	148	154	159	164	169	175	180	185	191	196	201	207	212
5' 2"	93	98	104	109	115	120	126	131	137	142	148	153	159	164	170	175	181	186	191	197	202	208	213	219
5' 3"	96	102	107	113	119	124	130	136	141	147	153	158	164	169	175	181	186	192	198	203	209	215	220	226
5' 4"	99	105	111	117	122	128	134	140	146	152	157	163	169	175	181	187	192	198	204	210	216	222	227	233
5' 5"	102	108	114	120	126	132	138	144	150	156	162	168	174	180	186	192	198	204	210	216	222	229	235	241
5' 6"	105	112	118	124	130	136	143	149	155	161	167	174	180	186	192	198	205	211	217	223	229	236	242	248
5' 7"	109	115	121	128	134	141	147	153	160	166	173	179	185	192	198	204	211	217	224	230	236	243	249	256
5' 8"	112	118	125	132	138	145	151	158	165	171	178	184	191	197	204	211	217	224	230	237	244	250	257	263
5' 9"	115	122	129	136	142	149	156	163	169	176	183	190	197	203	210	217	224	230	237	244	251	258	264	271
5' 10"	119	126	133	139	146	153	160	167	174	181	188	195	202	209	216	223	230	237	244	251	258	265	272	279
5' 11"	122	129	136	143	151	158	165	172	179	187	194	201	208	215	222	230	237	244	251	258	265	273	280	287
6'	125	133	140	148	155	162	170	177	184	192	199	207	214	221	229	236	243	251	258	266	273	280	288	295
6' 1"	129	137	144	152	159	167	174	182	190	197	205	212	220	228	235	243	250	257	265	273	281	288	296	303
6' 2"	132	140	148	156	164	171	179	187	195	203	210	218	226	234	242	249	257	265	273	281	288	296	304	312
6' 3"	136	144	152	160	168	176	184	192	200	208	216	224	232	240	248	256	264	272	280	288	296	304	312	320
6' 4"	140	148	156	164	173	181	189	197	206	214	222	230	238	247	255	263	271	280	288	296	304	312	321	329

SOURCE: National Heart, Lung, and Blood Institute. 1998. *Clinical Guidelines on the Identification, Evaluation, and Treatment of Overweight and Obesity in Adults: The Evidence Report.* Bethesda, MD: National Institutes of Health.

LABORATORY ACTIVITIES

Current BMI: _____ Target BMI: _____ Target body weight (from chart): _____

Alternative/additional goals:

Note: You can calculate target body weight from target BMI more precisely by using the following formula: (1) convert your height measurement to meters, (2) square your height measurement, (3) multiply this number by your target BMI to get your target weight in kilograms, and (4) convert your target weight from kilograms to pounds:

1. Height _____ in. × 0.0254 m/in. = height _____ m

2. Height _____ m × height _____ m = _____ m^2

3. Target BMI _____ × height _____ m = target weight _____ kg

4. Target weight _____ kg × 2.2 lb/kg = target weight _____ lb

Instructions: Target Body Weight from Target Body Fat Percentages

Use the following formula to determine the target body weight that corresponds to your target percent body fat.

Current percent body fat: _____ Target percent body fat: _____

Formula	*Example: 180-lb male,* *current percent body fat of 24%, goal of 21%*
1. To determine the fat weight in your body, multiply your current weight by percent body fat (determined through skinfold measurements and expressed as a decimal).	180 lb × 0.24 = 43.2 lb
2. Subtract the fat weight from your current weight to get your current fat-free weight.	180 lb − 43.2 lb = 136.8 lb
3. Subtract your target percent body fat from 1 to get target percent fat-free weight.	1 − 0.21 = 0.79
4. To get your target body weight, divide your fat-free weight by your target percent fat-free weight.	136.8 lb ÷ 0.79 = 173 lb

Note: You can express weight in either pounds or kilograms, as long as you use the unit of measurement consistently.

1. Current body weight _____ × percent body fat _____ = fat weight _____

2. Current body weight _____ − fat weight _____ = fat-free weight _____

3. 1 − target percent body fat _____ = target percent fat-free weight _____

4. Fat-free weight _____ ÷ target percent fat-free weight _____ = target body weight _____

Setting a Goal

Based on these calculations and other factors (including heredity, individual preference, and current health status), select a target weight or range of weights for yourself.

Target body weight: _____

Putting Together a Complete Fitness Program

LOOKING AHEAD...

After reading this chapter, you should be able to

- List the steps for putting together a personal fitness program.

- Describe strategies for maintaining a fitness program over the long term.

- Tailor a fitness program to accommodate different life stages and special health concerns.

TEST YOUR KNOWLEDGE

1. Which of the following physical activities is considered a high-intensity exercise?
   a. hiking uphill
   b. singles tennis
   c. jumping rope

2. Older adults should avoid exercise to protect themselves against falls and injuries. True or false?

3. Swimming is a total fitness activity that develops all the components of health-related fitness. True or false?

See answers on the next page.

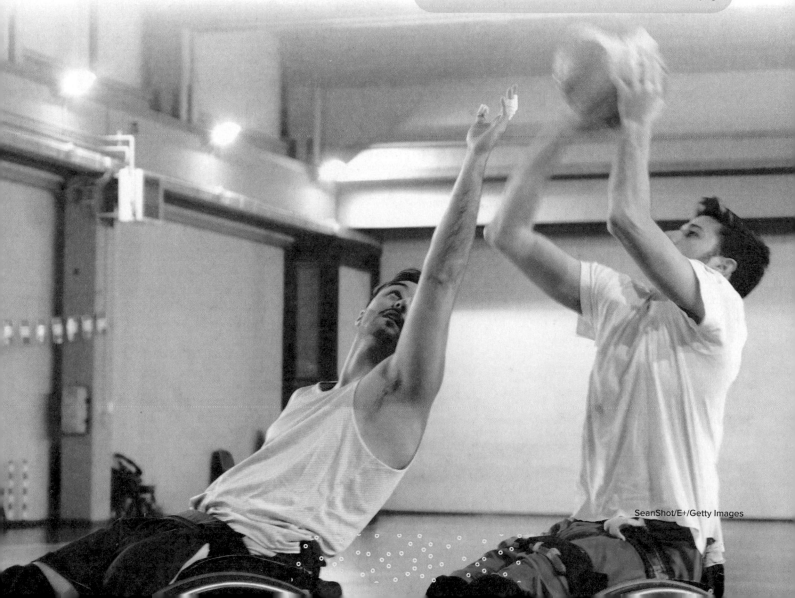

SeanShot/E+/Getty Images

U nderstanding the benefits of physical fitness, as explained in earlier chapters, is the first step toward creating a well-rounded exercise program. The next challenge is to choose activities and combine them into a program that develops all the components of fitness and helps you stay motivated. This chapter presents a step-by-step plan for creating and maintaining a well-rounded fitness program. At the end of this chapter, you'll find sample programs based on popular activities. These programs provide structure that can be helpful if you're beginning an exercise program for the first time.

DEVELOPING A PERSONAL FITNESS PLAN

If you're ready to create a complete fitness program based on the activities you enjoy most, begin by preparing the program plan and agreement in Lab 7.1. By carefully developing your plan and signing an agreement, you'll increase your chances of success. The step-by-step procedure outlined here will guide you through the steps of Lab 7.1 to create an exercise program that's right for you. (See Figure 7.1 for a sample personal fitness program plan and agreement.)

If you'd like additional help in setting up your program, choose one of the sample programs at the end of this chapter. Sample programs are provided for walking/jogging, bicycling, swimming, and rowing. They include detailed instructions for starting a program and developing and maintaining fitness.

1. Set Goals

Ask yourself, "What do I want from my fitness program?" Develop different types of goals—general and specific, long term and short term. General or long-term goals might include lowering your risk for chronic disease, improving posture, having more energy, or improving the fit of your clothes.

It's also a good idea to develop some specific, short-term goals based on measurable factors. Specific goals might be

- Raising cardiorespiratory capacity ($\dot{V}O_{2max}$) by 10%
- Reducing the time it takes you to jog two miles from 22 minutes to 19 minutes
- Increasing the number of push-ups you can do from 15 to 25
- Lowering your BMI from 26 to 24.5

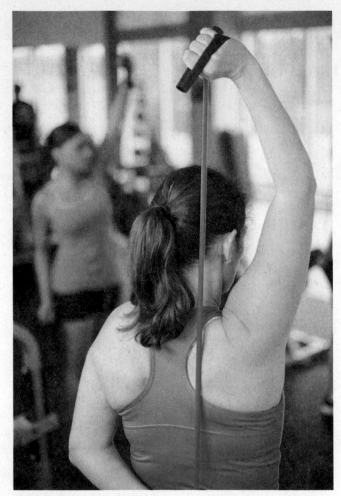

Fitness Tip An overall fitness program includes activities to develop all the components of physical fitness. Remember that you don't need to go to the gym for all your fitness activities. For example, research shows that, especially for young women, resistance bands are just as effective as weight machines or free weights for increasing muscular strength.

yellowdog/Cultura/Getty Images

Having specific goals will allow you to track your progress and enjoy the measurable changes brought about by your fitness program. Break your specific goals into several smaller steps (mini-goals), such as those shown in Figure 7.1. For example, instead of dwelling on losing 20 or 30 pounds, try losing 2 pounds. Remember, yard by yard is hard; inch by inch is a cinch. (For detailed discussions of goals and goal setting in a behavior change or fitness program, refer back to Chapters 1 and 2.)

Physical fitness assessment tests—as described in Chapters 3, 4, 5, and 6—are essential to determining your goals. They help you decide which types of exercise you should emphasize, and they help you understand the relative difficulty of attaining specific goals. If you have health problems, such as high blood pressure, heart disease, obesity, or serious joint or muscle disabilities, see your physician before taking assessment tests. Measure your progress by taking these tests about every three months.

A. I [Tracie Kaufman] am contracting with myself to follow a physical
   (name)
   fitness program to work toward the following goals:

Specific or short-term goals

1. Improving cardiorespiratory fitness by raising my $\dot{V}O_{2max}$ from 34 to 37 ml/kg/min
2. Improving upper body muscular strength and endurance rating from fair to good
3. Improving body composition (from 28% to 25% body fat)
4. Improving my tennis game (hitting 20 playable shots in a row against the ball machine)

General or long-term goals

1. Developing a more positive attitude about myself
2. Improving the fit of my clothes
3. Building and maintaining bone mass to reduce my risk of osteoporosis
4. Increasing my life expectancy and reducing my risk for diabetes and heart disease

B. **My program plan is as follows:**

Activities	Components (Check X)					Time	Frequency (Check X)							Intensity*
	CRE	MS	ME	F	BC		M	Tu	W	Th	F	S	S	
Swimming	X	X	X	X	X	35min	X		X		X			140–170 bpm
Tennis	X	X	X	X	X	90min						X		RPE } 4–6
Weight training		X	X	X	X	30min		X		X		X		see Lab 4.3
Stretching				X		25min	X		X		X	X		—

*List your target heart rate range or an RPE value if appropriate.

C. My program will begin on [Sept.] [21] My program includes the following schedule
   of mini-goals. For each step in my program, I will give myself the reward listed.

Completing 2 full weeks of program	Oct.	5	movie with friends
(mini-goal 1)			(reward)
$\dot{V}O_{2max}$ of 35 ml/kg/min	Nov.	2	new app or game
(mini-goal 2)			(reward)
Completing 10 full weeks of program	Nov.	30	new sweater
(mini-goal 3)			(reward)
Percent body fat of 27%	Dec.	22	weekend away
(mini-goal 4)			(reward)
$\dot{V}O_{2max}$ of 36 ml/kg/min	Jan.	18	new app or game
(mini-goal 5)			(reward)

D. My program will include the addition of physical activity to my daily routine (such
   as climbing stairs or walking to class):

1. Walking to and from campus job
2. Taking the stairs to dorm room instead of elevator
3. Bicycling to the library instead of driving
4. Taking a drop-in fitness class at the campus recreation center

E. My program will include the following strategies for reducing sedentary time:

1. Setting "move" reminders on phone and laptop
2. Moving during television commercial breaks or between programs
3. Standing or walking during phone calls

F. I will use the following tools to monitor my program and my progress toward
   my goals:

I'll use a chart that lists the number of laps and minutes I swim and the
charts for strength and flexibility from Labs 4.3 & 5.2.

I sign this contract as an indication of my personal commitment to reach my goal.

_____ Tracie Kaufman _____   [Sep.] [10]
                (your signature)

I have recruited a helper who will witness my contract and
swim with me three days per week
(list any way your helper will participate in your program)

_____ Russell Walker _____   [Sep.] [10]
                (witness's signature)

Figure 7.1 A sample personal fitness program plan and agreement.

Table 7.1 — Examples of Aerobic Activities and Their Intensities

MODERATE-INTENSITY ACTIVITIES	VIGOROUS-INTENSITY ACTIVITIES
• Walking briskly (3 miles per hour or faster, but not race-walking)	• Race-walking, jogging, or running
• Water aerobics	• Swimming laps
• Bicycling slower than 10 miles per hour	• Singles tennis
• Doubles tennis	• Cardio dance and other group fitness
• Social dancing	• Bicycling 10 miles per hour or faster
• General gardening	• Jumping rope
• Washing car	• Heavy gardening (continuous digging or hoeing)
• Fly fishing	• Hiking uphill or with a heavy backpack
• Round of golf	• **Interval training, Arc Trainer,** or **elliptical trainer:** 4 to 6 intervals of 30 seconds at maximum intensity, 3 minutes rest between intervals
• Frisbee	

SOURCE: Adapted from the Centers for Disease Control and Prevention. 2017. *Physical Activity Recommendations & Guidelines.* (https://www.cdc.gov/physicalactivity/resources/recommendations.html).

2. Select Activities

If you have already chosen activities and created separate program plans for different fitness components in Chapters 3, 4, and 5, you can put those plans together into a single program. It's usually best to include exercises to develop each of the health-related components of fitness. The components (with abbreviations used in Figure 7.1, section B) are as follows:

- Cardiorespiratory endurance (CRE) is developed by activities that use continuous rhythmic movements of large-muscle groups, like those in the legs (see Chapter 3).

- Muscular strength and endurance (MS and ME) are developed by strength training against resistance (see Chapter 4).

- Flexibility (F) is developed by stretching the major muscle groups (see Chapter 5).

- Healthy body composition (BC) can be developed by combining a sensible diet and a program of regular exercise, including cardiorespiratory endurance exercise to burn calories and resistance training to build muscle mass (see Chapter 6).

Table 7.1 shows the intensity levels of several popular activities that promote health. Check the intensity levels of the activities you're considering to make sure the program you put together will help you achieve your goals.

If you select activities you enjoy and that support your commitment rather than activities that turn exercise into a chore, your program will provide plenty of incentive for continuing. Consider the following factors in making your choices:

- *Fun and interest.* Your fitness program is much more likely to be successful if you choose activities that you currently engage in and enjoy. Often you can modify your current activities to fit your fitness program. If you want to add a new activity to your program, try it for a while before committing to it.

- *Your current skill and fitness level.* Although many activities are appropriate for beginners, some sports and activities require a certain level of skill to obtain fitness benefits. For example, if you are a beginning tennis player, you will probably not be able to sustain rallies long enough to develop cardiorespiratory endurance. A better choice might be a walking program while you improve your tennis game. To build skill for a particular activity, consider taking a class or getting some instruction from a physical activity coach or fellow participant.

- *Time and convenience.* You are more likely to maintain a long-term exercise program if you can easily fit exercise into your daily routine. As you consider activities, think about whether a special location or facility is required. Can you participate in the activity close to your home, school, or job? Are the necessary facilities available at convenient times (see Lab 7.2)? Can you participate in the activity year-round, or will you need to find an alternative during the summer or winter? Would a home treadmill make you more likely to exercise regularly?

- *Cost.* Some sports and activities require equipment, fees, or some type of membership investment. If you are on a tight budget, limit your choices to free or inexpensive activities. Investigate the facilities on your campus, which you may be able to use at little or no cost. Many activities require no equipment beyond an appropriate pair of shoes. Chapter 4 provides examples of resistance exercises you can do at home without equipment.

- *Special health needs.* If you have a particular health problem, choose activities that will conform to your needs and enhance your ability to cope. Ask your physician how to tailor an exercise program to your needs and goals. See the section "Exercise Guidelines for Life Stages and People with Special Health Concerns" later in this chapter.

TERMS

interval training Repeated bouts of intense exercise followed by rest (e.g., on a running track, sprint the straightaways and walk the turns for one to two miles).

Arc Trainer A weight-bearing, stationary exercise device that exercises the lower body muscles in a crescent-shape pattern.

elliptical trainer A weight-bearing stationary exercise device that works the lower body muscles in an elliptical pattern.

3. Set a Target Frequency, Intensity, and Time (Duration) for Each Activity

The next step is to apply the FITT-VP principle and set a starting frequency, intensity, and time (duration), volume, and progression for each type of activity you've chosen (see the summary in Figure 7.2 and the sample in Figure 7.1).

Cardiorespiratory Endurance Exercise As noted in earlier chapters, based on over 50 years of research on exercise and health, the U.S. Department of Health and Human Services concluded that most health benefits occur with at least 150 minutes per week of moderate-intensity physical activity (such as brisk walking) or 75 minutes per week of vigorous-intensity activity (such as jogging). Additional benefits occur with more exercise. An appropriate frequency for cardiorespiratory endurance exercise is three to five days per week. For intensity, note your target heart rate zone or RPE (rating of perceived exertion) value. Your target total workout time (duration) should be about 20–60 minutes per day, depending on the intensity of the activity. You can exercise in a single session or in multiple sessions of 10 or more minutes. New research on high-intensity interval training suggests that you can exercise for shorter durations if you train at maximal intensities; be sure to choose an intensity and volume of activity that is safe and appropriate for you.

Muscular Strength and Endurance Training At least two nonconsecutive days per week of strength training is recommended. As described in Chapter 4, a general fitness strength training program includes one or more sets of 8–12 repetitions of 8–10 exercises that work all major muscle groups. For intensity, choose a weight that is heavy enough to fatigue your muscles but not so heavy that you cannot complete the full number of repetitions with proper form. Exercises that use body weight for resistance also build strength and muscle endurance. A note of caution: Years of weight training can lead to stiffer blood vessels. Some studies show that doing aerobics after weight training helps to prevent blood vessel stiffening.

Flexibility Training Stretches should be performed at least two or three days per week (daily is most effective), when the muscles are warm. The stretches should work all major muscle groups. For each exercise, stretch to the point of slight tension or mild discomfort, and hold the stretch for 10–30 seconds; do 2–4 repetitions of each exercise.

4. Set Up a System of Mini-Goals and Rewards

To keep your program on track, set up a system of goals and rewards. Break your specific goals into several steps, and set a target date for each step. For example, if one goal of an 18-year-old male student's program is to improve upper-body strength and endurance, he could use the push-up test in Lab 4.2 to set intermediate goals. If he can perform 15 push-ups (for a rating of "very poor"), he might set intermediate goals of 17, 20, 25, and 30 push-ups (for a final rating of "fair"). By allowing several weeks between mini-goals and by specifying rewards, he'll be able to

	Cardiorespiratory endurance training	Strength training	Flexibility training
Frequency	3–5 days per week	2–3 nonconsecutive days per week	2–3 days per week (minimum); 5–7 days per week (ideal)
Intensity	55/65–90% of maximum heart rate	Sufficient resistance to fatigue muscles	Stretch to the point of tension
Time	20–60 minutes in sessions lasting 10 minutes or more	Duration of training sufficient to reach target volume	Hold stastic stretches for 10–30 seconds
Type	Continuous rhythmic activities using large muscle groups	Resistance exercises for all major muscle groups	Stretching exercises for all major joints
Volume	Equivalent of at least 150 minutes or 1,000 or more calories per week of moderate-intensity activity, consistent with individual fitness status and goals	8–12 repetitions of each exercise, 1 or more sets (2–4 sets recommended for most adults), with rest intervals of 2–3 minutes between sets (volume = resistance × sets × reps)	2–4 repetitions for a total stretching time of 60 seconds for each exercise
Progression	Gradually increase volume (frequency, intensity, and/or time) to achieve health and fitness goals; increasing intensity is most important for increasing fitness	Gradually increase resistance, number of sets, or frequency of training to achieve goals; intensity is the most important factor promoting improvements in strength and power	Stretch regularly to build and maintain normal range of motion; avoid excessive flexibility

Figure 7.2   A summary of the FITT-VP principle for the health-related components of fitness.
SOURCE: Adapted from American College of Sports Medicine. 2018. *ACSM's Guidelines for Exercise Testing and Prescription,* 10th ed. Philadelphia, PA: Wolters Kluwer Health.

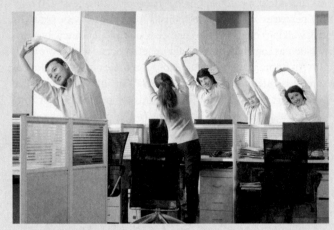
track his progress and reward himself as he moves toward his final goal. Reaching a series of small goals is more satisfying than working toward a single, more challenging goal that may take months to achieve. For more on choosing rewards, see Chapter 1 and Activity 4 in the Behavior Change Workbook at the end of the text.

5. Include Lifestyle Physical Activity and Strategies to Reduce Sedentary Time in Your Program

Daily physical activity is a simple but important way to improve your overall wellness. As part of your fitness program plan, specify ways to be more active during your daily routine, say, by taking the stairs up to class rather than taking an elevator. In addition, develop specific strategies to reduce the amount of time you spend being sedentary (see the box "The Importance of Reducing Sedentary Time"). You may find it helpful to first use a health journal to track your activities for several days. Review the records in your journal, identify routine opportunities to be more active, and add these to your program plan in Lab 7.1.

6. Develop Tools for Monitoring Your Progress

A record that tracks your daily progress will help remind you of your ongoing commitment to your program and give you a sense of accomplishment. Figure 7.3 shows you how to create a general program log and record the activity type, frequency, and times (durations). Or you can complete specific activity logs like those in Labs 3.2, 4.3, and 5.2 in addition to, or instead of, a general log. Post your log in a place where you'll see it often as a reminder and as an incentive for improvement. If you have specific, measurable goals, you can also graph your weekly or

Name   Tracie Kaufman

Enter time, distance, or another factor (such as heart rate or perceived exertion) to track your progress.

Activity/Date	M	Tu	W	Th	F	S	S	Weekly Total	M	Tu	W	Th	F	S	S	Weekly Total
1 Swimming	800 yd		725 yd		800 yd			2325 yd	800 yd		800 yd		850 yd			2450 yd
2 Tennis					90 min			90 min						95 min		95 min
3 Weight Training		X		X		X				X		X			X	
4 Stretching	X		X		X	X			X			X	X	X	X	

Figure 7.3   A sample program log.

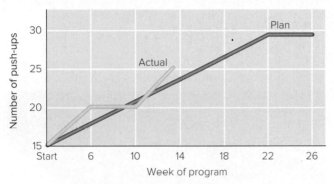

Figure 7.4   A sample program progress chart.

monthly progress toward each goal (Figure 7.4). To monitor the overall progress of your fitness program, you may choose to reassess your fitness every three months or so during the improvement phase of your program. Because the results of different fitness tests vary, be sure to compare results for the same assessments over time.

7. Make a Commitment

Your final step in planning your program is to make a commitment by signing an agreement. Find a witness for your agreement—preferably someone who will be actively involved in your program. Keep your agreement in a visible spot to remind you of your commitment.

PUTTING YOUR PLAN INTO ACTION

After you've developed a detailed plan and signed your agreement, you are ready to begin your fitness program. Refer to the specific training suggestions provided in Chapters 2, 3, 4, and 5 for advice on beginning and maintaining your program. Many people find it easier to plan a program than to put their plan into action and stick with it. Adherence to healthy lifestyle programs has become an important area of study for psychologists and health researchers. The guidelines here and in the next section reflect research into strategies that help people stick with an exercise program.

- *Start slowly and increase fitness gradually.* Overzealous exercising can cause discouraging discomforts and injuries. Your program is meant to last a lifetime. The important first step is to break your established pattern of inactivity. Be patient and realistic. After your body has adjusted to your starting level of exercise, slowly increase the amount of overload. Small increases are the key—achieving a large number of small improvements will eventually result in substantial gains in fitness. It's usually best to increase duration and frequency before increasing intensity.

- *Find an exercise buddy.* The social side of exercise is an important factor for many regular exercisers. Working out with a friend will make exercise more enjoyable and increase your chances of sticking with your program. Find an exercise partner who shares your goals and general fitness level. On days when a partner isn't available, a smartphone or MP3 player can be your workout buddy; see the box "Digital Motivation" for more information.

- *Ask for support from others.* Consistent exercise requires the support of important people in your life, such as parents, spouse, partner, and friends. Talk with them about your program, and let them know the importance of exercise and wellness in your life. Exercise needs to be a critical component of your day (just like sleeping and eating). Good communication will help others become more supportive of and enthusiastic about the time you spend on your wellness program.

- *Vary your activities.* You can make your program more fun over the long term if you participate in a variety of activities that you enjoy. You can also add interest by varying the routes you take when walking, playing with different tennis partners, or switching to a new volleyball or basketball court. Varying your activities, a strategy known as *cross-training,* has other benefits. It can help you develop balanced, total-body fitness. For example, by alternating running with swimming, you build both upper- and lower-body strength. Cross-training can reduce the risk of injury and overtraining because the same muscles, bones, and joints are not continuously subjected to the stresses of the same activity. You can cross-train either by choosing different activities on different days or by alternating activities within a single workout.

WELLNESS IN THE DIGITAL AGE
Digital Motivation

If you ever have trouble getting inspired to work out, motivation may be as close as your smartphone.

Since the iPhone's advent, dozens of interactive motivational applications ("apps") have been developed for use on smart cell phones. Coaching and motivational recordings are available for use on MP3 players, as well. These apps and recordings can substitute for an exercise partner when your workout buddy isn't around and can inspire you to keep your program on track. Some smartphone apps can monitor your workouts, track your progress, and even provide on-the-spot coaching to help you keep going.

Here are just a few examples of low-cost or free smartphone apps that can help you keep exercising:

- **Nike Training Club (http://www.nike.com/us/en_us/c/nike-plus/training-app).** This training app designs programs according to your goals and experience. Goals include "get lean"—high-intensity cardio exercise to promote weight loss; "get toned"—lightweight training and interval training; "get strong"—weight training to build strength and muscle mass; and "get focused"—15-minute workouts that target specific areas of the body. The app shows specific exercises, paces, and repetitions for the person exercising. It also has tools for motivating you to exercise, such as workout music and a clock that keeps track of the workout time. It is a digital personal trainer at an affordable price.

- **The Beast Sensor (https://www.thisisbeast.com/).** The Beast combines a wearable accelerometer with a smartphone app that tracks sets, reps, acceleration, force, and power. This is an excellent system for monitoring and promoting intense weight-training workouts.

- **Cyclemeter (https://abvio.com/cyclemeter/).** Use this highly motivational app for cycling, running, and walking. It brings detailed statistics to your workouts by keeping track of peak and average speed, caloric expenditure, rest times, elevation changes, and environmental conditions. You can store the results on the cloud or e-mail them to yourself, friends, or social media. You can also integrate the app with a heart rate monitor. The GPS function gives you a map or satellite view of your route.

- **Endomondo (https://www.endomondo.com).** This app uses GPS to keep track of routes used during running, walking, cycling, skating, or cross-country skiing. It also helps people share their workouts with social media, which promotes social accountability as a way to stick with the program.

- **Fitbit (https://www.fitbit.com/app).** This wearable device tracks daily step count, heart rate, sleep quality, nutrition, and energy expenditure and is compatible with a wide variety of devices. It also keeps track of your progress and encourages you to reach your goals.

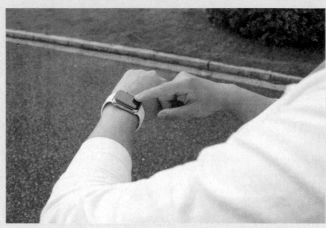

Yusuke Saito/123RF

- *Cycle the duration and intensity of your workouts.* Olympic athletes use a technique called periodization of training, meaning that they vary the duration and intensity of their workouts. Sometimes they exercise very intensely; other times they train lightly or rest. You can use the same technique to improve fitness more quickly and make your training program more varied and enjoyable. For example, if your program consists of walking, weight training, and stretching, pick one day a week for each activity to train a little harder or longer than you normally do. If you usually walk two miles at 16 minutes per mile, increase the pace to 15 minutes per mile once a week. If you lift weights twice a week, train more intensely during one of the workouts by using more resistance or performing multiple sets.

- *Adapt to changing environments and schedules.* Most people are creatures of habit and have trouble adjusting to change. Don't use bad weather or a new job as an excuse to give up your exercise program. If you walk in the summer, put on a warm coat and walk in the winter as well. If you can't go out because of darkness, join a gym and walk on a treadmill. Review the results of Lab 2.2 on overcoming barriers to activity to develop additional strategies.

- *Expect fluctuations and lapses.* On some days, your progress will be excellent, but on others, you'll barely be able to drag yourself through your scheduled activities. Don't let off-days or lapses discourage you or make you feel guilty (see the box "Getting Your Fitness Program Back on Track").

- *Choose other healthy lifestyle behaviors.* Exercise provides huge benefits for your health, but other behaviors are also important. Choose a nutritious diet, and avoid harmful habits like smoking and overconsumption of alcohol. Stay hydrated with water or other healthy beverages (see the box "Choosing Healthy Beverages"). Don't skimp on sleep, which has a mutually beneficial relationship with exercise. Physical activity improves sleep, and adequate sleep can improve physical performance.

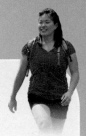

Lapses are a normal part of any behavior change program. The important point is to move on and avoid becoming discouraged. Try again and keep trying. Know that continued effort will lead to success. Here are some tips to help you keep going:

- Don't judge yourself too harshly, especially in comparison with others. Some people make faster gains in fitness than others. Focus on the improvements you've already made from your program and how good you feel after exercise—both physically and mentally.

- Visualize what it will be like to reach your goals. Keep these images in mind as an incentive to stick with your program.

- Use your exercise journal to identify thoughts and behaviors that are causing noncompliance. Devise strategies to combat these problematic patterns. If needed, change your environment or find more social support. For example, call a friend to walk with you, or keep exercise clothes in your car or backpack.

- Make changes in your plan and your reward system to help renew enthusiasm for and commitment to your program. Try changing fitness activities or your exercise schedule. Build in more opportunities to reward yourself.

- Plan ahead for difficult situations. Think about what circumstances might make it tough to keep up your fitness routine. Develop strategies to increase your chances of sticking with your program. For example, figure out ways to continue your program during vacation, travel, bad weather, and so on.

- If you're in a bad mood or just don't feel like exercising, remind yourself that physical activity is probably the one thing you can do that will make you feel better. Even if you can only do half your scheduled workout, you'll boost your energy, improve your mood, and help keep your program on track.

EXERCISE GUIDELINES FOR LIFE STAGES AND PEOPLE WITH SPECIAL HEALTH CONCERNS

Physical activity is beneficial for people of all ages and for many people with special health concerns.

Exercise Guidelines for Life Stages

A fitness program may need to be adjusted to accommodate the requirements of different life stages.

Children and Adolescents Lack of physical activity has led to alarming increases in overweight and obesity in children and adolescents. If you have children or are in a position to influence children, keep these guidelines in mind:

- Provide opportunities for children and adolescents to exercise every day. Minimize sedentary activities, such as watching television. Children and adolescents should aim for at least 60 minutes of moderate activity every day. Less fit kids should start with 30 minutes a day until their fitness improves and they can exercise longer.

- During family outings, choose dynamic activities. For example, go for a walk or park away from a mall and then walk to the stores.

- For children younger than 12, emphasize skill development and fitness rather than excellence in competitive sports. For adolescents, combine participation and training in lifetime sports with traditional, competitive sports.

- Make sure children are developmentally capable of participating in an activity. For example, catching skills are difficult for young children because their nervous system is not developed

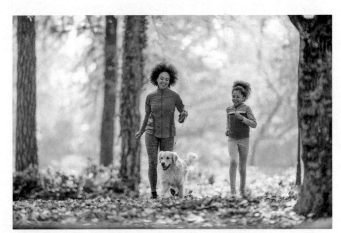

Fitness Tip People of all ages benefit from exercise. By including their children, not only do parents set a positive example that can lead to a lifetime of physical activity, but both parent and child also will have an exercise buddy.

Skynesher/E+/Getty Images

enough to fully master the skill. Gradually increase the complexity of the skill once the child has mastered the simpler skill.

- Make sure children get plenty of water when exercising in the heat. Make sure they are dressed properly when exercising in the cold.

Pregnant Women Exercise is important during pregnancy, but women should be cautious because some types of exercise can pose increased risk to the mother and the unborn child. The following guidelines are consistent with the recommendations of the American College of Obstetrics and Gynecology:

- See your physician about possible modifications needed for your particular pregnancy.

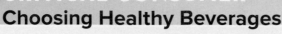

It's important to stay hydrated at all times, but especially when you are exercising. Too little water intake can leave you feeling fatigued, reduce your body's performance, and leave you vulnerable to heat-related sicknesses in hot weather. But *what* you drink is as significant as how much you drink, both when you are exercising and when you are going about your normal routine.

The Great Water Controversy

Wherever you see people exercising, you will see bottled water in abundance. For several years, a debate has been raging about the quality and safety of commercially bottled water. Manufacturing, bottling, shipping, and disposal processes pollute. Moreover, bottled water is no better for you than regular tap water. Some bottled waters may actually be bad for you, as explained below. To make matters worse, bottled water costs up to 1,900 times more than tap water.

In a 2011 analysis of 173 bottled water products, the Environmental Working Group found 38 contaminants in 10 popular brands of bottled water. Contaminants included heavy metals such as arsenic, pharmaceutical residues and other pollutants commonly found in urban wastewater, as well as a variety of industrial chemicals. Bottled-water companies are notoriously secretive about their products. Overall, 18% of bottled waters failed to list the location of their source, and 32% disclosed nothing about the treatment or purity of the water.

Many commercially bottled water products are, in fact, tap water drawn from municipal water systems. Such revelations have caused the Food and Drug Administration (FDA) to require bottlers to put statements on their products' labels, identifying them as having been drawn from a standard water supply. These products, priced many times higher than water from a residential tap, provide no benefit over standard tap water.

An even bigger issue is that plastic water bottles have become a huge environmental problem: Billions of bottles now pile up in landfills and float in the world's oceans. Some types of plastic take years to biodegrade, and many kinds of plastic

bottles will never decompose. Newer types of plastic bottles can decompose significantly faster than older bottles, but fast-degrading plastics have not yet come into widespread use in the bottled-water industry.

Experts say that when you're exercising, the cheapest and safest way to stay hydrated is to drink filtered tap water. If you need to carry water with you, buy a reusable container (preferably made of stainless steel) that you can clean after each use. If you drink from plastic bottles, be sure they are recyclable and dispose of them by recycling.

Other Choices

Instead of water, many people choose to drink sodas, juice, tea, or flavored water. While these kinds of beverages have their place, it's important not to drink them too often or in large amounts, especially if they are high in sugar or caffeine. Sugary drinks add empty calories to your diet, and caffeine is a psychoactive drug with a variety of side effects.

Regular (nondiet) sodas are now the leading source of calories in the American diet; most people don't count the calories from beverages as part of their daily caloric intake, leading them to underestimate their total intake. For this reason and others, many experts believe that soda consumption is a major factor in the increasing levels of obesity, metabolic syndrome, diabetes, and other chronic diseases among Americans.

If you're concerned that the liquid portion of your diet is not as healthy as it should be, choose water, fat-free milk, or unsweetened herbal tea more often. Avoid regular soda, sweetened bottled iced tea, flavored water, and fruit beverages made with little fruit juice. To make water more appealing, try adding slices of citrus fruit with sparkling water. With some imagination, you can make sure you stay hydrated without consuming excess calories, spending money unnecessarily, or hurting the environment.

SOURCE: Environmental Working Group. 2017. "Bottled water scorecard" (http://www.ewg.org/health/report/Bottled Water/Bottled-Water-Scorecard /Search).

- Continue mild to moderate exercise routines at least three times a week. (For most women, this means maintaining an exercise heart rate of 100–160 beats per minute.) Avoid exercising vigorously or to exhaustion, especially in the third trimester. Monitor exercise intensity by assessing how you feel rather than by monitoring your heart rate; ratings of perceived exertion (RPE) levels of 2–4 (fairly light to somewhat hard) are appropriate.

- Favor non- or low-weight-bearing exercises such as swimming or cycling over weight-bearing exercises, which can carry increased risk of injury.

- Avoid exercise in a supine position—lying on your back—after the first trimester. This position restricts blood flow to the uterus. Also avoid prolonged periods of motionless standing.

- Avoid exercise that could cause loss of balance, especially in the third trimester, and exercise that might injure the

abdomen, stress the joints, or carry a risk of falling (such as contact sports, vigorous racquet sports, skiing, and in-line skating).

- Avoid activities involving extremes in barometric pressure, such as scuba diving and mountain climbing.

- Especially during the first trimester, drink plenty of fluids and exercise in well-ventilated areas to avoid heat stress.

- Do three to five sets of 10 Kegel exercises daily. These exercises call for tightening the muscles of the pelvic floor for 5–15 seconds per repetition. Kegel exercises are thought to help prevent incontinence (involuntary loss of urine) and speed recovery after giving birth.

- After giving birth, resume prepregnancy exercise routines gradually, based on how you feel.

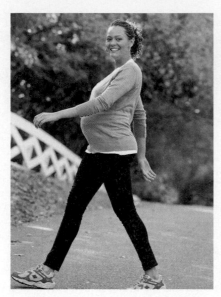

Fitness Tip Moderate-intensity activities such as walking, swimming, and low-impact group exercise are safe for most women during pregnancy. In addition to improving fitness, physical activity and exercise may also have medical benefits for a pregnant woman, including reduced risk of gestational diabetes and excessive weight gain.

Ariel Skelley/Blend Images/Getty Images

Older Adults Older people readily adapt to endurance exercise and strength training. Exercise principles are the same as for younger people, but some specific guidelines apply:

- Follow the same guidelines for aerobic exercise as younger adults, but judge intensity on a 10-point scale of perceived exertion rather than by heart rate.

- For strength training, use a lighter weight and perform more (10–15) repetitions than young adults.

- Perform flexibility exercises at least two days per week for at least 10 minutes. Exercises that improve balance should also be performed two days per week.

- Drink plenty of water and avoid exercising in excessively hot or cold environments. Wear clothes that speed heat loss in warm environments and prevent heat loss in cold environments.

- Warm up slowly and carefully. Increase intensity and duration of exercise gradually.

- Cool down slowly, continuing very light exercise until the heart rate is below 100.

- If you have physical disabilities or limitations and cannot meet the recommendation of at least 150 minutes per week of moderate-intensity exercise, do as much exercise as you can.

Exercise Guidelines for People with Special Health Concerns

As emphasized throughout the text, regular, appropriate exercise is safe and beneficial for everyone. In fact, for many people with special health concerns, the risks associated with not exercising are far greater than those associated with a moderate program of regular exercise.

The fitness recommendations made throughout this book are intended for the general population and can serve as basic guidelines for any exercise program. If you have a chronic health condition, however, you may need to modify your exercise program to accommodate your situation. This section presents precautions and recommendations for people with a variety of special health concerns.

These recommendations, however, are not intended to replace a physician's advice. If you have a special health concern, talk to your physician before starting any exercise program. For additional information about these and other health concerns, visit the website for Exercise Is Medicine: Rx for Health Series (https://www.exerciseismedicine.org/support_page.php/rx-for-health-series).

Arthritis

- Begin an exercise program as early as possible in the course of the disease.

- Warm up thoroughly before each workout to loosen stiff muscles and lower the risk of injury.

- For cardiorespiratory endurance exercise, avoid high-impact activities that may damage arthritic joints. Consider swimming, water walking, or other exercise that can be done in a warm pool.

- Strength train the whole body. Pay special attention to muscles that support and protect affected joints. For example, build the quadriceps, hamstrings, and calf muscles to support and protect arthritic knees. Start with small amounts of weight and gradually increase the intensity of your workouts.

- Perform flexibility exercises daily to maintain joint mobility.

Asthma

- Exercise regularly. Acute attacks are more likely to occur if you exercise only occasionally.

- Carry medication during workouts and avoid exercising alone. Use your inhaler as recommended by your physician.

- Warm up and cool down slowly to reduce the risk of acute attacks.

- When starting an exercise program, choose self-paced endurance activities, especially those involving interval training (short bouts of exercise followed by a rest period). Gradually increase the intensity of your cardiorespiratory endurance workouts.

- Educate yourself about situations that can trigger an asthma attack and act accordingly when exercising. For example, cold, dry air can trigger or worsen an attack, as can pollen, dust, and polluted air. To avoid attacks in dry air, drink water before, during, and after a workout to moisten your airways. In cold weather, cover your mouth with a mask or scarf to warm and humidify the air you breathe. Also, avoid outdoor activities during pollen season or when the air is polluted or dusty.

Diabetes

- Don't begin an exercise program unless your diabetes is under control and you have discussed exercise safety with your physician. Because people with diabetes have an increased risk for heart disease, an exercise stress test may be recommended.

- Don't exercise alone. Wear a bracelet that identifies you as someone with diabetes.

- If you take insulin or another medication, adjust the timing and amount of each dose as needed. Work with your physician and check your blood sugar level regularly so that you can learn to balance your energy intake and output and your medication dosage.

- To prevent abnormally rapid absorption of injected insulin, inject it over a muscle that will not be exercised, and wait at least an hour before exercising.

- Check your blood sugar before, during, and after exercise. Adjust your diet and insulin dosage as needed. Keep high-carbohydrate foods on hand during a workout. Avoid exercise if your blood sugar level is above 250 mg/dl; if your blood sugar level is below 100 mg/dl, eat some carbohydrate-rich food before exercising.

- If you have poor circulation or numbness in your extremities, check your skin regularly for blisters and abrasions, especially on your feet. Avoid high-impact activities and wear comfortable shoes.

- For maximum benefit and minimum risk, choose moderate-intensity activities.

Heart Disease and Hypertension

- Check with your physician about exercise safety before increasing your activity level. Your doctor may recommend that you take an exercise stress test before starting your program.

- Exercise at moderate intensity rather than high intensity. Keep your heart rate below the level at which abnormalities appear on an exercise stress test.

- Warm up and cool down gradually. Every warm-up and cool-down session should last at least 10 minutes.

- Monitor your heart rate during exercise, and stop if you experience dizziness or chest pain.

- If your physician prescribes nitroglycerin, carry it with you during exercise. If you take a beta-blocker to manage hypertension, use RPE rather than heart rate to monitor your exercise intensity (beta-blockers reduce heart rate). Exercise at an RPE level of "fairly light" to "somewhat hard." Your breathing should be unlabored, and you should be able to talk during exercise.

- Don't hold your breath when exercising. Doing so can cause sudden, steep increases in blood pressure. Take special care during weight training and do not lift heavy loads. Exhale during the exertion phase of each lift.

- Increase exercise frequency, intensity, and time very gradually.

Obesity

- For maximum benefit and minimum risk, begin by choosing low- to moderate-intensity activities. Increase intensity

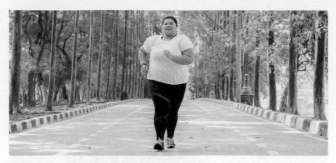

Fitness Tip The amount of physical activity needed to maintain a healthy weight varies from person to person. If you are overweight and starting an exercise program, begin with a low volume of moderate-intensity, low-impact activities. Increase overload gradually to allow your body to adjust—and to set yourself up for long-term success.

Creativa Images/Shutterstock

slowly as your fitness improves. Studies of overweight people show that exercising at moderate to high intensities causes more fat loss than training at low intensities.

- People who want to lose weight or maintain weight loss should exercise moderately for 60 minutes or more every day. To get the benefit of 60 minutes of exercise, you can exercise all at once or divide your total activity time into sessions of 10, 20, or 30 minutes.

- Choose non- or low-weight-bearing activities such as swimming, water exercises, cycling, or walking. Low-impact activities are less likely to cause joint problems or injuries.

- Stay alert for symptoms of heat-related problems during exercise (as described in Chapter 3). Obese people are vulnerable to heat intolerance.

- Ease into your exercise program, and increase overload gradually. Increase time and frequency of exercise before increasing intensity.

- Include strength training in your fitness program to build or maintain muscle mass.

- Include as much lifestyle physical activity in your daily routine as possible.

Osteoporosis

- For cardiorespiratory endurance activities, exercise at the maximum intensity that causes no significant discomfort. If possible, choose low-impact, weight-bearing exercises to help safely maintain bone density. (See Chapter 8 for strategies for building and maintaining bone density.)

- To prevent fractures, avoid any activity or movement that stresses the back or carries a risk of falling.

- Include weight training in your exercise program to improve strength and balance and to reduce the risk of falls and fractures. Always use proper exercise technique and avoid lifting heavy loads.

- Include muscle-strengthening exercises three days per week.

- Include bone-strengthening exercises, such as jumping, at least three days per week, if they are safe for you. If you already have bone loss, avoid high-impact activities. Also include balance exercises such as tai chi, which can help prevent falls.

COMMON QUESTIONS ANSWERED

Q **Should I exercise every day?**

A Some daily exercise is beneficial, but if you train intensely every day without giving yourself a rest, you will likely injure yourself or overtrain. When strength training, for example, rest at least 48 hours between workouts before exercising the same muscle group. For cardiorespiratory endurance exercise, rest or exercise lightly the day after an intense or lengthy workout. Balancing the proper amount of rest and exercise will help you feel better and improve your fitness faster.

Q **If exercise is so good for my health, why hasn't my physician ever mentioned it to me?**

A A recent study by the American College of Sports Medicine (ACSM) suggests that most people would benefit from getting a physician's advice about exercising. According to the study, 65% of patients said they would be more interested in exercising if their physicians suggested it. About 40% of physicians said they talk to their patients about exercise.

To encourage physicians and patients to talk more often about exercise and its benefits, the ACSM and the American Medical Association have launched the Exercise Is Medicine program. The program advises physicians to give more guidance to patients about exercise and suggests that everyone try to exercise at least five days each week. For more information on the program, visit www.exerciseismedicine.org.

SUMMARY

• Steps for putting together a complete fitness program include (1) setting realistic goals; (2) selecting activities to develop all the health-related components of fitness; (3) setting a target frequency, intensity, and time (duration) for each activity; (4) setting up a system of mini-goals and rewards; (5) making lifestyle physical activity and strategies to reduce sedentary time a part of the daily routine; (6) developing tools for monitoring progress; and (7) making a commitment.

• In selecting activities, consider fun and interest, your current skill and fitness levels, time and convenience, cost, and any special health concerns.

• Keys to beginning and maintaining a successful program include starting slowly, increasing intensity and duration gradually, finding a buddy, varying the activities and intensity of the program, and expecting fluctuations and lapses.

• Regular exercise is appropriate and beneficial for people in all stages of life, although program modifications may be necessary for safety.

• Regular exercise is also appropriate and beneficial for people with special health concerns such as arthritis, asthma, diabetes, heart disease and hypertension, obesity, and osteoporosis, if adapted to the particular condition.

FOR FURTHER EXPLORATION

American Academy of Orthopaedic Surgeons. Provides information about injuries, treatment, and rehabilitation, along with exercise guidelines for people with bone, muscle, and joint pain.

http://www.aaos.org

American Congress of Obstetricians and Gynecologists. Provides guidelines for promoting a healthy pregnancy and postpartum recovery, including exercise during pregnancy.

http://www.acog.org

American Diabetes Association. Promotes diabetes education, research, and advocacy; includes guidelines for diet and exercise for people with diabetes.

http://www.diabetes.org

American Heart Association. Includes information on fitness for kids as well as diet, exercise, fitness, and weight management for adults.

http://www.americanheart.org

For additional listings, see Chapters 2, 3, 4, 5, and 6.

SELECTED BIBLIOGRAPHY

American College of Sports Medicine. 2018. *ACSM's Guidelines for Exercise Testing and Prescription,* 10th ed. Philadelphia: Wolters Kluwer.

American College of Sports Medicine. 2013. *ACSM's Resource Manual for Guidelines for Exercise Testing and Prescription,* 7th ed. Philadelphia: Wolters Kluwer/Lippincott Williams & Wilkins Health.

Bangsbo, J., et al. 2019. Copenhagen consensus statement 2019: Physical activity and ageing. *British Journal Sports Medicine.* Published online.

Biswas, A., et al. 2015. Sedentary time and its association with risk for disease incidence, mortality, and hospitalization in adults: A systematic review and meta-analysis. *Annals of Internal Medicine* 162: 123–132.

Brody, L., and C. Hall. 2017. *Therapeutic Exercise,* 4th ed. Philadelphia: Wolters Kluwer.

Canadian Society for Exercise Physiology. 2011. *Public Health Agency of Canada Physical Activity Guidelines* (www.publichealth.gc.ca5).

Carlson, S. A., et al. 2015. Inadequate physical activity and health care expenditures in the United States. *Progress in Cardiovascular Diseases* 57(4): 315–323.

Chou, C. H., et al. 2019. High-intensity interval training enhances mitochondrial bioenergetics of platelets in patients with heart failure. *International Journal Cardiology* 274: 214–220.

DeFina, L. F., et al. 2015. Physical activity versus cardiorespiratory fitness: Two (partly) distinct components of cardiovascular health? *Progress in Cardiovascular Diseases* 57(4): 324–329.

Fahey, T., and M. Fahey. 2014. Nutrition, physical activity, and the obesity epidemic: Issues, policies, and solutions (1960s–present). In T. Oliver, ed., *The Guide to U.S. Health and Health Care Policy,* pp. 363–374. New York: DWJ Books.

Foulds, H. J. 2017. High volume physical activity and cardiovascular risk. *American Journal of Hypertension.* 30(4): 353–354.

Francois, M. E., et al. 2017. Similar metabolic response to lower- versus upper-body interval exercise or endurance exercise. *Metabolism* 68:1–10.

Harrington, R. A., et al. 2015. More than 10 million steps in the right direction: Results from the first American Heart Association scientific sessions walking challenge. *Progress in Cardiovascular Diseases* 57(4): 296–298.

Heinrich, K. M., et al. 2014. High-intensity compared to moderate-intensity training for exercise initiation, enjoyment, adherence, and intentions: An intervention study. *BMC Public Health* 14: 789.

Hills, A. P., et al. 2015. Supporting public health priorities: Recommendations for physical education and physical activity promotion in schools. *Progress in Cardiovascular Diseases* 57(4): 368–374.

Imboden, M. T., et al. 2018. Cardiorespiratory fitness and mortality in healthy men and women. *Journal American College Cardiology* 72(19): 2283–2292.

Joyner, M. J. 2017. Exercise and trainability. *Journal of Physiology.* Published online.

Kim, Y., et al. 2018. The combination of cardiorespiratory fitness and muscle strength, and mortality risk. *European Journal Epidemiology* 33(10): 953–964.

Koohsari, M. J., et al. 2015. Public open space, physical activity, urban design and public health: Concepts, methods and research agenda. *Health & Place* 33: 75–82.

Lavie, C. J., et al. 2019. Sedentary behavior, exercise, and cardiovascular health. *Circulation Research* 124(5): 799–815.

Leskinen, T., and U. M. Kujala. 2015. Health-related findings among twin pairs discordant for leisure-time physical activity for 32 years: The TWINACTIVE Study synopsis. *Twin Research in Human Genetics* 18(3): 266–272.

Liu, J. X., et al. 2019. The effects of high-intensity interval training versus moderate-intensity continuous training on fat loss and cardiometabolic health in pediatric obesity: A protocol of systematic review and meta-analysis. *Medicine* 98(10): e14751.

Lyden, K., et al. 2015. Discrete features of sedentary behaviors impact cardiometabolic risk factors. *Medicine and Science in Sports and Exercise* 47(5): 1079–1086.

Mabire, L., et al. 2017. The influence of age, sex and body mass index on the effectiveness of brisk walking for obesity management in adults. A systematic review and meta-analysis. *Journal of Physical Activity and Health* 7: 1–46.

Malina, R. M. 2015. Physical activity, health and nutrition. *World Review of Nutrition and Dietetics* 113: 68–71.

Manas, A., et al. 2019. Can physical activity offset the detrimental consequences of sedentary time on frailty? A moderation analysis in 749 older adults measured with accelerometers. *Journal American Medical Directors Association* 20(5): 834–638.

Marques, A., et al. 2015. Do students know the physical activity recommendations for health promotion? *Journal of Physical Activity and Health* 12(2): 253–256.

Marzetti, E., et al. 2017. Physical activity and exercise as countermeasures to physical frailty and sarcopenia. *Aging Clinical and Experimental Research* 29(1): 35–42.

Melanson, E. L. 2017. The effect of exercise on non-exercise physical activity and sedentary behavior in adults. *Obesity Reviews* 18(Suppl. 1): 40–49.

Muntaner-Mas, A., et al. 2019. A systematic review of fitness apps and their potential clinical and sports utility for objective and remote assessment of cardiorespiratory fitness. *Sports Medicine* 49(4): 587–600.

Myers, J., et al. 2015. Physical activity and cardiorespiratory fitness as major markers of cardiovascular risk: Their independent and interwoven importance to health status. *Progress in Cardiovascular Diseases* 57(4): 306–314.

Pedersen, B. K. 2019. Which type of exercise keeps you young? *Current Opinions Clinical Nutrition Metabolic Care* 22(2): 167–173.

Petersen, B. A., et al. 2017. Low load, high repetition resistance training program increases bone mineral density in untrained adults. *Journal of Sports Medicine and Physical Fitness* 57(1–2): 70–76.

Rivera-Torres, S., et al. 2019. Adherence to exercise programs in older adults: Informative report. *Gerontology Geriatrics Medicine* 5: 2333721418823604.

Romieu, I. 2017. Energy balance and obesity. *Cancer Causes and Control* 28(3): 247–258.

Rowlands, A. V. 2015. Physical activity, inactivity, and health. *Pediatric Exercise Science* 27(1): 21–25.

Sjogren, P., et al. 2014. Stand up for health—Avoiding sedentary behaviour might lengthen your telomeres: Secondary outcomes from a physical activity RCT in older people. *British Journal of Sports Medicine* 48(19): 1407–1409.

Slimani, M., et al. 2018. A meta-analysis to determine strength training related dose-response relationships for lower-limb muscle power development in young athletes. *Frontiers of Physiology* 9: 1155.

Soares-Miranda, L., et al. 2014. Physical activity and heart rate variability in older adults: The Cardiovascular Health Study. *Circulation* 129(21): 2100–2110.

Strain, T., et al. 2019. Physical activity surveillance through smartphone apps and wearable trackers: Examining the UK potential for nationally representative sampling. *Journal Medical Internet Research Mhealth Uhealth* 7(1): e11898.

U.S. Department of Health and Human Services. 2018. *Physical Activity Guidelines for Americans.* Washington, DC: U.S. Department of Health and Human Services.

Valle, C. G., et al. 2015. Physical activity in young adults: A signal detection analysis of Health Information National Trends Survey (HINTS) 2007 data. *Journal of Health Communication* 20(2): 134–146.

Viana, R. B., et al. 2019. Is interval training the magic bullet for fat loss? A systematic review and meta-analysis comparing moderate-intensity continuous training with high-intensity interval training (HIIT). *British Journal Sports Medicine.* Published online.

White, D. K., et al. 2015. Do short spurts of physical activity benefit cardiovascular health? The CARDIA Study. *Medicine and Science in Sports and Exercise* 47(11): 2353–2358.

Zhou, M., et al. 2018. Tai chi improves brain metabolism and muscle energetics in older adults. *Journal of Neuroimaging* 28(4): 359–364.

SAMPLE PROGRAMS FOR POPULAR ACTIVITIES

The following sections present four sample programs based on different types of cardiorespiratory activities—walking/jogging, bicycling, swimming, and rowing. Each sample program includes regular cardiorespiratory endurance exercise, resistance training, and stretching. Read the descriptions of the programs you're considering, and decide which will work best for you based on your present routine, the potential for enjoyment, and adaptability to your lifestyle. If you choose one of these programs, complete the personal fitness program plan in Lab 7.1, just as if you had created a program from scratch.

No program will produce enormous changes in your fitness level in the first few weeks. Follow the specifics of the program for three to four weeks. Then, if the exercise program doesn't seem suitable, make adjustments to adapt it to your particular needs. But retain the basic elements of the program that make it effective for developing fitness.

GENERAL GUIDELINES

The following guidelines can help make the activity programs more effective for you:

• *Frequency and time.* To improve physical fitness, exercise for 20–60 minutes at least three times a week.

• *Intensity.* To work effectively for cardiorespiratory endurance training or to improve body composition, raise your heart rate into its target zone. Monitor your pulse or use rates of perceived exertion to monitor your intensity. If you've been sedentary, begin very slowly. Give your muscles a chance to adjust to their increased workload. It's probably best to keep your heart rate below target until your body has had time to adjust to new demands. At first you may not need to work very hard to keep your heart rate in its target zone, but as your cardiorespiratory endurance improves, you will probably need to increase intensity.

• *Interval training.* Some of the sample programs involve continuous activity. Others rely on interval training, which calls for alternating a relief interval with exercise (walking after jogging, for example, or coasting after biking uphill). Interval training is an effective method of progressive overload and improves fitness rapidly (see Chapter 3).

• *Resistance training and stretching guidelines.* For the resistance training and stretching parts of the program, remember the general guidelines for safe and effective exercise. See the summary of guidelines in Figure 7.2

• *Warm-up and cool-down.* Begin each exercise session with a 10-minute warm-up. Begin your activity at a slow pace, and work up gradually to your target heart rate. Always slow down gradually at the end of your exercise session to bring your system back to its normal state. It's a good idea to do stretching exercises to increase your flexibility *after* cardiorespiratory exercise or strength training because your muscles will be warm and ready to stretch.

Follow the guidelines presented in Chapter 3 for exercising in hot or cold weather. Drink enough liquids to stay adequately hydrated, particularly in hot weather.

• *Record keeping.* After each exercise session, record your daily distance or time on a progress chart.

WALKING/JOGGING SAMPLE PROGRAM

Walking is the perfect exercise. It increases longevity; builds fitness; expends calories; prevents weight gain; and protects against heart disease, stroke, and back pain. You don't need to join a gym, and you can walk almost anywhere. People who walk 30 minutes five times per week will lose an average of 5 pounds in 6–12 months—without dieting, watching what they eat, or exercising intensely.

Jogging takes walking to the next level. Jogging only 75 minutes per week will increase fitness, promote weight control, and provide health benefits that will prevent disease and increase longevity. Your ultimate goal for promoting wellness is to walk at a moderate intensity for 150–300 minutes per week or jog at 70% effort or more for 75–150 minutes per week.

It isn't always easy to distinguish among walking, jogging, and running. For clarity and consistency, we'll consider walking to be any on-foot exercise of less than 5 miles per hour, jogging any pace between 5 and 7.5 miles per hour, and running any pace faster than that. The faster your pace or the longer you exercise, the more calories you burn (Table 1). The greater the number of calories burned, the higher the potential training effects of these activities. Table 2 contains a sample walking/jogging program.

Equipment and Technique

These activities require no special skills, expensive equipment, or unusual facilities. Comfortable clothing, well-fitted walking or running shoes (see Chapter 3), and a stopwatch or ordinary watch with a second hand are all you need.

When you advance to jogging, use proper technique:

• Run with your back straight and your head up. Look straight ahead, not at your feet. Shift your pelvis forward and tuck your buttocks in.

• Hold your arms slightly away from your body. Your elbows should be bent so that your forearms are parallel to the ground. You may cup your hands, but do not clench your fists. Allow your arms to swing loosely and rhythmically with each stride.

• Let your heel hit the ground first in each stride. Then roll forward onto the ball of your foot and push off for the next stride.

Table 1

Estimated Calories Expended by a 165-pound Adult at Different Intensities of Walking and Jogging for 150 and 300 minutes per week (min/wk)

	SPEED (MILES/HOUR)	SPEED (MINUTES/MILE)	CALORIES EXPENDED EXERCISING 150 MIN/WK	CALORIES EXPENDED EXERCISING 300 MIN/WK
	Rest	—	190	380
WALKING	2.5	24	565	1,130
	3.0	20	620	1,240
	4.0	15	940	1,880
	4.3	14	1,125	2,250
JOGGING	5.0	12	1,500	3,000
	6.0	10	1,875	3,750
	7.0	8.6	2,155	4,310
RUNNING	8.0	6.7	2,530	5,060
	10.0	6	3,000	6,000

NOTE: Heavier people will expend slightly more calories, while lighter people will expend slightly fewer

SOURCE: Adapted from Physical Activity Guidelines Advisory Committee. 2008. *Physical Activity Guidelines Advisory Committee Report.* Washington, DC: U.S. Department of Health and Human Services.

Table 2 | Sample Walking/Jogging Fitness Program

DAY	ACTIVITIES
Monday	• **Walking/jogging:** Walk briskly for 30 minutes or jog for 25 minutes. • **Stretching:** Stretch major muscle groups for 10 minutes after exercise. Do each exercise two times; hold stretch for 10–30 seconds.

Tuesday	• **Resistance workout:** Using body weight for resistance, perform the following exercises:
	  • Push-ups: 2 sets, 20 reps per set
	  • Pull-ups: 2 sets, 5 reps per set
	  • Unloaded squats: 2 sets, 10 reps per set
	  • Curl-ups: 2 sets, 20 reps per set
	  • Side bridges: 3 sets, 10-second hold (left and right sides)
	  • Spine extensions: 3 sets, 10-second hold (left and right sides)

Wednesday	• Repeat Monday activities.
Thursday	• Repeat Tuesday activities.
Friday	• Repeat Monday activities.
Saturday	• Rest.
Sunday	• Rest.

If you find this difficult, you can try a more flat-footed style, but don't land on the balls of your feet. More of a forefoot landing is recommended in barefoot running or with minimal footwear.

• Keep your steps short by allowing your foot to strike the ground in line with your knee. Keep your knees bent at all times.

• Breathe deeply through your mouth. Try to use your abdominal muscles rather than just your chest muscles to take deep breaths.

• Stay relaxed.

Find a safe, convenient place to walk or jog. Exercise on a trail, path, or sidewalk to stay clear of bicycles and cars. Make sure your clothes are brightly colored so that others can see you easily.

Beginning a Walking/Jogging Program

Start slowly if you have not been exercising, are overweight, or are recovering from an illness or surgery. At first, walk for 15 minutes at a slow pace, below your target heart rate zone. Gradually increase to 30-minute sessions. You will probably cover 1–2 miles. At the beginning, walk every other day.

You can gradually increase to walking five days per week or more if you want to expend more calories (which is helpful if you want to change body composition). Depending on your weight, you will expend ("burn") 90–135 calories during each 30-minute walking session. To increase the calories that you expend, walk for a longer time or for a longer distance instead of sharply increasing speed.

Start at the level of effort that is most comfortable for you. Maintain a normal, easy pace and stop to rest as often as you need to. Never prolong a walk past the point of comfort. When walking with a friend (a good motivator), let a comfortable conversation be your guide to pace. If you find that you cannot carry on a conversation without getting out of breath, you are walking too quickly.

Once your muscles have become adjusted to the exercise program, increase the duration of your sessions by no more than 10% each week. Keep your heart rate just below your target zone. Don't be discouraged by a lack of immediate progress, and don't try to speed things up by overdoing it. Remember that pace and heart rate can vary with the terrain, the weather, and other factors.

Advanced Walking

Advanced walking involves walking more quickly for longer times. You should feel an increased perception of effort, but the exercise intensity should not be too stressful. Vary your pace to allow for intervals of slow, medium, and fast walking. Keep your heart rate toward the lower end of your target zone with brief periods in the upper levels. At first, walk for 30 minutes and increase your walking time gradually until eventually you reach 60 minutes at a brisk pace and can walk 2–4 miles. Try to walk at least five days per week. Vary your program by changing the pace and distance or by walking routes with different terrains and views. You can expect to burn 200–350 calories or more during each advanced walking session.

Making the Transition to Jogging

Increase the intensity of exercise by gradually introducing jogging into your walking program. During a 2-mile walk, for example, periodically jog for 100 yards and then resume walking. Increase the number and distance of your jogging segments until you can jog continuously for the entire distance. More physically fit people may be capable of jogging without walking first. However, people unaccustomed to jogging should initially combine walking with short bouts of jogging.

A good strategy is to exercise on a 400-meter track at a local high school or college. Begin by covering 800 meters—jogging the straightaways and walking the turns. Progress to walking 200 meters (half lap) and jogging 200 meters; jogging 400 meters and walking 200 meters; jogging 800 meters, walking 200 meters; and jogging 1200 meters, walking 200 meters. Continue until you can jog 2 miles without stopping.

During the transition to jogging, adjust the ratio of walking to jogging to keep within your target heart rate zone as much as possible. Most people who sustain a continuous jogging or running program will find that they can stay within their target heart rate zone with a speed of 5.5–7.5 miles per hour (8–11 minutes per mile). Exercise at least every other day. Increasing frequency by doing other activities on alternate days will place less stress on the weight-bearing parts of your lower body than will a daily program of walking/jogging.

Developing Muscular Strength and Endurance and Flexibility

Walking, jogging, and running provide muscular endurance workouts for your lower body; they also develop muscular strength of the lower body to a lesser degree. If you'd like to increase your speed and performance, you might want to focus your program on lower-body exercises. (Don't neglect upper-body strength. It is important for overall wellness.) For flexibility, pay special attention to the hamstrings and quadriceps, which are not worked through their complete range of motion during walking or jogging. Strength training, particularly body-building, can sometimes decrease flexibility, so stretching is particularly important for people who lift weights.

Staying with Your Walking/Jogging Program

Health experts have found that simple motivators such as using a pedometer, walking a dog, parking farther from the office or grocery store, or training for a fun run help people stay with their programs. Use a pedometer or GPS exercise device to track your progress and help motivate you to increase distance and speed. Accurate pedometers for walking, such as those made by Omron, Yamax, and New-Lifestyles, cost $20–$40 and are accurate to about 5%. Sophisticated GPS-based devices and apps made by Polar, Garmin, and Nike keep track of your exercise speed and distance via satellite, monitor heart rate, and store data that can be downloaded wirelessly to your computer or their own websites. Several of these units can be plugged in to programs such as Google Earth, which give you a satellite view of your walking or jogging route.

A pedometer can also help you increase the number of steps you walk each day. Most sedentary people take only 2,000 to 3,000 steps per day. Adding 1,000 steps per day and increasing gradually until you reach 10,000 steps can increase fitness and help you manage your weight.

BICYCLING SAMPLE PROGRAM

Bicycling can also lead to large gains in physical fitness. For many people, cycling is a pleasant and economical alternative to driving and a convenient way to build fitness.

Equipment and Technique

Cycling has its own special array of equipment, including helmets, lights, safety gear, and biking shoes. The bike is the most expensive item, ranging from about $100 to $1,000 or more. Avoid making a large investment until you're sure you'll use your bike regularly. While investigating what the marketplace has to offer, rent or borrow a bike. Consider your intended use of the bike. Most cyclists who are interested primarily in fitness are best served by a sturdy road bike rather than a mountain bike or sport bike. Stationary cycles are good for rainy days and areas that have harsh winters.

Clothing for bike riding shouldn't be restrictive or binding; nor should it be so loose that it catches the wind and slows you down. Shirts that wick moisture away from your skin and padded biking shorts make a ride more comfortable. Wear glasses or goggles to protect your eyes from dirt, small objects, and irritation from wind. Wear a pair of well-padded gloves if your hands tend to become numb while riding or if you begin to develop blisters or calluses.

To avoid saddle soreness and injury, choose a soft or padded saddle, and adjust it to a height that allows your legs to almost reach full extension while pedaling. To prevent backache and neck strain, warm up thoroughly and periodically shift the position of your hands on the handlebars and your body in the saddle. Keep your arms relaxed and don't lock your elbows. To protect your knees from strain, pedal with your feet pointed straight ahead or very slightly inward, and don't pedal in high gear for long periods.

Bike riding requires a number of precise skills that practice makes automatic. If you've never ridden before, consider taking a course. In fact, many courses are not just for beginners. They'll help you develop skills in braking, shifting, and handling emergencies, as well as teach you ways of caring for and repairing your bike. An **e-bike** is a good choice for people who commute to work or want some help climbing hills or riding long distances. For safe cycling, follow these rules:

- Always wear a helmet.
- Keep on the correct side of the road. Bicycling against traffic is usually illegal and always dangerous.
- Obey all the same traffic signs and signals that apply to autos.
- On public roads, ride in single file, except in low-traffic areas (if the law permits). Ride in a straight line; don't swerve or weave in traffic.
- Be alert; anticipate the movements of other traffic and pedestrians. Listen for approaching traffic that is out of your line of vision.
- Slow down at street crossings. Check both ways before crossing.
- Use hand signals—the same as for automobile drivers—if you intend to stop or turn. Use audible signals to warn those in your path.
- Maintain full control. Avoid anything that interferes with your vision. Don't jeopardize your ability to steer by carrying anything (including people) on the handlebars.
- Keep your bicycle in good shape. Brakes, gears, saddle, wheels, and tires should always be in good condition.
- See and be seen. Use a headlight at night and equip your bike with rear reflectors. Use side reflectors on pedals, front and rear. Wear light-colored clothing or use reflective tape at night; wear bright colors or use fluorescent tape by day.
- Be courteous to other road users. Anticipate the worst and practice preventive cycling.
- Use a rear-view mirror.

e-bike Electrically assisted bike.   TERMS

Developing Cardiorespiratory Endurance

Cycling is an excellent way to develop and maintain cardiorespiratory endurance and a healthy body composition.

FITT-VP—frequency, intensity, time, type, volume, progression:

If you've been inactive for a long time, begin your cycling program at a heart rate that is 10–20% below your target zone. Beginning cyclists should pedal at about 80–100 revolutions per minute; adjust the gear so that you can pedal at that rate easily. You can equip your bicycle with a cycling computer that displays different types of useful information, such as speed, distance traveled, heart rate, altitude, and revolutions per minute.

Once you feel at home on your bike, try cycling 1 mile at a comfortable speed, and then stop and check your heart rate. Increase your speed gradually until you can cycle at 12–15 miles per hour (4–5 minutes per mile), a speed fast enough to bring most new cyclists' heart rate into their target zone. Allow your pulse rate to be your guide: More highly fit individuals may need to ride faster to achieve their target heart rate. Cycling for at least 20 minutes three days per week will improve your fitness.

At the beginning:

It may require several outings to get the muscles and joints of your legs and hips adjusted to this new activity. Begin each outing with a 10-minute warm-up. When your muscles are warm, stretch your hamstrings and your back and neck muscles. Until you become a skilled cyclist, select routes with the fewest hazards and avoid heavy automobile traffic.

As you progress:

Interval training is also effective with bicycling. Simply increase your speed to near maximum intensity for periods of 30 seconds to 2 minutes. Then ride more slowly for 2–3 minutes. Alternate the speed intervals and slow intervals for a total of 20–60 minutes, depending on your level of fitness. Biking over hilly terrain is also a form of interval training. Progress through a combination of increased speed or increased distance until you reach your fitness goals.

Developing Muscular Strength and Endurance and Flexibility

Bicycling develops a high level of endurance and a moderate level of strength in the muscles of the lower body. If one of your goals is to increase your cycling speed and performance, be sure to include exercises for the quadriceps, hamstrings, and buttocks muscles in your strength training program. For flexibility, pay special attention to the hamstrings and quadriceps, which are not worked through their complete range of motion during bike riding, and to the muscles in your lower back, shoulders, and neck.

SWIMMING SAMPLE PROGRAM

Swimming works every major muscle group in the body. It increases upper-and lower-body strength, promotes cardiovascular fitness, and is excellent for rehabilitating athletic injuries and preventing day-to-day aches and pains. It promotes weight control; builds powerful lungs, heart, and blood vessels; and promotes metabolic health. People weigh only 6-10 pounds in the water, so swimming places less stress on the knees, hips, and back than do jogging, hiking, volleyball, or basketball.

Swimming is one of the most popular recreational and competitive sports in the world. More than 120 million Americans swim regularly. More than 165,000 of these are competitive age-group swimmers (ages 5-18), and more than 30,000 competitors are over 19 years of age. You don't need a backyard pool to swim. Almost every town and city in America has a public pool. Pools are standard in many health clubs, YMCAs, and schools. Ocean and lake swimming may be options in the summer. High-tech wet suits make it possible to swim outdoors even in the middle of winter in many parts of the country.

Training Methods

Improved fitness from swimming depends on the quantity, quality, and frequency of training. Most swimmers use interval training to increase swimming fitness, speed, and endurance. Interval training calls for repeated fast swims at fixed distances followed by rest. Continuous distance or endurance training builds stamina and mental toughness. Interval and distance training each play important and different roles in improving fitness for swimming. Interval training improves overall swimming speed and the ability to swim fast at the beginning of a swim. Endurance training helps to maintain a faster average pace during a swim without becoming overly fatigued. Endurance training becomes more important when you want to compete in long, open-water swims or triathlons.

In swimming workouts, however, quality is better than quantity. Thirty years ago, elite swimmers from East Germany sometimes swam as much as 20,000 meters in a single workout (more than 12 miles). Recent studies found that competitive athletes who swam 4,000-6,000 meters per workout produced results similar to those who swam much farther. Likewise, recreational swimmers can improve fitness, strength, and power by swimming 1,000-2,000 meters (approximately 1,100-2,200 yards) per workout. Swim fast to get maximum benefits, but maintain good technique to maximize efficiency and minimize the risk of injury.

Interval training:

Interval training increases sprinting speed so that you can accelerate faster at the beginning of a swim. It also helps the body cope with metabolic waste products so that you can maintain your speed during the workout. To increase speed, swim intervals between 25 and 200 meters (or yards) at 80-90% effort. An example of a beginning program might be to swim 4 sets of 50 meters using the sidestroke at 70% of maximum effort, with a 1-minute rest between sets. A more advanced program would be to swim 10 sets of 100 meters using the freestyle stroke at 85-95% maximum effort with 30 seconds of rest between sets.

Endurance training:

Include longer swims—1,000 meters or more at a time—to build general stamina for swimming. Endurance training will improve aerobic capacity and help your cells use fuels and clear metabolic wastes. This will allow you to swim faster and longer. Longer swims promote metabolic health and build physical fitness.

Cross-training:

Cross-training combines more than one type of endurance exercise, such as swimming and jogging, in your program at a time. It also includes exercises that build strength, power, and skill. It is a good training method for people who prefer swimming but don't have daily access to a swimming pool or open water. Including multiple exercises, such as swimming and running, stair stepping, cycling, weight training exercises, and calisthenics, adds variety to the program. It also prepares you for a greater variety of physical challenges. See Chapter 3 for a discussion of cross-training and a description of typical workouts.

Technique: The Basic Swimming Strokes for General Conditioning

The best strokes for conditioning are the freestyle and sidestroke. Competitive athletes also swim the breaststroke, butterfly, and backstroke (but not the sidestroke). Learning efficient swimming strokes helps increase enjoyment and results in better workouts. Take a class from the Red Cross, local recreation department, or private coach if you are not a strong swimmer or need help with the basic strokes.

Freestyle:

While freestyle technically includes any unregulated stroke (such as the sidestroke), it generally refers to the front (Australian) crawl or overhand stroke. Freestyle is the fastest stroke and is best for general conditioning. Swim this stroke in a prone (face-down) position with arms stretched out in front and legs extended to the back. Move through the water by pulling first with the right arm and then with the left, while performing a kicking motion generated from the hips. During the stroke, rotate the thumb and palm 45 degrees toward the bottom of the pool. Pull in a semicircle downward toward the center of the body with the elbow higher than the hand. When the hand reaches the beginning of the ribcage, push the palm backward underneath the body as far as possible. Don't begin to stroke with the other hand until the first stroke is completed. Maximize the distance with each stroke by pulling fully and maintaining good posture.

The crawl uses a flutter kick, which involves moving the legs alternately with the force generated from the hips and a slight bend of the knees. Maintain a neutral spine during the stroke. A strong kick is important to minimize body roll during the stroke. For this reason, some of your training should include kicking without using the arms.

Breathing is almost always a problem for novice swimmers. Don't hold your breath! You will fatigue rapidly if you have poor air exchange during swimming. Breathe by turning the head to the side of a recovering stroke. Do not lift the head out of the water. Exhale continuously through the nose and mouth between breaths. Beginners should breathe on the same side following each stroke cycle (left and right arm strokes).

Sidestroke:

Even novices can get a good workout with minimal skill using the sidestroke. This is a good choice for beginners because you keep your head out of water and can swim great distances without fatigue. Lie in the water on your right side and stretch your right arm and hand in front of you in the direction you want to swim and place your left hand across your chest. Draw your right arm toward you, pulling at the water until your hand reaches your waist. At the same time, make a scissors kick with your legs. Repeat the stroke as your forward speed slows. Swim half the distance on your right side and the rest on your left side.

Beginning Swim Program

Take swimming lessons from a certified teacher or coach if you are a nonswimmer or have not used swimming as your primary form of exercise. A swim teacher can help you develop good technique, make more rapid progress, and avoid injuries.

To assess your starting fitness, take the 12-minute swim test described in Lab 3.1. Use the swim test table to help you measure progress in your program. Take the test every one or two months to help establish short-term goals.

Start your program by swimming one length (one-half lap) at a time, using either freestyle or sidestroke. If you can't swim the length of a standard pool (25 meters or yards), begin by swimming the width. As soon as you can, swim one length of the pool, rest for 30 seconds, and then repeat. Build up your capacity until you can swim 20 lengths with a short rest interval between each length. If you start your program with the sidestroke, try to switch to the freestyle stroke as quickly as you can.

Increase the distance of each swim to a full lap (50 meters or yards) with 30–60 seconds of rest between laps. Build up until you can swim 20 sets of 50-meter swims with 30 seconds of rest between sets. Gradually increase the distance of each set to 100-meter swims. You are ready for the next level when you can swim 10 sets of 100 meters with 30 seconds of rest between sets.

Swimming Program for Higher Levels of Fitness

This program includes a warm-up, specific conditioning drills for strokes and kicking, and a cool-down. It involves interval training three days a week and distance training two days per week.

Warm up before each workout by swimming 2–4 laps at an easy pace. It is also a good idea to warm up your legs and hips by holding on to the side of the pool and gently moving your legs using a flutter-kick motion. At the end of the workout, cool down by swimming 100–200 meters at a slow pace.

On Monday, Wednesday, and Friday, do interval training. Your goal is to swim intervals totaling 2,000 meters per workout (20 sets of 100 meters each) at a fast pace with 30 seconds of rest between each set, or interval (i.e., swim 100 meters, rest,

swim 100 meters, rest, etc.). Every fifth interval, swim 25 meters using your legs alone, with your arms extended in front of you. Have someone watch you during the legs-only swims to make sure you are kicking mainly from the hips and maintaining a neutral spine. Add variety to your interval training workouts by using gloves, swim paddles, or fins.

If you are unable to do the interval workout at first, modify it by increasing rest intervals, decreasing speed, or decreasing the number of sets as you gradually increase the volume and intensity.

On Tuesday and Thursday, do distance training. Swim 1,000–2,000 meters continuously at a comfortable pace. Although distance days will help develop endurance, they are used mainly to help you recover from intense interval training days.

Rest on Saturday and Sunday. Rest is very important to help your muscles and metabolism recover and build fitness. Rest will also prevent overtraining and overuse injuries. Include two rest days per week. Rest days can be consecutive (such as Saturday and Sunday) or interspersed during the normal workout schedule.

Integrating Swimming into a Total Fitness Program

You will develop fitness best and maintain interest in continuing your exercise program by varying the structure of your workouts. Incorporate kick boards, pull-buoys, hand paddles, and fins into some of your training sessions. Cross-training is a good option for developing well-rounded fitness. Swimming results in moderate gains in strength and large gains in endurance.

Because swimming is not a weight-bearing activity and is not done in an upright position, it elicits a lower heart rate per minute. Therefore, swimmers need to adjust their target heart rate zone. To calculate your target heart rate for swimming, use this formula:

Maximum swimming heart rate (MSHR) = 205 − age

Target heart rate zone = 65−90% of MSHR

For example, a 19-year-old swimmer would calculate his or her target heart rate zone for swimming as follows:

MSHR: 205 − 19 = 186 bpm

65% intensity: 0.65 × 186 = 121 bpm

90% intensity: 0.90 × 186 = 167 bpm

Swimming does not preserve bone density as you age, so swimmers are advised to include weight training in their exercise program. Perform at least one set of 10 repetitions for 8–10 exercises that use the major muscle groups in the body. To improve swimming performance, include exercises that work key muscles. For example, if you primarily swim the freestyle stroke, include exercises to increase strength in your shoulders, arms, upper back, and hips. Training the muscles you use during swimming can also help prevent injuries. In your flexibility training, pay special attention to the muscles you use during swimming, particularly the shoulders, hips, and back. Table 3 shows a basic sample swimming program that incorporates all these types of exercises.

Table 3	Sample Swimming Program

DAY	ACTIVITIES
Monday	• **Warm-up:** Swim 100–200 meters (2–4 laps of a standard pool) at an easy pace. • **Intervals:** Swim 10–20 sets of 100-meter swims at 90% effort, with 30 seconds of rest between sets. After every 5 sets, swim 25 meters using your legs alone. • **Cool-down:** Swim 100–200 meters at a slow pace. • **Weight training:** Do at least 1 set of 10 repetitions of 8–10 exercises that work the body's major muscle groups. • **Flexibility:** Do standard stretching exercises for the shoulders, chest, back, hips, and thighs.
Tuesday	• **Distance:** Swim 1,000–2,000 meters continuously at a comfortable pace.
Wednesday	• Repeat Monday activities.
Thursday	• Repeat Tuesday activities.
Friday	• Repeat Monday activities.
Saturday	• **Rest.**
Sunday	• **Rest.**

ROWING MACHINE SAMPLE PROGRAM

Rowing is a whole-body exercise that overloads the cardiorespiratory system and strengthens the major muscles of the body. The beauty and serenity of rowing on flat water in the morning is indescribable, but few people have access to a lake and rowing shell. Fortunately, sophisticated rowing machines simulate the rowing motion and make it possible to do this exercise at the fitness center or at a health club.

Modern rowing machines are very much like the real thing. They provide resistance with hydraulic pistons, magnets, air, or water. The best machines are solid and comfortable, provide a steady stroke, and allow you to maintain a neutral spine so that you don't injure your back. Many rowing machines come with LCD displays that show heart rate, stroke rate, power output, and estimated caloric expenditure. They are also preprogrammed with workouts for interval training, cardiovascular conditioning, and moderate-intensity physical activity. Good rowing mechanics are essential because, if done incorrectly, rowing can cause severe overuse injuries that can damage the back, hips, knees, elbows, and shoulders.

Technique: Basic Rowing Movement

Most of the power for rowing comes from the thigh and hip muscles and finishes with a pulling motion with the upper body. Maintain a neutral spine (that is, with normal curves) during the movement. Hinge at the hips and not at the back during the rowing motion.

The rowing movement includes the following phases:

• *The catch.* The catch involves sliding the seat forward on the track with arms straight as far as you can while keeping the spine neutral.

• *The drive.* The drive begins by pushing with the legs and keeping your arms straight.

• *The finish.* Finish by leaning back slightly (still maintaining a neutral spine) and pulling the handle to your abdomen.

• *The recovery.* Recover by extending your arms forward, hinging forward at the hips with a neutral spine, and sliding forward again on the seat for another "catch."

Training Methods

Your rowing program should include both continuous training and interval training. Continuous training calls for rowing for a specific amount of time—typically 20–90 minutes without stopping. Most people enjoy rowing at about 70% of maximum heart rate.

Interval training involves a series of exercise bouts followed by rest. The method manipulates distance, intensity, repetitions, and rest. An example of an interval workout would be to row for 8 sets of 4-minute exercise bouts at 85% effort with 2 minutes of rest between intervals, or sets. During interval training, changing one factor affects the others. For example, if you increase the intensity of exercise, you will need more rest between intervals and won't be able to do as many repetitions. High-intensity exercise builds fitness best but also increases the risk of injury and loss of motivation. Make intervals challenging but not so difficult that you get injured or discouraged.

Beginning Rowing Program

During the first few workouts, start conservatively by rowing for 10 minutes at a rate of about 20 strokes per minute with a moderate resistance. Exercise at about 60% effort. Do this workout three times during the first week. The movement is deceptively easy and invigorating. You are, however, using all the major muscle groups in the body and are probably not ready for a more intense exercise program.

After the first workout, do a series of 5-minute intervals during the first few weeks of training. For example, row for 5 minutes, rest 3 minutes, row 5 minutes, then rest 3 minutes. Build up until you can do 4–6 repetitions of 5-minute exercise intervals, resting only 1 minute between sets. Gradually, increase the time for each interval to 15 minutes and vary the rowing cadence from 20 to 25 strokes per minute. Your first short-term goal is to complete 30 minutes of continuous rowing without stopping.

Rowing Program for Higher Levels of Fitness

Vary your training methods after you can row continuously for 30 minutes, gain some fitness, and are used to the technique. Alternate between interval training and distance training. Doing both will help you develop fitness rapidly and improve rowing efficiency. A good strategy is to row continuously at about 70% effort for 30–60 minutes three days per week and practice interval training at 80–90% effort for two days per week. Do resistance and flexibility training two or three days per week. A basic but complete rowing machine program that includes continuous and interval training as well as resistance and flexibility exercises is shown in Table 4.

Table 4	Sample Rowing Machine Fitness Program

DAY	ACTIVITIES
Monday	• **Warm-up:** Row at low intensity for 2 minutes. • **Continuous rowing:** Row for 30 minutes at 70% effort (20–22 strokes per minute). • **Weight training (1–2 sets of 10 repetitions):** Squats, leg curls, bench press, lat pulls, raises, biceps curls, triceps extensions, curl-ups, side bridge (10 seconds per side), spine extensions (10 seconds per side). • **Stretching:** Do static stretching exercises for the shoulders, chest, back, hips, and thighs. Hold each stretch for 10–30 seconds.
Tuesday	• **Warm-up:** Row at low intensity for 2 minutes. • **Continuous rowing:** Row at 60–70% of maximum effort for 5 minutes. Rest for 3 minutes. • **Interval rowing:** Row 6 sets, for 5 minutes per set, at 25 strokes per minute (90% effort) Rest for 3 minutes between intervals.
Wednesday	• **Warm-up:** Row at low intensity for 2 minutes. • **Continuous rowing:** Row for 45 minutes at 70% effort (20–22 strokes per minute). • **Stretching:** Repeat Monday stretches.
Thursday	• **Warm-up:** Row at low intensity for 2 minutes. • **Continuous rowing:** Row for 30 minutes at 70% effort (20–22 strokes per minute). • **Weight training (1–2 sets of 10 repetitions):** Repeat Monday weight training exercises.
Friday	• **Warm-up:** Row at low intensity for 2 minutes. • **Continuous rowing:** Row for 30 minutes at 70% effort (20–22 strokes per minute). • **Stretching:** Repeat Monday stretches.
Saturday	• **Rest.**
Sunday	• **Rest.**

Name _____ Section _____ Date _____

LAB 7.1 A Personal Fitness Program Plan and Agreement

A. I, _____ , am making an agreement with myself to follow a physical fitness program
(name)
to work toward the following goals:

Specific or short-term goals (include current status for each):

1. _____

2. _____

3. _____

4. _____

General or long-term goals:

1. _____

2. _____

3. _____

4. _____

B. My program plan is as follows:

Activities	Components (Check ✓)					Frequency (Check ✓)							Intensity*	Time (duration)
	CRE	MS	ME	F	BC	M	Tu	W	Th	F	Sa	Su		

*Conduct activities for achieving CRE goals in your target range for heart rate or RPE.

C. My program will begin on _____. My program includes the following schedule of mini-goals. For each step in my program,
(date)
I will give myself the reward listed.

_____ _____ _____
(mini-goal 1)   (date)   (reward)

_____ _____ _____
(mini-goal 2)   (date)   (reward)

_____ _____ _____
(mini-goal 3)   (date)   (reward)

_____ _____ _____
(mini-goal 4)   (date)   (reward)

_____ _____ _____
(mini-goal 5)   (date)   (reward)

LABORATORY ACTIVITIES

D. My program will include the addition of physical activity to my daily routine (such as climbing stairs or walking to class):

1. _____
2. _____
3. _____
4. _____

E. My program will include the following strategies for reducing sedentary time:

1. _____
2. _____
3. _____
4. _____

F. I will use the following tools to monitor my program and my progress toward my goals (list any charts, graphs, or journals you plan to use):

_____
_____
_____

I sign this agreement as an indication of my personal commitment to reach my goal.

_____   _____
(your signature)   (date)

I have recruited a helper who will witness my agreement and _____

_____
_____
(list any way your helper will participate in your program)

_____   _____
(witness's signature)   (date)

Name _____ Section _____ Date _____

LAB 7.2   Getting to Know Your Fitness Facility

To help create a successful training program, take time to learn more about the fitness facility you plan to use.

Basic Information

Name and location of facility: _____

Hours of operation: _____

Times available for general use: _____

Times most convenient for your schedule: _____

Can you obtain an initial session or consultation with a trainer to help you create a program? _____ yes _____ no

If so, what does the initial planning session involve? _____

_____

Are any of the staff certified? Do any have special training? If yes, list/describe: _____

_____

What types of equipment are available for the development of cardiorespiratory endurance? Briefly list/describe: _____

_____

_____

_____

Are any group activities or classes available? If so, briefly describe: _____

_____

_____

What types of weight training equipment are available for use? _____

_____

Yes	No	
_____	_____	Is there a fee for using the facility? If so, how much? $ _____
_____	_____	Is a student ID required for access to the facility?
_____	_____	Do you need to sign up in advance to use the facility or any of the equipment?
_____	_____	Is there typically a line or wait to use the equipment during the times you use the facility?
_____	_____	Is there a separate area with mats for stretching and/or cool-down?
_____	_____	Do you need to bring your own towel?
_____	_____	Are lockers available? If so, do you need to bring your own lock? _____ yes _____ no
_____	_____	Are showers available? If so, do you need to bring your own soap and shampoo? _____ yes _____ no
_____	_____	Is drinking water available? (If not, be sure to bring your own bottle of water.)

LABORATORY ACTIVITIES

What other amenities, such as vending machines or saunas, are available at the facility? Briefly list/describe: _____

_____

_____

Information about Equipment

Fill in the specific equipment and exercise(s) that you can use to develop cardiorespiratory endurance and each of the major muscle groups. For cardiorespiratory endurance, list the type(s) of equipment and a sample starting workout: frequency, intensity, time, and other pertinent information (such as a setting for resistance or speed). For muscular strength and endurance, list the equipment and exercises, and indicate the order in which you'll complete them during a workout session. You can also combine aerobics and strength exercises by performing high-repetition kettlebell swings. Remember, you don't have to use equipment—you can use body weight or elastic bands as resistance.

Cardiorespiratory Endurance Equipment

Equipment	Sample Starting Workout

Muscular Strength and Endurance Equipment

Order	Muscle Groups	Equipment	Exercise(s)
	Neck		
	Chest		
	Shoulders		
	Upper back		
	Front of arms		
	Back of arms		
	Buttocks		
	Abdomen		
	Lower back		
	Front of thighs		
	Back of thighs		
	Calves		
	Whole body		
	Other:		

Nutrition

LOOKING AHEAD...

After reading this chapter, you should be able to

- List the essential nutrients and describe their functions.

- Describe the U.S. government dietary guidelines and the benefits of following them.

- Describe guidelines for diets that are plant based and for special population groups.

- Explain how to use food labels and other consumer tools to make informed choices about foods.

- Create a personal food plan that will promote wellness.

TEST YOUR KNOWLEDGE

1. All adults should consume one serving each of fruits and vegetables every day. True or false?

2. Candy is the leading source of added sugars in the American diet. True or false?

3. Which of the following is not a whole grain?
   a. brown rice
   b. wheat flour
   c. popcorn

See answers on the next page.

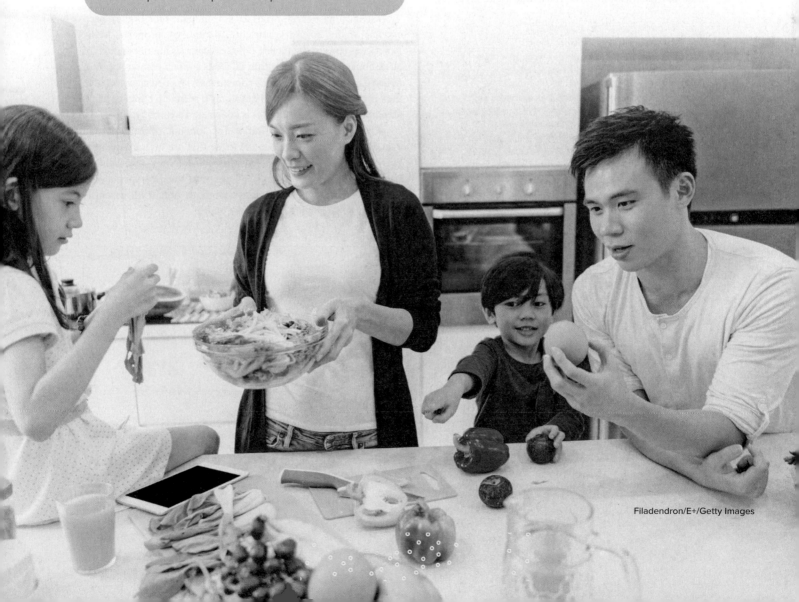

Filadendron/E+/Getty Images

Choosing a dietary pattern that provides the nutrients you need while limiting the substances linked to risk factors for disease should be an important part of your daily life. This chapter explains the basic principles of **nutrition**. It introduces the six classes of essential nutrients and discusses their role in the functioning of the body. You'll also find guidelines that you can use to design a healthy eating plan, and practical tools and advice to help you apply the guidelines to your life.

NUTRITIONAL REQUIREMENTS: COMPONENTS OF A HEALTHY DIET

You probably think about your diet in terms of the foods you like to eat. But more important for your health are the nutrients contained in those foods. The **essential nutrients** your body requires are proteins, fats, carbohydrates, vitamins, minerals, and water. The word *essential* means that you must get these substances from food because your body is unable to manufacture them, or at least not fast enough or in sufficient amounts to meet your physiological needs. The six classes of nutrients, along with their functions and major sources, are listed in Table 8.1.

The body needs some essential nutrients in relatively large amounts; these **macronutrients** include proteins, fats, carbohydrates,

and water. **Micronutrients**, such as vitamins and minerals, are required in much smaller amounts. Your body obtains nutrients through the process of **digestion**, which breaks down food into compounds that can be absorbed and the body can use (Figure 8.1). A diet that provides enough essential nutrients is vital because they provide energy, help build and maintain body tissues, and help regulate body functions.

Calories

The energy in foods is expressed as **kilocalories**. One kilocalorie represents the amount of heat it takes to raise the temperature of one liter of water 1°C. A person needs about 2,000 kilocalories a day to meet his or her energy needs. Although technically inaccurate, people refer to kilocalories as *calories,* which is a much smaller energy unit: 1 kilocalorie contains 1,000 calories. This text uses the familiar word *calorie* to stand for the larger energy unit; you'll also find *calorie* used on food labels.

Of the six classes of essential nutrients, three supply energy:

- Fat = 9 calories per gram
- Protein = 4 calories per gram
- Carbohydrate = 4 calories per gram

Alcohol, though not an essential nutrient, also supplies energy, providing 7 calories per gram.

Just meeting energy needs is not enough. Our bodies need enough of the essential nutrients to function properly. Many Americans consume sufficient or excess calories but not enough of all essential nutrients. Practically all foods contain combinations of nutrients, although foods are sometimes classified according to their predominant nutrients. For example, spaghetti contains small amounts of other nutrients, but is considered a carbohydrate food.

Nutrient density is an important concept related to food energy: Nutrient-dense foods are those that are high in essential nutrients but may be relatively low in calories. You can think of your daily calorie intake as a budget—you need to spend your calories wisely on nutrient-dense foods to obtain all essential nutrients while staying within your budget.

Answers (Test Your Knowledge)

1. **False.** For someone consuming 2,000 calories per day, about three servings each (2½ cups of vegetables and 2 cups of fruit) are recommended daily.
2. **False.** Regular (nondiet) sodas are the leading source of added sugars. Together with other beverages, they account for 47% of the added sugars in the American diet, and added sugars contribute an average of 13% of the total calories in American diets (more for children and teens). Each 12-ounce soda supplies about 10 teaspoons of sugar, or nearly 10% of the calories in a 2,000-calorie diet.
3. **b.** Unless labeled "whole wheat," wheat flour is processed to remove the bran and germ and is not a whole grain.

Table 8.1	The Six Classes of Essential Nutrients	
NUTRIENT	FUNCTION	MAJOR SOURCES
Proteins	Form important parts of muscles, bone, blood, enzymes, some hormones, and cell membranes; repair tissue; regulate water and acid-base balance; help in growth; supply energy	Meat, fish, poultry, eggs, milk, legumes, nuts
Carbohydrates	Supply energy to cells in brain, nervous system, and blood; supply energy to muscles during exercise	Grains (breads and cereals), fruits, vegetables, milk
Fats	Supply energy; insulate, support, and cushion organs; provide medium for absorption of fat-soluble vitamins	Animal foods, grains, nuts, seeds, fish, vegetables
Vitamins	Promote (initiate or speed up) specific chemical reactions within cells	Abundant in fruits, vegetables, and grains; also found in meat and dairy products
Minerals	Help regulate body functions; aid in growth and maintenance of body tissues; act as catalysts for release of energy	Found in most food groups
Water	Provides medium for chemical reactions; transports chemicals; regulates temperature; removes waste products	Fruits, vegetables, liquids

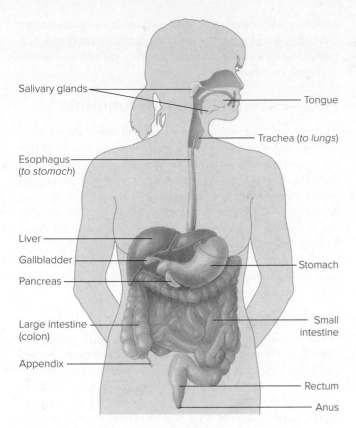

Salivary glands

Tongue

Trachea (*to lungs*)

Esophagus
(*to stomach*)

Liver

Gallbladder

Pancreas

Stomach

Large intestine
(colon)

Small
intestine

Appendix

Rectum

Anus

Figure 8.1   The digestive system. Food is broken down partially in the mouth, then further in the stomach by acids and other secretions and chemicals. Most absorption of nutrients occurs in the small intestine. Bacteria in the digestive tract, called gut flora, also help with digestion. The large intestine reabsorbs excess water; the remaining solid wastes are collected in the rectum and excreted through the anus.

Proteins—The Basis of Body Structure

Proteins form important parts of the body's main structural components: muscles and bones. Proteins also form important parts of blood, enzymes, cell membranes, and some hormones. When consumed, proteins also provide energy for the body (4 calories per gram).

Amino Acids The building blocks of proteins are called **amino acids**. Twenty common amino acids are found in food. Nine of these are essential (sometimes called indispensable). As long as foods supply certain nutrients, the body can produce the other 11 amino acids.

Complete and Incomplete Proteins Individual protein sources are considered "complete" if they supply all the essential amino acids in adequate amounts and "incomplete" if they do not. Meat, fish, poultry, eggs, milk, cheese, and soy provide complete proteins. Incomplete proteins, which come from plant sources such as nuts and **legumes** (dried beans and peas), are good sources of most essential amino acids but are usually low in one or more.

Certain combinations of vegetable proteins, such as wheat and peanuts in a peanut butter sandwich or rice and beans, allow each vegetable protein to make up for the amino acids missing in

the other protein. The combination yields a complete protein. It was once believed that vegetarians had to complement their proteins at each meal to receive the benefit of a complete protein. Now we know that proteins consumed throughout the course of the day can complement each other as part of a pool of amino acids the body can draw from to produce proteins. Plant-based diets should include a variety of vegetable protein sources to make sure all the essential amino acids are gotten in adequate amounts. (Healthy plant-based diets are discussed later in the chapter.)

Recommended Protein Intake The Food and Nutrition Board of the Institute of Medicine has established goals to help ensure adequate intake of protein as well as the other macronutrients (Figure 8.2). Protein intake goals can be calculated by multiplying your body weight in pounds by 0.36. So, if you weigh 125 pounds, you should consume at least 45 grams of protein per day, and if you weigh 180 pounds, adequate intake will be 65 grams. Table 8.2 lists some popular food items and the amount of protein each provides; labels on packaged foods show how much protein there is in each serving.

Most Americans meet or exceed the protein intake needed for adequate nutrition. If you consume substantially more protein than your body needs, the extra energy from protein is synthesized into fat for storage or burned for energy requirements, depending on your overall energy intake.

Consuming some protein above the amount needed for adequate nutrition is not harmful; suggested daily intake limits have been set as a proportion of overall calories rather than as specific amounts. The Food and Nutrition Board's recommended

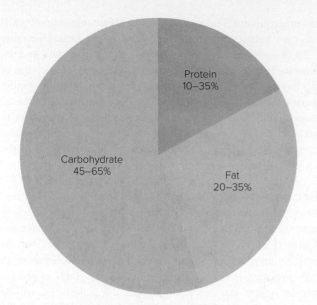

Figure 8.2 Acceptable Macronutrient Distribution Ranges (AMDRs) for protein, fat, and carbohydrate for adults age 19 and older, expressed as percentages of total daily calories.

NOTES: The lower ends of the ranges here represent the minimum intake necessary to meet essential nutrient needs. Individuals can allocate total daily energy intake among the three classes of macronutrients to suit individual preferences; goals for the three macronutrients must total 100%. To translate percentage goals into daily intake goals expressed in calories and grams, multiply the appropriate percentages by total daily energy intake and then divide the results by the corresponding calories per gram. For example, a fat limit of 35% applied to a 2,200-calorie diet would be calculated as follows: 0.35 × 2,200 = 770 calories of total fat; 770 ÷ 9 calories per gram = 86 grams of total fat.

SOURCE: Food and Nutrition Board, Institute of Medicine. 2002. *Dietary Reference Intakes for Energy, Carbohydrate, Fiber, Fat, Fatty Acids, Cholesterol, Protein, and Amino Acids.* Washington, DC: National Academies Press.

Table 8.2	Protein Content of Common Food Items

ITEM	PROTEIN (GRAMS)
3 ounces lean meat, poultry, or fish	20–27
¼ cup (3 ounces) tofu	7
1 cup cooked beans (black, white, pinto)	15–17
1 cup yogurt	8–13
1 ounce cheese (cheddar, Swiss)	6–8
½–1 cup cereals	1–6
1 egg cooked	6
1 cup ricotta cheese	28
1 cup milk	8
1 ounce nuts	2–6

NOTE: For the specific protein content of a food, check the food label or the searchable U.S. Department of Agriculture food composition database (https://ndb.nal.usda.gov/ndb/search).

SOURCE: U.S. Department of Agriculture, Agricultural Research Service. 2015. USDA National Nutrient Database for Standard Reference, Release 27. Nutrient Data Laboratory Home Page. (http://www.ars.usda.gov/ba/bhnrc/ndl; retrieved June 24, 2015).

amount is called Acceptable Macronutrient Distribution Ranges (AMDRs). Keeping intakes within the recommended range provides adequate intake of essential nutrients and reduces the risk of chronic disease.

Fats—Essential in Small Amounts

At 9 calories per gram, fats, also known as *lipids,* are the most concentrated source of energy. The fats stored in your body represent usable energy, help insulate your body, and support and cushion your organs. Fats in the diet help your body absorb fat-soluble vitamins, and they add flavor and texture to foods. Fats are the major fuel for the body during rest and light activity. Two fats—linoleic acid and alpha-linolenic acid, also called the essential fatty acids—are necessary components of the diet (Table 8.3). They are used to make compounds that regulate body functions such as the maintenance of blood pressure, vision, and the progress of a healthy pregnancy.

Types and Sources of Fats Food fats are usually composed of both **saturated** and **unsaturated** fatty acids (see Table 8.3). The dominant type of fatty acid determines the fat's characteristics. Saturated fats come mostly from animal products—red meats (hamburger, steak, roasts), whole milk, cheese, hot dogs, and lunchmeats—but are also found in tropical oils (coconut and palm oils). They are usually solid at room temperature. Most unsaturated fats in foods come from plant sources and are liquid at room temperature.

Depending on their structure, unsaturated fatty acids are further divided into *monounsaturated* and *polyunsaturated* fats. Olive, canola, safflower, and peanut oils contain mostly monounsaturated fatty acids. Soybean, corn, and cottonseed oils contain mostly polyunsaturated fatty acids. You may sometimes see polyunsaturated fats described more specifically by chemical structure as either omega-3 or omega-6 fats.

Hydrogenation and Trans Fats When unsaturated vegetable oils undergo the chemical process of **hydrogenation**, the result is a more solid fat from a liquid oil. The mixture contains both saturated and unsaturated fatty acids. Hydrogenation also changes some unsaturated fatty acids into **trans fatty acids**—unsaturated fatty acids with an atypical shape that affects their behavior in the body.

TERMS

saturated fats Fatty acids found mostly in animal products and tropical oils; usually solid at room temperature.

unsaturated fats Fatty acids found primarily in plant foods; usually liquid at room temperature.

hydrogenation A process by which hydrogens are added to unsaturated fats, increasing the degree of saturation and turning liquid oils into solid fats. Hydrogenation produces a mixture of saturated fatty acids and standard and trans forms of unsaturated fatty acids.

trans fatty acid A type of unsaturated fatty acid produced during the process of hydrogenation; trans fats have an atypical shape that affects their chemical activity.

Table 8.3 | Types of Fatty Acids

TYPE OF FATTY ACID	FOUND IN[a]
Saturated	• Animal fats (especially fatty meats and poultry fat and skin) • Butter, cheese, and other high-fat dairy products • Palm and coconut oils
Trans	• Some frozen pizza • Some types of popcorn • Deep-fried fast foods • Stick margarines, shortening • Packaged cookies and crackers • Processed snacks and sweets
Monounsaturated	• Olive, canola, and safflower oils • Avocados, olives • Peanut butter (without added fat) • Many nuts, including almonds, cashews, pecans, and pistachios
Polyunsaturated—omega-3[b]	• Fatty fish, including salmon, white albacore tuna, mackerel, anchovies, and sardines • Compared to fish, lesser amounts are found in walnut, flaxseed, canola, and soybean oils; tofu; walnuts; flaxseeds; and dark green leafy vegetables
Polyunsaturated—omega-6[b]	• Corn, soybean, and cottonseed oils (often used in margarine, mayonnaise, and salad dressings)

[a] Food fats contain a combination of types of fatty acids in various proportions. For example, soybean oil is composed mainly of polyunsaturated fatty acids (64%) but also contains monounsaturated (22%) and saturated (14%) fatty acids. Food fats are categorized here according to their predominant fatty acids.

[b] The essential fatty acids are polyunsaturated: Alpha-linolenic acid is an omega-3 fatty acid, and linoleic acid is an omega-6 fatty acid. Most Americans consume adequate amounts of essential fatty acids and should focus on limiting unhealthy fats.

Food manufacturers use hydrogenation to increase the stability of an oil so that it can be reused for deep frying, to improve the texture of certain foods (to make pie crusts flakier, for example), and to extend the shelf life of foods made with oil. In general, the more solid a hydrogenated oil is, the more saturated or trans fats it contains. For example, hard stick margarines typically contain more saturated and trans fats than soft tub or squeeze margarines.

Small amounts of trans fats occur naturally in animal fat, particularly beef, lamb, and dairy products, but a majority of trans fats in the American diet are artificial and come from partially hydrogenated oils. Many baked and fried foods are prepared with hydrogenated vegetable oils, which means they can be relatively high in saturated and trans fatty acids. The leading sources of trans fats in the American diet are fried fast foods such as French fries and fried chicken (typically fried in vegetable shortening rather than oil), baked and snack foods, and stick margarine.

Fats and Health Scientists are still unraveling the complex effects that individual types of fats and overall dietary patterns have on health and the risk for specific diseases. Most health experts agree on the dangers of artificial trans fats because of their double-negative effect on heart health: They raise levels of **low-density lipoprotein (LDL)**—"bad" cholesterol—and they also lower **high-density lipoprotein (HDL)**—"good" cholesterol. Consuming trans fats appears to increase the risk for both cardiovascular disease and type 2 diabetes. As awareness of these health risks has grown, cities and states have banned the use of trans fats in restaurants and food prepared for retail sale, and food manufacturers have reduced the amount of trans fats they use. And the Food and Drug Administration (FDA) required that all food

manufacturers stop using trans fats by June 2018, although some foods produced prior to the ban can be distributed through 2021. Even with the new law, it is important to check ingredient labels for partially hydrogenated oils: As long as a product has no more than half a gram of trans fats, the label may claim zero.

What about other types of fats? Many studies have examined the effects of dietary fat intake on blood **cholesterol** levels and the risk of heart disease. Although not all researchers agree, federal dietary guidelines, as well as those from the American Heart Association and the American College of Cardiology, strongly advise lowering saturated fat intake for reducing cardiovascular disease risk, especially for those people with risk factors for heart disease.

Continued research on the health risks and benefits of individual fats is ongoing. For example, do saturated fats in beef, butter, milk, and chocolate all have the same effect on heart disease risk? And what are the health effects of shifts in the intake of particular fats within the overall context of the diet? Dietary fat affects health in other ways besides heart disease risk. Diets

---

TERMS

low-density lipoprotein (LDL) A lipoprotein containing a moderate amount of protein and a large amount of cholesterol; "bad" cholesterol.

high-density lipoprotein (HDL) A lipoprotein containing relatively little cholesterol that helps transport cholesterol out of the arteries; "good" cholesterol.

cholesterol A waxy substance found in the blood and cells and needed for synthesis of cell membranes, vitamin D, and hormones.

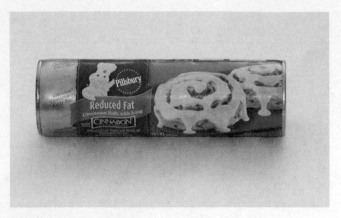

Wellness Tip An isolated focus on reducing dietary fat intake contributed to an explosion in the availability of processed foods promoted as being low in fat, such as the reduced-fat cinnamon rolls shown here. Many of these choices, however, are high in refined grains and added sugars and are not healthy choices. Focus on your overall dietary pattern and limit your intake of saturated fats, processed grains, and added sugars. Choose unsaturated fats, whole grains, fruits, and vegetables.

Diana Haronis/Moment Mobile/Getty Images

high in fatty red meat are associated with an increased risk of certain forms of cancer, especially colon cancer.

Recommended Fat Intake What does all this mean for you? Although more research is needed on the precise effects of different types and amounts of fat on overall health, evidence suggests that most people benefit from keeping their saturated fat intake within recommended intake levels and avoiding all artificial trans fats. But dietary patterns are more important for health than a focus on a single nutrient. The fats in your diet are found in foods that contain other nutrients, and the foods you consume are in the context of your overall diet. Increased body weight, aging, and sex are more important for predicting negative health events than is eating one kind of dietary fat rather than another.

The U.S. Department of Agriculture recommends that Americans limit their intake of saturated fat to less than 10% of total calories per day—but that they do so in the context of a healthy dietary pattern that emphasizes vegetables, fruits, whole grains, low-fat or nonfat dairy, seafood, legumes, and nuts. The pattern should also be low in red and processed meats,

sugar-sweetened foods and drinks, and refined grains. Healthy dietary patterns are described in detail later in the chapter.

Carbohydrates—A Key Source of Energy

Carbohydrates ("carbs") supply energy to body cells. Some cells, such as those in the brain and other parts of the nervous system and in the blood, prefer the carbohydrate **glucose** for fuel. During high-intensity exercise, muscles also use carbohydrates for fuel.

Simple and Complex Carbohydrates Carbohydrates are classified into two groups: simple and complex (Table 8.4). *Simple carbohydrates* consist of the single sugar molecules (monosaccharides) and the double sugars (disaccharides). Three important monosaccharides are glucose, fructose, and galactose. Glucose, the most common of the sugars, is used by both animals and plants for energy. Fructose is a very sweet sugar that is found in fruits, and galactose is the sugar in milk.

The disaccharides, pairs of single sugars, include sucrose (table sugar: fructose + glucose), maltose (malt sugar: glucose + glucose), and lactose (milk sugar: galactose + glucose). Simple carbohydrates add sweetness to foods. They are found naturally in fruits and milk and are added to soft drinks, fruit drinks, candy, and desserts. There is no evidence that any type of simple carbohydrate is more nutritious than others.

Complex carbohydrates include starches and most types of dietary fiber. Starches are found in a variety of plants, especially grains (wheat, rye, rice, oats, barley, and millet), legumes (dried beans, peas, and lentils), and tubers (potatoes and yams). Most other vegetables contain a mix of complex and simple carbohydrates. Fiber, which is discussed later in this chapter, is found in fruits, vegetables, and grains.

During digestion, your body breaks down carbohydrates into simple sugar molecules, such as glucose, for absorption. When glucose is in the bloodstream, the pancreas releases the hormone insulin, which allows cells to take up glucose and use it for energy and fat storage. The liver and muscles also take up glucose and store it in the form of a starch called **glycogen**. The muscles use glucose from glycogen as fuel during endurance events or long workouts. Some people have problems controlling their blood glucose levels, a disorder called diabetes mellitus.

Table 8.4	Simple and Complex Carbohydrates in Foods
SIMPLE CARBOHYDRATES ("SUGARS")	**COMPLEX CARBOHYDRATES**
Single sugar molecules (monosaccharides)	Starches (long, complex chains of sugar molecules)
- glucose (common in foods)	- grains (wheat, rye, rice, oats, barley, millet), dried corn
- fructose (fruits)	- legumes (dry beans, peas, and lentils)
- galactose (milk)	- tubers and other vegetables (potatoes, yams, corn)
Double sugar molecules (disaccharides; pairs of single sugars)	Fiber (nondigestible carbohydrates)
- sucrose or table sugar (fructose + glucose)	- soluble (oats, barley, legumes, some fruits and vegetables)
- maltose or malt sugar (glucose + glucose)	- insoluble (wheat bran, vegetables, whole grains)
- lactose or milk sugar (galactose + glucose)	

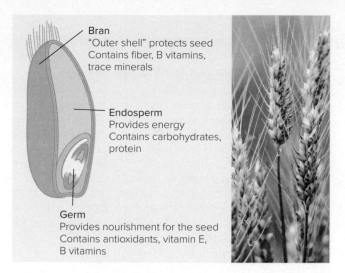

Bran
"Outer shell" protects seed
Contains fiber, B vitamins,
trace minerals

Endosperm
Provides energy
Contains carbohydrates,
protein

Germ
Provides nourishment for the seed
Contains antioxidants, vitamin E,
B vitamins

Figure 8.3 The parts of a whole grain kernel.
Lynx/iconotec.com/Glowimages

Refined versus Whole Grains Complex carbohydrates can be further divided into refined, or processed, carbohydrates and unrefined carbohydrates, or whole grains. Before they are processed, all grains are **whole grains**, consisting of an inner layer of germ, a middle layer called the endosperm, and an outer layer of bran (Figure 8.3). During processing, the germ and bran are often removed, leaving just the starchy endosperm. The refinement of whole grains transforms whole-wheat flour into white flour, brown rice into white rice, and so on.

Refined grains usually retain all the calories of their unrefined counterparts, but they tend to be less nutrient dense—lower in fiber, vitamins, minerals, and other beneficial compounds. Refined-grain products are often enriched or fortified with vitamins and minerals, but many of the nutrients lost in processing are not replaced.

Whole grains tend to take longer to chew and digest than refined ones; whole grains also generally enter the bloodstream more slowly. This slower digestive pace makes you feel full sooner and for a longer period. A slower rise in blood glucose levels after eating unrefined complex carbohydrates may help in the management of diabetes. Whole grains are also high in dietary fiber (discussed later).

Consumption of whole grains has been linked to a reduced risk of heart disease, diabetes, and cancer, and plays an important role in gastrointestinal health and body weight management. For all these reasons, whole grains are recommended over those that have been refined. See the box "Choosing More Whole-Grain Foods" for tips on increasing your intake of whole grains.

Glycemic Index and Glycemic Response Some foods such as table sugar and white bread cause a quick and dramatic rise in glucose and insulin levels, while others cause a slower and lower rise. A food that rapidly and significantly raises blood glucose levels is said to have a high **glycemic index**. Insulin and glucose levels rise following a meal or snack containing any type of carbohydrate.

Basing food choices on the glycemic index is difficult, for one, because whatever else you eat with a high-carbohydrate food will change the blood-sugar effect. But for people with particular health concerns, such as diabetes, the glycemic index may be important. In addition to the type of carbohydrate in the food, the total amount of carbohydrate in the diet is important for diabetes management. The easiest way to moderate the effects shown by the glycemic index, therefore, is to choose an overall dietary pattern that includes a variety of whole grains and vegetables daily and limits foods that are high in refined grains and added sugars.

Added Sugars *Added sugars* are sugars that are added to foods by food manufacturers or individuals; they include white sugar, brown sugar, high-fructose corn syrup, and other sweeteners added to most processed foods. (Naturally occurring sugars in fruit and milk are not considered added sugars.) Foods high in added sugar are generally high in calories and low in nutrients and fiber, thus providing "empty calories." High intake of added sugars from foods and beverages is associated with dental caries ("cavities"), excess body weight, and increased risk of type 2 diabetes, and may also increase risk for hypertension, stroke, and heart disease.

Added sugars currently contribute about 250–300 calories in the typical daily American diet, representing about 13–17% of total energy intake. A limit of 10% is suggested by the U.S. Department of Agriculture (USDA) and other organizations; even lower intakes may be needed to meet all nutrient needs at a given level of calorie intake. Major sources of sugar in the U.S. diet are sugar-sweetened beverages, snacks, and sweets. Due to updated food labeling regulations, added sugars are beginning to appear on food labels as manufacturers adopt the new label format.

To decrease added sugars from your diet, reduce your consumption of sugar-sweetened beverages (soft drinks, sweetened fruit drinks, sweetened sports beverages), sweet snacks, and desserts. The sugars in your diet should come mainly from whole fruits, which are excellent sources of vitamins and minerals, and from low-fat or fat-free milk and other dairy products, which are high in protein and calcium.

Recommended Carbohydrate Intake On average, Americans consume 200–300 grams of carbohydrate per day—well above the 130 grams needed to meet the body's requirement

carbohydrate An essential nutrient; sugars, starches, and dietary fiber are all carbohydrates.

glucose A simple sugar circulating in the blood that can be used by cells to fuel adenosine triphosphate (ATP) production.

glycogen A complex carbohydrate stored principally in the liver and skeletal muscles; the major fuel source during most forms of intense exercise. Glycogen is the storage form of glucose.

whole grain The entire edible portion of a grain (such as wheat, rice, or oats), including the germ, endosperm, and bran; processing removes parts of the grain, often leaving just the endosperm.

glycemic index A measure of how and how high a particular food raises blood sugar levels.

TERMS

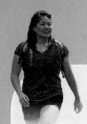

TAKE CHARGE
Choosing More Whole-Grain Foods

What Are Whole Grains?

The first step in adding more whole grains into your diet is to correctly identify them. The following are whole grains:

- whole wheat
- whole-grain corn
- whole rye
- popcorn
- whole oats
- brown rice
- oatmeal
- whole-grain barley

Other choices include bulgur (cracked wheat), farro, millet, kasha (roasted buckwheat kernels), quinoa, wheat and rye berries, amaranth, wild rice, graham flour, whole-grain kamut, whole-grain spelt, and whole-grain triticale.

Wheat flour, unbleached flour, enriched flour, and degerminated corn meal are not whole grains. Wheat germ and wheat bran are also not whole grains, but they are the constituents of wheat typically left out when wheat is processed and so are healthier choices than regular wheat flour, which typically contains just the grain's endosperm.

Checking Packages for Whole Grains

To find packaged foods—such as bread or pasta—that are rich in whole grains, read the list of ingredients and check for special health claims related to whole grains. The *first* item in the list of ingredients should be one of the whole grains in the preceding list. Product names and food color can be misleading. *When in doubt, always check the list of ingredients and make sure "whole" is the first word in the list.*

The FDA allows manufacturers to include special health claims for foods that contain 51% or more whole-grain ingredients. Such products may contain a statement such as the following on their packaging:

- "Rich in whole grain"
- "Made with 100% whole grain"
- "Diets rich in whole-grain foods may help reduce the risk of heart disease and certain cancers."

However, many whole-grain products will not carry such claims. This is one more reason to check the ingredient list to make sure you're buying a product made from one or more whole grains.

---

for essential carbohydrate. The AMDR for carbohydrates is 45–65% of total daily calories, which is about 225–325 grams of carbohydrate for someone who consumes 2,000 calories per day. The focus should be on consuming a variety of foods rich in complex carbohydrates, especially whole grains, and reducing intake of added sugars. Some athletes can benefit from high-carbohydrate diets; nutritional recommendations for athletes are discussed later in the chapter.

Fiber—A Closer Look

Dietary fiber is the term given to nondigestible carbohydrates naturally present in plants such as whole grains, fruits, legumes, and vegetables. Instead of being digested, fiber moves through the intestinal tract and provides bulk for feces in the large intestine, which in turn facilitates elimination. In the large intestine, bacteria break down some types of fiber into acids and gases, which explains why consuming too much fiber can lead to intestinal gas. Even though humans don't digest fiber, we need it for good health.

Types of Fiber There are two types of fiber: soluble and insoluble (Table 8.5). Both types are important for health. **Soluble (viscous) fiber** such as that found in oat bran or legumes can delay stomach emptying, slow the movement of glucose into the blood after eating, and reduce absorption of cholesterol. Soluble fiber dissolves or swells in water (like oatmeal that gets soft). In contrast, **insoluble fiber** does not dissolve in water. It increases fecal bulk and helps prevent constipation, hemorrhoids, and other digestive disorders. We can find

insoluble fiber in all plants, and especially in wheat bran or psyllium seed.

The Food and Nutrition Board gives three other descriptions of fiber:

- Dietary fiber (as mentioned) refers to the nondigestible carbohydrates (and the noncarbohydrate substance lignin) that are naturally present in plants such as grains, fruits, legumes, and vegetables.

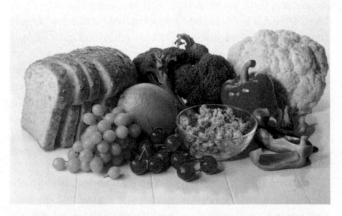

Wellness Tip To reduce the risk of chronic disease and maintain intestinal health, daily fiber intake of 38 grams for men and 25 grams for women is recommended. Americans currently consume about half this amount. Fruits, vegetables, and whole grains are excellent sources of carbohydrates and fiber. Drink plenty of water to get the most health benefits from the fiber you consume.

Smneedham/Photolibrary/Getty Images

Table 8.5	Types, Effects, and Sources of Dietary Fiber	
	SOLUBLE FIBER	INSOLUBLE FIBER
Physiological effects	• Slows digestion and nutrient absorption • Helps prevent a rapid rise in blood glucose following a meal • Improves blood cholesterol levels	• Adds bulk to stool • Helps food pass more quickly through the digestive tract • Helps prevent constipation
Examples of food sources	Oat bran, barley, nuts, legumes, apples, berries	Whole wheat and other whole grains, wheat bran, vegetables

- **Functional fiber** refers to nondigestible carbohydrates that have been either isolated from natural sources or synthesized in a laboratory and then added to a food product or dietary supplement.

- **Total fiber** refers to the sum of dietary and functional fiber in your diet.

A high-fiber diet can help reduce the risk of type 2 diabetes, heart disease, and pulmonary disease, as well as improve gastrointestinal health and aid in the management of metabolic syndrome and body weight. Some studies have linked high-fiber diets with a reduced risk of colon and rectal cancer. Other studies have suggested that it is the total dietary pattern—one rich in fruits, vegetables, and whole grains—that may be responsible for this reduction in risk. A high-fiber diet has also been linked to healthier gut bacteria, which in turn may reduce the risk of obesity and improve immune function.

Sources of Fiber All plant foods contain some dietary fiber. Fruits, legumes, oats (especially oat bran), and barley all contain the viscous types of fiber that help lower blood glucose and cholesterol levels. Wheat (especially wheat bran), cereals, grains, and vegetables are all good sources of cellulose and other fibers that help prevent constipation. Psyllium, which is often added to cereals or used in fiber supplements and laxatives, improves intestinal health and helps control glucose and cholesterol levels. The processing of packaged foods can remove fiber, so it's important to depend on fresh fruits and vegetables and foods made from whole grains as your main fiber sources.

Vitamins—Organic Micronutrients

Vitamins are organic (carbon-containing) substances required in small amounts to regulate various processes within living cells (Table 8.6). Humans need 13 vitamins; of these, 4 are fat soluble (A, D, E, and K) and 9 are water soluble (C and the B vitamins, thiamin, riboflavin, niacin, vitamin B-6, folate, vitamin B-12, biotin, and pantothenic acid).

Solubility affects how a vitamin is absorbed, transported, and stored in the body. The water-soluble vitamins are absorbed directly into the bloodstream. Excess amounts of water-soluble vitamins are generally removed by the kidneys and excreted in urine. Fat-soluble vitamins require a more complex absorptive process. They are usually carried in the blood by special proteins and are stored in the liver and in fat tissues rather than excreted.

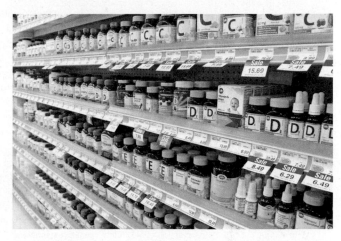

Wellness Tip Vitamin and mineral supplements are popular, but they are not usually necessary for healthy people who eat a balanced diet.

Niloo138/123RF

Functions of Vitamins Many vitamins help chemical reactions take place. They provide no energy to the body directly but help release the energy stored in carbohydrates, proteins, and fats. Other vitamins are critical in the production of red blood cells and the maintenance of the nervous, skeletal, and immune systems. Some vitamins act as **antioxidants**, which help preserve

---

TERMS

dietary fiber Nondigestible carbohydrates and lignin that are intact in plants.

soluble (viscous) fiber Fiber that dissolves in water or is broken down by bacteria in the large intestine.

insoluble fiber Fiber that does not dissolve in water and is not broken down by bacteria in the large intestine.

functional fiber Nondigestible carbohydrates either isolated from natural sources or synthesized; these may be added to foods and dietary supplements.

total fiber The total amount of dietary fiber and functional fiber in the diet.

vitamins Carbon-containing substances needed in small amounts to help promote and regulate chemical reactions and processes in the body.

antioxidant A substance that protects against the breakdown of food or body constituents by free radicals; antioxidants' actions include binding oxygen, donating electrons to free radicals, and repairing damage to molecules.

Table 8.6   Facts about Vitamins

VITAMIN AND RECOMMENDED INTAKES*	IMPORTANT DIETARY SOURCES	MAJOR FUNCTIONS	SIGNS OF PROLONGED DEFICIENCY	TOXIC EFFECTS OF MEGADOSES
FAT SOLUBLE				
Vitamin A Men: 900 µg Women: 700 µg	Liver, milk, butter, cheese, fortified margarine; carrots, spinach, and other orange and deep green vegetables and fruits	Maintenance of vision, skin, linings of the nose, mouth, digestive, and urinary tracts, immune function	Night blindness; dry, scaling skin; increased susceptibility to infection; loss of appetite; anemia; kidney stones	Liver damage, miscarriage and birth defects, headache, vomiting and diarrhea, vertigo, double vision, bone abnormalities
Vitamin D Men: 15 µg Women: 15 µg	Fortified milk and margarine, fish oils, butter, egg yolks (sunlight on skin also produces vitamin D)	Development and maintenance of bones and teeth; promotion of calcium absorption	Rickets (bone deformities) in children; bone softening, loss, fractures in adults	Kidney damage, calcium deposits in soft tissues, depression, death
Vitamin E Men: 15 mg Women: 15 mg	Vegetable oils, whole grains, nuts and seeds, green leafy vegetables, asparagus, peaches	Protection and maintenance of cellular membranes	Red blood cell breakage and anemia, weakness, neurological problems, muscle cramps	Relatively nontoxic but may cause excess bleeding or formation of blood clots
Vitamin K Men: 120 µg Women: 90 µg	Green leafy vegetables; smaller amounts widespread in other foods	Production of factors essential for blood clotting and bone metabolism	Hemorrhaging	None reported
WATER SOLUBLE				
Biotin Men: 30 µg Women: 30 µg	Cereals, yeast, egg yolks, soy flour, liver; widespread in foods	Synthesis of fat, glycogen, and amino acids	Rash, nausea, vomiting, weight loss, depression, fatigue, hair loss	None reported
Folate Men: 400 µg Women: 400 µg	Green leafy vegetables, yeast, oranges, whole grains, legumes, liver	Amino acid metabolism, synthesis of RNA and DNA, new cell synthesis	Anemia, weakness, fatigue, irritability, shortness of breath, swollen tongue	Masking of vitamin B-12 deficiency
Niacin Men: 16 mg Women: 14 mg	Eggs, poultry, fish, milk, whole grains, nuts, enriched breads and cereals, meats, legumes	Conversion of carbohydrates, fats, and proteins into usable forms of energy	Pellagra (symptoms include diarrhea, dermatitis, inflammation of mucous membranes, dementia)	Flushing of skin, nausea, vomiting, diarrhea, liver dysfunction, glucose intolerance
Pantothenic acid Men: 5 mg Women: 5 mg	Animal foods, whole grains, broccoli, potatoes; widespread in foods	Metabolism of fats, carbohydrates, and proteins	Fatigue, numbness and tingling of hands and feet, gastrointestinal disturbances	None reported
Riboflavin Men: 1.3 mg Women: 1.1 mg	Dairy products, enriched breads and cereals, lean meats, poultry, fish, green vegetables	Energy metabolism; maintenance of skin, mucous membranes, nervous system structures	Cracks at corners of mouth, sore throat, skin rash, hypersensitivity to light, purple tongue	None reported
Thiamin Men: 1.2 mg Women: 1.1 mg	Whole-grain and enriched breads and cereals, organ meats, lean pork, nuts, legumes	Conversion of carbohydrates into usable forms of energy; maintenance of appetite and nervous system function	Beriberi (symptoms include muscle wasting, mental confusion, anorexia, enlarged heart, nerve changes)	None reported
Vitamin B-6 Men: 1.3 mg Women: 1.3 mg	Eggs, poultry, fish, whole grains, nuts, soybeans, liver, kidney, pork	Metabolism of amino acids and glycogen	Anemia, convulsions, cracks at corners of mouth, dermatitis, nausea, confusion	Neurological abnormalities and damage
Vitamin B-12 Men: 2.4 µg Women: 2.4 µg	Meat, fish, poultry, fortified cereals, cheese, eggs, milk	Synthesis of blood cells; other metabolic reactions	Anemia, fatigue, nervous system damage, sore tongue	None reported
Vitamin C Men: 90 mg Women: 75 mg	Peppers, broccoli, brussels sprouts, spinach, citrus fruits, strawberries, tomatoes, potatoes, cabbage, other fruits and vegetables	Maintenance and repair of connective tissue, bones, teeth, cartilage; promotion of healing; aid in iron absorption	Scurvy, anemia, reduced resistance to infection, loosened teeth, joint pain, poor wound healing, hair loss, poor iron absorption	Urinary stones in some people, acid stomach from ingesting supplements in pill form, nausea, diarrhea, headache, fatigue

*Recommended intakes for adults ages 19–30; to calculate your personal Dietary Reference Intakes (DRIs) based on age, sex, and other factors, visit the Interactive DRI website (http://fnic.nal.usda.gov/fnic/interactiveDRI).

SOURCES: National Academy of Sciences. 1998: *Dietary Reference Intakes for Thiamin, Riboflavin, Niacin, Vitamin B6, Folate, Vitamin B12, Pantothenic Acid, Biotin and Choline*; National Academy of Sciences. 2000. *Dietary Reference Intakes for Vitamin C, Vitamin E, Selenium, and Carotenoids*; National Academy of Sciences. 2001. *Dietary Reference Intakes for Vitamin A, Vitamin K, Arsenic, Boron, Chromium, Copper, Iodine, Iron, Manganese, Molybdenum, Nickel, Silicon, Vanadium, and Zinc*; National Academy of Sciences. 2011. *Dietary Reference Intakes for Calcium and Vitamin D*; Ross, A. C. 2012. *Modern Nutrition in Health and Disease*. Lippincott Williams & Wilkins.

the health of cells. Key vitamin antioxidants include vitamin E, vitamin C, and the vitamin A precursor beta-carotene. (Antioxidants are described later in the chapter.)

Sources of Vitamins The human body must obtain most of the vitamins it requires from foods. Vitamins are abundant in fruits, vegetables, and grains. In addition, many processed foods, such as flour and breakfast cereals, contain added vitamins. Vitamin B-12 is found only in foods that are fortified or that come from animal sources. A few vitamins are made in the body: The skin makes vitamin D when it is exposed to sunlight, and intestinal bacteria make vitamin K. Nonetheless, you still need to get vitamin D and vitamin K from foods (see Table 8.6).

Vitamin Deficiencies and Excesses If your diet lacks a particular vitamin, characteristic symptoms of deficiency can develop (see Table 8.6). For example, vitamin A deficiency can cause night blindness, and people whose diets lack vitamin B-12 can develop anemia. Vitamin deficiency diseases are relatively rare in the United States because vitamins are readily available from our food supply. However, many Americans consume lower-than-recommended amounts of several vitamins, including vitamins A and D. Nutrient intake that is consistently below recommended levels can have adverse effects on health even if it is not low enough to cause a deficiency disease. For example, low intake of folate increases a woman's chance of giving birth to a baby with a neural tube defect (a congenital malformation of the central nervous system). Low intake of folate and vitamins B-6 and B-12 has been linked to increased heart disease risk; low vitamin D intake may harm bone health.

Extra vitamins in the diet can be harmful, especially when taken as supplements. For example, vitamin A plays an important role in bone growth, but too much vitamin A can trigger bone loss and an increase in the risk of fracture. Megadoses of fat-soluble vitamins are particularly dangerous because the excess is stored in the body rather than excreted, increasing the risk of toxicity. Even when supplements are not taken in excess, relying on them for an adequate intake of vitamins can be problematic. There are many substances in foods other than vitamins and minerals that have important health effects. Later, this chapter discusses specific recommendations for vitamin intake and when a supplement is advisable. For now, keep in mind that it's best to get most of your vitamins from foods rather than supplements.

The vitamins and minerals in foods can be easily lost or destroyed during storage or cooking. To retain their value, eat or process vegetables immediately after buying them. If you can't do this, store them in a cool place, covered to retain moisture—either in the refrigerator (for a few days) or in the freezer (for a longer term). To reduce nutrient losses during food preparation, minimize the amount of water used and the total cooking time. Develop a taste for a crunchier texture in cooked vegetables. Baking, steaming, broiling, grilling, and microwaving are all good methods of preparing vegetables.

Minerals—Inorganic Micronutrients

Minerals are inorganic (non-carbon-containing) elements you need in relatively small amounts to help regulate body functions, aid in the growth and maintenance of body tissues, and help release energy (Table 8.7). There are about 17 essential minerals. The major minerals, those that the body needs in amounts exceeding 100 milligrams (mg) per day, include calcium, phosphorus, magnesium, sodium, potassium, and chloride. The essential trace minerals, which you need in minute amounts, include copper, fluoride, iodine, iron, selenium, and zinc.

Characteristic symptoms develop if an essential mineral is consumed in a quantity too small or too large for good health. For example, most Americans consume the mineral sodium in excess as part of dietary salt. The majority of sodium Americans consume comes from processed foods and restaurant meals. High sodium consumption raises blood pressure, and thus the risk for heart disease and stroke; reducing dietary salt has become an important public health initiative. The good news is that blood pressure begins to decrease within weeks of lowering sodium intake.

Minerals commonly lacking in the American diet include iron, calcium, magnesium, and potassium. Low potassium intake is considered a public health concern because it is linked to high blood pressure and heart disease; you can improve your potassium intake by choosing a dietary pattern rich in fruits, vegetables, and legumes. Iron-deficiency **anemia** is a problem in some age groups, and researchers fear poor calcium intakes in childhood are sowing the seeds for future **osteoporosis**, especially in women. See the box "Eating for Healthy Bones" to learn more.

Water—Vital but Often Ignored

Water is the major component in both foods and the human body: You are composed of about 50–60% water. Your need for other nutrients, in terms of weight, is much less than your need for water. You can live up to 50 days without food but only a few days without water.

Water is distributed all over the body, among lean and other tissues and in blood and other body fluids. Water is used in the digestion and absorption of food and is the medium in which most chemical reactions take place within the body. Some water-based fluids, such as blood, transport substances around the body; other fluids serve as lubricants or cushions. Water also helps regulate body temperature.

---

minerals Inorganic compounds needed in relatively small amounts for the regulation, growth, and maintenance of body tissues and functions.

TERMS

anemia A deficiency in the oxygen-carrying material in the red blood cells.

osteoporosis A condition in which the bones become extremely thin and brittle and break easily; due largely to insufficient calcium intake.

Table 8.7 — Facts about Selected Minerals

MINERAL AND RECOMMENDED INTAKES*	IMPORTANT DIETARY SOURCES	MAJOR FUNCTIONS	SIGNS OF PROLONGED DEFICIENCY	TOXIC EFFECTS OF MEGADOSES
Calcium Men: 1,000 mg Women: 1,000 mg	Milk and milk products, tofu, fortified orange juice and bread, green leafy vegetables, bones in fish	Formation of bones and teeth; control of nerve impulses, muscle contraction, blood clotting	Stunted growth in children, bone mineral loss in adults; urinary stones	Kidney stones, calcium deposits in soft tissues, inhibition of mineral absorption, constipation
Fluoride Men: 4 mg Women: 3 mg	Fluoridated water, tea, marine fish eaten with bones	Maintenance of tooth and bone structure	Higher frequency of tooth decay	Increased bone density, mottling of teeth, impaired kidney function
Iodine Men: 150 µg Women: 150 µg	Iodized salt, seafood, processed foods	Essential part of thyroid hormones, regulation of body metabolism	Goiter (enlarged thyroid), cretinism (birth defect)	Depression of thyroid activity, hyperthyroidism in susceptible people
Iron Men: 8 mg Women: 18 mg	Meat and poultry, fortified grain products, dark green vegetables, dried fruit	Component of hemoglobin, myoglobin, and enzymes	Iron-deficiency anemia, weakness, impaired immune function, gastrointestinal distress	Nausea, diarrhea, liver and kidney damage, joint pains, sterility, disruption of cardiac function, death
Magnesium Men: 400 mg Women: 310 mg	Widespread in foods and water (except soft water); especially found in grains, legumes, nuts, seeds, green vegetables, milk	Transmission of nerve impulses, energy transfer, activation of many enzymes	Neurological disturbances, cardiovascular problems, kidney disorders, nausea, growth failure in children	Nausea, vomiting, diarrhea, central nervous system depression, coma; death in people with impaired kidney function
Phosphorus Men: 700 mg Women: 700 mg	Present in nearly all foods, especially milk, cereal, peas, eggs, meat	Bone growth and maintenance, energy transfer in cells	Impaired growth, weakness, kidney disorders, cardiorespiratory and nervous system dysfunction	Drop in blood calcium levels, calcium deposits in soft tissues, bone loss
Potassium Men: 4,700 mg Women: 4,700 mg	Meats, milk, fruits, vegetables, grains, legumes	Nerve function and body water balance	Muscular weakness, nausea, drowsiness, paralysis, confusion, disruption of cardiac rhythm	Cardiac arrest
Selenium Men: 55 µg Women: 55 µg	Seafood, meat, eggs, whole grains	Defense against oxidative stress; regulation of thyroid hormone action	Muscle pain and weakness, heart disorders	Hair and nail loss, nausea and vomiting, weakness, irritability
Sodium Men: 1,500 mg Women: 1,500 mg	Salt, soy sauce, fast food, processed foods, especially lunch meats, canned soups and vegetables, salty snacks, processed cheese	Body water balance, acid-base balance, nerve function	Muscle weakness, loss of appetite, nausea, vomiting; deficiency rarely seen	Edema, hypertension in sensitive people
Zinc Men: 11 mg Women: 8 mg	Whole grains, meat, eggs, liver, seafood (especially oysters)	Synthesis of proteins, RNA, and DNA; wound healing; immune response; ability to taste	Growth failure, loss of appetite, impaired taste acuity, skin rash, impaired immune function, poor wound healing	Vomiting, impaired immune function, decline in blood HDL levels, impaired copper absorption

*Recommended intakes for adults ages 19–30; to calculate your personal DRIs based on age, sex, and other factors, visit the Interactive DRI website (http://fnic.nal.usda.gov/fnic/interactiveDRI).

SOURCES: National Academy of Sciences. 1997. *Dietary Reference Intakes for Calcium, Phosphorous, Magnesium, Vitamin D, and Fluoride;* National Academy of Sciences. 2001. *Dietary Reference Intakes for Vitamin A, Vitamin K, Arsenic, Boron, Chromium, Copper, Iodine, Iron, Manganese, Molybdenum, Nickel, Silicon, Vanadium, and Zinc;* National Academy of Sciences. 2005. *Dietary Reference Intakes for Water, Potassium, Sodium, Chloride, and Sulfate;* National Academy of Sciences. 2011. *Dietary Reference Intakes for Calcium and Vitamin D;* Ross, A. C. 2012. *Modern Nutrition in Health and Disease.* Lippincott Williams & Wilkins.

Water is contained in almost all foods, particularly in liquids, fruits, and vegetables. The foods and beverages you consume provide 80–90% of your daily water intake; the remainder is generated through metabolism. You lose water in urine, feces, and sweat and through evaporation from your lungs.

About 20% of daily water intake comes from food. Most people can make up the rest and maintain a healthy water balance by consuming beverages at meals and drinking fluids in response to thirst.

The Food and Nutrition Board has set levels of adequate water intake to maintain hydration. Under these guidelines, men need to consume about 3.7 total liters of water, with 3.0 liters (about 13 cups) coming from beverages; women need 2.7 total liters, with 2.2 liters (about 9 cups) coming from beverages. If you exercise vigorously or live in a hot climate, you need to consume additional fluids to maintain a balance between water consumed and water lost. Severe dehydration causes weakness and can lead to death.

Osteoporosis is a condition in which the bones become dangerously thin and fragile over time. An estimated 10 million Americans over age 50 have osteoporosis, and another 34 million are at risk. Women account for about 80% of osteoporosis cases.

Most of adult bone mass is built by age 18 in girls and 20 in boys. Bone density peaks between ages 25 and 35; after that, bone mass is lost over time. To prevent osteoporosis, the best strategy is to build as much bone as possible during your youth and do everything you can to maintain it as you age. Up to 50% of bone loss is determined by controllable lifestyle factors such as diet and exercise. Key nutrients in a healthy dietary pattern for bone health include the following:

- **Calcium.** Getting enough calcium is important throughout life to build and maintain bone mass. Milk, yogurt, and calcium-fortified orange juice, bread, and cereals are all good sources.

- **Vitamin D.** Vitamin D is necessary for bones to absorb calcium; a daily intake of 600 IU (15 µg) is recommended for individuals ages 1–70. Vitamin D can be obtained from foods and is manufactured by the skin when exposed to sunlight. Candidates for vitamin D supplements include people who eat few foods rich in vitamin D, get little sun (i.e., don't expose their face, arms, and hands to the sun for 5–15 minutes a few times each week), or live in higher latitudes where sunlight is weaker.

- **Vitamin K.** Vitamin K promotes the synthesis of proteins that help keep bones strong. Broccoli and leafy green vegetables are rich in vitamin K.

- **Other nutrients.** Other nutrients that may play an important role in bone health include vitamin C, magnesium, potassium, phosphorus, fluoride, manganese, zinc, copper, and boron.

Several dietary substances may have a *negative* effect on bone health, especially if consumed in excess. These include alcohol, sodium, caffeine, and retinol (a form of vitamin A). Drinking lots of soda, which often replaces milk in the diet, has been shown to increase the risk of bone fracture in teenage girls.

The effect of protein on bone mass depends on other nutrients: Protein helps build bone as long as calcium and vitamin D intake are adequate. But if calcium and vitamin D are low, high protein intake can lead to bone loss.

Weight-bearing aerobic exercise helps maintain bone mass throughout life, and strength training improves bone density, muscle mass, strength, and balance. Drinking alcohol only in moderation, not smoking, and managing depression and stress are also important for maintaining strong bones. For people who develop osteoporosis, a variety of medications are available to treat the condition.

SOURCES: Movassagh, E. Z., and H. Vatanparast. 2017. "Current evidence on the association of dietary patterns and bone health: A scoping review," *Advances in Nutrition* 8(1): 1–16; Institute of Medicine of the National Academies. 2010. *Dietary Reference Intakes for calcium and vitamin D* (http://www.iom.edu/~/media/Files/Report%20Files/2010/Dietary-Reference-Intakes-for-Calcium-and-Vitamin-D/Vitamin%20D%20and%20Calcium%202010%20Report%20Brief.pdf).

Other Substances in Food

Many substances in food are not essential nutrients but may influence health.

Antioxidants When the body uses oxygen or breaks down certain fats or proteins as a normal part of metabolism, substances called **free radicals** are produced. A free radical is a chemically unstable molecule that reacts with fats, proteins, and DNA, damaging cell membranes and mutating genes. Free radicals have been implicated in aging, cancer, cardiovascular disease, and other degenerative diseases like arthritis. Environmental factors such as cigarette smoke, exhaust fumes, radiation, excessive sunlight, certain drugs, and stress can increase free radical production.

Antioxidants found in foods can block the formation and action of free radicals and repair the damage they cause. Some essential nutrients, such as vitamin C, vitamin E, and selenium, are also antioxidants. Antioxidants such as carotenoids are found in yellow, orange, and dark green leafy vegetables. In general, fruits and vegetables have a high antioxidant value, as do herbs, spices, berries, nuts, and chocolate.

Phytochemicals Antioxidants fall into the broader category of **phytochemicals**, substances found in plant foods that may help prevent chronic disease. For example, certain substances found in soy foods may help lower cholesterol levels. Sulforaphane, a compound isolated from broccoli and other **cruciferous vegetables**, may render some carcinogenic compounds harmless. Allyl sulfides, a group of chemicals found in garlic and onions, appear to boost the activity of immune cells. Phytochemicals found in whole grains are associated with a reduced risk of cardiovascular disease, diabetes, and cancer. Carotenoids found in green vegetables may help preserve eyesight with age. Further research on phytochemicals may extend the role of nutrition to the prevention and treatment of many chronic diseases.

TERMS

free radical An electron-seeking compound that can react with fats, proteins, and DNA, damaging cell membranes and mutating genes in its search for electrons; produced through chemical reactions in the body and by exposure to environmental factors such as sunlight and tobacco smoke.

phytochemical A naturally occurring substance found in plant foods that may help prevent and treat chronic diseases such as heart disease and cancer; *phyto* means "plant."

cruciferous vegetables Vegetables of the cabbage family, including cabbage, broccoli, brussels sprouts, kale, and cauliflower; the flower petals of these plants form the shape of a cross, hence the name.

To get phytochemicals, eat a variety of fruits, vegetables, and unprocessed grains rather than relying on supplements. Like many vitamins and minerals, isolated phytochemicals may be harmful if taken in high doses. Another reason to get your phytochemicals from food is that their health benefits may be the result of chemical substances working in combination. The role of phytochemicals in disease prevention is discussed further in Chapter 12.

❓ Ask Yourself

QUESTIONS FOR CRITICAL THINKING AND REFLECTION

Experts say that two of the most important factors in a healthy diet are eating the "right" kinds of carbohydrates and eating the "right" kinds of fats. Based on what you've read so far in this chapter, which are the "right" carbohydrates and the "right" fats? How would you say your own diet stacks up when it comes to carbs and fats?

NUTRITIONAL GUIDELINES: PLANNING YOUR DIET

Scientific and government groups have created a number of useful tools to help people design healthy diets.

The guidelines discussed in this section are the **Dietary Reference Intakes (DRIs)**, Daily Values, Dietary Guidelines for Americans, and MyPlate.

Dietary Reference Intakes (DRIs)

The Food and Nutrition Board establishes dietary standards, or recommended intake levels, for Americans of all ages. The current set of standards, called Dietary Reference Intakes (DRIs), is frequently reviewed and updated as new nutrition-related information becomes available.

DRI Standards The DRIs include a set of four reference values used as standards for both recommended intakes and maximum safe intakes. The recommended intake of each nutrient is expressed as either a *Recommended Dietary Allowance* (RDA) or as an *Adequate Intake* (AI). An AI is set when there is not enough information available to set an RDA value. Regardless of the type of standard used, the DRIs represent the best available estimate of intakes for optimal health—for preventing both nutritional deficiencies and chronic diseases.

Used primarily in nutrition policy and research, the *Estimated Average Requirement* (EAR) is the average daily nutrient intake level estimated to meet the requirement of half the healthy individuals in a particular life stage and gender group. For example, a 2016 study shows that although most American infants under age 2 years meet their nutritional needs, 10% have an iron intake below the EAR. The *Tolerable Upper Intake Level* (UL) is the maximum daily intake that is unlikely to cause health problems in a healthy person. For example, the RDA for calcium for an 18-year-old female is 1,300 mg per day; the UL is 3,000 mg per day.

Because of a lack of data, ULs have not been set for all nutrients. This does not mean that people can tolerate long-term intakes of these vitamins and minerals above recommended levels. Like all chemical agents, nutrients can produce adverse effects if intakes are excessive. Furthermore, there is no established benefit from consuming nutrients at levels above the RDA or AI. The DRIs for many nutrients are found in Tables 8.6 and 8.7. For a personalized DRI report for your sex and life stage, visit the Interactive DRI website (http://fnic.nal.usda.gov/fnic/interactiveDRI).

Should You Take Vitamin or Mineral Supplements? High-dose vitamin and mineral supplements have been promoted as a way to prevent or delay the onset of many diseases, including heart disease and several kinds of cancer. These claims remain controversial. According to the latest research, a balanced diet of whole foods—not high-dose supplementation—is the best way to promote health and prevent disease.

While most Americans can get the vitamins and minerals they need by eating a varied diet, in setting the DRIs, the Food and Nutrition Board recommended supplements of particular nutrients for the following groups:

- Women who are capable of becoming pregnant should take 400 micrograms (μg) per day of folic acid (the synthetic form of the vitamin folate) from fortified foods or supplements in addition to folate from a varied diet. This level of folate intake reduces the risk of neural tube defects. Enriched breads, flours, corn meals, rice, noodles, and other grain products are fortified with folic acid. Folate is found naturally in green leafy vegetables, legumes, oranges, and strawberries.

- People over age 50 should eat foods fortified with vitamin B-12, take B-12 supplements, or both to meet the majority of the DRI of 2.4 μg of B-12 daily.

- Because of the oxidative stress caused by smoking, smokers should get 35 mg *more* vitamin C per day than the RDA set for their age and sex, and this extra amount can easily be obtained from foods.

Supplements may also be recommended in other cases. Women with heavy menstrual flows may need extra iron. Older people, people with dark skin, and people exposed to little sunlight may need extra vitamin D. Some plant-based diets may need supplemental calcium, iron, zinc, and vitamin B-12. People with other diets may benefit from taking supplements based on their lifestyle, physical condition, medicines, or dietary habits.

Although dietary supplements are sold over the counter, the question of whether to take supplements is a serious one.

Dietary Reference Intakes (DRIs) An **TERMS** umbrella term for four types of nutrient standards: Adequate Intake (AI), Estimated Average Requirement (EAR), and Recommended Dietary Allowance (RDA) are levels of intake considered adequate to prevent nutrient deficiencies and reduce the risk of chronic disease; Tolerable Upper Intake Level (UL) is the maximum daily intake that is unlikely to cause health problems.

Some vitamins and minerals are dangerous when ingested in excess, as described previously in Tables 8.6 and 8.7. Large doses of particular nutrients can also cause health problems by affecting the absorption of other vitamins and minerals or interacting with medications. For all these reasons, you should think carefully about whether to take high-dose supplements, and consult a physician or registered dietitian.

Daily Values

The **Daily Values** are a simplified version of the RDA used on food labels and include standards for fat, cholesterol, carbohydrate, dietary fiber, and selected vitamins and minerals. The Daily Values represent appropriate intake levels for a 2,000-calorie diet. The percent Daily Value shown on a food label shows how that food contributes to your recommended daily intake. Food labels are described in detail later in the chapter.

Dietary Guidelines for Americans

To provide general guidance for choosing a healthy diet and reducing the risk of chronic diseases, the USDA and the U.S. Department of Health and Human Services jointly issue the **Dietary Guidelines for Americans**, which is revised every five years.

The Dietary Guidelines is designed to help Americans make healthy and informed food choices. The main objective of the *2015-2020 Dietary Guidelines* is to encourage healthy eating patterns and regular physical activity among Americans, two-thirds of whom are overweight or obese, yet undernourished in several key nutrients. The guidelines offer practical tips for how people can make shifts in their diet to integrate healthier choices. They also include findings on the broader environmental and social aspects of the American diet—that is, the "food environment."

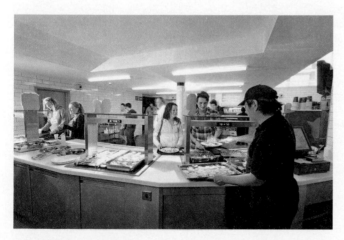

Wellness Tip About half of all American adults have one or more preventable chronic diseases that are related to poor eating habits and inactivity; these include high blood pressure, type 2 diabetes, cardiovascular disease, and certain forms of cancer. The food and portion size choices you make at every meal can influence your risk for, or management of, many health conditions.

Peter D Noyce/Alamy Stock Photo

Earlier versions of the Dietary Guidelines focused more on individual dietary components. However, people do not eat individual nutrients or single foods but rather foods in combination, to form an overall eating pattern that has cumulative effects on health. The *2015-2020 Dietary Guidelines* points out the large discrepancy between the recommendations and the actual American diet, which includes too few vegetables, fruits, high-fiber whole grains, low-fat milk and milk products, and seafood and too much added sugar, solid fat, refined grains, and sodium. Following these guidelines will promote health and reduce risk of diseases such as heart disease, cancer, diabetes, stroke, osteoporosis, and obesity.

General Recommendations The Dietary Guidelines offers five primary recommendations:

1. Follow a healthy eating pattern across the lifespan.
2. Focus on variety, nutrient density, and amount.
3. Limit calories from added sugars and saturated fats and reduce sodium intake.
4. Shift to healthier food and beverage choices.
5. Support healthy eating patterns for all.

All segments of our society, from families to restaurants, food producers to policymakers, have a responsibility in supporting healthy choices. A healthy eating pattern is not a rigid prescription, but rather an adaptable framework in which individuals can enjoy foods that meet their personal, cultural, and traditional preferences and fit within their budget and lifestyle. Adopting a healthy eating pattern and engaging in regular physical activity will go a long way toward improving health and reducing the risk of chronic disease in every life stage.

Building Healthy Eating Patterns A healthy eating pattern is one that meets nutrient needs while not exceeding calorie requirements. The three dietary patterns developed by the *2015-2020 Dietary Guidelines* focus on healthy eating and physical activity patterns:

- **Healthy U.S.-Style Pattern.** Based on the types and proportions of foods Americans typically consume, but in nutrient-dense forms and appropriate amounts.
- **Healthy Vegetarian Pattern.** Includes more legumes, processed soy products, nuts and seeds, and whole grains; it contains no meat, poultry, or seafood, but is close to the Healthy U.S.-Style Pattern in amounts of all other food groups. Dairy and eggs are still included because the majority of vegetarians eat them; however, the plan can be vegan with plant-based substitutions.

- **Healthy Mediterranean-Style Pattern.** Reflecting a dietary pattern associated with many cultures bordering the Mediterranean Sea, which includes more fruits and seafood and less dairy than the Healthy U.S.-Style Pattern. The Mediterranean diet has been associated with positive health outcomes such as lower rates of heart disease and total mortality.

All three patterns are based on amounts of food from different food groups (and subgroups) according to overall energy intake. They also share an emphasis on whole fruits, vegetables, whole grains, beans and peas, fat-free and low-fat milk and milk products, and healthy oils; they include less red meat and more seafood than the typical American diet. Healthy dietary patterns include oils, but they limit the amount of energy that people should consume from solid fats.

A fundamental principle of all healthy dietary patterns is that people should eat nutrient-dense foods so that they can obtain all the needed nutrients without exceeding their daily energy requirements. In addition, people should strive to get their nutrients from foods rather than from dietary supplements. Table 8.8 compares the three patterns for a 2,000-calorie diet. To see a more detailed breakdown of the recommendations for the three healthy dietary patterns, see the Nutrition Resources section at the end of the chapter.

Although the greatest emphasis of the Dietary Guidelines is on consuming an overall healthy eating pattern, specific recommendations have been set for dietary components of particular public health concern:

- Consume less than 10% of calories per day from added sugars. The current average intake among Americans is about 13–16%, with about half the total coming from sugar-sweetened beverages.

- Consume less than 10% of calories per day from saturated fats.

- Consume less than 2,300 mg per day of sodium. The current average intake among Americans is about 3,400 mg, most of it coming from processed foods.

- If you consume alcohol, do so in moderation—up to one drink per day for women and two drinks per day for men—and only if you are of legal drinking age.

In addition, the Dietary Guidelines stress that all Americans should strive to meet the federal physical activity guidelines and aim to achieve and maintain a healthy body weight.

Table 8.8　USDA Food Patterns at the 2,000-Calorie Level

FOOD GROUP	HEALTHY U.S.-STYLE PATTERN	HEALTHY VEGETARIAN PATTERN	HEALTHY MEDITERRANEAN-STYLE PATTERN
Vegetables	**2½ c-eq/day**	**2½ c-eq/day**	**2½ c-eq/day**
Dark green	1½ c-eq/wk	1½ c-eq/wk	1½ c-eq/wk
Red & orange	5½ c-eq/wk	5½ c-eq/wk	5½ c-eq/wk
Legumes (beans & peas)	1½ c-eq/wk	3 c-eq/wk*	1½ c-eq/wk
Starchy	5 c-eq/wk	5 c-eq/wk	5 c-eq/wk
Other	4 c-eq/wk	4 c-eq/wk	4 c-eq/wk
Fruit	**2 c-eq/day**	**2 c-eq/day**	**2½ c-eq/day**
Grains	**6 oz-eq/day**	**6½ oz-eq/day**	**6 oz-eq/day**
Whole grains	3 oz-eq/day	3½ oz-eq/day	3 oz-eq/day
Refined grains	3 oz-eq/day	3 oz-eq/day	3 oz-eq/day
Dairy	**3 c-eq/day**	**3 c-eq per day**	**2 c-eq per day**
Protein Foods	**5½ oz-eq/day**	**3½ oz-eq/day**	**6½ oz-eq/day**
Seafood	8 oz-eq/wk	n/a	15 oz-eq/wk
Meat, poultry, eggs	26 oz-eq/wk	3 oz-eq/wk (eggs)	26 oz-eq/wk
Nuts, seeds, soy products	5 oz-eq/wk	15 oz-eq/wk	5 oz eq/wk
Oils	**27 g/day**	**27 g/day**	**27 g/day**
Limit on calories for other uses (% of total calories)**	270 cal/day (14%)	290 cal/day (15%)	260 cal/day (13%)

NOTE: c-eq = cup-equivalent, the amount of a food or beverage product that is considered equal to 1 cup from the vegetables, fruits, or dairy food groups; oz-eq = ounce-equivalent, the amount of a food product that is considered equal to 1 ounce from the grain or protein food food groups.

*For the Vegetarian Pattern, half of total legume intake counts as vegetables and half as protein foods.

** If all food choices to meet food group recommendations are in nutrient-dense forms, a small number of calories remain within the overall calorie limit of the Pattern (i.e., limit on calories for other uses). Calories up to the specified limit can be used for added sugars, added refined starches, solid fats, or alcohol, or to eat more than the recommended amount of food in a food group.

SOURCES: U.S. Department of Health and Human Services, and U.S. Department of Agriculture. 2015. *2015–2020 Dietary Guidelines for Americans*, 8th ed. (http://health.gov/dietaryguidelines/2015/guidelines/); Food and Nutrition Board, Institute of Medicine. 2002. *Dietary Reference Intakes for Energy, Carbohydrate, Fiber, Fat, Fatty Acids, Cholesterol, Protein, and Amino Acids*. Washington, DC: National Academies Press.

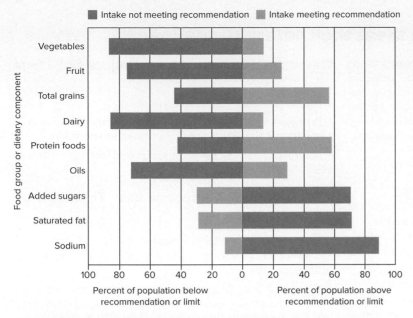

Legend: ■ Intake not meeting recommendation ■ Intake meeting recommendation

Y-axis (Food group or dietary component): Vegetables, Fruit, Total grains, Dairy, Protein foods, Oils, Added sugars, Saturated fat, Sodium

X-axis: 100 80 60 40 20 0 20 40 60 80 100

Percent of population below recommendation or limit | Percent of population above recommendation or limit

Figure 8.4 Dietary intakes compared to recommendations. The bars show the percentages of the U.S. population age 1 year and over who are below, at, or above each dietary goal or limit. The center (0) line is the goal or limit. For most people, meaning those represented by the orange sections of the bars, shifting toward the center line will improve eating patterns. For example, over 80% of people do not eat enough vegetables—they fall below the recommendation. Within the area of the graph demonstrating our consumption of foods we should limit—added sugars, saturated fat, and sodium—the orange bars show that over 80% of people exceed the recommended limit for sodium intake.

SOURCE: U.S. Department of Agriculture. "What we eat in America, NHANES 2007–2010, for average intakes by age-sex group. Healthy U.S.-style food patterns, which vary based on age, sex, and activity level, for recommended intakes and limits." (See 2015–2020 Dietary Guidelines for Americans, https://health.gov/dietaryguidelines/2015/guidelines/chapter-2/current-eating-patterns-in-the-united-states/).

Making Shifts to Align with Healthy Eating Patterns

The eating patterns of the U.S. population are low in vegetables, fruits, whole grains, dairy, seafood, and oil, while they are high in refined grains, added sugars, saturated fats, sodium, as well as meats, poultry, and eggs. Additionally, most Americans consume too many calories and do not meet the physical activity guidelines. For many of us, achieving a healthy eating pattern will require changes to our current food and beverage choices—shifts both within and between food groups. Figure 8.4 shows the lack of alignment between the typical eating patterns currently in the United States and those in the Dietary Guidelines. The box "Positive Changes to Meet the Dietary Guidelines" gives some strategies for shifting your behavior.

Planning and Budgeting for Healthy Eating

Are healthy food options available and affordable at your school and worksite? How far is it from your home to the nearest place to purchase fruits and vegetables? How many food advertisements are you exposed to daily? Factors such as these can have an enormous influence on your behavior—both positive and negative—sometimes without your awareness.

Students often complain that they cannot afford fruits and vegetables. But many also spend hundreds of dollars on unnecessary supplements, eating out, and fast foods. Buying groceries and eating at home is cheaper and gives you more control over the ingredients added to your food.

Before heading out to the store:

- Plan for a couple of meals and write down the necessary ingredients.
- Create a grocery list so that you do not spontaneously pick up prepackaged food, frozen meals, and desserts.
- Shop on a full stomach so that the chips and cookies do not tempt you.

At the store:

- Buy foods that take more prep work but save money—choose fresh fruits and vegetables instead of precut, bagged, and canned produce; make your own guacamole, bean dips, and salad dressings.
- Stock up on organic black beans, low-fat refried beans, whole-grain pasta, and other staples when they go on sale; buy in bulk.
- Alternate meats with other sources of protein (e.g., quinoa, nuts, tofu, and cottage cheese).

USDA's MyPlate

To help consumers put the Dietary Guidelines for Americans into practice, the USDA also issues the food guidance system known as **MyPlate**. MyPlate provides a simple graphic

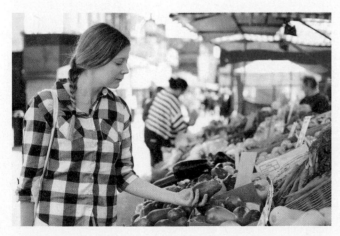

Wellness Tip Farmers' markets are an important way to bring healthy food choices to residents of inner cities. Support the establishment of farmers' markets in your community.

Michael Spring/123RF

MyPlate A food-group plan that provides practical advice to ensure a balanced intake of the essential nutrients.

TERMS

Positive Changes to Meet the Dietary Guidelines

Remember to focus on nutrient-dense options for the majority of your food choices: Use your calorie budget wisely. The tips here focus on the types of changes and swaps needed for the majority of Americans to move toward the dietary pattern recommended in the Dietary Guidelines.

Vegetables: Consume More Vegetables from All Subgroups

- Increase the vegetable content of mixed dishes while decreasing the amounts of other food components that you may overconsume—for example, cut the meat or cheese in half and double the vegetables in a soup, stew, or casserole.
- Always choose a green salad or a vegetable as a side dish. Incorporate vegetables into most meals and snacks.
- Replace foods high in calories, saturated fat, or sodium, such as some meats, poultry, cheeses, and snack foods, with vegetables.

Fruits: Increase Fruit Intake, Especially from Whole Fruits

- Choose more fruits as snacks, in salads, as side dishes, and as desserts in place of foods with added sugars such as cookies, pies, cakes, and ice cream.

Grains: Swap Whole Grains for Refined

- Shift from white to 100% whole-wheat breads, white to whole-grain pasta, and white to brown rice (see the section on whole grains earlier in the chapter).
- Cut back on refined-grain desserts and sweet snacks that are high in added sugars, solid fats, or both. Choose smaller portions and eat them less often. For healthy swaps, try plain popcorn instead of buttered and bread instead of a croissant or biscuit, for example.

Dairy: Increase Intake

- Drink fat-free or low-fat milk (or soy beverage) with meals; choose yogurt as a snack; or use yogurt as an ingredient in salad dressings, spreads, and other prepared dishes.
- Favor milk and yogurt for additional dairy servings; cheese has more sodium and saturated fat and less potassium, vitamin A, and vitamin D than milk and yogurt.

Protein: Add Variety and Make More Nutrient-Dense Choices

- Increase seafood intake if yours is low: Try seafood as the protein choice in meals twice per week in place of meat, poultry, or eggs—for example, a tuna sandwich or a salmon steak.
- Use legumes or nuts and seeds in mixed dishes instead of some meat or poultry—for example, bean chili instead of a mixed-meat dish or almonds instead of ham on a main-dish salad.

Oils: Increase Intake As You Reduce Solid Fats

- Use vegetable oil in place of butter, stick margarine, shortening, lard, or coconut oils when cooking.
- Increase intake of foods that naturally contain oils, such as seafood and nuts, in place of some meat and poultry.
- Choose options for salad dressings and spreads made with oils instead of solid fats.

Saturated Fats: Reduce to Less Than 10% of Calories per Day

- Substitute foods high in unsaturated fats for foods high in saturated fats; for example, use oils rather than solid fats for food preparation.
- Read food labels to identify the types of fats in prepared foods; compare and choose lower-fat forms of foods and beverages that contain solid fats (e.g., fat-free milk instead of 2% or whole).
- Adjust proportions of ingredients in mixed dishes to increase vegetables, whole grains, lean meat, and lower-fat cheeses in place of some of the fatty meat or regular cheeses.
- Consume foods higher in solid fats less often and in smaller portions.

Added Sugars: Reduce to Less Than 10% of Calories per Day

- Choose beverages with no added sugars, such as water, in place of sugar-sweetened beverages.
- Reduce portion sizes of sugar-sweetened beverages, and choose them less often.
- Limit servings and decrease portion sizes of grain-based and dairy desserts and sweet snacks.
- Choose unsweetened or no-sugar-added versions of canned fruit, fruit sauces, and yogurt.

Sodium: Reduce Intake

- Read food labels to compare sodium content, choosing products with less sodium.
- Choose fresh, plain frozen, or no-salt-added canned vegetables and fresh protein sources rather than processed meat and poultry.
- Eat at home more often; cooking from scratch allows you to control the sodium content.
- Limit sauces, mixes, and "instant" flavoring packs that come with rice and noodles; use your own flavorings based on herbs and spices rather than salt.

Physical Activity: Do More!

- Increase weekly physical activity, especially during commute time and leisure activities.
- Reduce sedentary time; take frequent exercise breaks.

SOURCE: U.S. Department of Health and Human Services and U.S. Department of Agriculture. 2015. *2015–2020 Dietary Guidelines for Americans,* 8th ed. (http://health.gov/dietaryguidelines/2015/guidelines).

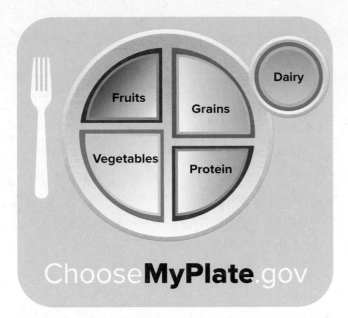

Figure 8.5 USDA's MyPlate. illustrates the five food groups that are building blocks for a healthy diet; visit ChooseMyPlate.gov for a personalized plan.

SOURCE: U.S. Department of Agriculture. MyPlate, 2011. (http://www.ChooseMyPlate .gov; retrieved April 17, 2015).

| Table 8.9 | USDA Estimated Daily Calorie Intake Levels to Maintain Energy Balance | | |

AGE (YEARS)	SEDENTARY*	MODERATELY ACTIVE**	ACTIVE†
FEMALE*			
16–18	1,800	2,000	2,400
19–25	2,000	2,200	2,400
26–30	1,800	2,000	2,400
31–50	1,800	2,000	2,200
51–60	1,600	1,800	2,200
61 & up	1,600	1,800	2,000
MALE			
16–18	2,400	2,800	3,200
19–20	2,600	2,800	3,000
21–25	2,400	2,800	3,000
26–35	2,400	2,600	3,000
36–40	2,400	2,600	2,800
41–45	2,200	2,600	2,800
46–55	2,200	2,400	2,800
56–60	2,200	2,400	2,600
61–65	2,000	2,400	2,600
66–75	2,000	2,200	2,600
76 & up	2,000	2,200	2,400

* A lifestyle that includes only the light physical activity associated with typical day-to-day life.

**A lifestyle that includes physical activity equivalent to walking about 1.5–3 miles per day at 3–4 miles per hour (30–60 minutes a day of moderate physical activity), in addition to the light physical activity associated with typical day-to-day life.

***Estimates for females do not include women who are pregnant or breastfeeding.

†Active means a lifestyle that includes physical activity equivalent to walking more than 3 miles per day at 3–4 miles per hour (60 or more minutes a day of moderate physical activity), in addition to the light physical activity associated with typical day-to-day life.

SOURCE: U.S. Department of Health and Human Services and U.S. Department of Agriculture. 2015. *2015–2020 Dietary Guidelines for Americans*, 8th ed. (http://health.gov/dietaryguidelines/2015/guidelines/); Food and Nutrition Board, Institute of Medicine. 2002. *Dietary Reference Intakes for Energy, Carbohydrate, Fiber, Fat, Fatty Acids, Cholesterol, Protein, and Amino Acids*. Washington, DC: National Academies Press.

showing how to use the five food groups to build a healthy plate at each meal (Figure 8.5). If you need to change your dietary pattern, use MyPlate to build a healthy eating style by focusing on variety, amount of food consumed, and nutrition. You can get a personalized version of MyPlate recommendations by visiting ChooseMyPlate.gov. Using the daily plan food feature, you can determine the amount of each food group you need based on your calorie allowance. Your plan is personalized based on your age, gender, weight, height, and level of physical activity.

MyPlate is available in Spanish, and it offers special recommendations for dieters, preschoolers aged 2–5, children aged 6–11, and pregnant and breastfeeding women. MyPlate On Campus is an initiative to allow students to become ambassadors of healthy eating and healthy lifestyles. MyPlate On Campus provides resources and practical guidelines for promoting health and wellness uniquely customized for students and the campus lifestyle.

Energy Intake and Portion Sizes To build a healthy eating style, base your food group goals on an appropriate level of energy intake. Table 8.9 provides guidance for determining an appropriate calorie intake for weight maintenance. Everyone is different, however, and the number of calories you need will vary depending on multiple factors, such as being overweight or underweight. You can set a rough calorie goal by tracking your food and calorie intake for at least several days (a longer tracking period improves accuracy). You should monitor your body weight over time, and adjust calorie intake and physical activity as needed to meet your personal weight goals. See Chapter 9 for much more on maintaining a healthy weight.

Most people underestimate the number of calories they consume and the size of their portions. See the box "Judging Portion Sizes" for strategies to improve the accuracy of your estimates. MyPlate doesn't use number of portions as the basis of recommendations; instead, amounts are listed in terms of cup-equivalents and ounce-equivalents. These units of measurement allow you to align servings of foods that differ—those that are concentrated versus those that are more airy or contain more water. For example, ½ cup of blueberries and ¼ cup of raisins both count as ½ cup-equivalent of fruit.

Next, let's take a look at each food group in MyPlate.

Studies have shown that most people underestimate the size of their food portions, in many cases by as much as 50%. If you need to retrain your eye, try using measuring cups and spoons and an inexpensive kitchen scale when you eat at home. With a little practice, you'll learn the difference between 3 and 8 ounces of chicken or meat, and what a half-cup of rice really looks like. For quick estimates, use the following equivalents:

- 1 teaspoon of margarine = one die
- small cookie or cracker = a poker chip
- 2 tablespoons of peanut butter = a ping-pong ball

- ¼ cup nuts = a golf ball
- 1- to 2-ounce muffin or roll = a plum or large egg
- 1½ ounces of cheese = your thumb, four dice stacked together
- 2-ounce bagel = a hockey puck or yo-yo
- 3 ounces of chicken or meat = a deck of cards
- 1 medium potato = a computer mouse
- ½ cup of cooked rice, pasta, or potato = ½ baseball
- 1 cup of cereal flakes = a fist
- 1 medium fruit (apple or orange) = a baseball

Vegetables: Vary Your Veggies Together, fruits and vegetables should make up half your plate. Vegetables contain carbohydrates, dietary fiber, vitamin C, folate, potassium, and many other nutrients, and they are naturally low in calories and fat. A 2,000-calorie diet should include 2½ cups of vegetables daily. Each of the following counts as 1 cup-equivalent from the vegetable group:

- 1 cup raw or cooked vegetables
- 2 cups raw leafy salad greens
- 1 cup vegetable juice

Because vegetables vary in the nutrients they provide, eat a variety to obtain maximum nutrition. The USDA recommends weekly servings from the five subgroups within the vegetables group (see Table 8.8). Eat vegetables from several subgroups each day.

- *Dark-green vegetables* (examples: broccoli, bok choy, romaine lettuce, spinach, collards, kale)
- *Red and orange vegetables* (examples: tomatoes, carrots, sweet potatoes, red peppers, winter squash)
- *Beans and peas* (examples: green beans and green peas; lentils; black, kidney, navy, pinto, white, and soybeans). This subgroup includes dried beans and peas (legumes), which because of their protein content can be counted in the vegetable group or in the protein group as plant-based sources of protein.
- *Starchy vegetables* (examples: corn, potatoes, green peas)
- *Other vegetables* (examples: artichokes, asparagus, beets, cauliflower, green beans, head lettuce, onions, mushrooms, zucchini)

Fruits: Focus on Whole Fruits Fruits are rich in carbohydrates, dietary fiber, and many vitamins, especially vitamin C. A 2,000-calorie diet should include 2 cups of fruits daily. Each of the following counts as 1 cup-equivalent of fruit:

- 1 cup fresh, canned, or frozen fruit
- 1 cup fruit juice (100% juice)
- 1 small whole fruit
- ½ cup dried fruit

Choose whole fruits often; they are higher in fiber and often lower in calories than fruit juices. Fruit *juices* typically contain more nutrients and less added sugar than fruit *drinks*. Choose canned fruits packed in 100% fruit juice or water rather than in syrup.

Grains: Make Half Your Grains Whole Grains Foods from this group are usually low in fat and rich in complex carbohydrates, dietary fiber (if grains are unrefined), and many vitamins and minerals. A 2,000-calorie diet should include 6 ounce-equivalent servings each day, and half of those servings should be whole grains, such as whole-grain bread, whole-wheat pasta, high-fiber cereal, or brown rice. The following count as 1 ounce-equivalent:

- 1 slice of bread
- 1 small (2½-inch diameter) muffin
- 1 cup ready-to-eat cereal flakes
- ½ cup cooked cereal, rice, grains, or pasta
- 1 6-inch tortilla

Choose foods that are typically made with little fat or added sugar (bread, rice, pasta) over those that are high in fat and added sugar (croissants, chips, cookies, doughnuts).

Dairy: Move to Low-Fat and Fat-Free Dairy This group includes all milk and milk products such as yogurt and cheeses, as well as lactose-free and lactose-reduced products. Soy milk (calcium-fortified) is also part of the dairy group. Those consuming 2,000 calories per day should include 3 cups of milk or the equivalent daily. Each of the following counts as 1 cup-equivalent:

- 1 cup milk or yogurt
- ½ cup ricotta cheese
- 1½ ounces natural cheese
- 2 ounces processed cheese

Protein Foods: Vary Your Protein Routine This group includes meat, poultry, fish, dried beans and peas, eggs, nuts, seeds, and processed soy products. A 2,000-calorie diet should include 5½ ounce-equivalents daily. Each of the following counts as 1 ounce-equivalent:

- 1 ounce cooked lean meat, poultry, or fish
- ¼ cup cooked beans (legumes) or tofu
- 1 egg
- 1 tablespoon peanut butter
- ½ ounce nuts or seeds

Choose lean meats and skinless poultry, and become aware of your serving sizes. Choose at least one serving of plant proteins, such as black beans, lentils, or tofu, every day. Include at least 8 ounces of cooked seafood per week and select a variety of protein foods to improve nutrient intake and health benefits. Plant-based options in the protein foods group include beans and peas, processed soy products, and nuts and seeds.

Other Foods Our diets also include oils, solid fats, and added sugars. Although oils are not a food group, they do provide essential nutrients and are included in USDA food patterns. Solid fats and added sugars do not provide essential nutrients.

OILS Oils and soft margarines include vegetable oils and soft vegetable oil table spreads that have no trans fats. Oils and fats that are

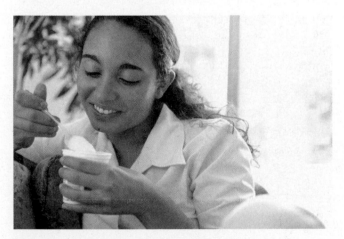

Wellness Tip Research shows that some protein-rich foods can give you a quick mental boost, which can be helpful before an exam.

Marc Romanelli/The Image Bank/Getty Images

liquid at room temperature and come from many plants and fish sources are included. Oils are major sources of vitamin E and unsaturated fatty acids, including the essential fatty acids, but they are not a food group. A 2,000-calorie diet should include 6 teaspoons of oils per day. One teaspoon is the equivalent of the following:

- 1 teaspoon vegetable oil or soft margarine
- 1 tablespoon salad dressing or light mayonnaise

Foods that are mostly oils include nuts, olives, avocados, and some fish. The following portions include about 1 teaspoon of oil: 8 large olives, ⅙ medium avocado, ½ tablespoon peanut butter, and ⅓ ounce roasted nuts. Food labels can help you identify the type and amount of fat in various foods.

SOLID FATS AND ADDED SUGARS If you choose nutrient-dense foods from all food groups, you will have a small proportion of your daily calorie budget left to "spend." For those wanting to maintain weight, these calories may be used to increase the amount of food from a food group; to consume foods that are not in the lowest-fat form or that contain added sugars; to add oil, fat, or sugars to foods; or to consume alcohol. People who are trying to lose weight and improve their health should limit solid fats and added sugars. As described earlier, making better beverage choices is a key strategy for reducing intake of added sugars. Sodas, energy drinks, and sports drinks contribute added sugars but few nutrients to the American diet. The differences in nutrients between soda and other beverages are shown in Figure 8.6. The average American consumes nearly 800 calories daily from solid fats and added sugars—far higher than the recommended limits.

DASH Eating Plan

Other food-group plans have been proposed by a variety of experts and organizations, some to address the needs of special populations. One well-studied alternative is DASH, which stands for Dietary Approaches to Stop Hypertension. As its name suggests, the DASH eating plan was developed to help people lower high blood pressure and it is tailored with special attention to sodium and other nutrients of concern for managing blood pressure. Refer to Figure 4 in the Nutrition Resources at the end of the chapter for more information on DASH.

The Vegetarian Alternative

Vegetarians choose a diet with one essential difference from the diets described previously—they eliminate or restrict foods of animal origin (meat, poultry, fish, eggs, milk). Plant-based diets tend to be lower in total calories and calories from fat, saturated fat, cholesterol, and animal protein and higher in complex carbohydrates, dietary fiber, potassium, folate, vitamins C and E,

vegetarian Someone who follows a diet that restricts or eliminates foods of animal origin. **TERMS**

Nutrient	Recommended Daily Intake* 2,000 calories	Orange Juice 168 calories % Daily	Nutrient value	Low-Fat (1%) Milk 150 calories % Daily	Nutrient value	Regular Cola 152 calories % Daily	Nutrient value	Bottled Iced Tea 150 calories % Daily	Nutrient value
Carbohydrate	300 g	14%	40.5 g	6%	18 g	13%	38 g	13%	37.5 g
Added sugars	32 g					119%	38 g	108%	34.5 g
Fat	65 g			6%	3.9 g				
Protein	55 g			22%	12 g				
Calcium	1,000 mg	3%	33 mg	45%	450 mg	1%	11 mg		
Potassium	4,700 mg	15%	710 mg	12%	570 mg	<1%	4 mg		
Vitamin A	700 µg	4%	30 µg	31%	216 µg				
Vitamin C	75 mg	193%	145.5 mg	5%	3.6 mg				
Vitamin D	5 µg			74%	3.7 µg				
Folate	400 µg	40%	160 µg	5%	20 µg				

Bars show percentage of recommended daily intake or limit

*Recommended intakes and limits appropriate for a 19-year-old woman consuming 2,000 calories per day.

Figure 8.6 Nutrient density of 12-ounce portions of selected beverages. Color bars represent percentage of recommended daily intake or limit for each nutrient.

carotenoids, and phytochemicals. Individuals who follow a plant-based diet generally have a lower body mass index than those who do not. And plant-based dietary patterns are associated with lower mortality rates. Some people adopt a plant-based diet for health reasons, whereas others do so out of concern for the environment, for financial reasons, or for reasons related to ethics or religion.

Types of Plant-Based Diets There are various plant-based styles. The wider the variety of the diet eaten, the easier it is to meet nutritional needs.

- *Vegans* eat only plant foods.
- *Lacto-vegetarians* eat plant foods and dairy products.
- *Lacto-ovo-vegetarians* eat plant foods, dairy products, and eggs.

Others can be categorized as partial vegetarians, semi-vegetarians, or pescovegetarians. These people eat plant foods, dairy products, eggs, and usually a small selection of poultry, fish, and other seafood. Many other people choose vegetarian meals frequently but are not strictly vegetarian.

A Plant-Based Food Plan Table 8.8 outlines the USDA's Healthy Vegetarian diet plan for a 2,000-calorie diet (refer to Figure 2 in the Nutrition Resources at the end of the chapter for information on other calorie levels). Configuring MyPlate for vegetarians requires only a few key modifications: For the protein group, vegetarians can focus on the nonmeat choices of dry beans and peas, nuts, seeds, eggs, and soy foods like tofu. Vegans

and other vegetarians who do not eat or drink any dairy products must find other rich sources of calcium. Fruits, vegetables, and whole grains are healthy choices for people following all types of vegetarian diets.

People following a more plant-based diet may choose to include meat alternatives—foods that approximate the taste and texture of meat but are made from vegetarian ingredients like soy, gluten, or legumes. They may mimic beef patties, sausages, chicken strips, and similar animal foods. Recently developed products like the Impossible Burger and the Beyond Burger are

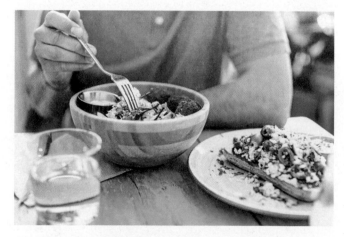

Wellness Tip Variety is the key to maintaining a healthy balanced vegetarian diet. Choose nutrient-dense foods rich in calcium, iron, zinc, and vitamins D and B-12.

VioletaStoimenova/E+/Getty Images

promoted as especially meat-like and even "bleed" like beef. As with any processed food, consider the overall nutritional profile of meat alternatives you select. (See Chapter 15 for more on the potential environmental benefits of meat alternatives.)

A healthy vegetarian diet, emphasizing a wide variety of plant foods, will supply all the essential amino acids. Choosing minimally processed and unrefined foods will maximize nutrient value and provide ample dietary fiber. Plant foods alone can provide all needed nutrients except vitamin B-12 and possibly vitamin D, calcium, iron, and zinc. Strategies for getting these and other nutrients include the following:

- *Vitamin B-12* is found naturally only in animal foods. If dairy products and eggs are limited or avoided, B-12 can be found in fortified foods such as ready-to-eat cereals, soy beverages, meat substitutes, special yeast products, and supplements.

- *Vitamin D* can be obtained by spending 5–15 minutes a day in the sun, by consuming vitamin D-fortified products like ready-to-eat cereals and soy or rice milk, or by taking a supplement.

- *Calcium* is found in legumes, tofu processed with calcium, dark-green leafy vegetables, nuts, tortillas made from lime-processed corn, fortified orange juice, soy milk, bread, and other foods.

- *Iron* is found in whole grains, fortified bread and breakfast cereals, dried fruits, leafy green vegetables, nuts and seeds, legumes, and soy foods. The iron in plant foods is more difficult for the body to absorb than the iron from animal sources. Eating or drinking a good source of vitamin C with most meals is helpful because vitamin C improves iron absorption.

- *Zinc* is found in whole grains, nuts, legumes, and soy foods.

If you are a vegetarian, remember that it's especially important to eat as wide a variety of foods as possible to ensure that all your nutritional needs are satisfied. Vegetarian diets for children, teens, and pregnant and lactating women warrant professional guidance.

Functional Foods

The American diet contains numerous *functional foods*. Two of the earliest functional foods introduced in the United States were iodized salt and milk fortified with vitamins A and D. More recently, manufacturers began fortifying breads and grains with folic acid to reduce the incidence of neural tube defects.

Although the definition of functional foods continues to evolve, this term generally refers to foods containing components that may provide positive health benefits. They include foods that are fortified, enriched, or enhanced, or that contain dietary components with additional potential to benefit health. Other examples of functional foods are calcium-fortified orange juice, margarine enriched with sterols or stanols to lower the risk of heart disease, energy bars for improved athletic performance, and vitamin B-12-enriched soy milk for vegetarians.

Dietary Challenges for Various Population Groups

Certain population groups should be aware of special dietary challenges.

Children and Teenagers Parents with young children can provide a variety of healthy food options. For example, parents can add vegetables to casseroles and fruit to cereal, or offer fruit and vegetable juices or plain yogurt or fruit shakes instead of sugary drinks. Many children and teenagers enjoy eating at fast-food restaurants, but they should be encouraged to select the healthiest menu choices and to balance the day's diet with low-fat, nutrient-rich foods. Allowing children to help prepare meals is another good way to encourage good eating habits.

College Students Foods that are convenient for college students are not always the healthiest choices. Students who eat in buffet-style dining halls, cafeterias, and snack bars can easily overeat, and the foods offered are not necessarily high in nutrients or low in fat. The same is true of meals at fast-food restaurants. However, it is possible to make healthy eating both convenient and affordable. See the tips in the box "Eating Strategies for College Students."

Pregnant and Breastfeeding Women Good nutrition is essential to a healthy pregnancy. Nutrition counseling before conception can help women establish a balanced eating plan and healthy body weights for a healthy pregnancy. During pregnancy and while breastfeeding, women are often advised to take a nutrient supplement in addition to following a special diet, as recommended by MyPlate's Daily Checklist for Moms.

To reduce the risk of neural tube defects in the fetus, the U.S. Public Health Service recommends that all women of childbearing age get 400 µg of folic acid daily from fortified foods or supplements.

Older Adults Nutrient needs change as people age. Older adults tend to become less active and may not need as many calories to maintain body weight. At the same time, the absorption of some nutrients tends to be lower in older adults because of age-related changes in the digestive tract. For these reasons, older adults should focus on eating nutrient-dense foods.

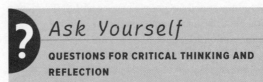

? *Ask Yourself*

QUESTIONS FOR CRITICAL THINKING AND REFLECTION

What factors influence your food choices—convenience, cost, availability, habit? Do you ever consider nutritional content or nutritional recommendations like those found in MyPlate? If not, how big a change would it be for you to think of nutritional content first when choosing food? Is it something you could do easily?

Eating Wherever

- Eat a colorful, varied diet. The more colorful your diet is, the more varied and rich in fruits and vegetables it will be. Fruits and vegetables are typically inexpensive, delicious, nutritious, and nutrient-dense.

- Eat breakfast. You'll have more energy in the morning and be less likely to grab an unhealthy snack later on.

- Choose healthy snacks—fruits, vegetables, whole grains, and cereals.

- Drink low- or nonfat milk, water, mineral water, or 100% fruit juice more often than soft drinks or sweetened beverages.

- Pay attention to portion sizes. Enjoy your food, but eat less.

- Combine physical activity with healthy eating.

- Plan to eat meals with friends and family members who choose healthy foods and can provide support and inspiration.

Eating in the Dining Hall

- Choose a meal plan that includes breakfast.

- Decide what you want to eat before you get in line, and stick to your choices.

- Build your meals around whole grains and vegetables. Ask for small servings of meat and high-fat main dishes.

- Choose leaner poultry, fish, or bean dishes rather than high-fat meats and fried entrees.

- Ask that gravies and sauces be served on the side; limit your intake.

- Choose broth-based or vegetable soups rather than cream soups.

- At the salad bar, load up on leafy greens, beans, and fresh vegetables. Avoid mayonnaise-coated salads, bacon, croutons, and high-fat dressings. Put dressing on the side; dip your fork into it rather than pouring it over the salad.

- Choose fruit for dessert rather than cookies or cakes.

Eating in Fast-Food Restaurants

- Most fast-food chains can provide a brochure with the nutritional content of their menu items. Ask for it, or check the restaurant's website for nutritional information. Order small single burgers with no cheese instead of double burgers with many toppings. If possible, get them broiled instead of fried.

- Ask for items to be prepared without mayonnaise, tartar sauce, sour cream, or other high-fat sauces. Ketchup, mustard, and fat-free mayonnaise or sour cream are better choices and are available at many fast-food restaurants.

- Choose whole-grain buns or bread for sandwiches.

- Choose chicken items made from chicken breast, not processed chicken.

- Order vegetable pizzas without extra cheese.

- If you order French fries or onion rings, get the smallest size and/or share them with a friend. Better yet, get a salad or a fruit cup instead.

- For food truck meals, use the same strategies suggested for fast-food restaurants—choose lean proteins and ask for condiments on the side. If your favorite food truck doesn't have healthy options, ask that they be added to the menu.

Eating on the Run

- When you need to eat in a hurry, remember that you can carry healthy foods in your backpack or a small insulated lunch sack (with a frozen gel pack to keep fresh food from spoiling).

- Carry items that are small and convenient but nutritious, such as fresh fruits or vegetables, nuts and dried fruit, whole-wheat buns or muffins, snack-size cereal boxes, and water.

- Make healthy choices at vending machines such as water or 100% fruit juice for beverages and whole-grain crackers or pretzels, nuts, seeds, baked chips, low-fat popcorn, and low-fat granola bars as snacks.

For example, foods fortified with vitamin B-12 and/or B-12 supplements are recommended for people over age 50. Calcium and vitamin D intake can be inadequate; therefore, physicians may suggest supplementation to reduce bone loss and risk of osteoporosis. Antioxidants from fruits and vegetables are important in older adults to reduce age-related changes in vision and cognitive functioning. Because constipation is a common problem, consuming foods high in dietary fiber and drinking enough fluids are important goals.

Athletes Key dietary concerns for athletes are meeting increased energy and fluid requirements for training and making healthy food choices throughout the day. For more on this topic, see the box "Do Athletes Need a Different Diet?"

People with Special Health Concerns Many Americans have special health concerns that affect their dietary needs. For example, people with diabetes benefit from a well-balanced diet that is low in simple sugars, high in complex carbohydrates, and relatively rich in monounsaturated fats. People with high blood pressure need to limit their sodium consumption and control their weight. If you have a health problem or concern that may require a special diet, discuss your situation with a physician or registered dietitian.

If you exercise vigorously and frequently or if you are an athlete in training, you likely have increased energy and fluid requirements. Research supports the following recommendations for athletes:

- **Energy intake.** Someone engaged in a vigorous training program may have energy needs as high as 6,000 calories per day—far greater than the energy needs of a moderately active person. Athletes must consume enough calories to fuel their training and all basic body functions. Weight loss can be a sign of insufficient energy intake, but body systems may adjust in ways that disrupt hormonal and metabolic functioning without changes in body weight. Other signs that an athlete may need more calories include recurrent injuries and illnesses, decreased performance, and psychological symptoms such as irritability and depression.

    Athletes who need to maintain low body weight and fat (such as gymnasts, skaters, and wrestlers) need to get enough calories and nutrients while avoiding unhealthy eating patterns such as bulimia. The combination of low body fat, high physical activity, and disordered eating habits—and, in women, amenorrhea—is associated with osteoporosis, stress fractures, and other injuries. If keeping your weight and body fat low for athletic reasons is important to you, seek dietary advice from a qualified dietitian and make sure your physician is aware of your eating habits. See Chapter 6 for more on problems associated with low body fat.

- **Carbohydrates.** Carbohydrates are the principal fuels used during exercise at intensities above 65% of maximum effort. Endurance athletes involved in competitive events lasting longer than 90 minutes may benefit from increasing carbohydrate intake to 60–70% of their total calories. Specifically, the American College of Sports Medicine (ACSM) recommends that athletes consume 2.7–5.5 grams per pound of body weight daily, depending on their weight, sport, and other nutritional needs. This increase should come in the form of complex carbohydrates, and athletes should take care that high consumption of carbohydrate does not lead to underconsumption of other nutrients.

High carbohydrate intake builds and maintains glycogen stores in the muscles, resulting in greater endurance and delayed fatigue during competitive events or long workouts. The ACSM recommends that before exercise an active adult or athlete eat a meal or snack that is relatively high in carbohydrates, moderate in protein, and low in fat and fiber. Carbohydrates (e.g., low-sugar sports beverages and gels) consumed during prolonged athletic events provide fluid, electrolytes, and glucose to help fuel muscles and can extend the availability of glycogen stored in muscles. Eating carbohydrates 30 minutes, two hours, and four hours after exercise can help replenish glycogen stores in the liver and muscles.

- **Fat.** The ACSM recommends that athletes follow the general public health guidelines for dietary fat intake.

- **Protein.** For endurance and strength-trained athletes, the ACSM recommends eating 0.54–0.91 grams of protein per pound of body weight each day, which is considerably higher than the standard DRI of 0.36 gram per pound. This level of protein is easily obtainable from foods; in fact, most Americans eat more protein than they need every day. A balanced diet can provide the protein most athletes need.

    There is no evidence that consuming supplements containing vitamins, minerals, protein, or specific amino acids builds muscle or improves sports performance. Strength and muscle are built with exercise, not extra protein, and carbohydrates provide the fuel needed for muscle-building exercise. Some research suggests spreading your protein intake across the day, every three or four hours (for example, breakfast, lunch, afternoon snack, and dinner).

- **Fluids.** If you exercise heavily or live in a hot climate, you should drink extra fluids to maximize performance and prevent heat illness. For a strenuous endurance event, prepare yourself the day before by drinking plenty of fluids. The ACSM recommends drinking 2–3 milliliters (~½ a teaspoon) of fluid per pound of body weight about four hours before the event. During the event, take in enough fluids to compensate for fluid loss due to sweating; the amount required depends on the individual and his or her sweat rate. Afterward, drink enough to replace lost fluids—about 16–24 ounces for every pound of weight lost.

    Water is a good choice for fluid replacement for events lasting 60–90 minutes. For longer workouts or events, a sports drink can be a good choice. These contain water, electrolytes, and carbohydrates and can provide some extra energy as well as replace electrolytes like sodium lost in sweat.

SOURCES: Thomas, D. T., et al. 2016. "American College of Sports Medicine joint position statement. Nutrition and athletic performance," *Medicine and Science in Sports and Exercise* 48(3): 543–568; Clark, N. 2016. *Weight and protein: Hot topics at the ACSM annual meeting* (http://www.acsm.org /public-information/acsm-blog/2016/06/10/weight-and-protein-hot-topics -at-the-acsm-annual-meeting).

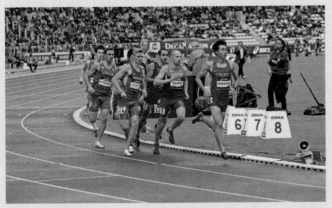

Denys Kuvaiev/123RF

NUTRITIONAL PLANNING: MAKING INFORMED CHOICES ABOUT FOOD

Knowing about nutrition is a good start to making sound choices about food. It also helps if you can interpret food labels, make wise choices about dietary supplements, understand food additives, and avoid foodborne illnesses and environmental contaminants.

Food Labels

All processed foods regulated by either the FDA or the USDA include standardized nutrition information on their labels. Every food label shows serving sizes and the amount of many nutrients in each serving, including saturated fat, protein, dietary fiber, and sodium. To make informed choices about food, learn to read and understand food labels (see the box "Using Food Labels").

Food label regulations also require that foods meet strict definitions if their packaging includes terms such as *light, low-fat,* or *high-fiber* (Table 8.10). Health claims such as "good source of dietary fiber" or "low in saturated fat" on packages are regulated and can be signals that a product can be wisely included in your diet.

Food labels are not required on fresh meat, poultry, fish, fruits, and vegetables (many of these products are not packaged). You can get information on the nutrient content of these items online. Also, supermarkets may have posters or pamphlets

listing the nutrient contents of unpackaged foods. In Lab 8.3, you compare foods using the information on their labels.

Calorie Labeling: Restaurants and Vending Machines

As of May 2018, calorie information is required on restaurant menus, vending machines, and signs near the food in chain restaurants and similar retail food establishments (those with 20 or more locations). Chain restaurants are also required to provide more detailed nutrition information about their menu.

Dietary Supplements

Dietary supplements include vitamins, minerals, amino acids, herbs, enzymes, and other compounds. Although dietary supplements are sold over the counter and are often thought of as safe and natural, they may contain powerful bioactive chemicals that can have toxic effects if consumed in excess.

In the United States, dietary supplements are not legally considered drugs and are not regulated like drugs. Before they are approved by the FDA and put on the market, drugs undergo clinical studies to determine safety, effectiveness, side effects and risks, possible interactions with other substances, and appropriate dosages. The FDA does not authorize or test dietary supplements, and manufacturers are not required to demonstrate either safety or

Table 8.10	Food Package Nutrient Claims
CLAIM	WHAT IT MEANS
Healthy*	A food that is low in total fat or has predominantly mono- and/or polyunsaturated fats; has no more than 360–480 mg of sodium and 60 mg of cholesterol; and provides 10% or more of the Daily Value for vitamin A, vitamin C, vitamin D, protein, calcium, iron, potassium, or dietary fiber
Light or lite	33% fewer calories or 50% less fat than a similar product
Reduced or fewer	At least 25% less of a nutrient than a similar product; can be applied to fat ("reduced fat"), saturated fat, cholesterol, sodium, and calories
Extra or added	10% or more of the Daily Value per serving when compared to what a similar product has
Good source	10–19% of the Daily Value for a particular nutrient per serving
High, rich in, or excellent source of	20% or more of the Daily Value for a particular nutrient per serving
Low calorie	40 calories or less per serving
High fiber	5 grams or more of fiber per serving
Good source of fiber	2.5–4.9 grams of fiber per serving
Fat-free	Less than 0.5 gram of fat per serving
Low-fat	3 grams of fat or less per serving
Saturated or trans fat-free	Less than 0.5 gram of saturated fat and 0.5 gram of trans fatty acids per serving
Low saturated fat	1 gram or less of saturated fat per serving and no more than 15% of total calories
Low sodium	140 mg or less of sodium per serving
Very low sodium	35 mg or less of sodium per serving
Lean	Cooked seafood, meat, or poultry with less than 10 grams of fat, 4.5 grams or less of saturated fat, and less than 95 mg of cholesterol per serving
Extra lean	Cooked seafood, meat, or poultry with less than 5 grams of fat, 2 grams of saturated fat, and 95 mg of cholesterol per serving

*To reflect current scientific understanding and public health concerns, in 2016, the FDA updated the criteria for the "healthy" claim to also allow it for foods that are not low in total fat but instead have a fat profile makeup of predominantly unsaturated fats; the FDA also added potassium and vitamin D to the list of nutrients covered by the claim. Additional changes to the "healthy" claim are being considered.

NOTE: The FDA has not yet defined nutrient claims relating to carbohydrates, so foods labeled low- or reduced-carbohydrate do not conform to any approved standard.

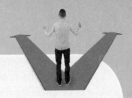

The "Nutrition Facts" section of a food label is designed to help consumers make food choices based on the nutrients that are most important to good health. In addition to listing nutrient content by weight, the label puts the information in the context of a daily diet of 2,000 calories, with the understanding that your calorie needs may be higher or lower depending on your age, gender, height, weight, and physical activity level.

Food labels use uniform serving sizes. This means that if you look at different brands of salad dressing, for example, you can compare calories and fat content based on the serving amount. Food label serving sizes, however, may be larger or smaller than USDA serving size equivalents.

The Nutrition Facts label had been in use without major changes since the 1990s. Based on research into how consumers use food labels as well as changes to the nutrients of most concern to Americans, the FDA announced changes to the look and content of the label in 2016. Some new features include:

- Adding added sugars, vitamin D, and potassium to all labels; Vitamins A and C will no longer be required because deficiencies in these vitamins are rare today

- Removing the listing for "Calories from Fat" because research shows the type of fat is more important than the number of grams

- Revising Daily Values for certain nutrients to reflect the latest recommendations

- Updating serving size labeling for certain packages to be more realistic and to reflect amounts typically eaten at one time

- Refreshing the design to highlight calorie content and serving size and to make other parts of the label easier to read

During the transition period, you will see either the current or the new label on products. All manufacturers are required to use the new labels by 2021.

SOURCE: U.S. Food and Drug Administration. 2019. *Changes to the Nutrition Facts Label.* (https://www.fda.gov/Food/GuidanceRegulation/GuidanceDocumentsRegulatoryInformation/LabelingNutrition/ucm385663.htm).

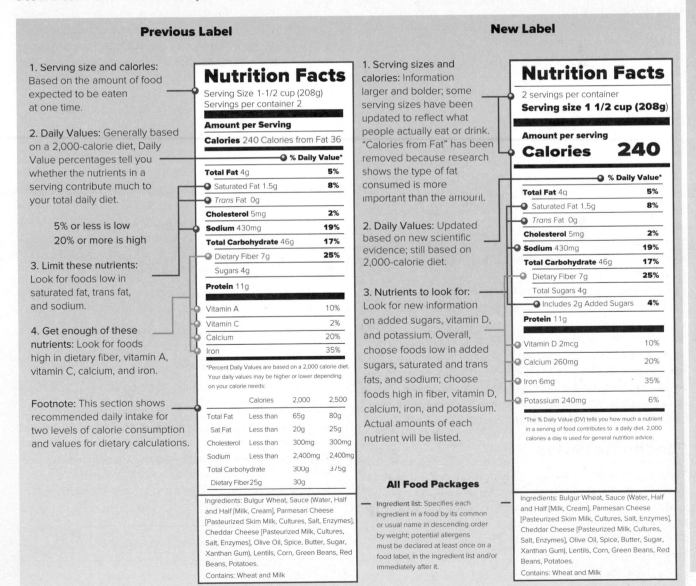

effectiveness before these products are marketed. Although dosage guidelines exist for some of the compounds in dietary supplements, dosages for many are not well established.

Large doses of some dietary supplements can cause health problems by affecting the absorption of certain vitamins or minerals or interacting with medications. Garlic supplements, for example, can cause bleeding if taken with anticoagulant (blood-thinning) medications. Some supplements can have side effects. St. John's wort, for example, increases the skin's sensitivity to sunlight and may decrease the effectiveness of oral contraceptives, drugs used to treat HIV infection, and many other medications. For this reason, ask your doctor or a dietitian before taking any high-dosage supplement.

Drugs and supplements are also manufactured quite differently: FDA-approved medications are standardized for potency, and they require quality control and proof of purity. Dietary supplement manufacturing is not as closely regulated, and there is no guarantee that a product contains a given ingredient at all, let alone in the appropriate amount. The potency of herbal supplements can vary widely due to differences in growing and harvesting conditions, preparation methods, and storage. Contamination and misidentification of plant compounds are also potential problems.

In an effort to provide consumers with more reliable and consistent information about supplements, the FDA has developed labeling regulations. Labels similar to those found on foods are now required for dietary supplements. For more information, see the box "Using Dietary Supplement Labels."

Food Additives

Have you ever read the ingredients of your favorite processed or packaged food? Today, approximately 3,000 substances are intentionally added to foods to maintain or improve nutritional quality, to maintain freshness, to help in processing or preparation, or to alter taste or appearance. The most widely used additives in foods are sugar, salt, and corn syrup; these three, plus citric acid, baking soda, vegetable colors, mustard, and pepper, account for 98% by weight of all food additives used in the United States.

Food additives pose no significant health hazard to most people because the levels used are well below any that could produce toxic effects. One additive of potential concern for some people is sulfites, used to keep vegetables from turning brown; sulfites can cause severe reactions in some people, and the FDA strictly limits their use and requires clear labeling on any food containing them. Monosodium glutamate (MSG) has been said to cause headaches and other symptoms for 40 years, but no consistent evidence supports these claims.

Foodborne Illness

Many people worry about additives or pesticide residues in their food, but a greater threat comes from microorganisms that cause foodborne illnesses. Raw or undercooked animal products, such as chicken, hamburger, and oysters, pose the greatest risk, although in recent years contaminated fruits and vegetables have been catching up.

The Centers for Disease Control and Prevention (CDC) estimates that 48 million illnesses, 128,000 hospitalizations, and 3,000 deaths occur each year in the United States due to foodborne contaminants. One out of six people contract a foodborne disease each year. Symptoms include diarrhea, vomiting, fever, pain, headache, and weakness. Although the effects of foodborne illness are usually not serious, children, pregnant women, and elderly people are more at risk for severe complications such as rheumatic diseases, seizures, blood poisoning, and death. Young children and older adults are more likely to have severe complications or to die from foodborne illnesses. In all, 13% of infections, 24% of hospitalizations, and 57% of deaths due to foodborne illnesses occurred among adults age 65 and over.

Causes of Foodborne Illnesses Most cases of foodborne illness are caused by **pathogens**, disease-causing microorganisms that contaminate food, usually from improper handling. Eight known pathogens contribute to the vast majority of illnesses, hospitalizations, and deaths related to foodborne illness, most notably *Salmonella* (most often found in eggs, on vegetables, and on poultry); norovirus (most often found in salad ingredients and shellfish); *Campylobacter jejuni* (most often found in meat and poultry); *Toxoplasma* (most often found in meat); *Escherichia coli* (*E. coli*) O157:H7 (most often found in meat and water); *Listeria monocytogenes* (most often found in lunch meats, sausages, and hot dogs); and *Clostridium perfringens* (most often found in meat and gravy). The most frequent causes of infection and hospitalizations are norovirus and *Salmonella*.

Although pathogens are usually destroyed during cooking, the U.S. government is taking steps to bring down levels of contamination by improving national testing and surveillance. Raw meat and poultry products are now sold with safe-handling and cooking instructions, and all packaged, unpasteurized fresh fruit and vegetable juices carry warnings about potential contamination.

Although foodborne illness outbreaks associated with food-processing plants make headlines, most cases of illness trace back to poor food handling in the home or in restaurants. The FDA encourages people to follow four basic food safety principles:

- *Clean* hands, food contact surfaces, and vegetables and fruits.
- *Separate* raw, cooked, and ready-to-eat foods while shopping, storing, and preparing foods.
- *Cook* foods to a safe temperature.
- *Chill* (refrigerate) perishable foods promptly.

Avoid certain high-risk foods, including raw (unpasteurized) milk, cheeses, and juices; raw or undercooked seafood, meat, poultry, and eggs; and raw sprouts. These precautions are especially important for pregnant women, young children, older adults, and people with weakened immune systems or certain chronic diseases. For more information on food safety, see the box "Safe Food Handling."

---

pathogen A microorganism that causes disease. **TERMS**

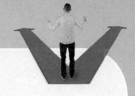

In addition to basic information about the product, labels must include a "Supplement Facts" panel, modeled after the Nutrition Facts panel used on food labels (see the sample label). Under the Dietary Supplement Health and Education Act (DSHEA) and food labeling laws, supplement labels can make three types of health-related claims:

- *Nutrient-content claims, such as* "high in calcium," "excellent source of vitamin C," or "high potency." The claims "high in" and "excellent source of" mean the same as they do on food labels. A "high potency" single-ingredient supplement must contain 100% of its Daily Value; a "high potency" multi-ingredient product must contain 100% or more of the Daily Value of at least two-thirds of the nutrients present for which Daily Values have been established.

- *Health claims,* if they have been evaluated by the FDA. Health claims may be either "authorized" or "qualified." Authorized claims have significant supporting scientific evidence; an example is the association between adequate calcium intake and reduced risk of osteoporosis. A qualified claim is based on less evidence and must include a disclaimer. The FDA does not itself test for safety or ensure a supplement works.

- *Structure-function claims,* such as "antioxidants maintain cellular integrity" or "this product enhances energy levels." Because these claims are not reviewed by the FDA, they must carry a disclaimer (see the sample label).

Tips for Choosing and Using Dietary Supplements

- Check with your physician before taking a supplement. Many are not meant for children, older people, women who are pregnant or breastfeeding, people with chronic illnesses or upcoming surgery, or people taking prescription or over-the-counter medications. When you visit your doctor, bring a list of all dietary supplements you are taking. Do not take mega-doses (more than double DRI levels) without your doctor's approval.

- Follow the cautions, instructions for use, and dosage given on the label.

- Look for the U.S. Pharmacopeial Convention (USP) verification mark on the label, indicating that the product meets minimum safety and purity standards developed under the Dietary Supplement Verification Program by the USP. The USP mark means that the product (1) contains the ingredients stated on the label, (2) has the declared amount and strength of ingredients, (3) will dissolve effectively, (4) has been screened for harmful contaminants, and (5) has been manufactured using safe, sanitary, and well-controlled procedures. The Natural Products Association has a self-regulatory testing program for its members; other, smaller associations and labs, including consumerlab.com, also test and rate dietary supplements.

- Choose brands made by nationally known food and drug manufacturers or "house brands" from large retail chains. Due to their size and visibility, such sources are likely to have high manufacturing standards.

- If you experience side effects, stop using the product and contact your physician. Report any serious reactions to the FDA's MedWatch monitoring program (1-800-FDA-1088 or online at http://www.fda.gov/Safety/MedWatch/default.htm).

For More Information about Dietary Supplements

FDA: https://www.fda.gov/food/dietary-supplements
NIH Office of Dietary Supplements: https://ods.od.nih.gov
USDA: https://www.nal.usda.gov/fnic/dietary-supplements
U.S. Pharmacopeial Convention: http://www.usp.org

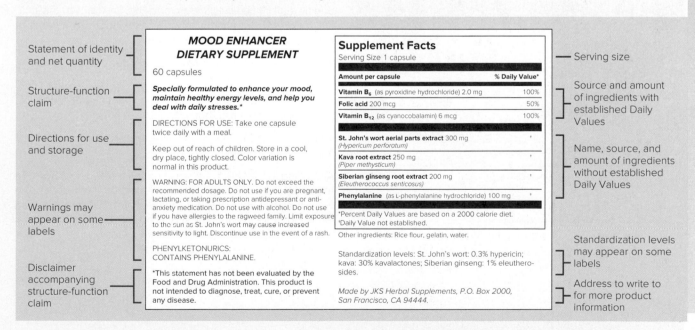

Statement of identity and net quantity

Structure-function claim

Directions for use and storage

Warnings may appear on some labels

Disclaimer accompanying structure-function claim

MOOD ENHANCER DIETARY SUPPLEMENT

60 capsules

Specially formulated to enhance your mood, maintain healthy energy levels, and help you deal with daily stresses.*

DIRECTIONS FOR USE: Take one capsule twice daily with a meal.

Keep out of reach of children. Store in a cool, dry place, tightly closed. Color variation is normal in this product.

WARNING: FOR ADULTS ONLY. Do not exceed the recommended dosage. Do not use if you are pregnant, lactating, or taking prescription antidepressant or anti-anxiety medication. Do not use with alcohol. Do not use if you have allergies to the ragweed family. Limit exposure to the sun as St. John's wort may cause increased sensitivity to light. Discontinue use in the event of a rash.

PHENYLKETONURICS: CONTAINS PHENYLALANINE.

*This statement has not been evaluated by the Food and Drug Administration. This product is not intended to diagnose, treat, cure, or prevent any disease.

Supplement Facts
Serving Size 1 capsule

Amount per capsule	% Daily Value*
Vitamin B₆ (as pyroxidine hydrochloride) 2.0 mg	100%
Folic acid 200 mcg	50%
Vitamin B₁₂ (as cyanocobalamin) 6 mcg	100%
St. John's wort aerial parts extract 300 mg *(Hypericum perforatum)*	†
Kava root extract 250 mg *(Piper methysticum)*	†
Siberian ginseng root extract 200 mg *(Eleutherococcus senticosus)*	†
Phenylalanine (as L-phenylalanine hydrochloride) 100 mg	†

*Percent Daily Values are based on a 2000 calorie diet.
†Daily Value not established.

Other ingredients: Rice flour, gelatin, water.

Standardization levels: St. John's wort: 0.3% hypericin; kava: 30% kavalactones; Siberian ginseng: 1% eleutherosides.

Made by JKS Herbal Supplements, P.O. Box 2000, San Francisco, CA 94444.

Serving size

Source and amount of ingredients with established Daily Values

Name, source, and amount of ingredients without established Daily Values

Standardization levels may appear on some labels

Address to write to for more product information

Shopping

- Don't buy food in containers that leak, bulge, or are severely dented. Refrigerated foods should be cold, and frozen foods should be solid.

- Check the food label for an expiration date and for safe-handling instructions.

- Place meat, poultry, and seafood in plastic bags, and separate foods in grocery cart.

- Select cold and frozen foods last to ensure they stay refrigerated until just before checkout.

Storing Food

- Store raw meat, poultry, fish, and shellfish in containers in the refrigerator so that the juices don't drip onto other foods. Keep these items away from other foods, surfaces, utensils, and serving dishes to prevent cross-contamination.

- Store eggs in the coldest part of the refrigerator, not in the door, and use them within three to five weeks.

- Keep hot foods hot (140°F or above) and cold foods cold (40°F or below); harmful bacteria can grow rapidly between these two temperatures. Refrigerate foods within two hours of

purchase or preparation and within one hour if the air temperature is above 90°F. Freeze foods at or below 0°F. Use or freeze fresh meats within three to five days and fresh poultry, fish, and ground meat within one to two days. Use refrigerated leftovers within three to four days.

Preparing Food

- Thoroughly wash your hands with warm soapy water for 20 seconds before and after handling food, especially raw meat, fish, shellfish, poultry, or eggs.

- Make sure counters, cutting boards, dishes, utensils, and other equipment are thoroughly cleaned with hot soapy water before and after use. Wash dishcloths and kitchen towels frequently.

- Use separate cutting boards for meat, poultry, and seafood and for foods that will be eaten raw, such as fruits and vegetables. Replace cutting boards once they become worn or develop hard-to-clean grooves.

- Thoroughly rinse and scrub fruits and vegetables with a brush (but not with soap or detergent), or peel off the skin.

- Don't eat raw animal products, including raw eggs in home-made hollandaise sauce, eggnog, or cookie dough.

- Thaw frozen food in the refrigerator, in cold water, or in the microwave, not on the kitchen counter. Cook foods immediately after thawing.

Cooking

- Cook foods thoroughly, especially beef, poultry, fish, pork, and eggs; cooking kills most microorganisms. Use a food thermometer to ensure that foods are cooked to a safe temperature. Hamburgers should be cooked to 160°F. Turn or stir microwaved food to make sure it is heated evenly throughout.

- Cook stuffing separately from poultry; or wash poultry thoroughly, stuff immediately before cooking, and transfer the stuffing to a clean bowl immediately after cooking. The temperature of cooked stuffing should reach 165°F.

- Cook eggs until they're firm, and fully cook foods containing eggs.

- To protect against *Listeria,* reheat ready-to-eat foods like hot dogs until steaming hot.

- Because of possible contamination with *E. coli* 0157:H7 and *Salmonella,* avoid raw sprouts.

According to the USDA, "When in doubt, throw it out." Even if a food looks and smells fine, it may not be safe. If you aren't sure that a food has been prepared, served, and stored safely, don't eat it. For more information, visit Foodsafety.gov.

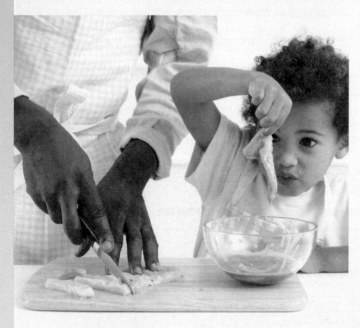

Dave King/Dorling Kindersley/Getty Images

Treating Foodborne Illness If you think you may be having a bout of foodborne illness, drink plenty of clear fluids to prevent dehydration, and rest to speed recovery. To prevent further contamination, wash your hands often and always before handling food until you recover. A fever higher than 102°F, blood in the stool, or dehydration deserves a physician's evaluation or a trip to your school's health clinic, especially if the symptoms persist for more than two or three days. In cases of suspected botulism—characterized by symptoms such as double vision, paralysis, dizziness, and vomiting—consult a physician immediately.

Irradiated Foods

Food irradiation is the treatment of foods with gamma rays, X-rays, or high-voltage electrons to kill potentially harmful pathogens, including bacteria, parasites, insects, and fungi that cause foodborne illness. It also reduces spoilage and extends shelf life. For example, irradiated strawberries stay unspoiled in the refrigerator up to three weeks, versus only three to five days for untreated berries. Even though irradiation has been generally endorsed by agencies such as the World Health Organization, the CDC, and the American Medical Association, few irradiated foods are currently on the market due to consumer resistance and skepticism. Studies indicate that when consumers are given information about the process of irradiation and the benefits of irradiated foods, most want to purchase them.

 All primary irradiated foods (meat, vegetables, and so on) are labeled with the flowerlike radura symbol and a brief information label; spices and foods that are merely ingredients do not have to be labeled. Proper handling of irradiated foods is still critical for preventing foodborne illness.

Environmental Contaminants and Organic Foods

Contaminants are present in the food-growing environment. Environmental contaminants include various minerals, antibiotics, hormones, pesticides, and industrial chemicals. Safety regulations attempt to keep our exposure to contaminants at safe levels, but monitoring is difficult, and many substances (such as pesticides) persist in the environment long after being banned from use.

Organic Foods Concern about pesticides and other environmental contaminants prompts many to choose **organic** foods. To be certified as organic, foods must meet strict production, processing, handling, and labeling criteria. Organic crops are grown without the use of conventional pesticides and must meet limits on pesticide residues. The use of synthetic fertilizers, genetic engineering, ionizing radiation, and sewage sludge is prohibited. For meat, milk, eggs, and other animal products to be certified organic, animals must be given organic feed and access to the outdoors and may not be given antibiotics or growth hormones. Products can be labeled "100% organic" if they contain all organic ingredients and "organic" if they contain at least 95% organic ingredients; all such products may carry the USDA organic seal. A product with at least 70% organic ingredients can be labeled "made with organic ingredients" but cannot use the USDA seal.

Organic foods, however, are not necessarily free of chemicals. They may be contaminated with pesticides used on neighboring lands or on foods transported in the same train or truck. However, they tend to have lower levels of pesticide residues than conventionally grown crops. Some experts recommend that consumers who want to buy organic fruits and vegetables spend their money on those that carry lower pesticide residues than their conventional counterparts (the "dirty dozen"): apples, bell peppers, celery, cherries, imported grapes, nectarines, peaches, pears, potatoes, red raspberries, spinach, and strawberries. Experts also recommend buying organic beef, poultry, eggs, dairy products, and baby food. Fruits and vegetables that carry little pesticide residue, whether grown conventionally or organically, include asparagus, avocados, bananas, broccoli, cauliflower, corn, kiwi, mangoes, onions, papaya, pineapples, and peas. All foods are subject to strict pesticide limits; the debate about the health effects of small amounts of residue is ongoing.

Whether organic foods are better for your health cannot be said for certain, but organic farming is better for the environment. Benefits include sustainable farming practices, preservation of biodiversity, healthier soil, protection of water supplies, reduced use of fossil fuels, improved animal welfare, protection of ecosystems, and safer conditions for farmworkers. Buying organic food, buying locally grown foods, and participating in a community garden are ways to support food production that benefits and sustains the environment.

Guidelines for Fish Consumption You may have heard reports of possible mercury contamination in fish. Overall, however, fish and shellfish are healthy sources of protein, omega-3 fats, and other nutrients, and experts continue to encourage consumption of both wild-caught and farmed fish. Prudent choices can minimize the risk of any possible negative health effects. High mercury concentrations are most likely to be found in predator fish—large fish that eat smaller fish. Mercury can cause brain damage to fetuses and young children. According to FDA and Environmental Protection Agency (EPA) guidelines, women who are or who may become pregnant and nursing mothers should follow these guidelines to minimize their exposure to mercury:

- Do not eat shark, swordfish, king mackerel, or tilefish.
- Eat 8–12 ounces each week of a variety of fish and shellfish that are lower in mercury, such as shrimp, canned light tuna, salmon, pollock, and catfish. Limit consumption of albacore tuna to 6 ounces per week.
- Check advisories about the safety of recreationally caught fish from local lakes, rivers, and coastal areas. If no information is available, limit consumption to 6 ounces per week.

The same guidelines apply to children, although they should consume smaller servings.

A PERSONAL PLAN

No single type of diet provides optimal health for everyone. Many cultural dietary patterns can meet people's nutritional requirements. Customize your food plan based on your age, gender, weight, activity level, medical risk factors, and personal tastes.

Assessing and Changing Your Diet

The first step in planning a healthy diet is to examine what you currently eat. Labs 8.1 and 8.2 help you analyze your current diet and compare it with optimal dietary goals.

To put your plan into action, use the behavioral self-management techniques and tips described in Chapter 1. If you identify several changes you want to make, focus on one at a time. You might start, for example, by substituting water for sugar-sweetened beverages. When you become used to that, you can try substituting whole-wheat bread for white bread. The information on eating behavior in Lab 8.1 will help you identify and change unhealthy patterns of eating.

Staying Committed to a Healthy Diet

Beyond knowledge and information, you also need support in difficult situations. Keeping to your plan is easiest when you choose and prepare your own food at home. Advance planning is the key: mapping out meals and shopping appropriately, cooking in advance when possible, and preparing enough food for leftovers. A tight budget does not necessarily make it difficult to eat healthy meals. When you are eating out, consider your food choices and portion sizes carefully.

Strategies like these are helpful, but small changes cannot transform a fundamentally high-sugar, high-calorie meal into a moderate, healthful one. Often, the best advice is to bypass a cinnamon roll with thick white icing for a flavorful but low-sugar option. Many selections offered in ethnic restaurants are healthy choices (refer to the "Ethnic Foods" box for suggestions).

TIPS FOR TODAY AND THE FUTURE

Opportunities to improve your diet present themselves every day, and small changes add up.

RIGHT NOW YOU CAN
- Substitute a healthy snack for an unhealthy one.
- Drink a glass of water and put a bottle of water in your backpack for tomorrow.
- Plan to make healthy selections when you eat out, such as choosing steamed vegetables instead of French fries, or salmon instead of steak.

IN THE FUTURE YOU CAN
- Visit the MyPlate website at ChooseMyPlate.gov and use the online tools to create a personalized nutrition plan.
- Learn to cook healthier meals. There are hundreds of free websites and low-cost cookbooks that provide recipes for healthy dishes.

SUMMARY

- The six classes of nutrients are proteins, fats, carbohydrates, vitamins, minerals, and water.

- Nutrients are essential to humans when the body cannot produce them and must be gotten through food. Nutrients in foods provide energy, measured in kilocalories (commonly called calories); build and maintain body tissues; and regulate body functions.

- Protein, an important component of body tissue, is composed of amino acids; nine are essential to good health. Foods from animal sources provide complete proteins. Plants provide incomplete proteins.

- Fats, a major source of energy, also insulate the body and cushion the organs. Just 3–4 teaspoons of vegetable oil per day supply the essential fats. Unsaturated fats should be favored over saturated fats. Trans fats should be avoided.

- Carbohydrates provide energy to the brain, nervous system, and blood and to muscles during high-intensity exercise. Naturally occurring simple carbohydrates and unrefined complex carbohydrates should be favored over added sugars and refined carbohydrates.

- Fiber includes plant substances that are impossible for the human body to digest. It helps reduce cholesterol levels and promotes the passage of wastes through the intestines.

- The 13 essential vitamins are organic substances that promote specific chemical and cell processes and act as antioxidants. The 17 known essential minerals are inorganic substances that regulate body functions, aid in growth and tissue maintenance, and help in the release of energy from food. Deficiencies in vitamins and minerals can cause severe symptoms over time, but excess doses are also dangerous.

DIVERSITY MATTERS
Ethnic Foods

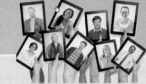

Over the past decades, as people have come to the United States from many countries, Thai, Vietnamese, Afghani, Ethiopian, and Moroccan eateries, to name a few, have sprung up in cities and towns and near universities. For many of us, trying new foods is a fun, social, and usually delicious experience. Each cuisine arises from its local geography and the plants and animals available there. Each also evolves from cultural beliefs regarding food and health, as well as from historical events like trade, war, and immigration. For example, the cuisine of the United States began with English dishes that settlers brought to the colonies, and it was influenced later by foods and recipes of American Indians, African slaves, and immigrants from other countries in Europe as well as from Asia, Mexico, and Central America. These influences continue to shape American cuisine today.

By exploring world cuisines, you can learn about new cultures, new foods, and new flavor combinations. As you experiment, you will also want to keep healthy eating in mind, and you can do so by choosing dishes that are steamed, poached, boiled, roasted, grilled, broiled, stewed, lightly stir-fried, or broth-based—and by minimizing those that are fried, deep-fried, breaded, or cooked in butter, cream, or cheese sauces. The following table points you to healthy choices from a variety of ethnic cuisines.

	Choose More Often	Choose Less Often
Chinese	Hoisin sauce, oyster sauce, wine sauce, plum sauce, velvet sauce, or hot mustard Fresh fish and seafood, skinless chicken, tofu Mixed vegetables, Chinese greens	Crab rangoon Crispy (Peking) duck or chicken Sweet-and-sour dishes made with breaded and deep-fried meat, poultry, or fish
Greek	Shish kabobs (souvlaki) Dolmas (grape leaves) stuffed with rice Tzatziki (yogurt, cucumbers, and garlic) Tabouli (bulgur-based salad)	Saganaki (fried cheese) Pies such as spanakopita and tyropita Deep-fried falafel (chickpea patties)
Indian	Dishes prepared masala (curry), tandoori (roasted in a clay oven), or tikke (pan roasted); kebabs Raita (yogurt and cucumber salad) and other yogurt-based dishes and sauces Dal (lentils), pullao or pilau (basmati rice)	Ghee (clarified butter) Korma (meat in cream sauce) Samosas, pakoras (fried dishes) Poori, bhatura, or paratha (fried breads) Molee and other coconut milk-based dishes
Italian	Pasta primavera or pasta, polenta, risotto, or gnocchi with marinara, red or white wine, white or red clam, or light mushroom sauce Dishes that are grilled or prepared cacciatore (tomato-based sauce) or piccata (lemon sauce) Cioppino (seafood stew) Vegetable soup, minestrone or fagioli (beans)	Antipasto (smoked meats) Dishes that are prepared alfredo, frito (fried), crema (creamed), alla panna (with cream), or carbonara (egg, cheese, and bacon)
Japanese	Dishes prepared nabemono (boiled), shabu-shabu (in boiling broth), mushimono (steamed), nimono (simmered), yaki (broiled), or yakimono (grilled) Sushi or domburi (mixed rice dish)	Tempura (battered and fried) Agemono (deep fried) Katsu (fried pork cutlet) Sukiyaki Fried tofu
Mexican	Soft corn or wheat tortillas Refried beans, nonfat or low-fat; rice and beans Ceviche (fish marinated in lime juice) Gazpacho, menudo, or black bean soup	Crispy, fried tortillas Refried beans made with lard Fried ice cream
Moroccan	Couscous, harira (tomatoes, lentils, chickpeas and lamb), Zaalouk (cooked eggplant and tomatoes with olive oil), B'ssara (bean soup made with olive oil)	Makouda (deep-fried), Chebakia (deep-fried), Sfinge (doughnuts)
Thai	Satay (skewered and grilled meats) Fish sauce, basil sauce, chili or hot sauces Bean thread noodles, Thai salad	Coconut milk soup Mee-krob (crispy noodles)

COMMON QUESTIONS ANSWERED

Q MyPlate recommends such large amounts of vegetables and fruit. How can I possibly eat that many servings without gaining weight?

A First, consider your typical portion sizes; you may be closer to meeting the recommendations than you think. Many people consume large servings of foods and underestimate the size of their portions. For example, a large banana may contain the equivalent of a cup of fruit. Likewise, a small salad may easily contain one cup of leafy greens and count as one-half cup of vegetables. Use a measuring cup or a food scale for a few days to train your eye to accurately estimate food portion sizes. The ChooseMyPlate .gov website includes charts of portion-size equivalents for each food group.

If you need to increase your overall intake of fruits and vegetables, look for healthy substitutions. If you are like most Americans, you are consuming more than the recommended number of calories from added sugars and solid fats; trim some of these calories to make room for additional servings of fruits and vegetables. Your beverage choices may be a good place to start. Do you routinely consume regular sodas,

sweetened energy or fruit drinks, or whole milk? One regular 12-ounce soda contains the equivalent of about 150 calories of added sugars; an 8-ounce glass of whole milk provides about 75 calories as discretionary fats. Substituting water or low-fat milk would free up calories for additional servings of fruits and vegetables. A half-cup of carrots, tomatoes, apples, or melon has only about 25 calories; you could consume six cups of these foods for the calories in one can of regular soda. Substituting lower-fat condiments for full-fat butter, mayonnaise, and salad dressing is another good way to trim calories to make room for additional servings of nutrient-rich fruits and vegetables.

Also consider your portion sizes and/or the frequency with which you consume foods high in discretionary calories: You may not need to eliminate a favorite food—instead, just cut back. For example, cut your consumption of fast-food fries from four times a week to once a week, or reduce the size of your ice cream dessert from a cup to one-half cup. High-sugar treats should be consumed infrequently and in small amounts.

For additional help on improving food choices to meet dietary recommendations, visit ChooseMyPlate.gov and the family-friendly chart of "We Can! Go, Slow, and Whoa" foods at the site for the National Heart, Lung, and Blood Institute (http://

www.nhlbi.nih.gov/health/public/heart /obesity/wecan/downloads/gswtips.pdf).

Q What exactly are genetically modified foods? Are they safe? How can I recognize them on the shelf, and how can I know when I'm eating them?

A Genetic engineering involves altering the characteristics of a plant, animal, or microorganism by adding, rearranging, or replacing genes in its DNA; the result is a genetically modified (GM) organism. New DNA may come from related species of organisms or from entirely different types of organisms. Many GM crops are already grown in the United States. For example, more than 90% of U.S. soybean crops have been genetically modified; some GM corn crops have also been modified to carry genes for herbicide or pest resistance. Products made with GM organisms include juice, soda, nuts, tuna, frozen pizza, spaghetti sauce, canola oil, chips, salad dressing, and soup.

The potential benefits of GM foods cited by supporters include improved yields overall and in difficult growing conditions, increased disease resistance, improved

---

- Water aids in digestion and food absorption, allows chemical reactions to take place, serves as a lubricant or cushion, and helps regulate body temperature.

- Foods contain other substances, such as phytochemicals, that may not be essential nutrients but that may protect against chronic diseases.

- The Dietary Reference Intakes, Daily Values, Dietary Guidelines for Americans, and MyPlate food guidance system provide standards and recommendations for getting all essential nutrients from a varied, balanced diet and for eating in ways that protect against chronic disease.

- The *2015–2020 Dietary Guidelines for Americans* presents five guidelines: (1) Follow a healthy eating pattern across the lifespan; (2) focus on variety, nutrient density, and amount; (3) limit calories from added sugars and saturated fats and reduce sodium intake; (4) shift to healthier food and beverage choices; and (5) support healthy eating patterns for all.

- Choosing the right amount of foods from each group in MyPlate every day helps ensure the appropriate amounts of calories and necessary nutrients.

- A vegan diet requires special planning but can meet all human nutritional needs.

- Different population groups, such as college students and athletes, face special dietary challenges and should plan their diets to meet their particular needs.

- Consumers can get help applying nutritional principles by reading the standardized labels that appear on all packaged foods and on dietary supplements.

- Although nutritional basics are well established, no single diet provides wellness for everyone. Individuals should focus on their particular needs and adapt general dietary principles to meet them.

nutritional content, lower prices, and less use of pesticides. Critics of biotechnology argue that unexpected effects may occur: Gene manipulation could elevate levels of naturally occurring toxins or allergens, permanently change the gene pool and reduce biodiversity, and produce pesticide-resistant insects through the transfer of genes. In 2000, a form of GM corn approved for use only in animal feed was found to have commingled with other varieties of corn and to have been used in human foods; this mistake sparked fears of allergic reactions and led to recalls. Opposition to GM foods is strong in Europe; in many developing nations that face food shortages, responses to GM crops are more positive.

In 2016, the National Academy of Sciences released a report stating that there is no proof that GM food on the market is unsafe but that changes are needed to better regulate these foods and assess potential problems, especially as the related technologies and techniques change. Labeling has been another major concern. Surveys indicate that the majority of Americans want to know if their foods contain GM organisms. However, under current rules, the FDA requires special labeling only when a food's composition is changed significantly or when a known allergen is introduced. For example, soybeans that contain a gene from a peanut would have to be labeled because peanuts are a common allergen. The only foods guaranteed not to contain GM ingredients are those certified as organic.

Q How can I tell if I'm allergic to a food?

A A true food allergy is a reaction of the body's immune system to a food or food ingredient, often a protein. This immune reaction can occur within minutes of ingesting the food, resulting in symptoms such as hives, diarrhea, difficulty breathing, or swelling of the lips or tongue. The most severe response is a systemic reaction called anaphylaxis, which involves a potentially life-threatening drop in blood pressure. Food allergies affect only about 2% of the adult population and approximately 5% of infants and young children. People with food allergies, especially children, are more likely to have asthma or other allergic conditions.

Just eight foods account for more than 90% of the food allergies in the United States: cow's milk, eggs, peanuts, tree nuts (walnuts, cashews, and others), soy, wheat, fish, and shellfish. Food manufacturers are now required to state the presence of these eight allergens in plain language in the list of ingredients on food labels.

Many people who believe they have food allergies may actually suffer from a food intolerance, a much more common source of adverse food reactions that typically involves problems with metabolism rather than with the immune system. The body may not be able to adequately digest a food or the body may react to a particular food compound. Food intolerances have been attributed to lactose (milk sugar), gluten (a protein in some grains), tartrazine (yellow food coloring), sulfites, MSG, and the sweetener aspartame. Although symptoms of a food intolerance may be similar to those of a food allergy, they are typically more localized and not life threatening. Many people with food intolerance can safely and comfortably consume small amounts of the food that affects them.

If you suspect you have a food allergy or intolerance, a good first step is to keep a food diary. Note everything you eat or drink, any symptoms you develop, and how long after eating that the symptoms appear. Then make an appointment with your physician to go over your diary and determine if any additional tests are needed. People at risk for severe allergic reactions must diligently avoid trigger foods and carry medications to treat anaphylaxis.

FOR FURTHER EXPLORATION

Academy of Nutrition and Dietetics. Provides a wide variety of educational materials on nutrition.

http://www.eatright.org

American Heart Association: Recipes. Provides basic information about nutrition, tips for shopping and eating out, and heart-healthy recipes.

https://recipes.heart.org

FDA: Food. Offers information and interactive tools about topics such as food labeling, food additives, dietary supplements, and foodborne illness.

http://www.fda.gov/food/default.htm

Food Safety Hotlines. Provide information on the safe purchase, handling, cooking, and storage of food.

https://www.foodsafety.gov/contact.html

Forks over Knives. Shares articles by doctors from Cleveland Clinic and Cornell University on plant-based diets; also includes recipe ideas.

http://www.forksoverknives.com

Fruits and Veggies—More Matters. Hosted by the Produce for Better Health Foundation; promotes the consumption of fruits and vegetables every day.

http://www.fruitsandveggiesmorematters.org/

Gateways to Government Nutrition Information. Provides access to government resources relating to food safety, including consumer advice and information on specific pathogens.

http://www.foodsafety.gov

http://www.nutrition.gov

Harvard School of Public Health: The Nutrition Source. Provides knowledge for healthy eating, including advice on interpreting news on nutrition, and suggestions for building a healthy diet.

http://www.hsph.harvard.edu/nutritionsource

International Food Information Council. Food Insight. Provides information on food safety and nutrition for consumers, journalists, and educators.

http://www.foodinsight.org/

MedlinePlus: Nutrition. Provides links to information from government agencies and major medical associations on a variety of nutrition topics.

http://www.nlm.nih.gov/medlineplus/nutrition.html

MyPlate. Provides personalized dietary plans and many tips for developing a healthy eating style. The site also includes suggestions for healthy eating on a budget and tips for college students.

http://www.ChooseMyPlate.gov

National Academies' Food and Nutrition Board. Provides information about the Dietary Reference Intakes and related guidelines.

http://www.nationalacademies.org/hmd/About-HMD/Leadership-Staff /HMD-Staff-Leadership-Boards/Food-and-Nutrition-Board.aspx

National Institutes of Health: Osteoporosis and Related Bone Diseases National Resource Center. Provides information about osteoporosis prevention and treatment; includes a special section on men and osteoporosis.

http://www.niams.nih.gov/Health_Info/Bone/

National Osteoporosis Foundation. Provides information on the causes, prevention, detection, and treatment of osteoporosis.

http://www.nof.org

USDA Center for Nutrition Policy and Promotion. Includes information on the Dietary Guidelines and MyPlate.

http://www.cnpp.usda.gov

USDA Food and Nutrition Information Center. Provides a variety of materials relating to the Dietary Guidelines, food labels, MyPlate, and many other topics.

http://www.nal.usda.gov/fnic

USDA Hotline. Use this hotline for questions about meat and poultry.

800-535-4555

Vegetarian Resource Group. Provides information and links for vegetarians and people interested in learning more about vegetarian diets.

http://www.vrg.org

USDA Nutrient Data Laboratory. Provides nutrient breakdowns of individual food items.

http://www.ars.usda.gov/ba/bhnrc/ndl

See also the resources listed in Chapters 9, 11, and 12.

SELECTED BIBLIOGRAPHY

Adebamowo, S. N., et al. 2015. Association between intakes of magnesium, potassium, and calcium and risk of stroke: 2 cohorts of US women and updated meta-analyses. *American Journal of Clinical Nutrition* 101(6): 1269–1277.

Afshin, A., et al. 2017. The prospective impact of food pricing on improving dietary consumption: A systematic review and meta-analysis. *PLoS One* 12(3): e0172277.

Ahluwalia, N., et al. 2016. Usual nutrient intakes of US infants and toddlers generally meet or exceed Dietary Reference Intakes: Findings from NHANES 2009–2012. *American Journal of Clinical Nutrition* 104(4): 1167–1174.

American Diabetes Association. 2019. *Glycemic Index and Diabetes* (http://www.diabetes .org/food-and-fitness/food/what-can-i-eat/understanding-carbohydrates/glycemic -index-and-diabetes.html?loc=ff-slabnav).

American Heart Association. 2015. *Diet and Lifestyle Recommendations* (http://www .heart.org/heartorg/gettinghealthy/diet-and-lifestyle-recommendations_ucm _305855_article.jsp).

Bailey, R. L., V. L. Fulgoni, A. E. Cowan, and P. C. Gaine. 2018. Sources of added sugars in young children, adolescents, and adults with low and high Intakes of added sugars. *Nutrients, 10*(1): 102.

Bowman, S. A., et al. 2018. Food patterns equivalents intakes by Americans: What we eat in America, NHANES 2003–2004 and 2015–2016. Food Surveys Research Group. *Dietary Data Brief,* No. 20.

Centers for Disease Control and Prevention. 2017. *Know Your Limit for Added Sugars* (https://www.cdc.gov/nutrition/data-statistics/know-your-limit-for-added-sugars .html).

Centers for Disease Control and Prevention. 2018. *Burden of Foodborne Illness: Findings* (https://www.cdc.gov/foodborneburden/2011-foodborne-estimates.html).

Centers for Disease Control and Prevention. 2018. *Food Safety* (http://www.cdc.gov /foodsafety/).

Centers for Disease Control and Prevention. 2018. *Sodium: The Facts* (http://www.cdc .gov/salt/pdfs/Sodium_Fact_Sheet.pdf).

Chowdhury, R., et al. 2014. Association of dietary, circulating, and supplement fatty acids with coronary risk: A systematic review and metaanalysis. *Annals of Internal Medicine* 160(6): 398–406.

Denny, S. 2016. *Get the Facts on Dietary Guidelines, MyPlate, and Food Labels. Academy of Nutrition and Dietetics* (http://www.eatright.org/resource/food/nutrition/dietary -guidelines-and-myplate/get-the-facts).

Fitch, C., and K. S. Keim; Academy of Nutrition and Dietetics. 2012. Position of the Academy of Nutrition and Dietetics: Use of nutritive and nonnutritive sweeteners. *Journal of the Academy of Nutrition and Dietetics* 112(5): 739–758.

Food and Nutrition Board, Institute of Medicine. 2005. *Dietary Reference Intakes for Energy, Carbohydrate, Fiber, Fat, Fatty Acids, Cholesterol, Protein, and Amino Acids.* Washington, DC: National Academies Press.

Food and Nutrition Board, Institute of Medicine. 2005. *Dietary Reference Intakes for Water, Potassium, Sodium, Chloride, and Sulfate.* Washington, DC: National Academies Press.

Harvard Medical School. 2018. *The Truth About Fats: The Good, the Bad, and the In-Between* (http://www.health.harvard.edu/staying-healthy/the-truth-about-fats -bad-and-good).

Hedrick, V. E., et al. 2017. Dietary quality changes in response to a sugar-sweetened beverage-reduction intervention: Results from the Talking Health randomized controlled clinical trial. *American Journal of Clinical Nutrition* 105(4): 824–833.

Hellmuth, J., G. D. Rabinovici, and B. L. Miller. 2019. The rise of pseudomedicine for dementia and brain health. *JAMA* 321(6): 543–544.

Hooper, L., et al. 2015. Reduction in saturated fat intake for cardiovascular disease. *Cochrane Database of Systematic Reviews* 6:CD011737.

Insel, P., et al. 2016. *Nutrition,* 6th ed. Burlington, MA: Jones & Bartlett.

Jackson, S. L., et al. 2016. Prevalence of excess sodium intake in the United States— NHANES, 2009–2012. *MMWR* 64(52): 1393–1397.

Jessri, M., W. Y. Lou, and M. R. L'Abbé. 2016. 2015 Dietary Guidelines for Americans is associated with a more nutrient-dense diet and lower risk of obesity. *American Journal of Clinical Nutrition* 104(5): 1378–1392.

Katz, D. L., and S. Meller. 2014. Can we say what diet is best for health? *Annual Review of Public Health* 35: 83–103.

Kirwan, J. P., et al. 2016. A whole-grain diet reduces cardiovascular risk factors in overweight and obese adults: A randomized controlled trial. *Journal of Nutrition* 146(11): 2244–2251.

Li, W., et al. 2016. Dietary phytochemical and cancer chemoprevention: A perspective on oxidative stress, inflammation, and epigenetics. *Chemical Research in Toxicology* 29(12): 2071–2095.

Martinez-González, M. A., E. Ros, and R. Estruch. 2018. Primary prevention of cardiovascular disease with a Mediterranean diet. *New England Journal of Medicine* 379(14): 1388–1389.

Melina, V., W. Craig, and S. Levin. 2016. Position of the Academy of Nutrition and Dietetics: Vegetarian diets. *Journal of the Academy of Nutrition and Dietetics* 116(12): 1970–1980.

Micha, R., et al. 2017. Association between dietary factors and mortality from heart disease, stroke, and type 2 diabetes in the United States. *Journal of the American Medical Association* 317(9): 912–924.

National Academy of Sciences. 2016. *Genetically Engineered Crops: Experience and Prospects* (https://www.nap.edu/catalog/23395/genetically-engineered-crops -experiences-and-prospects?utm_source=NAP_embed_book_widget&utm _medium=widget&utm_campaign=Widget_v4&utm_content=23395).

National Institutes of Health. Osteoporosis and Related Bone Diseases. National Resource Center. 2015. *Vitamin A and Bone Health* (http://www.niams.nih.gov /Health_Info/Bone/Bone_Health/Nutrition/vitamin_a.asp).

Obayashi, Y., and Y. Nagamura. 2016. Does monosodium glutamate really cause headache? A systematic review of human studies. *The Journal of Headache and Pain* 17: 54.

Orlich, M. J., et al. 2015. Vegetarian dietary patterns and the risk of colorectal cancers. *JAMA Internal Medicine* 175(5): 767–776.

Rodriguez, L. A., et al. 2016. Added sugar intake and metabolic syndrome in U.S. adolescents. *Public Health Nutrition* 19(13): 2424–2434.

Rosinger, A., et al. 2017. Sugar-sweetened beverage consumption among U.S. adults, 2011–2014. *National Center for Health Statistics Data Brief,* No. 270: 1–8.

Ross, S. M. 2015. Cardiovascular disease mortality: The deleterious effects of excess dietary sugar intake. *Holistic Nursing Practice* 29(1): 53–57.

Sacks, F. M., et al. 2017. Dietary fats and cardiovascular disease: A presidential advisory from the American Heart Association. *Circulation* 136: e1–e23.

Sirsikar, S., and A. Sirsikar. 2015. Prevention and management of postmenopausal osteoporosis. *International Journal of Innovative and Applied Research* 3(6): 5–26.

Sonnenburg, E. D., et al. 2016. Diet-induced extinctions in the gut microbiota compound over generations. *Nature* 529(7585): 212–215.

Strate, L. L., et al. 2017. Western dietary pattern increases, whereas prudent dietary pattern decreases, risk of incident diverticulitis in a prospective cohort study. *Gastroenterology* S0016-5085(17)30006-9.

Tufts Health & Nutrition Letter. 2019. *The Healthy-Aging Diet: What You Eat Can Help You Live Healthier and Longer. A Special Report.* Medford, MA: Tufts University Health News.

U.S. Department of Agriculture. 2015. *Biotechnology Frequently Asked Questions (FAQs)* (http://www.usda.gov/wps/portal/usda/usdahome?contentid=BiotechnologyFAQs .xml&navid=AGRICULTURE).

U.S. Department of Agriculture. 2015. *Scientific Report of the 2015 Dietary Guidelines Advisory Committee* (http://www.health.gov/dietaryguidelines/2015-scientificreport).

U.S. Department of Agriculture. 2016. *Adoption of Genetically Engineered Crops in the U.S.* (https://www.ers.usda.gov/data-products/adoption-of-genetically-engineered -crops-in-the -us.aspx).

U.S. Department of Agriculture, Agricultural Research Service. 2018. *Energy Intakes: Percentages of Energy from Protein, Carbohydrate, Fat, and Alcohol, by Gender and Age, What We Eat in America, NHANES 2015–2016.* Washington, DC: USDA.

U.S. Department of Health and Human Services and U.S. Department of Agriculture. 2015. *2015-2020 Dietary Guidelines for Americans,* 8th ed. (http://health.gov /dietaryguidelines/2015/guidelines/).

U.S. Food and Drug Administration. 2015. *FDA Cuts Trans Fats in Processed Foods* (https://humansciences.okstate.edu/fcs/site-files/research/FDA-Cuts-Trans-Fat-in -Processed-Food.pdf).

U.S. Food and Drug Administration. 2018. *Calorie Labeling on Restaurant Menus and Vending Machines: What You Need to Know* (https://www.fda.gov/food/labeling nutrition/ucm436722.htm).

U.S. Food and Drug Administration. 2018. *Changes to the Nutrition Facts Label* (https://www .fda.gov/Food/GuidanceRegulation/GuidanceDocumentsRegulatoryInformation /LabelingNutrition/ucm385663.htm).

U.S. Food and Drug Administration. 2018. *Food Allergies: What You Need to Know* (http://www.fda.gov/Food/IngredientsPackagingLabeling/FoodAllergens /ucm079311.htm).

U.S. Food and Drug Administration. 2018. *"Healthy" on Food Labeling* (https://www .fda.gov/food/guidanceregulation/guidancedocumentsregulatoryinformation /labelingnutrition/ucm520695.htm).

Vos, M. S., et al. 2016. Added sugars and cardiovascular risk in children: A scientific statement from the American Heart Association. *Circulation* 22.

Wang, D. D., et al. 2016. Association of specific dietary fats with total and cause-specific mortality. *JAMA Internal Medicine* 176(8): 1134–1145.

Wang, X., et al. 2014. Fruit and vegetable consumption and mortality from all causes, cardiovascular disease, and cancer: Systematic review and dose-response meta-analysis of prospective cohort studies. *BMJ* 349: g4490.

Whelton, P. K., et al. 2018. 2017 Guideline for High Blood Pressure in Adults: A report of the American College of Cardiology/American Heart Association Task Force on Clinical Practice Guidelines. *Journal of the American College of Cardiology* 71: e127–e248.

Wu, L., and D. Sun. 2017. Adherence to Mediterranean diet and risk of developing cognitive disorders: An updated systematic review and meta-analysis of prospective cohort studies. *Scientific Reports* 7: 41317.

Zong, G., et al. 2016. Intake of individual saturated fatty acids and risk of coronary heart disease in US men and women: Two prospective longitudinal cohort studies. *BMJ* 355: i5796.

Calorie level of pattern	1,600	1,800	2,000	2,200	2,400	2,600	2,800	3,000
Food Group	**Daily amount** of food from each group (vegetable and protein foods subgroup amounts are per week)							
Fruits	1.5 c	1.5 c	2 c	2 c	2 c	2 c	2.5 c	2.5 c
Vegetables	2 c	2.5 c	2.5 c	3 c	3 c	3.5 c	3.5 c	4 c
Dark-green veg	1.5 c/wk	1.5 c/wk	1.5 c/wk	2 c/wk	2 c/wk	2.5 c/wk	2.5 c/wk	2.5 c/wk
Red/Orange veg	4 c/wk	5.5 c/wk	5.5 c/wk	6 c/wk	6 c/wk	7 c/wk	7 c/wk	7.5 c/wk
Beans and peas	1 c/wk	1.5 c/wk	1.5 c/wk	2 c/wk	2 c/wk	2.5 c/wk	2.5 c/wk	3 c/wk
Starchy veg	4 c/wk	5 c/wk	5 c/wk	6 c/wk	6 c/wk	7 c/wk	7 c/wk	8 c/wk
Other veg	3.5 c/wk	4 c/wk	4 c/wk	5 c/wk	5 c/wk	5.5 c/wk	5.5 c/wk	7 c/wk
Grains	5 oz eq	6 oz eq	6 oz eq	7 oz eq	8 oz eq	9 oz eq	10 oz eq	10 oz eq
Whole grains	3 oz eq	3 oz eq	3 oz eq	3.5 oz eq	4 oz eq	4.5 oz eq	5 oz eq	5 oz eq
Other grains	2 oz eq	3 oz eq	3 oz eq	3.5 oz eq	4 oz eq	4.5 oz eq	5 oz eq	5 oz eq
Protein foods	5 oz eq	5 oz eq	5.5 oz eq	6 oz eq	6.5 oz eq	6.5 oz eq	7 oz eq	7 oz eq
Meat poultry, eggs	23 oz eq/wk	23 oz eq/wk	26 oz eq/wk	28 oz eq/wk	31 oz eq/wk	31 oz eq/wk	33 oz eq/wk	33 oz eq/wk
Seafood	8 oz eq/wk	8 oz eq/wk	8 oz eq/wk	9 oz eq/wk	10 oz eq/wk	10 oz eq/wk	10 oz eq/wk	10 oz eq/wk
Nuts, seeds, soy	4 oz eq/wk	4 oz eq/wk	5 oz eq/wk	5 oz eq/wk	5 oz eq/wk	5 oz eq/wk	6 oz eq/wk	6 oz eq/wk
Dairy	3 c	3 c	3 c	3 c	3 c	3 c	3 c	3 c
Oils	22 g	24 g	27 g	29 g	31 g	34 g	36 g	44 g
Limit on calories for other uses (calories and % of calories)*	130 cal (8%)	170 cal (9%)	270 cal (14%)	280 cal (13%)	350 cal (15%)	380 cal (15%)	400 cal (14%)	470 cal (16%)

Food group amounts shown in cup (c) or ounce equivalents (oz eq). Oils, solid fats, and added sugars are shown in grams (g).
Quantity equivalents for each food group are:
- Grains, 1 ounce equivalent is: ½ cup cooked rice, pasta, or cooked cereal; 1 ounce dry pasta or rice; 1 slice bread; 1 cup ready-to-eat cereal flakes.
- Fruits and vegetables, 1 cup equivalent is: 1 cup raw or cooked fruit or vegetable, 1 cup fruit or vegetable juice, 2 cups leafy salad greens.
- Protein Foods, 1 ounce equivalent is: 1 ounce lean meat, poultry, or seafood; 1 egg; ¼ cup cooked beans or tofu; 1 Tbsp peanut butter; ½ ounce nuts/seeds.
- Dairy, 1 cup equivalent is: 1 cup milk or yogurt, 1½ ounces natural cheese such as cheddar cheese or 2 ounces of processed cheese.

*All foods are assumed to be in nutrient-dense forms, lean or low-fat, and prepared without added fats, sugars, refined starches, or salt. If all food choices to meet food group recommendations are in nutrient-dense forms, a small number of calories remain within the overall calorie limit of the Pattern. Calories up to the specified limit can be used for added sugars, added refined starches, solid fats, alcohol, or to eat more than the recommended amount of food in a food group. The overall eating pattern also should not exceed the limits of less than 10% of calories from added sugars and less than 10% of calories from saturated fats. At most calorie levels, amounts that can be accommodated are less than these limits. For adults of legal drinking age who choose to drink alcohol, a limit of up to one drink per day for women and up to two drinks per day for men within limits on calories for other uses applies; and calories from protein, carbohydrate, and total fats should be within the Acceptable Macronutrient Distribution Ranges (AMDRs).

Figure 1.   Healthy U.S.-Style Food Patterns

SOURCE: U.S. Department of Health and Human Services and U.S. Department of Agriculture. 2015. *2015–2020 Dietary Guidelines for Americans,* 8th ed. (http://health.gov /dietaryguidelines/2015/guidelines).

Calorie level of pattern	1,600	1,800	2,000	2,200	2,400	2,600	2,800	3,000
Food Group	Daily amount[a] of food from each group (vegetable and protein foods subgroup amounts are per week)							
Fruits	1.5 c	1.5 c	2 c	2 c	2 c	2 c	2.5 c	2.5 c
Vegetables	2 c	2.5 c	2.5 c	3 c	3 c	3.5 c	3.5 c	4 c
Dark-green veg	1.5 c/wk	1.5 c/wk	1.5 c/wk	2 c/wk	2 c/wk	2.5 c/wk	2.5 c/wk	2.5 c/wk
Red/Orange veg	4 c/wk	5.5 c/wk	5.5 c/wk	6 c/wk	6 c/wk	7 c/wk	7 c/wk	7.5 c/wk
Beans and peas[b]	1 c/wk	1.5 c/wk	1.5 c/wk	2 c/wk	2 c/wk	2.5 c/wk	2.5 c/wk	3 c/wk
Starchy veg	4 c/wk	5 c/wk	5 c/wk	6 c/wk	6 c/wk	7 c/wk	7 c/wk	8 c/wk
Other veg	3.5 c/wk	4 c/wk	4 c/wk	5 c/wk	5 c/wk	5.5 c/wk	5.5 c/wk	7 c/wk
Grains	5.5 oz eq	6.5 oz eq	6.5 oz eq	7.5 oz eq	8.5 oz eq	9.5 oz eq	10.5 oz eq	10.5 oz eq
Whole grains	3.5 oz eq	3.5 oz eq	3.5 oz eq	4 oz eq	4.5 oz eq	5 oz eq	5.5 oz eq	5.5 oz eq
Other grains	2 oz eq	3 oz eq	3 oz eq	3.5 oz eq	4 oz eq	4.5 oz eq	5 oz eq	5 oz eq
Protein foods	2.5 oz eq	3 oz eq	3.5 oz eq	4 oz eq	4 oz eq	5 oz eq	5 oz eq	5.5 oz eq
Beans and peas[b]	4 oz eq/wk	6 oz eq/wk	6 oz eq/wk	8 oz eq/wk	8 oz eq/wk	10 oz eq/wk	10 oz eq/wk	12 oz eq/wk
Eggs	3 oz eq/wk	3 oz eq/wk	3 oz eq/wk	3 oz eq/wk	3 oz eq/wk	3 oz eq/wk	4 oz eq/wk	4 oz eq/wk
Nuts and seeds	5 oz eq/wk	6 oz eq/wk	7 oz eq/wk	8 oz eq/wk	9 oz eq/wk	10 oz eq/wk	11 oz eq/wk	12 oz eq/wk
Tofu/processed soy	5 oz eq/wk	6 oz eq/wk	7 oz eq/wk	8 oz eq/wk	9 oz eq/wk	10 oz eq/wk	11 oz eq/wk	12 oz eq/wk
Dairy	3 c	3 c	3 c	3 c	3 c	3 c	3 c	3 c
Oils	22 g	24 g	27 g	29 g	31 g	34 g	36 g	44 g
Limit on calories for other uses (calories and % of calories)c	180 cal (11%)	190 cal (11%)	290 cal (15%)	330 cal (15%)	390 cal (16%)	390 cal (15%)	400 cal (14%)	440 cal (15%)

[a]Food group amounts shown in cup (c) or ounce equivalents (oz eq). Oils, solid fats, and added sugars are shown in grams (g).
  Quantity equivalents for each food group are:
   • Grains, 1 ounce equivalent is: ½ cup cooked rice, pasta, or cooked cereal; 1 ounce dry pasta or rice; 1 slice bread; 1 cup ready-to-eat cereal flakes.
   • Fruits and vegetables, 1 cup equivalent is: 1 cup raw or cooked fruit or vegetable, 1 cup fruit or vegetable juice, 2 cups leafy salad greens.
   • Protein Foods, 1 ounce equivalent is: 1 ounce lean meat, poultry, or seafood; 1 egg; ¼ cup cooked beans or tofu; 1 tbsp peanut butter; ½ ounce nuts/seeds.
   • Dairy, 1 cup equivalent is: 1 cup milk or yogurt, 1½ ounces natural cheese (e.g. cheddar cheese) or 2 ounces of processed cheese.

[b]About half of total beans and peas are shown as vegetables, in cup eqs, and half as protein foods, in ounce eqs. To determine total weekly beans and peas in cup eq, add the amount in vegetables plus the amount in protein food (in ounce eqs) divided by four. (For example, for 2,000-calorie level, 1.5 c/wk + (6 oz eq/wk ÷ 4) = 3 c eq/wk.)

[c]All foods are assumed to be in nutrient-dense forms, lean or low-fat, and prepared without added fats, sugars, refined starches, or salt. If all food choices to meet food group recommendations are in nutrient-dense forms, a small number of calories remain within the overall calorie limit of the Pattern. Calories up to the specified limit can be used for added sugars, added refined starches, solid fats, alcohol, or to eat more than the recommended amount of food in a food group. The overall eating pattern also should not exceed the limits of less than 10% of calories from added sugars and less than 10% of calories from saturated fats. At most calorie levels, amounts that can be accommodated are less than these limits. For adults of legal drinking age who choose to drink alcohol, a limit of up to one drink per day for women and up to two drinks per day for men within limits on calories for other uses applies; and calories from protein, carbohydrate, and total fats should be within the Acceptable Macronutrient Distribution Ranges (AMDRs).

	1,600	1,800	2,000	2,200	2,400	2,600	2,800	3,000
Total beans/peas	2 c eq/wk	3 c eq/wk	3 c eq/wk	4 c eq/wk	4 c eq/wk	5 c eq/wk	5 c eq/wk	6 c eq/wk

Figure 2. Healthy Vegetarian Patterns.
SOURCE: U.S. Department of Health and Human Services and U.S. Department of Agriculture. 2015. *2015–2020 Dietary Guidelines for Americans,* 8th ed. (http://health.gov /dietaryguidelines/2015/guidelines).

Calorie level of pattern	1,600	1,800	2,000	2,200	2,400	2,600	2,800	3,000
Food Group	**Daily amount** of food from each group (vegetable and protein foods subgroup amounts are per week)							
Fruits	1.5 c	2 c	2.5 c	2.5 c	2.5 c	2.5 c	3 c	3 c
Vegetables	2 c	2.5 c	2.5 c	3 c	3 c	3.5 c	3.5 c	4 c
Dark-green veg	1.5 c/wk	1.5 c/wk	1.5 c/wk	2 c/wk	2 c/wk	2.5 c/wk	2.5 c/wk	2.5 c/wk
Red/Orange veg	4 c/wk	5.5 c/wk	5.5 c/wk	6 c/wk	6 c/wk	7 c/wk	7 c/wk	7.5 c/wk
Beans and peas	1 c/wk	1.5 c/wk	1.5 c/wk	2 c/wk	2 c/wk	2.5 c/wk	2.5 c/wk	3 c/wk
Starchy veg	4 c/wk	5 c/wk	5 c/wk	6 c/wk	6 c/wk	7 c/wk	7 c/wk	8 c/wk
Other veg	3.5 c/wk	4 c/wk	4 c/wk	5 c/wk	5 c/wk	5.5 c/wk	5.5 c/wk	7 c/wk
Grains	5 oz eq	6 oz eq	6 oz eq	7 oz eq	8 oz eq	9 oz eq	10 oz eq	10 oz eq
Whole grains	3 oz eq	3 oz eq	3 oz eq	3.5 oz eq	4 oz eq	4.5 oz eq	5 oz eq	5 oz eq
Other grains	2 oz eq	3 oz eq	3 oz eq	3.5 oz eq	4 oz eq	4.5 oz eq	5 oz eq	5 oz eq
Protein foods	5.5 oz eq	6 oz eq	6.5 oz eq	7 oz eq	7.5 oz eq	7.5 oz eq	8 oz eq	8 oz eq
Meat, poultry, eggs	23 oz eq/wk	23 oz eq/wk	26 oz eq/wk	28 oz eq/wk	31 oz eq/wk	31 oz eq/wk	33 oz eq/wk	33 oz eq/wk
Seafood	11 oz eq/wk	15 oz eq/wk	15 oz eq/wk	16 oz eq/wk	16 oz eq/wk	17 oz eq/wk	17 oz eq/wk	17 oz eq/wk
Nut seeds, soy	4 oz eq/wk	4 oz eq/wk	5 oz eq/wk	5 oz eq/wk	5 oz eq/wk	5 oz eq/wk	6 oz eq/wk	6 oz eq/wk
Dairy	2 c	2 c	2 c	2 c	2 c	2.5 c	2.5 c	2.5 c
Oils	22 g	24 g	27 g	29 g	31 g	34 g	36 g	44 g
Limit on calories for other uses (calories and % of calories)*	140 cal (9%)	160 cal (9%)	260 cal (13%)	270 cal (12%)	300 cal (13%)	330 cal (13%)	350 cal (13%)	430 cal (14%)

Food group amounts shown in cup (c) or ounce equivalents (oz eq). Oils, solid fats, and added sugars are shown in grams (g).
Quantity equivalents for each food group are:
- Grains, 1 ounce equivalent is: ½ cup cooked rice, pasta, or cooked cereal; 1 ounce dry pasta or rice; 1 slice bread; 1 cup ready-to-eat cereal flakes.
- Fruits and vegetables, 1 cup equivalent is: 1 cup raw or cooked fruit or vegetable, 1 cup fruit or vegetable juice, 2 cups leafy salad greens.
- Protein Foods, 1 ounce equivalent is: 1 ounce lean meat, poultry, or seafood; 1 egg; ¼ cup cooked beans or tofu; 1 Tbsp peanut butter; ½ ounce nuts/seeds.
- Dairy, 1 cup equivalent is: 1 cup milk or yogurt, 1½ ounces natural cheese such as cheddar cheese or 2 ounces of processed cheese.

*All foods are assumed to be in nutrient-dense forms, lean or low-fat, and prepared without added fats, sugars, refined starches, or salt. If all food choices to meet food group recommendations are in nutrient-dense forms, a small number of calories remain within the overall calorie limit of the Pattern. Calories up to the specified limit can be used for added sugars, added refined starches, solid fats, alcohol, or to eat more than the recommended amount of food in a food group. The overall eating pattern also should not exceed the limits of less than 10% of calories from added sugars and less than 10% of calories from saturated fats. At most calorie levels, amounts that can be accommodated are less than these limits. For adults of legal drinking age who choose to drink alcohol, a limit of up to one drink per day for women and up to two drinks per day for men within limits on calories for other uses applies; and calories from protein, carbohydrate, and total fats should be within the Acceptable Macronutrient Distribution Ranges (AMDRs).

Figure 3. Healthy Mediterranean-Style Patterns.
SOURCE: U.S. Department of Health and Human Services and U.S. Department of Agriculture. 2015. *2015–2020 Dietary Guidelines for Americans,* 8th ed. (http://health.gov/dietaryguidelines/2015/guidelines).

Food groups	Number of servings per day (or per week, as noted)				Serving sizes and notes
	1,600 calories	2,000 calories	2,600 calories	3,100 calories	
Grains	6	6–8	10–11	12–13	1 slice bread, 1 oz dry cereal, $1/2$ cup cooked rice, pasta, or cereal; choose whole grains
Vegetables	3–4	4–5	5–6	6	1 cup raw leafy vegetables, $1/2$ cup cooked vegetables, $1/2$ cup vegetable juice
Fruits	4	4–5	5–6	6	$1/2$ cup fruit juice, 1 medium fruit, $1/4$ cup dried fruit, $1/2$ cup fresh, frozen, or canned fruit
Low-fat or fat-free dairy foods	2–3	2–3	3	3–4	1 cup milk; 1 cup yogurt, $11/2$ oz cheese; choose fat-free or low-fat types
Meat, poultry, fish	3–6	6 or less	6	6–9	1 oz cooked meats, poultry, or fish: select only lean; trim away visible fats; broil, roast, or boil instead of frying; remove skin from poultry
Nuts, seeds, legumes	3 servings per week	4–5 servings per week	1	1	$1/3$ cup or $11/2$ oz nuts, 2 Tbsp or $1/2$ oz seeds, $1/2$ cup cooked dry beans/peas, 2 Tbsp peanut butter
Fats and oils	2	2–3	3	4	1 tsp soft margarine, 1 Tbsp low-fat mayonnaise, 2 Tbsp light salad dressing, 1 tsp vegetable oil; DASH has 27% of calories as fat (low in saturated fat)
Sweets	0	5 servings/ week or less	2	2	1 Tbsp sugar, 1 Tbsp jelly or jam, $1/2$ cup sorbet, 1 cup lemonade; sweets should be low in fat

Figure 4.   The DASH Eating Plan.

SOURCE: National Institutes of Health, and National Heart, Lung, and Blood Institute. *Your Guide to Lowering Your Blood Pressure with DASH.* 2006. (http://www.nhlbi.nih.gov/health/public/heart/hbp/dash/new_dash.pdf).

Name _____ **Section** _____ **Date** _____

LAB 8.1 Your Daily Diet versus MyPlate

Make three photocopies of the worksheet in this lab and use them to keep track of everything you eat for three consecutive days. Break down each food item into its component parts, and list them separately in the column labeled "Food." Then enter the portion size you consumed in the correct food-group column. For example, a turkey sandwich might be listed as follows: whole-wheat bread, 2 oz-equiv of whole grains; turkey, 2 oz-equiv of meat/beans; tomato, ⅓ cup other vegetables; romaine lettuce, ¼ cup dark-green vegetables; 1 tablespoon mayonnaise dressing, 1 teaspoon (4.5 g) oils. It can be challenging to track values for added sugars and oils and fats, but use food labels to be as accurate as you can. Additional guidelines for counting discretionary calories can be found at ChooseMyPlate.gov.

For vegetables, enter your portion sizes in both the "Total" column and the column corresponding to the correct subgroup; for example, the spinach in a spinach salad would be entered under "Dark Green" and carrots would be entered under "Red & Orange." For the purpose of this three-day activity, you will compare only your total vegetable consumption against MyPlate guidelines; as described in the chapter, vegetable subgroup recommendations are based on weekly consumption. However, it is important to note which vegetable subgroups are represented in your diet; over a three-day period, you should consume several servings from each of the subgroups.

Date: _____

Food	Grains (oz-eq)		Vegetable (cups)						Fruits (cups)	Milk (cups)	Protein Foods (oz-eq)	Oils (g)	Discretionary Calories	
	Whole	Other	Total	Dark Green	Red & Orange	Beans & Peas	Starchy	Other					Solid Fats (g)	Added Sugars (g)
Daily Total														

LABORATORY ACTIVITIES

Next, average your daily intake totals for the three days and enter them in the following chart. For example, if your three daily totals for the fruit group were 1 cup, 1½ cups, and 2 cups, your average daily intake would be 1½ cups. Fill in the recommended intake totals that apply to you from ChooseMyPlate.gov or your chosen dietary pattern from the Nutrition Resources section.

MyPlate Food Group	Recommended Daily Amounts or Limits	Your Actual Average Daily Intake
Grains (total)	oz-eq	oz-eq
Whole grains	oz-eq	oz-eq
Other grains	oz-eq	oz-eq
Vegetables (total)	cups	cups
Fruits	cups	cups
Milk	cups	cups
Protein foods	oz-eq	oz-eq
Oils	tsp	tsp
Solid fats	g	g
Added sugars	g/tsp	g/tsp

Using Your Results

How did you score? How close is your diet to that recommended by MyPlate? Are you surprised by the amount of food you are consuming from each food group or from added sugars and solid fats?

What should you do next? If the results of the assessment indicate that you could boost your level of wellness by improving your diet, set realistic goals for change. Do you need to increase or decrease your consumption of any food groups? List any areas of concern below, along with a goal for change and strategies for achieving the goal you've set. If you see that you are falling short in one food group, such as fruits or vegetables, but have many foods that are rich in discretionary calories from solid fats and added sugars, try decreasing those items in favor of an apple, a bunch of grapes, or some baby carrots. Think carefully about the reasons behind your food choices. For example, if you eat doughnuts for breakfast every morning because you feel rushed, make a list of ways to save time to allow for a healthier breakfast.

Problem: _____

Goal: _____

Strategies for change: _____

_____

_____

Problem: _____

Goal: _____

Strategies for change: _____

_____

_____

Problem: _____

Goal: _____

Strategies for change: _____

_____

_____

Enter the results of this lab in the Preprogram Assessment column in Appendix B. If you've set goals and identified strategies for change, begin putting your plan into action. After several weeks of your program, complete this lab again and enter the results in the Postprogram Assessment column of Appendix B. How do the results compare?

Name _____ **Section** _____ **Date** _____

LAB 8.2 Dietary Analysis

You can complete this activity using either a nutrition analysis software program or information about the nutrient content of foods available online; see the For Further Exploration section and Nutritional Content of Popular Items from Fast-Food Restaurants for recommended websites. Connect users can track and analyze their food intake using the dietary analysis tool NutritionCalc Plus; launch it by clicking on the NutritionCalc Plus link on the Resources list from your Connect class home page. (This lab asks you to analyze one day's diet. For a more complete and accurate assessment of your diet, analyze the results from several different days, including a weekday and a weekend day.)

DATE _____										DAY: M Tu W Th F Sa Su			
Food	Amount	Calories	Protein (g)	Carbohydrate (g)	Dietary fiber (g)	Fat, total (g)	Saturated fat (g)	Sodium (mg)	Vitamin D (µg)	Calcium (mg)	Iron (mg)	Potassium (mg)	
Recommended totals*			10–35%	45–65%	25–38 g	20–35%	<10%	≤2300 mg	µg	mg	mg	mg	
Actual totals**		cal	g / %	g / %	g	g / %	g / %	mg	µg	mg	mg	mg	

*Fill in the appropriate DRI values for vitamin D, calcium, iron, and potassium from Tables 8.6 and 8.7 or by visiting the Interactive DRI website (http://fnic.nal.usda.gov/fnic/interactiveDRI).

**Total the values in each column. Protein and carbohydrate provide 4 calories per gram; fat provides 9 calories per gram. For example, if your day's total energy intake was 2,000 calories, including 270 grams of carbohydrate, you would calculate your percentage of total calories from carbohydrate as follows: (270 g × 4 cal/g) ÷ 2,000 = 54%. Percentages may not total 100% due to rounding.

LABORATORY ACTIVITIES

Using Your Results

How did you score? How close is your diet to that recommended in this chapter? Are you surprised by any of the results of this assessment?

What should you do next? Enter the results of this lab in the Preprogram Assessment column in Appendix B. If your daily diet meets all the recommended intakes, congratulations—and keep up the good work. If the results of the assessment pinpoint areas of concern, then work with your food record to determine what changes you could make to meet all the guidelines. Make changes, additions, and deletions until it conforms to all or most of the guidelines. Or, if you prefer, start from scratch to create a day's diet that meets the guidelines. Use the following chart to experiment and record your final, healthy sample diet for one day. Then put what you learned from this exercise into practice in your daily life. After several weeks of your program, complete this lab again and enter the results in the Postprogram Assessment column of Appendix B. How do the results compare?

DATE _____   DAY: M Tu W Th F Sa Su

Food	Amount	Calories	Protein (g)	Carbohydrate (g)	Dietary fiber (g)	Fat, total (g)	Saturated fat (g)	Sodium (mg)	Vitamin D (µg)	Calcium (mg)	Iron (mg)	Potassium (mg)
Recommended totals*			10–35%	45–65%	25–38 g	20–35%	< 10%	≤ 2300 mg	µg	mg	mg	mg
Actual totals**		cal	g / %	g / %		g	g / %	g / %	µg	mg	mg	mg

Name _____ **Section** _____ **Date** _____

LAB 8.3   Informed Food Choices

Part I Using Food Labels

Choose three food items to evaluate. You might want to select three similar items, such as regular, low-fat, and nonfat salad dressing, or three very different items. Record the information from their food labels in the following table. Include all available values; items marked with an asterisk (*) may not appear on a label, depending on which version of the label is in use on the foods you evaluate.

Food Items			
Serving size			
Total calories	cal	cal	cal
Total fat—grams	g	g	g
—% Daily Value	%	%	%
Saturated fat—grams	g	g	g
—% Daily Value	%	%	%
Trans fat—grams	g	g	g
Cholesterol	mg	mg	mg
Sodium—milligrams	mg	mg	mg
—% Daily Value	%	%	%
Total carbohydrate—grams	g	g	g
—% Daily Value	%	%	%
Dietary fiber—grams	g	g	g
—% Daily Value	%	%	%
Total sugars—grams	g	g	g
*Added sugars—grams	g	g	g
—% Daily Value	%	%	%
Protein—grams	g	g	g
*Vitamin A—% Daily Value	%	%	%
*Vitamin C—% Daily Value	%	%	%
*Vitamin D—% Daily Value	%	%	%
Calcium—% Daily Value	%	%	%
Iron—% Daily Value	%	%	%
*Potassium—% Daily Value	%	%	%

How do the items you chose compare? You can do a quick nutrient check by totaling the Daily Value percentages for nutrients you should limit (saturated fat, sodium, added sugars) and the nutrients you should favor (dietary fiber, vitamins, minerals) for each food. Which food has the largest percent Daily Value sum for nutrients to limit? For nutrients to favor?

Food Items			
Calories	cal	cal	cal
% Daily Value total for nutrients to limit (saturated fat, sodium, added sugars)	%	%	%
% Daily Value total for nutrients to favor (fiber, vitamins, minerals)	%	%	%

LABORATORY ACTIVITIES

Part II Evaluating Fast Food

Use the nutritional information available from fast-food restaurants to complete the chart on this page for the last fast-food meal you ate. Add up your totals for the meal. Compare the values for fat, protein, carbohydrate, and sodium content for each food item and for the meal as a whole with the levels suggested by the Dietary Guidelines for Americans. Calculate the percent of total calories derived from fat, saturated fat, protein, and carbohydrate using the formulas given.

To get fast-food nutritional information, ask for a nutrition information brochure when you visit the restaurant, or visit restaurant websites:

- Arby's (http://www.arbysrestaurant.com)

- Burger King (http://www.burgerking.com)

- Domino's Pizza (http://www.dominos.com)

- Jack in the Box (http://www. jackinthebox.com)

- KFC (http://www.kfc.com)

- McDonald's (http://www.mcdonalds.com)

- Subway (http://www.subway.com)

- Taco Bell (http://www.tacobell.com)

- Wendy's (http://www.wendys.com).

If you haven't recently been to a fast-food restaurant, fill in the chart for any sample meal you might eat.

FOOD ITEMS								
	Dietary Guidelines							Total**
Serving size (g)		g	g	g	g	g	g	g
Calories		cal	cal	cal	cal	cal	cal	cal
Total fat—grams		g	g	g	g	g	g	g
—% calories*	20–35%	%	%	%	%	%	%	%
Saturated fat—grams		g	g	g	g	g	g	g
—% calories*	<10%	%	%	%	%	%	%	%
Protein—grams		g	g	g	g	g	g	g
—% calories*	10–35%	%	%	%	%	%	%	%
Carbohydrate—grams		g	g	g	g	g	g	g
—% calories*	45–65%	%	%	%	%	%	%	%
Sodium†	800 mg	mg	mg	mg	mg	mg	mg	mg

*To calculate the percent of total calories from each food energy source (fat, carbohydrate, protein), use the following formula:

$$\frac{\text{(number of grams of energy source)} \times \text{(number of calories per gram of energy source)}}{\text{(total calories in serving of food item)}}$$

(**NOTE:** Fat and saturated fat provide 9 calories per gram; protein and carbohydrate provide 4 calories per gram.) For example, the percent of total calories from protein in a 150-calorie dish containing 10 grams of protein is

$$\frac{\text{(10 grams of protein)} \times \text{(4 calories per gram)}}{\text{(150 calories)}} = \frac{40}{150} = 0.27, \text{ or } 27\% \text{ of total calories from protein}$$

**For the Total column, add up the total grams of fat, carbohydrate, and protein contained in your sample meal and calculate the percentages based on the total calories in the meal. (Percentages may not total 100% due to rounding.) For cholesterol and sodium values, add up the total number of milligrams.

†Recommended daily limit of sodium is divided by 3 here to give an approximate recommended limit for a single meal.

SOURCE: Insel, P. M., W. T. Roth, C. E. Insel. 2016. "Wellness Worksheet 66," *Core Concepts in Health,* 14th ed. New York: McGraw-Hill.

Design elements: Evidence for Exercise box (shoes and stethoscope): Vstock LLC/Tetra Images/Getty Images; Take Charge box (lady walking): VisualCommunications/E+/Getty Images; Critical Consumer box (man): Sam74100/iStock/Getty Images; Diversity Matters box (holding devices): Robert Churchill/iStockphoto/Rawpixel Ltd/Getty Images; Wellness in the Digital Age box (Smart Watch): Hong Li/DigitalVision/Getty Images

CHAPTER 9

Weight Management

LOOKING AHEAD...

After reading this chapter, you should be able to

- Explain the health risks associated with overweight and obesity.

- Explain the factors that may contribute to a weight problem.

- Describe lifestyle factors that contribute to weight gain and loss.

- Identify and describe the symptoms and health risks of eating disorders.

- Design a personal plan for successfully managing body weight.

TEST YOUR KNOWLEDGE

1. About what percentage of American adults are overweight?
   a. 20%
   b. 40%
   c. 70%

2. The consumption of low-calorie sweeteners has helped Americans control their weight. True or false?

3. Approximately what percentage of female high school and college students have either anorexia or bulimia?
   a. <1%
   b. 2–4%
   c. 7–10%

See answers on the next page.

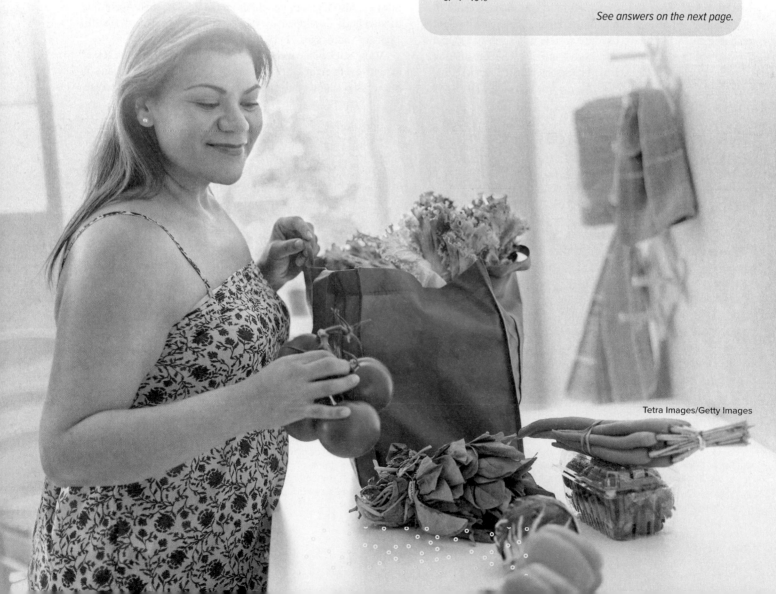

Tetra Images/Getty Images

Amelia is a 19-year-old college sophomore who rarely thought about her weight until her jeans got too tight. Since she began college, she has gained 14 pounds. Amelia decided to step up her exercise, playing volleyball and jogging a few times a week and taking the stairs instead of the elevator. But after several months, she'd lost only two pounds. What was she doing wrong?

When Amelia enrolled in a nutrition class and was asked to analyze her diet, it became clearer. For breakfasts, she usually grabbed a muffin or sweet roll and orange juice; for lunch, a sandwich on white bread, soda, and potato chips; and dinners were often pizza or pasta with a small side salad. Her diet was convenient but dominated by sugar and refined carbohydrates. Amelia began changing her diet, by replacing refined flours with whole grains, substituting low-fat milk or whole fruits for OJ, eating more vegetables and less pasta, and limiting her sodas to once a week instead of every day. After these changes, her weight began dropping. Once she reached her target weight, she continued with her new diet and physical activities. So far she has avoided regaining the weight.

When it comes to losing weight, diet is more important than exercise. Physical activity plays a key role in preventing weight gain and maintaining weight loss; it can also boost weight loss in combination with calorie restriction. Aside from eating and exercise behaviors, what else is involved in weight management? In this chapter, we discuss the complex factors involved in weight management, which have become so relevant given the global crisis of obesity. We explore the body's internal weight-regulating mechanisms as well as external factors such as food marketing. We also introduce the major eating disorders.

Table 9.1	Obese Americans Age 20 and Older: 2018	
	OBESE (BMI ≥ 30)	
	% of population	
Both sexes	31.7	
Males	31.8	
Females	31.5	
Not Hispanic or Latino		
White males	31.3	
White females	29.1	
Black males	31.7	
Black females	44.9	
Asian males	11.3*	
Asian females	11.9*	
Hispanic or Latino males	35.2	
Hispanic or Latino females	36.1	

*The data for Asians are from 2011–2014.

SOURCE: National Center for Health Statistics. 2019. "Early release of selected estimates based on data from January–September 2018 National Health Interview Survey," *Obesity*. (https://public.tableau.com/views/FIGURE6_3/Dashboard6_3?:embed=y&:showVizHome=no&:embed=true).

rates are also high among children and adolescents: According to standards developed by the National Institutes of Health, 18.5% of youth, ages 12–19, are obese.

Many studies have confirmed that obesity and—to a lesser extent—overweight can shorten lives (Figure 9.1). Obesity is one of six major controllable risk factors for heart disease,

THE OVERWEIGHT AND OBESITY CRISIS

Over two-thirds of American adults are overweight, and about half of overweight adults fall into the higher-risk category of obese. This is a serious public health problem because being overweight or obese is linked to heart disease, type 2 diabetes, chronic liver disease, stroke, and other chronic diseases that can be fatal. The World Health Organization estimates that 2.2 billion people worldwide are overweight or obese. Obesity also affects emotional health, leading to anxiety from poor body image, social isolation, and discrimination.

Regardless of race, ethnicity, gender, or age, all U.S. population groups are affected by overweight and obesity. Table 9.1 shows the percentage of American adults who are obese, but

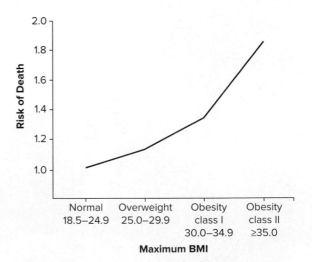

Figure 9.1 Weight history and all-cause mortality. Researchers followed more than 200,000 adults for 16 years and examined the relationship between an individual's maximum BMI over the period and subsequent mortality. A maximum BMI above the normal category was associated with an excess risk of death that increased with increasing BMI.

SOURCE: Yu, E., et al. 2017. "Weight history and all-cause and cause-specific mortality in three prospective cohort studies," *Annals of Internal Medicine* 166(2): 613–620.

Answers (Test Your Knowledge)

1. **c.** About 70% of American adults are overweight, including 36% who are obese.

2. **False.** Studies fail to show that low-calorie sweeteners help weight loss.

3. **b.** About 2–4% of female students suffer from bulimia or anorexia, and many more occasionally engage in behaviors associated with these eating disorders.

and, in addition to the conditions listed earlier, obesity increases the risk of cardiovascular disease (CVD), hypertension, certain forms of cancer, gallbladder disease, kidney disease, respiratory problems, joint diseases, skin problems, impaired immune function, and sleep disorders. Nearly 90% of people with type 2 diabetes are overweight when diagnosed.

Weight loss can have a significant positive impact on health. Even modest weight loss improves blood levels of good cholesterol (HDL), triglycerides, and glucose, as well as blood pressure. A weight loss of just 5–10% in obese individuals can reduce the risk of weight-related health conditions and increase life expectancy.

Assessing Weight

As described in Chapter 6, **overweight** is defined as total body weight above the recommended range for good health. **Obesity** is defined as a more serious degree of overweight that carries multiple health risks. Both terms, as determined by large-scale population surveys, are used to identify weight ranges that are associated with increased risk of certain diseases and health problems. The most important thing to consider for health is the proportion of the body's total weight that is fat—the percent body fat. For example, two men of the same height and weight may differ widely in percent body fat. If one has 12% body fat, and the other 22% body fat, only the second man's body composition is considered unhealthy. Assessment methods based on body weight alone are less accurate than those based on body fat, but they are commonly used because body weight is easier to measure than body fat.

Body mass index (BMI) is a measure of body weight that is useful for estimating a person's weight status (e.g., underweight, normal, or overweight) and for classifying the health risks of body weight. This measure is helpful when more sophisticated methods aren't available. BMI is often used in surveys and studies, and it is the basis for the population statistics presented in this chapter. BMI is a fairly accurate measure of the health risks of body weight for most average people. It is less accurate for muscular athletes, people under 5 feet tall, older adults with little muscle mass, and certain other groups. BMI is calculated by dividing body weight (in kilograms) by the square of body height (in meters); an alternative equation based on pounds and inches is the following:

$$BMI = (weight \div [height \times height]) \times 703$$

(Space for calculations and a complete BMI chart appear in Labs 6.1 and 6.2.)

BMI is combined with waist measurement to more accurately assess health risks. Waist measurement helps provide an assessment of body fat distribution. **Visceral fat**, fat stored around the internal organs, is more harmful to health than **subcutaneous fat**, fat stored under the skin. For classifying your health risks, use the combination of BMI and waist measurement in Table 9.2, or complete one of the more sophisticated body composition assessment methods presented in Chapter 6.

> **TERMS**
>
> **overweight** Body weight above the recommended range for good health; sometimes defined as a body mass index between 25 and 29.9, a measure of the proportion of weight to height.
>
> **obesity** Severely overweight, characterized by an excessive accumulation of body fat; may also be defined in terms of some measure of total body weight or a body mass index of 30 or more.
>
> **visceral fat** Fat located around major organs; also called *intra-abdominal fat*.
>
> **subcutaneous fat** Fat located under the skin.

Table 9.2	Body Mass Index, Waist Circumference, and Disease Risk			
			DISEASE RISK* RELATIVE TO NORMAL WEIGHT AND WAIST CIRCUMFERENCE	
	BMI (KG/M²)	OBESITY CLASS	MEN: WAIST 40 IN (102 CM) OR LESS / WOMEN: WAIST 35 IN (88 CM) OR LESS	MEN: WAIST >40 IN (102 CM) / WOMEN: WAIST >35 IN (88 CM)
Underweight	<18.5		–	–
Normal	18.5–24.9		–	–
Overweight	25.0–29.9	I	Increased	High
Obesity	30.0–34.9	II	High	Very high
	35.0–39.9	II+	Very high	Very high
Extreme Obesity	40.0+	III	Extremely high	Extremely high

*Disease risk for type 2 diabetes, hypertension, and cardiovascular disease.

NOTE: Increased waist circumference also can be a marker for increased risk, even in persons of normal weight.

SOURCE: Adapted from National Heart, Lung, and Blood Institute. 1998. *Clinical Guidelines on the Identification, Evaluation, and Treatment of Overweight and Obesity in Adults: The Evidence Report.* Bethesda, MD: National Institutes of Health; De Lorenzo, A. 2016. "New obesity classification criteria as a tool for bariatric surgery indication," *World Journal of Gastroenterology* 22(2): 681–703.

HOW DID I GET TO BE MY WEIGHT?

People vary in their ability to gain or lose weight. We all know someone who can eat large amounts of food without gaining weight while others will skip meals and never lose weight. Experts have developed theories and models that attempt to explain these individual variations. For decades we have heard that the best way to lose weight is through "energy balance" or "calories in, calories out." Drink a soda? Just jog off the calories. Exercise for an hour? Reward yourself with an ice cream sundae! But if the formula is so simple and easy to follow, why are so many of us obese or overweight and suffering a host of weight-related conditions?

In this section, we present several models that address factors complicating weight loss and maintenance, including the role of metabolism and hormonal responses to certain foods. Some factors are within our control, such as diet and exercise; genetic and environmental factors are not.

Energy Balance Model

Energy balance is the relationship between the amount of energy (calories) taken into the body through food and drink (energy in), and the amount of calories expended through metabolic and physical activity (energy out). If you burn the same amount of energy as you take in (a *neutral* energy balance), your weight can remain constant. The energy balance equation for many Americans today is tipped toward the energy-in side—a *positive energy balance* that promotes weight gain. This means that many people take in more calories than they expend. Even a very small positive energy balance can, over time, lead to significant gains in weight and fat. The opposite condition is a *negative energy balance,* which occurs when energy intake is less than energy use. To create a negative energy balance, the "calories in, calories out" model suggests you can burn more energy by increasing your level of physical activity and take in less energy by consuming fewer calories.

This model doesn't reflect other factors that may influence the balance. Specific calorie sources may promote weight gain in addition to their contribution of calories to the "energy in" side of the equation. For example, a portion of unsalted nuts and a candy bar may have the same number of calories, but because the body absorbs fewer calories from nuts than from other foods, nuts do not cause much weight gain.

Carbohydrate-Insulin Model

In the carbohydrate-insulin model, the primary cause of obesity is overeating refined carbohydrates, which trigger an insulin response. When we eat processed food and other sugars that elevate insulin levels, the calories get trapped inside fat cells. Consequently, fewer calories remain available in the bloodstream, which makes us feel hungry and contributes to overeating. Insulin stimulates fat tissues to absorb glucose and also decreases the release of fatty acids from fat cells; it inhibits production of ketones in the liver and promotes fat and glycogen deposition. To put it simply: The problem is not overeating, but eating the wrong kind of calories, which expands fat tissue.

Multi-Factor Model

A third model puts less responsibility on your daily choices than the first two models. While it recognizes that fat accumulation does indeed depend on how much energy is consumed versus expended, the model suggests that obesity is a multifaceted problem that also includes genetic, metabolic, hormonal, psychological, cultural, and socioeconomic factors.

Genetic Factors Scientists have so far identified more than 50 genes associated with obesity. Genes influence body size and shape, body fat distribution, and metabolic rate. Genetic factors also affect the ease with which weight is gained as a result of overeating and where on the body extra weight is added.

The *set-point theory* suggests that our bodies are designed to maintain a healthy and generally stable weight within a narrow range, or at a "set point," despite the variability in energy intake and expenditure. This theory is based on the idea that the rate at which our body burns calories adjusts according to the amount of food that we eat. Can we change our set point? It appears that when we maintain changes in our activity level and in our diets over a long period of time, our set point does change. Therefore, the set-point theory does not imply that we cannot maintain weight loss. However, physiological factors may make it easier to maintain a higher rather than a lower set point.

Fat Cells The amount of fat (adipose tissue) the body can store is a function of the number and size of fat (adipose) cells, which is influenced by both genetic and lifestyle factors. Some people are born with an above-average number of fat cells and thus have the potential for storing more energy as body fat. Overeating at critical times, such as in childhood, can cause the body to create more fat cells. If a person loses weight, fat cell content is depleted, but the number of fat cells may not decrease. Fat tissue is not a passive form of energy storage; rather, fat cells send out chemical signals in order to be replenished. These signals affect multiple organs and systems, including those controlling appetite, metabolism, and immunity.

Metabolism Metabolism is the sum of all the vital processes by which food energy and nutrients are made available to and used by the body. The largest component of metabolism, **resting metabolic rate (RMR)**, is the energy required to maintain vital body functions while the body is at rest, including respiration, heart rate, body temperature, and blood pressure.

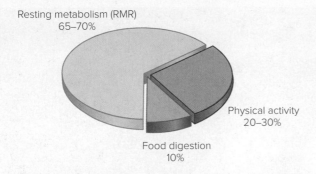

Resting metabolism (RMR)
65–70%

Physical activity
20–30%

Food digestion
10%

Figure 9.2   Where does food energy go? Energy in food you consume is expended through resting metabolism (maintaining vital body functions while at rest), physical activity, and digestion. Resting metabolism is the largest component of the "energy out" side of energy balance.

As shown in Figure 9.2, resting metabolism (RMR) accounts for about 65–70% of daily energy expenditure. The energy required to digest food accounts for up to an additional 10% of daily energy expenditure. The remaining 20–30% is expended during physical activity.

Genetics affects metabolic rate. Men, who have a higher proportion of muscle mass than women, have a higher RMR because muscle tissue is more metabolically active than fat, requiring more energy to support its activities. A higher RMR means that a person burns more calories while at rest and can therefore take in more calories without gaining weight. Some individuals inherit a higher or lower RMR than others; RMR may vary by as much as 25% among same-weight individuals.

A number of factors reduce metabolic rate, making weight management challenging. Low-calorie intake and weight loss reduce RMR. When energy intake declines and weight is lost, the body responds by trying to conserve energy, reducing both RMR and the energy required to perform physical tasks. In essence, the body "defends" the original starting weight. Consider two people of the same size and activity level who both currently weigh 150 pounds, but one of whom used to weigh 170 pounds; the individual who lost weight will need to consume fewer calories to maintain the 150-pound weight than the person who had always been at that weight. This physiological response of the body points to the importance of preventing weight gain in the first place.

Exercise can have a modest positive effect on RMR. As described in Chapters 3 and 4, exercise temporarily raises RMR, and resistance training can increase muscle mass, which in turn boosts metabolism. In one recent study, a regular resistance training program increased RMR by an average of 5% in healthy adults. While relatively small, this degree of increase in RMR can still be helpful over the long term in maintaining a healthy weight. Resistance training may also protect against age-related declines in RMR.

Hormones   Hormones play a role in the accumulation of body fat, especially for women. Hormonal changes at puberty, during pregnancy, and at menopause contribute to the amount and location of fat accumulation. For example, during puberty, hormones cause the development of secondary sex characteristics such as larger breasts, wider hips, and added fat under the skin. This addition of body fat at puberty is normal and healthy.

In addition to insulin, two other hormones thought to be linked to obesity are leptin and ghrelin. Secreted by the body's fat cells, leptin is carried to the brain, where it appears to let the brain know how big or small the body's fat stores are. With this information, the brain can regulate appetite and metabolic rate accordingly. Leptin levels are higher in people who are obese, but obesity may cause the body to be less responsive to leptin's signals. Low-calorie diets may reduce leptin and cause an increase in appetite.

The hormone ghrelin, released by the stomach, is responsible for increasing appetite. Ghrelin levels go up before eating and down for approximately 3 hours after a meal. Together with leptin, ghrelin also has a role in regulating body weight. Adequate sleep and a diet high in whole grains and protein lower ghrelin levels.

Researchers hope to use leptin, ghrelin, and other hormones to develop treatments for obesity based on appetite control. As most of us will admit, however, feelings of hunger may often *not* be the primary reason we overeat.

Gut Microbiota   The human intestine houses millions of bacteria that form the intestinal flora (gut flora). These bacteria help digest the foods you eat, and they produce some vitamins, such as vitamin K. Studies show that lean people differ from overweight people in the composition of their intestinal flora, suggesting that intestinal flora may be involved in the development of obesity. Diets high in processed foods have been linked to less diverse intestinal microbiota. Such diets have also been linked to a higher proportion of bacteria types associated with increased energy absorption and hormonal changes that increase appetite—both factors that can contribute to obesity.

Psychology, Culture, and Behavior   Many people have learned to use food as a means of coping with stress and negative emotions. Eating can provide a powerful distraction from difficult feelings—loneliness, anger, boredom, anxiety, shame, sadness, inadequacy. It can be used to combat low moods, low energy levels, and low self-esteem. When eating becomes the primary means of regulating emotions, **binge eating** or other unhealthy eating patterns can develop.

Obesity is strongly associated with socioeconomic status. The prevalence of obesity goes down as family income level goes up, especially among women and children. These differences may reflect greater access to unprocessed and low-calorie foods, to information about nutrition, and to physical activity among upper-income women. Upper-income women also may have acquired greater sensitivity and concern for a slim physical appearance. In contrast, the prevalence of obesity in some ethnic groups may reflect a greater acceptance of larger body types and different cultural values related to food choices in those groups.

> **binge eating**   A pattern of eating in which normal food consumption is interrupted by episodes of high consumption.
>
> **TERMS**

In some families and cultures, food is used as a symbol of love and caring. It is an integral part of social gatherings and celebrations. In such cases, it may be difficult to change established eating patterns because they are linked to cultural and family values.

Sleep In addition to diet and exercise habits, sleep is another health behavior that impacts weight management. Short sleep duration and sleep debt are associated with increased BMI and abdominal obesity, and researchers are still investigating how they might be linked. One possibility is that lack of sleep may affect hormone levels, appetite regulation, and metabolism. Short sleep duration is also associated with increased snacking and overall energy intake. Another factor is that use of multimedia devices may contribute to sleep deprivation and increase both energy intake and sedentary time. Getting adequate sleep is critical for overall wellness.

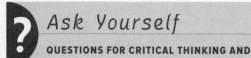

Ask Yourself

QUESTIONS FOR CRITICAL THINKING AND REFLECTION

Is anyone in your family overweight? If so, can you identify factors that may contribute to this weight problem, such as heredity, eating patterns, or psychosocial factors? Has the person tried to address the problem? How is the issue handled in your family? Do family members help the situation or make it worse?

Food Marketing and Public Policy The environment in which many Americans live and work can be "obesogenic"— meaning it encourages overconsumption of calories and discourages physical activity. This combination promotes weight gain rather than weight maintenance or loss. Food marketing and pricing, food production and distribution systems, and national agricultural policies all impact individual food choices.

The food industry promotes the sale of high-calorie processed foods at every turn. For example, vending machines offer mainly chocolate bars and unhealthy snacks, airlines offer complimentary soft drinks, and restaurants provide all-you-can-eat fried food buffets. Children are especially vulnerable to marketing that pushes ultra-processed foods high in sugar, salt, fat, and additives. Because they have a stronger preference for sweets than adults do, children are targeted from a young age and encouraged to make unhealthy choices.

Many experts observe that U.S. agricultural policy encourages farmers to produce corn and its by-product, high fructose corn syrup, at the expense of fruits and vegetables. As a result, over the past 30 years, the price of fruits and vegetables has risen much faster than the prices of other consumer goods, while the price of sugar, sweets, and carbonated drinks declined. Issues of price and availability of healthy food can have a profound effect on food choices. Low-income neighborhoods often have only fast-food venues offering high-calorie, highly processed foods.

Public policies can also have a positive influence. For example, the updated food labels and new regulations requiring chain restaurants and vending machine operators to post calorie

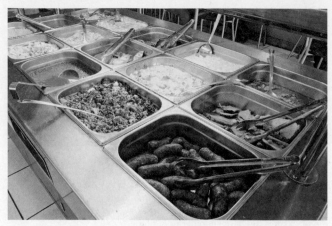

Wellness Tip Environmental factors can have a positive or negative influence on weight management. Identify key influences in your own environment. Develop strategies to take advantage of positive opportunities and to combat negative influences.
Luiz Ribeiro Ribeiro/123RF

information should help consumers make more informed choices. Other public health responses recommended by experts to support positive lifestyle choices for weight management include the following:

- Change food pricing to promote healthful options. For example, tax sugary beverages and offer incentives to farmers and food manufacturers to produce and market affordable healthy choices and smaller portion sizes.
- Limit advertising of unhealthy foods targeting children.
- Fund strategies to promote physical activity by creating more walkable communities, parks, and recreational facilities.

Rather than leaving all discussion to policy makers, public health experts are encouraging people to mobilize grassroots campaigns against the way food is currently distributed and marketed. Look around your community, school, and workplace: What aspects of the environment make it easier or more difficult to make healthy choices? What foods are available for purchase— and where and at what cost? Does the community environment and transportation system support walking or cycling, or is driving the only practical way to get around?

ADOPTING A HEALTHY LIFESTYLE FOR SUCCESSFUL WEIGHT MANAGEMENT

Are most weight problems lifestyle problems? Despite the growing prevalence of obesity in children and adolescents, many young adults get away with very unhealthy eating and exercise habits and don't develop a weight problem. But as the rapid growth of adolescence slows and family and career obligations increase, maintaining a healthy weight becomes a greater challenge. Slow weight gain is a major cause of overweight and obesity, so weight management is important for everyone, not just for people who are currently overweight. A good time to develop a lifestyle for successful weight management is during early adulthood, when healthy behavior patterns have a better chance of taking hold.

Adopt healthy behaviors you can maintain throughout your life. These behaviors include good eating habits, regular physical activity and exercise, strategies that help you think positively and manage your emotions effectively, and coping strategies for the stresses and challenges in your life.

Dietary Patterns and Eating Habits

In contrast to dieting, which involves some form of food restriction, the term *diet* refers to your daily food choices. Everyone has a diet, but not everyone is dieting. It's important to develop a diet that you enjoy and that enables you to maintain a healthy body composition. Follow the healthy U.S., Mediterranean, or vegetarian eating patterns, or DASH, discussed in Chapter 8; consult MyPlate for more information and tips. For weight management, pay special attention to total calories, portion sizes, energy and nutrient density, and eating habits.

Total Calories MyPlate suggests approximate daily energy intakes based on gender, age, and activity level. However, the precise number of calories needed to maintain weight will vary from one person to another based on heredity, fitness status, level of physical activity, and other factors. Focus more on your individual energy balance than on a general recommendation for daily calorie intake. To calculate your approximate daily caloric needs, complete Lab 9.1. If you choose to track calories, keep in mind that most people underestimate their energy intake and that energy needs change as body weight changes.

Just as important as tracking total energy intake for successful weight loss is choosing good sources of calories from fruits, vegetables, proteins, and unprocessed complex carbohydrates (see the box, "Are All Calories and Dietary Patterns Equal for Weight Loss?"). To maintain weight loss, you will probably have to continue some of the calorie restriction you used to lose the weight. Therefore, adopt a level of food intake that you can enjoy over the long term. For most people, maintaining weight loss is more difficult than losing the weight in the first place. To identify weight-loss goals and ways to meet them, complete Lab 9.2.

Portion Sizes Overconsumption of total calories is closely tied to portion sizes. Many Americans are unaware that the portion sizes of fast foods and of foods served at restaurants have increased, and most of us significantly underestimate the amount of food we eat (Figure 9.3). Studies have consistently found that people underestimate portion sizes by as much as 25%. When participants in one study were asked to report their food intake over the previous 24 hours, the majority underestimated their intake by about 600 calories. Another study showed that when people ordered from a restaurant menu that included calorie labels, they ate less. Limiting portion sizes is critical for weight management. For many people, concentrating on portion sizes is easier than counting calories. See Chapter 8 for more information and hints on choosing appropriate portion sizes.

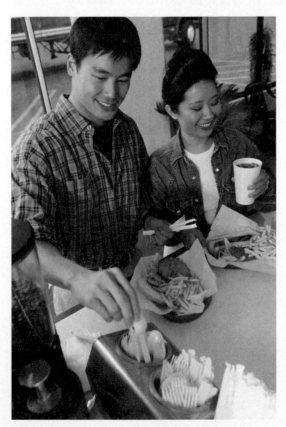

Wellness Tip If you think of fast food as your only available food option, you may find it difficult to make healthy lifestyle changes. When you do eat at a fast-food restaurant, pay special attention to your choices and your portion sizes. Choosing small instead of large fries can save 250 calories; water instead of a 12-ounce regular soda can save 150 calories. Over time, these kinds of calorie savings can add up!

Steve Mason/Photodisc/Alamy Stock Photo

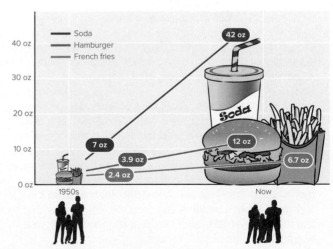

Figure 9.3 The new (ab)normal. Portion sizes have been growing. So have we. The average restaurant meal today is more than four times larger than in the 1950s. Adults today are, on average, 26 pounds heavier. To eat healthy, there are things we can do for ourselves and our community. Order the smaller meals on the menu, split a meal with a friend, or eat half and take the rest home. Ask the managers at favorite restaurants to offer smaller meals.

SOURCE: Centers for Disease Control and Prevention. "Making health easier." (http://MakingHealthEasier.org/TimeToScaleBack).

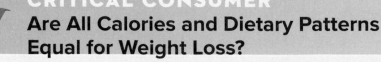

Many popular diets are promoted as the weight loss answer for all, but researchers continue to investigate the complex web of factors that influence the success or failure of efforts to lose weight and maintain that loss over time. Most researchers agree that total calorie intake is important, but preliminary evidence suggests some specific foods and eating patterns may help improve the odds for people trying to manage their weight.

Evaluating Dietary Composition: Balance of Protein, Carbohydrates, and Fats

Scientists are investigating whether particular patterns of macronutrient intake (e.g., higher protein, lower fat, or lower carbohydrate) are better for weight loss, for weight loss maintenance, and/or for improving health markers such as blood fat levels. How might macronutrient balance impact weight management? Two possible areas of influence are appetite and resting metabolic rate (RMR). Eating foods high in protein tends to make people feel fuller than eating foods high in fat or carbohydrate. This increase in satiety may help people refrain from overeating, thereby managing overall energy intake. On the flip side, foods high in simple sugars and refined carbohydrates may cause increased appetite (and eating) due to swings in the level of insulin.

One key challenge for weight-loss maintenance is the drop in RMR that follows weight loss. In some small, short-term studies, researchers compared the three dietary patterns—low fat, low glycemic index, and low carbohydrate—and the effect each had on RMR following weight loss. On average, the low-carbohydrate dietary pattern was associated with the smallest reduction in RMR. However, additional studies are needed to confirm the findings and determine their importance over a longer time period. An additional challenge is that extreme shifts in macronutrient balance are difficult for people to maintain over time.

How do various diets measure up over months and years? Researchers have not found significant differences. A study comparing weight loss among adults assigned to one of four reduced-calorie diets differing in percentages of protein, carbohydrate, and fat found that weight loss at two years was similar for all four diets (about nine pounds). However, weight loss was strongly associated with attendance at group sessions. Other studies have also found little difference in weight loss among popular reduced-calorie diets; most resulted in modest weight loss and reduced heart disease risk factors. The more closely people adhered to each diet, however, the more weight they lost. The American Heart Association notes that many dietary patterns can produce weight loss, and their latest guidelines list more than 15 approaches that can lead to weight loss if calories are reduced.

An interesting finding of multiple weight-loss and weight-maintenance studies is that people respond differently to different diets. So, for example, on a diet with a given balance of protein, carbohydrates, and fats, some people experience much greater weight loss than others. Similarly, changes in RMR after weight loss on different diets also vary. These findings point to individual differences in the factors affecting weight management—genetics, metabolism, hormones, and intestinal flora. Thus, there is no single diet that is for everyone. Researchers are trying to identify methods of matching people to an approach likely to be effective, but in the meantime, people can experiment with different dietary patterns to see what works best for them.

Making Quality Food Choices in Healthy Dietary Patterns

The typical American dietary pattern—high in sugary beverages, refined carbohydrates, red meat, and solid fats—is associated with obesity. For weight loss, choose high-quality calorie sources in a healthier dietary pattern; refer back to the patterns and food choices recommended in Chapter 8. Remember that there is more to foods than energy. Consume high-quality calorie sources, whatever dietary composition you choose. Nutrient-dense foods can help with both weight management and chronic disease prevention.

Maintaining Energy Balance Counts: The National Weight Control Registry

Important lessons can be drawn from the National Weight Control Registry—an ongoing study of people who have lost significant amounts of weight and kept it off. The participants (80% women, 20% men) in the registry lost 66 pounds and kept the weight off for more than five years. Nearly all participants use a combination of diet and exercise to manage their weight. Fifty-five percent of the participants chose a diet program to lose weight. Forty-five percent manage their weight on their own. Common strategies include eating breakfast, self-monitoring weight and food intake, and getting exercise of about one hour per day. The most common dietary pattern used by registry participants is low-fat/high-carbohydrate. Greater weight regain in this group of individuals came as a result of decreases in physical activity, fewer dietary restraints, less individual monitoring of body weight, and increased percentage of energy intake from fat. This study illustrates that to lose weight and keep it off, you must decrease daily calorie intake and increase daily physical activity—and continue to do so over your lifetime. Whatever dietary pattern you choose, make sure it contains high-quality, nutrient-dense foods and that it is a pattern you can maintain over the long term.

SOURCES: Hall, K. D., et al. 2016. "Energy expenditure and body composition changes after an isocaloric ketogenic diet in overweight and obese men," *American Journal of Clinical Nutrition* 104(2): 324–333; Ebeling, C. B., et al. 2012. "Effects of dietary composition on energy expenditure during weight-loss maintenance," *Journal of the American Medical Association* 307(24): 2627–2634; M. D. Jensen, et al. 2014. "AHA/ACC/TOC guideline for the management of overweight and obesity in adults: A report of the American College of Cardiology/American Heart Association Task Force on Practice Guidelines and the Obesity Society," *Circulation* 129(25 Suppl. 2): S102–S138; Thomas, J. G., et al. 2014. "Weight-loss maintenance for 10 years in the National Weight Control Registry," *American Journal of Preventive Medicine* 46(1): 17–23; Sacks, F. M., et al. 2009. "Comparison of weight loss diets with different compositions of fat, protein, and carbohydrates," *New England Journal of Medicine* 360: 859–873.

Table 9.3	Examples of Foods Low in Energy Density	
FOOD	AMOUNT	CALORIES
Carrot, raw	1 medium	25
Popcorn, air popped	2 cups	62
Apple	1 medium	72
Vegetable soup	1 cup	72
Plain oatmeal	½ cup	80
Fresh blueberries	1 cup	80
Corn on the cob (plain)	1 ear	80
Cantaloupe	½ melon	95
Light (fat-free) yogurt with fruit	6 oz.	100
Unsweetened applesauce	1 cup	100
Pear	1 medium	100
Sweet potato, baked	1 medium	120

Quality of Food Choices: Energy (Calorie) Density and Nutrient Density Experts also recommend that you pay attention to **energy density**—the number of calories per ounce or gram of weight in a food. Studies suggest that it isn't consumption of a certain amount of fat or calories in food that reduces hunger and leads to feelings of fullness and satisfaction. Rather, it is consumption of a certain weight of food. Foods that are low in energy density have more volume and bulk; that is, they are relatively heavy but have few calories (Table 9.3). For example, for the same 100 calories, you could eat 20 baby carrots or four pretzel twists. You are more likely to feel fuller after eating the serving of carrots because it weighs 10 times as much as the serving of pretzels (10 ounces versus 1 ounce). Fresh fruits and vegetables, with their high water and fiber content, are low in energy density, as are whole-grain foods. Fresh fruits contain fewer calories and more fiber than fruit juices or drinks. Meat, ice cream, potato chips, croissants, crackers, and cakes and cookies are examples of foods high in energy density.

As you decrease consumption of foods high in energy density, choose those that are also high in nutrient density—foods that are relatively low in calories but high in nutrients. Strategies for lowering the energy density of your diet while also increasing its nutrient density include the following:

- Eat fruit with breakfast and for dessert.
- Add extra vegetables to sandwiches, casseroles, stir-fry dishes, pizza, pasta dishes, and fajitas.
- Start meals with a bowl of broth-based soup; include a green salad or fruit salad.
- Snack on fresh fruits and vegetables rather than crackers, chips, or other energy-dense snack foods.

- Limit serving sizes of energy-dense foods such as butter, mayonnaise, cheese, chocolate, fatty meats, croissants, and snack foods that are fried, are high in added sugars (including reduced-fat products), or contain trans fat.
- Pay special attention to your beverage choices. Many sweetened drinks are low in nutrients and high in calories from added sugar.
- Limit processed foods, especially those high in added sugars and refined carbohydrates; these are usually energy dense, nutrient poor, and also high on the glycemic index.

Avoiding processed foods may be a particularly important strategy. In a 2019 study, researchers found that participants ate an average of about 500 more calories per day (and gained weight) when eating a diet of highly processed foods compared to a diet of unprocessed foods. The two diets were matched in terms of their macronutrient composition, and participants were allowed to consume as much or as little as they wanted. Researchers aren't sure exactly why the highly processed diet led to increased calorie consumption, but they did find different responses in levels of appetite-controlling hormones between the two diets. While on the diet of processed foods, people also ate faster, meaning they may have consumed more calories before their brain signaled they were full. The bottom line is that for both overall health and weight management, a diet of unprocessed foods is the best choice.

Eating Habits Equally important to weight management is eating small, frequent meals—including breakfast and snacks—on a regular schedule. Eating every 3–4 hours can help fuel healthy metabolism, maintain muscle mass, and prevent between-meal hunger that often leads to unhealthy snacking. Skipping meals leads to excessive hunger, feelings of deprivation, and increased vulnerability to binge eating or snacking. It is better to consume the majority of calories during the day rather than in the evening. Set some rules governing food choices. Breakfast rules might include choosing a high-fiber cereal that is low in added sugar with low-fat milk on most days, and saving pancakes and waffles for special occasions unless they are whole grain. A good goal is to eat in moderation; no foods need to be entirely off-limits, though some should be eaten judiciously.

Physical Activity and Exercise

According to the 2018 Physical Activity Guidelines, activity has a role in preventing weight gain, losing weight, and maintaining weight loss. Moderate-to-vigorous activity can prevent or minimize excessive weight gain and help you maintain weight in the healthy range. Avoiding weight gain is easier than losing weight, and if you are at a healthy weight, a lifetime exercise program can help keep you there. Your total daily energy expenditure in physical activity includes not just purposeful exercise but also what's called non-exercise activity thermogenesis (NEAT), which is the energy you use for daily activities such as walking to class, cooking, and cleaning. Even a small increase in activity level can help you maintain your weight; see the box "Be More Active During Screen Time" for suggestions.

TAKE CHARGE
Be More Active During Screen Time

Eleven: That's the number of hours per day a 2018 Nielsen report says average Americans spend with smartphones, computers, tablets, televisions, video games, and radios. And that's up more than an hour from 2015. Because much of our time spent with technology asks little of our bodies, excessive hours sitting in front of a screen, whether for work, study, or pleasure, contributes to the health risks of a sedentary lifestyle—and makes weight management more challenging. (See Chapters 2 and 7 for more on the dangers of sedentary time and suggestions for reducing it.)

You'll benefit from limiting the amount of time you spend sitting, but you can also incorporate some physical activity and boost NEAT even when engaged in screen time. Try some of the following suggestions.

Your working position and posture:

- If you can, alternate between a chair and a standing desk and/or a stability ball to avoid spending an extended period in the same position. Balancing on a stability ball works your back and core muscles; be sure to use good form at all times.

- When you do sit in a chair, tap your feet, fidget, wiggle, bounce, and dance in your chair. Any extra movements keep you more physically active.

- Follow the suggestions for posture in Chapter 5 to prevent stress on your joints.

Strength training in place—try some of the following or develop your own screen-time workout:

- *Leg extensions:* Extend one leg and rest the heel on the floor; lift your leg off the ground three inches or higher while keeping your back straight, and hold 5–10 seconds. Repeat with the other leg.

- *Air or chair squats:* Perform air squats as described in Chapter 4, or use a sturdy chair (without wheels) to indicate the bottom position of the squat. Don't lean forward or put your full weight on the chair as you lower into the squat position.

- *Desk, chair, or wall push-ups:* Place your hands on a sturdy surface and perform push-ups while keeping your body in a straight line; the lower the surface, the more difficult the exercise.

- *Press-ups:* Sit in a sturdy chair with armrests. Lean slightly forward and use your arms to push your body slowly off the seat; hold for a few seconds and release. Repeat.

- *Seated toe press:* Start with your feet flat on the floor and then push down with your toes as you raise your heels; hold the contraction of the calf muscles for several seconds, and then return to the starting position. Repeat.

- *Isometric chest press:* With elbows out to the side and palms together in front of your chest, press your hands and hold the position; relax and repeat. Be sure to breath throughout the contraction.

- *Isometric abdominals:* Use your abdominal muscles to pull your belly button toward your spine; hold the position, relax, and repeat. You can also do isometric contractions of your gluteals and many other muscle groups. Squeeze a tennis ball to develop grip strength.

- Add exercises that use a resistance band or small hand weights, such as arm curls; seated rows; front, side, and overhead arm raises; side and back leg raises; and knee curls.

Stretch and breathe:

- Try the upper-body stretches from Chapter 5 from a seated position: head turns and tilts, towel stretch, across-the-body and overhead stretch, upper-back stretch, and lateral stretch.

- Stretch your calves by extending your legs, one at a time, and pulling your toes back.

- Pull your shoulders back to open your chest; expand your abdomen as you breathe deeply.

SOURCES: Nielsen Company. 2018. *The Total Audience Report Q1 2018.* (https://www.nielsen.com/us/en/insights/news/2018/time-flies-us-adults-now-spend-nearly-half-a-day-interacting-with-media.html); Villablanca, P. A., et al. 2015. "Nonexercise activity thermogenesis in obesity management," *Mayo Clinic Proceedings* 90(4): 509–519; NIH National Institute on Aging. 2016. *Exercise and Physical Activity: Your Everyday Guide–Sample Exercises–Strength.* (https://www.nia.nih.gov/health/publication/exercise-physical-activity/sample-exercises-strength).

For people who are trying to lose weight, increasing activity can help burn additional calories but is generally less important than reducing calorie intake during the weight-loss phase. Studies comparing exercise, diet, and combination approaches show that for most people, calorie restriction is more effective than exercise alone, and a combination of the two yields the best results. Figure 9.4 shows the results of one such study; after 12 months, weight loss was greatest in the combination group, but diet alone produced significantly more weight loss than exercise alone. Part of the reason for this finding is that it is challenging to create a large negative energy balance with exercise alone. In addition, many people unconsciously compensate for calories burned during an exercise session—for example, by eating more or by engaging in less physical activity during the rest of the day.

Physical activity is especially important for weight loss maintenance. Many people who lose weight gain it back. As discussed in the section on metabolism, the body works against weight loss efforts, compensating by reducing RMR and increasing hunger signals, thereby pushing weight back toward its starting point. These challenges were illustrated in a follow-up study of contestants on *The Biggest Loser.* During the original competition, obese participants lost large amounts of weight through significant calorie restriction and intense exercise. As expected, RMR dropped as they lost weight and hormone levels shifted to increase hunger. But six years later, even after regaining most of the lost weight, RMR was still reduced, and reduced more than expected based on their new weights. Because the slowing of their metabolism persisted, they were burning fewer calories at rest than they did prior to

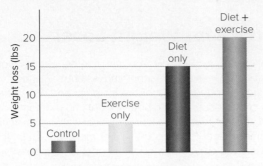

Figure 9.4 Effects of diet (calorie restriction), exercise, and a combination of diet and exercise on weight loss.
SOURCE: Foster-Schubert, K. E., et al. 2012. "Effect of diet and exercise, alone or combined, on weight and body composition in overweight-to-obese postmenopausal women," *Obesity* 20(8): 1628–1638.

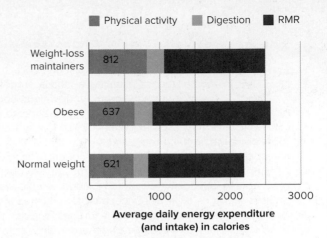

Average daily energy expenditure (and intake) in calories

Figure 9.5 Physical activity for weight maintenance. In a study comparing successful weight-loss maintainers to controls with normal body weight and obesity, higher physical activity among the maintenance group appeared to be the primary strategy for preventing weight regain. These findings were based on laboratory measurements of energy expenditure rather than often inaccurate self-reports of diet and exercise.
SOURCE: Ostendorf, D. M., et al. 2019. "Physical activity energy expenditure and total daily energy expenditure in successful weight loss maintainers," *Obesity* 27(3): 496–504.

weight loss. While most people don't follow an extreme program like these contestants, the difficulty of weight loss maintenance is universal. The news was not all bad, however. Participants had maintained an average weight loss of about 12%, along with better cholesterol profiles and other improved disease risk factors.

People who have successfully maintained weight loss over time engage in high levels of physical activity. Among *The Biggest Loser* contestants, less weight regain was strongly associated with physical activity levels—the greater the activity, the less the weight regain. In a 2019 study, researchers compared the energy expenditure of three groups: individuals who were overweight or obese, successful weight-loss maintainers, and normal body weight controls. The group who maintained weight loss burned (and consumed) a similar number of calories to the overweight/obese group, but they compensated and avoided weight regain by using significantly more calories in physical activity (Figure 9.5). Taken together, these and other findings suggest that physical activity is critical for avoiding weight regain.

How might physical activity and exercise help with weight loss maintenance? As described earlier, exercise can affect metabolism. When people exercise, they slightly increase their RMR—the number of calories their bodies burn at rest. A 2011 study of college-age men showed that following 45 minutes of vigorous exercise, the participants' resting metabolic rate remained elevated for 14 hours—during which the men burned an average of 200 additional calories while at rest or performing normal, everyday activities. While not everyone will have this significant of a response, any increase in RMR is helpful for weight management. Resistance training builds muscle mass, and more muscle translates into a higher metabolic rate. Resistance training can also help you maintain your muscle mass during weight loss, potentially lessening the associated drop in RMR.

People who have lost weight also have to contend with hormonal changes that increase hunger signals, making it difficult to maintain calorie restrictions. Moderate-intensity endurance exercise, if performed frequently for a relatively long duration, can burn a significant number of calories; increasing total energy expenditure through activity means more can be eaten without gaining weight. While some permanent calorie restriction is

typically needed, greater physical activity translates into less calorie restriction to maintain energy balance and weight loss. However, for energy expenditure through activity to help in weight management, you can't compensate for a workout by eating or sitting more.

The bottom line is that regular physical activity, maintained throughout life, is the best thing we can do for our health, and it also helps with weight management (see the box "What Is the Best Way to Exercise for Weight Loss?").

Thoughts and Emotions

The way you think about yourself and your world influences, and is influenced by, how you feel and how you act. In fact, research on people who struggle with their weight indicates that many suffer from low self-esteem, and the negative emotions that accompany it are significant problems. Often, people with low self-esteem compare the actual self to an internally held picture of the "ideal self," an image based on perfectionist goals and beliefs about how they and others should look. The more these two pictures differ, the larger the negative impact on self-esteem and the more likely the presence of negative emotions.

Besides the internal picture we hold of ourselves, all of us carry on an internal dialogue about events happening to us and around us. This *self-talk* can be either deprecating or positively motivating, depending on our beliefs and attitudes. Having realistic beliefs and goals and engaging in positive self-talk and problem solving support a healthy lifestyle. (Chapter 10 and Activity 11 in the Behavior Change Workbook at the end of the text include strategies for developing realistic self-talk.)

THE EVIDENCE FOR EXERCISE
What Is the Best Way to Exercise for Weight Loss?

If weight loss is your primary goal, the guidelines for planning a fitness program can vary depending on your weight, body composition, and current level of fitness. If you are obese or your fitness level is very low, start with a lower-intensity workout (55% of maximum heart rate), and stick with it until your cardiorespiratory fitness level improves enough to support short bouts of higher-intensity exercise. A study of 136 obese men and women found that those who included aerobic exercise in their regimens achieved a much better outcome than those who engaged only in resistance exercises: The aerobicizers achieved more cardiopulmonary fitness, reduced more abdominal and visceral fat, and improved their insulin sensitivity. Those who added resistance training (like using resistance bands or lifting weights) lost the most weight. On top of aerobics and resistance training, balance and flexibility exercises have been shown to reduce injury for obese people as well as any mobile person.

For weight loss to occur, exercise at lower intensities has to be offset by longer and/or more frequent exercise sessions. Experts recommend 60–90 minutes of daily exercise for anyone who needs to lose weight or maintain weight loss. If you cannot fit such a large block of activity into your daily schedule, break your workouts into short segments—as little as 10–15 minutes each. This approach is probably best for someone who has been sedentary because it allows the body to become accustomed to exercise at a gradual pace while preventing injury and avoiding strain on the heart.

Many research studies have shown that walking is an ideal form of exercise for losing weight and avoiding weight gain. A landmark 15-year study by the University of North Carolina at Charlotte showed that, over time, people who did not walk gained 18 pounds more than people who walked just 30 minutes per day. Those who regularly walked farther were better able to lose or maintain weight. Other studies found that people who walked 30 minutes five times per week lost an average of five pounds in 6–12 months, without dieting, watching what they ate, or exercising intensely. You can lose even more weight if you eat sensibly and walk farther and faster.

Regular walking is one of the simplest and most effective health habits for controlling body weight and promoting health. Even if you're sedentary, a few months of walking can increase your fitness level to the point where more vigorous types of exercise—and even greater health benefits—are possible.

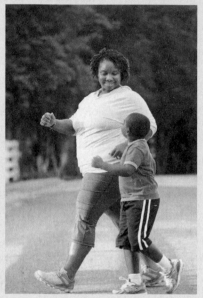

Ariel Skelley/Blend Images/Getty Images

SOURCES: Gordon-Larsen, P., et al. 2009. "Fifteen-year longitudinal trends in walking patterns and their impact on weight change," *American Journal of Clinical Nutrition* 89(1): 19–26; Higgins, J. P., and C. L. Higgins. 2016. "Prescribing exercise to help your patients lose weight," *Cleveland Clinic Journal of Medicine* 83(2): 141–150; Levine, J. A., et al. 2008. "The role of free-living daily walking in human weight gain and obesity," *Diabetes* 57(3): 548–554.

Coping Strategies

Appropriate coping strategies help you deal with the stresses of life; they are also an important lifestyle factor in weight management. Many people use drugs, alcohol, smoking, or gambling as ways to cope; others use eating. Those who overeat use food to alleviate loneliness or fatigue, as an antidote to boredom, or as a distraction from problems. Some people even overeat to punish themselves for real or imagined transgressions.

An interesting phenomenon regarding weight-loss interventions among college students has recently been observed: Groups of students who shared certain characteristics did better at losing and managing weight than did groups of dissimilar students. The study grouped students according to common psychosocial factors (such as emotional eating) that contribute to weight gain. These clusters of similar students were able to lose more weight and keep more weight off than were groups of students who did not share common dietary or psychosocial characteristics. The findings of this study may help shape group-oriented weight-loss programs in the future and contribute to an understanding of coping strategies.

For a summary of the components of weight management through healthy lifestyle choices, see the box "Lifestyle Strategies for Successful Weight Management."

APPROACHES TO OVERCOMING A WEIGHT PROBLEM

Each year, Americans spend more than $70 billion on various weight-loss plans and products. If you are overweight, you may already be creating a plan to lose weight and keep it off. You have many options.

Lifestyle Strategies for Successful Weight Management

Food Choices

- Focus on making good choices from each food group, eating a variety of foods, and balancing your food intake with your energy expenditure.

- Select foods with a *low energy* (calorie) density and a *high nutrient* density. Favor unprocessed over processed foods.

- Check labels for serving sizes, calories, and nutrients. Watch for hidden calories. Reduced-fat foods often have as many calories as their full-fat versions.

- Limit calories in the form of soda, fruit drinks, sports drinks, alcohol, and specialty coffees and teas. Water and nonfat or low-fat milk are good beverage choices.

- For very tempting high-calorie foods, eat small amounts under controlled conditions. Go out for a scoop of ice cream, for example, rather than buying half a gallon for your freezer.

Planning and Serving

- Periodically monitor your calorie intake and compare this to your calorie expenditure, noting where your energy balance is. Do you need to exercise more? Eat less?

- Don't go longer than three to four hours without eating, and consume the majority of your calories during the day rather than in the evening. Avoid late-night eating, a behavior specifically associated with weight gain among college students.

- Fix more meals yourself and eat out less often.

- Keep low-calorie snacks on hand to combat the "munchies." Fresh fruits and vegetables are good choices.

- When shopping, make a list and stick to it. Don't shop when you're hungry. Avoid aisles that contain problem foods.

- Pay attention to portion sizes. Use measuring cups and spoons and a food scale to become familiar with portion sizes.

- Serve meals on small plates and in small bowls to help you eat smaller portions without feeling deprived. (Research has shown that using a larger plate makes food portions appear smaller, so people serve themselves more food and overeat.)

- Eat only in specifically designated spots. Remove food from other areas of your home. When you eat, just eat. Don't do anything else.

- Eat slowly. It takes time for your brain to get the message that your stomach is full. Take small bites and chew food thoroughly. Pay attention to every bite, and enjoy your food.

Special Occasions

- When you eat out, choose a restaurant where you can make healthy food choices. Ask the server not to put bread and butter on the table before the meal, and request that sauces and salad dressings be served on the side. If portion sizes are large, take half your food home for a meal later in the week. Don't choose supersized meals.

- If offered food you don't want by friends or family, accept a small portion or politely decline.

Physical Activity and Stress Management

- Increase your level of daily physical activity as slowly as necessary based on your current fitness level.

- Begin an exercise program that includes cardiorespiratory endurance exercise, strength training, and stretching.

- Get six to eight hours of sleep a night.

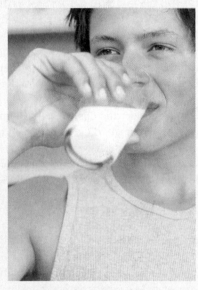

- Develop techniques for handling stress that don't involve food. See Chapter 10 for more on stress management.

- Develop strategies for coping with non-hunger cues to eat, such as boredom, sleepiness, or anxiety. Try calling a friend, taking a walk, or reading a magazine.

- Tell family members and friends that you're changing your eating and exercise habits. Ask them to be supportive.

Klaus Tiedge/Corbis/Getty Images

Doing It Yourself

If you need to lose weight, focus on adopting the healthy lifestyle described throughout this book. The "right" weight for you can evolve naturally. Combine modest cuts in energy intake with exercise, and avoid very-low-calorie diets.

Set Reasonable Goals According to the Centers for Disease Control and Prevention (CDC), reasonable weight loss for someone who is obese is 5–10% of body weight over 6 months. For example, for someone who weighs 200 pounds, a 5% weight loss would be 10 pounds. The person in this example may still be in the "overweight" or "obese" range, but this degree of weight loss can reduce the chronic-disease risks related to obesity. Modest weight loss can also be easier to maintain. Even more modest weight loss, in the 3–5% range, and the lifestyle changes used to achieve and maintain it, is likely to improve blood pressure, reduce cholesterol and glucose levels, and reduce the risk for diabetes.

Some diet plans have an initiation phase of rapid weight loss, such as 6–8 pounds for the first two weeks. Then the plans transition to a reduced weight loss of 0.5–2.0 pounds per week. Rapid weight loss not only relies on dramatic and unsustainable strategies such as dehydration, but it can also result in immediate and longer-term health problems, such as decreased bone density.

Don't try to lose weight more rapidly than 0.5–2.0 pounds per week, which will require a negative energy balance of at least 250–1,000 calories per day. Although this balance may help you lose weight at the start of a diet, some people need an even greater negative calorie balance as their metabolic rate slows: As described earlier in the chapter, your lower energy intake and loss of weight prompt the body to conserve energy and lower the RMR.

In general, a low-calorie diet provides 1,200–1,500 calories per day. Most low-calorie diets cause a rapid loss of body water at first. After this phase, weight loss declines, and dieters are often misled into believing that their efforts are not working. They give up, not realizing that the large initial fluid loss is not as significant as smaller fat losses occurring later in the diet.

The National Institutes of Health has a planning tool that provides individual energy-intake estimates for reaching a goal weight within a specific time period and maintaining it afterward (https://www.niddk.nih.gov/bwp). The tool can provide a starting point for planning, as well as a reality check on your goals.

Develop a Plan You Can Stick With Maintaining weight loss is usually a bigger challenge than losing weight. Without lifestyle changes, most weight lost during a period of dieting is regained. Weight management is a lifelong project. When planning a weight-management program, include strategies that you can maintain over the long term, both for food choices and for physical activity. If you want to use a digital tracking tool in your program, consider the tips in the box "Apps and Wearables for Weight Management." A registered dietitian or nutritionist can recommend a personalized plan when you want to lose weight on your own. For more strategies, refer to the section on "Adopting a Healthy Lifestyle for Successful Weight Management."

Diet Books

Many people who try to lose weight by themselves fall prey to one or more of the hundreds of diet books on the market. Although some books contain useful advice and motivational tips, most make empty promises. Look for books that advocate a balanced approach to diet plus exercise and sound nutritional advice. Reject those with any of the following:

- An approach based on an unbalanced way of eating, such as a high-carbohydrate-only diet or one focused on a single food, such as cabbage or grapefruit

- A claim that it is based on a "scientific breakthrough" or that it has the "secret to success"

- Gimmicks, such as matching eating to blood type, hyping insulin resistance as the cause of obesity, or combining foods in special ways to achieve weight loss

- Promises of quick weight loss or limits placed on the selection of healthy foods

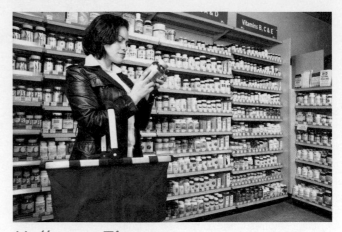

Wellness Tip Many plans and supplements claim to promote weight loss, but few have any research supporting their effectiveness for long-term weight management. If you're tempted to start taking an over-the-counter weight-loss supplement, do your homework first. Ask for your doctor's opinion, and check the FDA's supplement website at http://www.fda.gov/Food/DietarySupplements.

VStock LLC/Tanya Constantine/Tetra Images/Getty Images

Many diets cause weight loss if maintained. The real difficulty is finding a safe and healthy pattern of food choices and physical activity that results in long-term maintenance of a healthy body weight and reduced risk of chronic disease.

Dietary Supplements and Diet Aids

The number of dietary supplements and other weight-loss aids on the market has also increased in recent years. These products typically promise a quick and easy path to weight loss. Most of these products are marketed as dietary supplements and so are subject to fewer regulations than over-the-counter (OTC) medications. According to the Federal Trade Commission (FTC), more than half of advertisements for weight-loss products make representations that are likely to be false. And although the FTC will order companies to stop making baseless and bogus product claims when discovered, consumers are urged to critically evaluate any product that sounds too good to be true.

Potentially harmful hidden and undisclosed ingredients are a growing problem in products promoted for weight loss. Consumers may take a diet product that doesn't list quantities of approved prescription drug ingredients. In some cases the products also contain untested and unstudied ingredients or controlled substances (substances whose use is strictly regulated by the government). Such situations are common because the FDA cannot test for potentially harmful hidden ingredients in all products. Also, consumer advisories for tainted products identify only a small proportion of the potentially harmful products on the market.

The following sections describe some commonly marketed OTC products for weight loss.

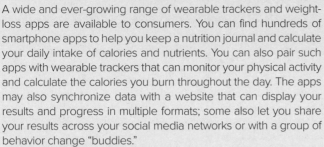

A wide and ever-growing range of wearable trackers and weight-loss apps are available to consumers. You can find hundreds of smartphone apps to help you keep a nutrition journal and calculate your daily intake of calories and nutrients. You can also pair such apps with wearable trackers that can monitor your physical activity and calculate the calories you burn throughout the day. The apps may also synchronize data with a website that can display your results and progress in multiple formats; some also let you share your results across your social media networks or with a group of behavior change "buddies."

Do these digital tools help with weight loss and weight maintenance? Research findings have been mixed. As with any health habit, tracking alone is unlikely to create permanent behavior change. Apps and wearables for weight management may be most effective when you pair tracking with evidence-based behavior-change techniques, such as reviewing goals, developing a specific action plan, planning for relapse prevention, and providing prompts, personalized feedback, rewards, and opportunities for motivational support. Pairing a digital tool with in-person or phone counseling from a health professional may further boost success.

If you decide to use a wearable and/or app to track diet and exercise for your weight-management program, consider the following:

- Does the app track what you want to track, and is it easy to use? Try it for a week or more: Did you stick with it?

- Does the app incorporate evidence-based behavior-change strategies? What does it offer besides tracking? Look for apps with motivation components (e.g., feedback, rewards and challenges, and a system of points or levels).

- If you want to share your results with friends on social media, is that functionality supported? Can you join other app users in a supportive group?

- How was the app developed? Has it undergone scientific evaluation? Were behavior-change or medical experts involved in its development? If users claim the app has provided some level of effectiveness or success, what evidence is provided to back up the claim? Satisfaction or popularity ratings do not necessarily reflect effectiveness for supporting weight loss.

Even with the help of digital devices and programs, weight management is still primarily a matter of personal effort, perseverance, and a commitment to lifestyle changes that last for life.

SOURCES: Abedtash, H., and R. J. Holden. 2017. "Systematic review of the effectiveness of health-related behavioral interventions using portable activity sensing devices (PASDs)," *Journal of the American Medical Informatics Association.* doi: 10.1093/jamia/ocx006; Ross, K. M., and R. R. Wing. 2016. "Impact of newer self-monitoring technology and brief phone-based intervention on weight loss: A randomized pilot study," *Obesity* 24(8): 1653–1659; Jakicic, J. M., et al. 2016. "Effect of wearable technology combined with lifestyle intervention on long-term weight loss: The IDEA randomized clinical trial," *JAMA* 316(11): 1161–1171; Flores Mateo, G., et al. 2015. "Mobile phone apps to promote weight loss and increase physical activity: A systematic review and meta-analysis," *Journal of Medical Internet Research* 17(11): E253.

Formula Drinks and Food Bars Canned diet drinks, powders used to make shakes, and diet food bars and snacks are meal replacements. They are designed to help you lose weight by substituting for some or all of your daily food intake. Meal replacements are convenient. However, most people find it difficult to use these products for long periods, and although they sometimes result in rapid short-term weight loss, the weight is typically regained because users don't learn to change their eating and lifestyle behaviors.

Herbal Supplements As described in Chapter 8, herbs are marketed as dietary supplements, and there is little information about effectiveness, proper dosage, drug interactions, and side effects. In addition, labels may not accurately reflect the ingredients and dosages present, and safe manufacturing practices are not guaranteed. Herbal supplements on the market today are described in Table 9.4.

Other Supplements Fiber is another common ingredient in OTC diet aids, promoted for appetite control. However, dietary fiber acts as a bulking agent in the large intestine, not the stomach, so it doesn't have a pronounced effect on appetite. In addition, many diet aids contain only 3 or fewer grams of fiber, which do not contribute much toward the recommended daily intake of 25–38 grams.

Other popular dietary supplements include conjugated linoleic acid, carnitine, chromium, pyruvate, calcium, B vitamins, chitosan, and a number of products labeled "fat absorbers," "fat blockers," or "starch blockers." Research has not found these products to be effective, and many have potentially adverse side effects.

Weight-Loss Programs

Weight-loss programs come in a variety of types, including noncommercial and commercial programs, websites, and clinical programs.

Noncommercial Support Organizations Noncommercial programs such as TOPS (Take Off Pounds Sensibly) and Overeaters Anonymous (OA) mainly provide group support. They do not advocate any particular diet, but they do recommend seeking professional advice for creating an individualized diet and exercise plan. Like Alcoholics Anonymous, OA is a 12-step program with a spiritual orientation that promotes abstinence from compulsive overeating. These types of programs are generally free.

Commercial Weight-Loss Programs Commercial weight-loss programs typically provide group support, nutrition education, physical activity recommendations, and behavior modification advice. Some also make packaged foods available to assist in following dietary advice.

Table 9.4 — Safety and Effectiveness of Common Over-the-Counter Weight-Loss Pills

INGREDIENT	PROPOSED MECHANISM OF ACTION	EVIDENCE OF EFFICACY	REPORTED ADVERSE EFFECTS
Alli (OTC form of orlistat)	Decreases absorption of dietary fat	Possible modest benefit; less effective than prescription strength form (Xenical)	Loose stools, gas with oily spotting, more frequent and hard to control bowel movements; reduced absorption of some nutrients; rare cases of liver damage
Bitter orange (synephrine)	Increased energy expenditure, mild appetite suppressant	Possible effect on resting metabolic rate; inconclusive effects on weight loss	Chest pain, anxiety, increased blood pressure and heart rate
Caffeine (as added caffeine or from guarana, kola nut, yerba mate, or other herbs)	Stimulates central nervous system, increases fat oxidation	Possible modest effect on body weight or decreased weight gain over time	Nervousness, jitteriness, vomiting, and tachycardia
Chitosan	Binds dietary fat in the digestive tract	Minimal effect on body weight	Bloating, flatulence, indigestion, constipation, nausea, heartburn
Chromium	Increases lean muscle mass; promotes fat loss; reduced hunger and fat cravings	Minimal effect on body weight and body fat	Headache, watery stools, constipation, weakness, vertigo, nausea, vomiting, hives
Conjugated linoleic acid	Promotes reduction in fat cells	Minimal effect on body weight and body fat	Abdominal pain, constipation, diarrhea, indigestion, and (possibly) adverse effects on blood lipid levels
Green tea extract	Increases energy expenditure and fat use, reduces fat absorption	Possible modest effect on body weight	Abdominal pain, constipation, nausea, increased blood pressure, liver damage
Guar gum	Acts as bulking agent in the gut, increases feelings of fullness	No effect on body weight	Abdominal pain, flatulence, diarrhea, nausea, cramps
Hoodia	Suppresses appetite, reduces food intake	Limited research, but no apparent effect on energy intake or body weight	Headache, dizziness, nausea, and vomiting
Pyruvate	Increases fat burning and energy expenditure	Possible minimal effect on body weight and body fat	Diarrhea, gas, bloating, and (possibly) decreased good cholesterol (HDL)
Raspberry ketone	Alters fat metabolism	Insufficient research to draw firm conclusions	None known

SOURCE: National Institutes of Health: Office of Dietary Supplements. 2019. *Dietary Supplements for Weight Loss: Fact Sheet for Health Professionals.* (https://ods.od.nih.gov/factsheets/WeightLoss-HealthProfessional)

A responsible and safe weight-loss program should have the following features:

- Healthy eating plans that reduce calories but do not exclude specific foods or food groups

- Tips on ways to increase moderate-intensity physical activity

- Tips on healthy habits that also keep your cultural needs in mind, such as lower-fat versions of your favorite foods

- A goal of slow and steady weight loss

- A recommendation for medical evaluation and care if you have health problems, are taking medication, or are planning to follow a special formula diet that requires monitoring by a doctor

- A plan to keep the weight off after you have lost it

- Information on all fees and costs, including those of supplements and prepackaged foods, as well as data on risks and expected outcomes of participating in the program

You should also consider whether a program fits your lifestyle and whether you are truly ready to make a commitment to it. A strong commitment and a plan for maintenance are especially important because only 10–15% of program participants maintain their weight loss; the rest gain back all they had lost or more.

One study of participants found that regular exercise was the best predictor of maintaining weight loss, and frequent television viewing was the best predictor of weight gain.

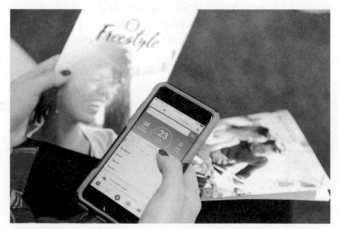

Wellness Tip Commercial weight-loss programs yield mixed results, but most provide nutritional counseling and support for people who are serious about losing weight. If the structure and support a program provides seem like something you'd like to try, be sure to evaluate the recommended dietary and activity patterns carefully.

Diane Bondareff/AP Images

Clinical Weight-Loss Programs Medically supervised clinical programs are usually located in a hospital or other medical setting. Designed to help those who are severely obese, these programs typically involve a closely monitored very-low-calorie diet. The cost of a clinical program is usually high, but insurance often covers part of the fee.

Prescription Drugs for Obesity

For a medicine to cause weight loss, it must (1) reduce energy consumption, (2) increase energy expenditure, and/or (3) interfere with energy absorption. The medications most often prescribed for weight loss are appetite suppressants that reduce feelings of hunger or increase feelings of fullness. Appetite suppressants usually work by increasing levels of catecholamine or serotonin, two brain chemicals that affect mood and appetite. Although some medications are approved only for short-term use, most experts agree that medications must be safe to use over the long term in order to be effective for treatment of obesity.

Appetite suppressants approved for long-term use include Belviq (lorcaserin), Qsymia (phentermine and topiramate extended-release), Contrave (bupropion and naltrexone), and Saxenda (liraglutide). All have potential side effects, such as sleeplessness, nervousness, euphoria, and increases in blood pressure and heart rate. Headaches, constipation or diarrhea, dry mouth, and insomnia are other side effects. If you are taking a prescription medication, discuss any concerns about side effects with your physician.

Orlistat lowers calorie consumption by blocking fat absorption in the intestines; it prevents about 30% of the fat in food from being digested. Similar to the fat substitute olestra, orlistat also reduces the absorption of fat-soluble vitamins and antioxidants. Therefore, a vitamin supplement is highly recommended for people taking orlistat. Side effects include severe liver injury, diarrhea, cramping, and other gastrointestinal problems if users do not follow a low-fat diet. Alli is a lower-dose version of orlistat that is sold over the counter.

Prescription medications work best in conjunction with behavior modification. Studies have generally found that appetite suppressants produce modest weight loss above the loss expected with nondrug obesity treatments. In a review published in 2016, researchers reported that people taking a prescription medication were two to three times more likely to have at least 5% weight loss than people taking a placebo. Individuals respond differently, however, and some lose more weight than others. Weight loss tends to level off or reverse after four to six months on a medication, and many people regain the weight they've lost when they stop taking the drug.

Prescription weight-loss drugs are not for people who want to lose only a few pounds. The latest federal guidelines advise people to try lifestyle modification for at least six months before trying drug therapy. Prescription drugs are recommended only for people who have been unable to lose weight with nondrug options and who have a BMI over 30 (or over 27 if an additional risk factor such as diabetes or high blood pressure is present). For severely obese people who have been unable to lose weight by other methods, prescription drugs may provide a good option.

Surgery

An estimated 7.7% of adult Americans age 20 and older have a BMI greater than 40, qualifying them as severely or morbidly obese. In 1975 in the U.S., 0.5% of men and 1.5% of women were severely obese. Forty years later, these percentages have jumped to 5.5% of men and 9.9% of women. Severe obesity is a serious medical condition that is often complicated by other health problems such as diabetes, sleep disorders, heart disease, and arthritis. Surgical intervention—known as *bariatric surgery*—may be necessary as a treatment of last resort. Bariatric surgery may be recommended for patients with a BMI greater than 40, or greater than 35 with obesity-related illnesses.

Due to the increasing prevalence of severe obesity, surgical treatment is becoming more common worldwide. Obesity-related health conditions, as well as risk of premature death, generally improve after surgical weight loss. Surgery, however, carries risks. Patients with poor cardiorespiratory fitness prior to surgery experience more postoperative complications, including stroke, kidney failure, and even death, than patients with higher fitness levels.

The goal is to promote weight loss by reducing the amount of food the patient can eat. Bariatric surgery modifies the gastrointestinal tract. One method partitions the stomach with staples or a band, while another modifies the way the stomach drains (gastric bypass). Potential complications from surgery include nutritional deficiencies, fat intolerance, nausea, vomiting, and reflux. As many as 10–20% of patients may require follow-up surgery to address complications.

Weight loss from surgery generally ranges between 40% and 70% of total body weight over the course of a year. The key to success is to have adequate follow-up and to stay motivated so that life behaviors and eating patterns are changed permanently.

The surgical technique of liposuction involves the removal of small amounts of fat from specific locations. Liposuction is not a method for treating obesity.

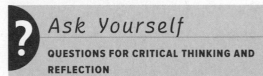

? Ask Yourself

QUESTIONS FOR CRITICAL THINKING AND REFLECTION

Why do you think some people continue to buy in to fad diets and weight-loss gimmicks, even though they are constantly reminded that the key to weight management is lifestyle change? Have you ever tried a fad diet or dietary supplement? If so, what were your reasons for trying it? What were the results?

Gaining Weight

Just as for losing weight, a program for weight gain should be gradual and should include both exercise and dietary changes. The foundation of a successful and healthy program for weight gain is a combination of strength training and in most cases a high-carbohydrate, high-protein diet that also contains healthy fats. Strength training will help you add weight as muscle rather than fat.

Energy balance is also important in a program for gaining weight. You need to consume more calories than your body requires in order to gain weight, but you need to choose those extra calories wisely. Fatty, sweet, high-calorie foods may seem like an obvious choice, but consuming additional calories as empty calories from solid fats and added sugars can jeopardize your health and your weight-management program. Your body is more likely to convert excess dietary fat into fat tissue than into muscle mass.

A better strategy is to consume additional calories as protein, healthy fats, and complex carbohydrates from whole grains, fruits, and vegetables. Add healthy calories from nutrient-dense, energy-dense foods such as nuts. A diet for weight gain should contain about 60–65% of total daily calories from carbohydrates. You probably do not need to be concerned with protein. Although protein requirements increase when you exercise, the protein consumption of most Americans is already well above the DRI.

To gain primarily muscle weight instead of fat, a gradual program of weight gain is your best bet. Try these strategies for consuming extra calories:

- Don't skip any meals. If you fill up too fast, try eating five or six smaller meals.

- Add two or three snacks to your daily eating routine. Try trail mix, smoothies, and nut butters on crackers.

- Try a sports drink or supplement that has at least 60% of calories from carbohydrates, as well as significant amounts of protein, vitamins, and minerals. (But don't use supplements to replace meals because they don't contain all of the components of food.)

Psychological Help

When concerns about body weight and shape have developed into an eating disorder, professional help is recommended. Therapists who help people with these disorders should have experience in weight management, body image issues, eating disorders, addictions, and abuse issues.

BODY IMAGE

The collective picture of the body as seen through the mind's eye, **body image** consists of perceptions, images, thoughts, attitudes, and emotions. A negative body image is characterized by dissatisfaction with the body in general or some part of the body in particular.

Developing a positive body image is an important aspect of psychological wellness and successful weight management. Dissatisfaction with body size and shape comes from external, cultural forces as well as internal, psychological perceptions that are specific to life stages. For example, a cultural ideal of female body shape in Western society has become progressively thinner,

> **body image** The mental representation a person holds about her or his body is influenced by cultural models and consists of perceptions, images, thoughts, attitudes, and emotions about the body.
>
> **TERMS**

whereas actual female body size continues to increase. How we individually perceive these norms and act on them, for example, by not eating enough or refusing to appear in a bathing suit, represents our psychological response.

Severe Body Image Problems

Poor body image can cause significant psychological distress. Preoccupation with a perceived defect in appearance can damage self-esteem and interfere with relationships. Adolescents and adults who have a negative body image are more likely to diet restrictively, eat compulsively, or develop some other form of disordered eating.

When dissatisfaction becomes extreme, the condition is called *body dysmorphic disorder (BDD)*. BDD affects about 2% of Americans, males and females in equal numbers. BDD usually begins before age 18 but can begin in adulthood. Sufferers are overly concerned with physical appearance, often focusing on slight flaws that are not obvious to others. Individuals with BDD may spend hours every day thinking about their flaws and looking at themselves in mirrors; they may desire and seek repeated cosmetic surgeries. BDD is related to obsessive-compulsive disorder and can lead to depression, social phobia, and suicide if left untreated. Medication and therapy can help people with BDD.

In some cases, body image may bear little resemblance to fact. A person with the eating disorder anorexia nervosa typically has a severely distorted body image, believing herself to be fat even when she has become emaciated (see the next section for more on anorexia). Distorted body image is also a hallmark of *muscle dysmorphia,* a disorder experienced by some bodybuilders and other active people who see themselves as small and out of shape despite being very muscular. People with muscle dysmorphia may let obsessive weight training interfere with their work and relationships. They may also use potentially dangerous muscle-building drugs.

To assess your body image, complete the body image self-test in Lab 9.3.

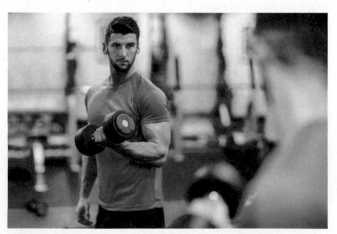

Fitness Tip Exercise is a healthy practice, but people with eating disorders or body image problems sometimes exercise excessively, building their lives around their workouts. Compulsive exercise can lead to injuries, low body fat, and other health problems. Track your exercise habits for a week; if they seem excessive and you can't seem to cut back, talk to a professional counselor or your doctor to find out if you have a body image problem.

Wavebreak Media Ltd/123RF

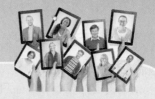

Body Image and Gender

Women are much more likely than men to be dissatisfied with their bodies, often wanting to be thinner. Body weight perception has been found to begin in girls as young as age 7 years. Approximately 50% of girls and undergraduate women report being dissatisfied with their bodies. Girls and women are much more likely than boys and men to diet, develop eating disorders, and become obese.

The image of the ideal woman presented in the media is often unrealistic and even unhealthy. In a review of BMI data for Miss America pageant winners since 1922, researchers noted a significant decline in BMI over time, with an increasing number of recent winners having BMIs in the "underweight" category. The average fashion model is four to seven inches taller and almost 50 pounds lighter than the average American woman. Most fashion models are thinner than 98% of American women.

Our culture may be promoting an unattainable masculine ideal as well. Researchers have found that males who form their ideals from media-generated images show a preference for thinness and muscularity. Researchers studying male action figures note that they have become increasingly muscular. Such media messages can be demoralizing; boys and men also suffer from body image problems, although not as commonly as girls and women.

Body Image and Ethnicity

Although some groups espouse thinness as an ideal body type, others, like many traditional African societies, prefer full-figured women's bodies, which are seen as symbols of health, prosperity, and fertility. African American teenage girls have a more positive body image than European American girls; in one survey, two-thirds of them defined beauty as "the right attitude," whereas European American girls were more preoccupied with weight and body shape. In another study about pressure to look like idealized images, Latina women reported the greatest pressure (over white or black women) to be physically attractive.

Nevertheless, recent evidence indicates that African American women are as likely to engage in disordered eating behavior—especially binge eating and vomiting—as their Latina, Native American, and European American counterparts. This finding underscores the complex nature of eating disorders and body image.

Avoiding Body Image Problems

To minimize your risk of developing a body image problem, keep the following strategies in mind:

- Focus on healthy habits and good physical health.

- Put concerns about physical appearance in perspective. Your worth as a human being does not depend on how you look.

- Practice body acceptance. You can influence your body size and type through lifestyle to some degree, but the fact is that some people are genetically designed to be bigger or heavier than others.

- Find things to appreciate in yourself besides an idealized body image. People who can learn to value other aspects of themselves are more accepting of the physical changes that occur naturally with age.

- View eating as a morally neutral activity—eating dessert isn't "bad" and doesn't make you a bad person.

- See the beauty and fitness industries for what they are. Realize that their goal is to prompt you to be dissatisfied with yourself so that you will buy their products.

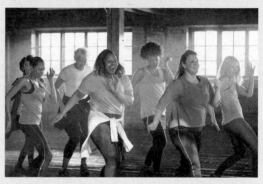
DigitalVision/Getty Images

SOURCES: Bruns, G. L. and M. M. Carter. 2015. "Ethnic differences in the effects of media on body image: The effects of priming with ethnically different or similar models," *Eating Behaviors* 17: 33–36; Haytko, D. L., et al. 2014. "Body image and ethnicity: A qualitative exploration," *Journal of Management and Marketing Research* 17; Webb, J. B., et al. 2013. "Do you see what I see: An exploration of inter-ethnic body size comparisons among college women," *Body Image* 10(3): 369–379.

Healthy Change and Acceptance

There are limits to the changes that can be made to body weight and body shape, both of which are influenced by heredity. Knowing when the limits to healthy change have been reached—and learning to accept those limits—is crucial for overall wellness. Women in particular tend to measure self-worth in terms of their appearance. When they don't measure up to an unrealistic cultural ideal, they see themselves as defective, and their self-esteem falls. The result can be negative body image, disordered eating, or even a full-blown eating disorder (see the box "Gender, Ethnicity, and Body Image."

Weight management is most successful in a positive and realistic atmosphere. For an obese person, losing as few as 10 pounds can reduce blood pressure and improve mood. The hazards of excessive dieting and overconcern about body weight need to be countered by a change in attitude. A reasonable weight must take into account a person's weight history, social circumstances, metabolic profile, and psychological well-being.

EATING DISORDERS

Problems with body weight and weight control are not limited to excessive body fat. A growing number of people, especially adolescent girls and young women, experience **eating disorders**. Eating disorders are characterized by severe disturbances in body image, eating patterns, and eating-related behavior. In the United States, it is estimated that 20 million women and 10 million men suffer from an eating disorder (anorexia nervosa, bulimia nervosa, and binge-eating disorder) some time in their lives. Many more people have abnormal eating habits and attitudes about food that disrupt their lives, even though these habits do not meet the criteria for a major eating disorder. To assess your eating habits, complete Lab 9.3.

Eating disorders are classified as mental disorders. Although many explanations for the development of eating disorders have been proposed, individuals with such disorders share one central feature: a dissatisfaction with body image and body weight. Such dissatisfaction is created by distorted thinking, including perfectionist beliefs, unreasonable demands for self-control, and excessive self-criticism. Dissatisfaction with body weight leads to dysfunctional attitudes about eating, such as fear of fat, preoccupation with food, and problematic eating behaviors.

Anorexia Nervosa

People with **anorexia nervosa** have an intense fear of gaining weight or becoming fat. Although they may express a great interest in food, they do not eat enough food to maintain a reasonable body weight. They may engage in compulsive behaviors or rituals that help them avoid eating. People with anorexia are typically introverted, emotionally reserved, and socially insecure. Their entire sense of self-esteem may be tied up in their evaluation of their body shape and weight. Approximately 1% of female adolescents have anorexia. Although it can occur earlier or later, anorexia typically develops during puberty and the late teenage years, with an average onset age of about 19 years.

Anorexia nervosa has been linked to a variety of medical complications, including disorders of the cardiovascular, gastrointestinal, and endocrine systems. Because of extreme weight loss, females with anorexia often stop menstruating. When body fat is virtually gone and muscles are severely wasted, the body turns to its organs in a desperate search for protein. Death can occur from heart failure caused by electrolyte imbalances. About 1 in 10 women with anorexia dies of starvation, cardiac arrest, or other medical complications—one of the highest death rates for any psychiatric disorder. Depression is also a serious risk, and about half the fatalities relating to anorexia are suicides.

Bulimia Nervosa

A person with **bulimia nervosa** engages in recurrent episodes of binge eating followed by **purging**. Bulimia is often difficult to recognize because sufferers conceal their eating habits and usually maintain a normal weight, although they may experience weight fluctuations of 10–15 pounds. Although bulimia usually begins in adolescence or young adulthood, it has begun to emerge at increasingly younger (11–12 years) and older (40–60 years) ages. The average age of onset is about 20 years.

A bulimic person may rapidly consume thousands of calories by binge eating; during a binge, bulimics feel as though they have lost control and cannot stop or limit how much they eat. This is followed by an attempt to get rid of the food by purging, usually by vomiting or using laxatives or diuretics. Some binge and purge only occasionally; others do so many times every day. Binges may be triggered by a major life change or other stressful event. Binge eating and purging may become a way of dealing with difficult feelings such as anger and disappointment.

The binge-purge cycle of bulimia places a tremendous strain on the body and can have serious health effects, including tooth decay, esophageal damage and chronic hoarseness, menstrual irregularities, depression, liver and kidney damage, and cardiac arrhythmia.

Binge-Eating Disorder

Binge-eating disorder (BED) affects 2.8% of American adults: 3.5% of women and 2% of men. It is characterized by uncontrollable eating without any compensatory purging behaviors. Common eating patterns are eating more rapidly than normal, eating until uncomfortably full, eating when not hungry, and preferring to eat alone. Uncontrolled eating is usually followed by weight gain and feelings of guilt, shame, and depression. Many people with binge-eating disorder mistakenly see rigid dieting as the only solution to their problem, but this usually causes feelings of deprivation and a return to overeating.

Compulsive overeaters rarely eat because of hunger. Instead, they use food to cope with stress, conflict, and other difficult

---

TERMS

eating disorder A serious disturbance in eating patterns or eating-related behavior, characterized by a negative body image and concerns about body weight or body fat.

anorexia nervosa An eating disorder characterized by a refusal to maintain body weight at a minimally healthy level and an intense fear of gaining weight or becoming fat; self-starvation.

bulimia nervosa An eating disorder characterized by recurrent episodes of binge eating and then purging to prevent weight gain.

purging The use of vomiting, laxatives, excessive exercise, restrictive dieting, enemas, diuretics, or diet pills to compensate for food that has been eaten and that the person fears will produce weight gain.

binge-eating disorder An eating disorder characterized by repeated episodes of eating large amounts of food in a short period of time; episodes are marked by feelings of lack of control.

Secrecy and denial are two hallmarks of eating disorders, so it can be hard to know if someone has anorexia or bulimia. Signs that someone may have anorexia include sudden weight loss, excessive dieting or exercise, guilt or preoccupation with food or eating, frequent weighing, fear of becoming fat despite being thin, and baggy or layered clothes to conceal weight loss. Signs that someone may have bulimia include excessive eating without weight gain; secretiveness about food (stealing, hiding, or hoarding food); self-induced vomiting (bathroom visits during or after a meal); swollen glands or puffy face; erosion of tooth enamel; and use of laxatives, diuretics, or diet pills to control weight.

If you decide to approach a friend with your concerns, here are some tips to follow:

- Find out about treatment resources in your community (see the "For Further Exploration" section for suggestions). You may want to consult a professional at your school clinic or counseling center about the best way to approach the situation.

- Arrange to speak with your friend in a private place, and allow enough time to talk.

- Express your concerns, with specific observations of your friend's behavior. Expect him or her to deny or minimize the problem and possibly to become angry with you. Stay calm and nonjudgmental, and continue to express your concern.

- Avoid giving simplistic advice about eating habits. Listen if your friend wants to talk, and offer your support and understanding. Give your friend the information you found about where he or she can get help, and offer to go along.

- If the situation is an emergency—if your friend has fainted, for example, or attempted suicide—call 9-1-1 for help immediately.

- If you are upset about the situation, consider talking to someone yourself. The professionals at the clinic or counseling center are there to help you. Remember, you are not to blame for another person's eating disorder.

---

emotions or to provide solace or entertainment. Binge eaters are almost always obese, so they face all the health risks associated with obesity. In addition, binge eaters may have higher-than-average rates of depression and anxiety.

Other Specified Feeding or Eating Disorders (OSFED)

Eating habits and body image run along a continuum from healthy to seriously disordered. Where an individual falls along that continuum can change depending on life stresses, illnesses, and many other factors. People with feeding or eating disorders that can cause significant distress or impairment, but do not meet the criteria for another feeding or eating disorder, may be classified as having "other specified feeding or eating disorders" (OSFED).

OSFED is a feeding or eating disorder that does not meet full diagnostic criteria for anorexia, bulimia, or binge-eating disorder. Examples of OSFED include atypical anorexia nervosa, a condition in which weight is not below normal; bulimia nervosa with less frequent bulimic episodes; purging disorder, a condition without binge eating; and night eating syndrome, in which the individual engages in excessive nighttime food consumption.

Ideally, our relationship to food should be a happy one. The biological urge to satisfy hunger is one of our most basic drives, and eating is associated with many pleasurable sensations. For some of us, food triggers pleasant memories of good times, family, holidays, and fun. But for too many people, food is a source of anguish rather than pleasure. In the lives of affected individuals, eating results in feelings of guilt and self-loathing rather than satisfaction, causing tremendous disruption.

How do you know if you have disordered eating habits (for example, skipping meals or avoiding vegetables) that can lead to the more serious eating disorder? When thoughts about weight and food dominate your life, you have a problem. If you're convinced that your worth as a person hinges on how you look and how much you weigh, it's time to get help. Self-induced vomiting or laxative use after meals, even if only once in a while, is reason for concern. Do you feel compelled to exercise excessively to compensate for what you've eaten? Do you routinely restrict your food intake and sometimes eat nothing in an effort to feel more in control? These are all danger signs and could mean that you are developing a serious problem. Lab 9.3 can help you determine whether you are at risk for an eating disorder.

Treating Eating Disorders

The treatment of eating disorders must address both problematic eating behaviors and the misuse of food to manage stress and emotions. Treatment for anorexia nervosa first involves averting a medical crisis by restoring adequate body weight; similarly, the first step for treating bulimia nervosa or binge-eating disorder involves stabilizing the eating patterns. Afterward, psychological aspects of the disorders can be addressed, such as identifying and changing the patterns of thinking that lead to disordered eating. Treatment usually involves a combination of psychotherapy, medication, and medical management. Friends and family members often want to know what they can do to help; for suggestions, see the box "If Someone You Know Has an Eating Disorder."

People with milder patterns of disordered eating may benefit from getting a nutrition checkup with a registered dietitian. A professional can determine appropriate body weight and calorie intake and offer advice on how to budget calories into a balanced, healthy diet.

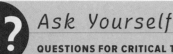

Ask Yourself

QUESTIONS FOR CRITICAL THINKING AND REFLECTION

Have you known someone you thought may be suffering from an eating disorder? How did you come to that conclusion?

TIPS FOR TODAY AND THE FUTURE

Many factors play into weight management, but you can focus on healthy, small portions of food and staying physically fit.

RIGHT NOW YOU CAN

- Assess your weight-management needs. Do you need to gain weight, lose weight, or stay at your current weight?
- List five things you can do to add more physical activity (not exercise) to your daily routine.
- Identify the foods you regularly eat that may be sabotaging your ability to manage your weight.

IN THE FUTURE YOU CAN

- Make an honest assessment of your body image. Is it accurate and fair, or is it unduly negative and unhealthy? If your body image presents a problem, consider getting professional advice on how to view yourself realistically.
- Keep track of your energy needs to determine whether your energy-balance is neutral. Use this information as part of your long-term weight-management efforts.

SUMMARY

- Excess body weight increases the risk of numerous diseases, particularly cardiovascular disease, cancer, and diabetes.

- The influence of heredity on weight can in many cases be overcome with attention to lifestyle factors.

- Physiological factors involved in the regulation of body weight and body fat include metabolic rate and hormones.

- Weight management involves more than a simple balance of energy in and energy out or an excess of insulin responses. It also includes genetic, metabolic, hormonal, psychological, cultural, and socioeconomic factors.

- Nutritional guidelines for weight management and wellness include controlling consumption of total calories, unhealthy fats, sugar, and refined carbohydrates; monitoring portion sizes and calorie density; increasing consumption of whole grains, fruits, and vegetables; and developing an eating schedule.

- Activity guidelines for weight control emphasize engaging in moderate-intensity physical activity for 60–90 minutes or more per day;

regular, prolonged endurance exercise and weight training can burn a significant number of calories while maintaining muscle mass.

- The sense of well-being that results from a well-balanced diet can reinforce commitment to weight control; improve self-esteem; and lead to realistic, as opposed to negative, self-talk. Those who are successfully managing their weight find strategies other than eating as means of coping with stress.

- In cases of extreme obesity, weight loss requires medical supervision; in less extreme cases, people can set up individual programs, getting guidance from reliable books or by joining a formal weight-loss program.

- Dissatisfaction with body image and body weight can lead to physical problems and serious eating disorders, including anorexia nervosa, bulimia nervosa, binge-eating disorder, and other specified feeding or eating disorders (OSFED).

FOR FURTHER EXPLORATION

Calorie Control Council. Includes a variety of interactive calculators, including an Exercise Calculator that estimates the calories burned from various forms of physical activity.

http://www.caloriecontrol.org

Centers for Disease Control and Prevention: Healthy Weight. Provides a variety of information and tools to help people assess their weight and plan healthy lifestyle changes.

http://www.cdc.gov/healthyweight

Frontline: Fat. Information from a PBS *Frontline* special that looked at how society, genetics, and biology have influenced our relationship with food and our current problems with obesity and eating disorders.

http://www.pbs.org/wgbh/pages/frontline/shows/fat

MedlinePlus: Obesity and Weight Control. Provides reliable information from government agencies and key professional associations.

http://www.nlm.nih.gov/medlineplus/obesity.html

http://www.nlm.nih.gov/medlineplus/weightcontrol.html

National Heart, Lung, and Blood Institute (NHLBI): Aim for a Healthy Weight. Provides information and tips on diet and physical activity, as well as a BMI calculator.

http://www.nhlbi.nih.gov/health/public/heart/obesity/lose_wt

Weight-control Information Network (WIN). A service of the National Institute of Diabetes and Digestive and Kidney Diseases, serves as an online clearinghouse of weight-management information.

http://win.niddk.nih.gov/

There are also many resources for people concerned about body image and eating disorders:

MedlinePlus: Eating Disorders

http://www.nlm.nih.gov/medlineplus/eatingdisorders.html

National Association of Anorexia Nervosa and Associated Disorders

http://www.anad.org

National Eating Disorders Association

http://www.nationaleatingdisorders.org

Women's Body Image and Health

http://www.womenshealth.gov/body-image/

See also the listings in Chapters 1, 6, and 8.

COMMON QUESTIONS ANSWERED

Q What's a healthy snack that will tide me over to the next meal without contributing to weight gain?

A Try nuts. They're delicious, easy to carry, and healthy! Studies routinely connect them with longevity and lower risk for heart disease, type 2 diabetes, metabolic syndrome, and certain cancers. Nuts are high in protein and fiber, nutrients such as magnesium, selenium, potassium, vitamins (E, K, and B-6), omega-3s, and antioxidants. Nuts are rich in unsaturated fats associated with heart health and disease prevention.

What about weight gain? Although high in fat and calories, healthy fats, along with high protein and fiber, make nuts a filling snack and can keep you from eating other, less healthy foods. In studies, consuming nuts in modest portions is not associated with weight gain, regardless of study participants' other dietary choices or restrictions; some studies even report that consuming nuts helps lose weight.

Aim for snacking on whole, unsalted nuts—roasted and unroasted—although "dry roasted" nuts are preferred because they are not roasted in oils. Avoid nuts in processed foods: Trail mix products can also contain candies, chocolate, pretzels, and excessive sodium; nuts as part of snack bars often come with added sugars and processed ingredients. Honey-roasted nuts can include 4–8 grams of added sugar, and salted nuts can have as high as 120 mg of sodium in a single serving.

The American Heart Association recommends about four 1.5-ounce servings of unsalted nuts per week. According to MyPlate, 1 ounce of nuts is equivalent to about 24 almonds, 48 pistachios, or 14 walnut halves. Check the packaging for serving size details. For maximum nutritional benefit, choose a variety of nuts—walnuts, almonds, pecans, macadamia nuts, and hazelnuts. Peanuts, which are technically legumes, can also be included in your healthy nut consumption.

Q How can I achieve a "perfect" body?

A The current cultural ideal of an ultratoned, ultrafit body is impossible for most people to achieve. A reasonable goal for body weight and body shape must take into account your heredity, weight history, social circumstances, metabolic rate, and psychological well-being. Don't set goals based on movie stars or fashion models. Modern photographic techniques can make people look much different on film or in magazines than they do in person. Many of these people are also genetically endowed with body shapes that are impossible for most of us to emulate. The best approach is to work with what you've got. Adopting a wellness lifestyle that includes regular exercise and a healthy diet will naturally result in the best possible body shape for you. Obsessively trying to achieve unreasonable goals can lead to problems such as eating disorders, overtraining, and injuries.

SELECTED BIBLIOGRAPHY

2018 Physical Activity Guidelines Advisory Committee. 2018. *2018 Physical Activity Guidelines Advisory Committee Scientific Report*. Washington, DC: U.S. Department of Health and Human Services.

American Academy of Child and Adolescent Psychiatry. 2016. *Obesity in Children and Teens* (http://www.aacap.org/AACAP/Families_and_youth/Facts_for_Families/FFF-Guide/Obesity-In-Children-And-Teens-079.aspx).

American Psychiatric Association. 2013. *Diagnostic and Statistical Manual of Mental Disorders* (5th ed.). Washington, DC: American Psychiatric Publishing.

Andreyeva, T., A. S. Tripp, and M. B. Schwartz. 2015. Dietary quality of Americans by Supplemental Nutrition Assistance Program participation status: A systematic review. *American Journal of Preventive Medicine* 49(4): 594–604.

Aristizabal, J. C., et al. 2015. Effect of resistance training on resting metabolic rate and its estimation by a duel-energy X-ray absorptiometry metabolic map. *European Journal of Clinical Nutrition* 69(7): 831–836.

Arora, T., et al. 2016. The impact of sleep debt on excess adiposity and insulin sensitivity in patients with early type 2 diabetes mellitus. *Journal of Clinical Sleep Medicine* 12(5): 673–680.

Baer, D. J., and J. A. Novotny. 2019. Metabolizable energy from cashew nuts is less than that predicted by Atwater factors. *Nutrients* 11(1): 33. doi.org/10.3390/nu11010033.

Boulangé, C. L., et al. 2016. Impact of the gut microbiota on inflammation, obesity, and metabolic disease. *Genome Medicine* 8: 42.

Bray, M. S., et al. 2016. NIH working group report—using genomic information to guide weight management: From universal to precision treatment. *Obesity* 24(1): 14–22.

Brown, P. 2016. Carbohydrate study leaves diet researchers divided. *MedPageToday* (http://www.medpagetoday.com/primarycare/dietnutrition/59012).

Cava, E., N. C. Yeat, and B. Mittendorfer. 2017. Preserving healthy muscle during weight loss. *Advances in Nutrition* 8(3): 511–519.

Cheung, P. C., et al. 2016. Childhood obesity incidence in the United States: A systematic review. *Childhood Obesity* 12(1): 1–11.

Doucet, É., K. McInis, and S. Mahmoodianfard. 2018. Compensation in response to energy deficits induced by exercise or diet. *Obesity Reviews* 19(S1). doi: https://doi.org/10.1111/obr.12783

Fothergill, E., et al. 2016. Persistent metabolic adaptation 6 years after "The Biggest Loser" competition. *Obesity* 24(8): 1612–1619.

Freedhoff, Y., and K. D. Hall. 2016. Weight loss diet studies: We need help not hype. *Lancet* 388(10047): 849–851.

Gardner, C. D., et al. 2018. Effect of low-fat vs. low-carbohydrate diet on 12-month weight loss in overweight adults and the association with genotype pattern or insulin secretion: The DIETFITS randomized clinical trial. *JAMA* 319(7): 667–679.

GBD 2015 Obesity Collaborators. 2017. Health effects of overweight and obesity in 195 countries over 25 years. *New England Journal of Medicine*. doi:10.1056/NEJMoa1614362.

Global BMI Mortality Collaboration. 2016. Body-mass index and all-cause mortality: Individual-participant-data meta-analysis of 239 prospective studies in four continents. *Lancet* 388(10046): 776–786.

Guo, J., et al. 2019. Objective vs. self-reported energy intake changes during low-carbohydrate and low-fat diets. *Obesity* 27(3): 420–426.

Hall, K. D., et al. 2016. Energy expenditure and body composition changes after an isocaloric ketogenic diet in overweight and obese men. *American Journal of Clinical Nutrition* 104(2): 324–333.

Hall, K. D., et al. 2019. Ultra-processed diets cause excess calorie intake and weight gain: A one-month inpatient randomized controlled trial of ad libitum food intake. *Cell Metabolism* 30: 1–11.

Hall, K. D., S. J. Guyenet, and R. L. Leibel. 2018. The carbohydrate-insulin model of obesity is difficult to reconcile with current evidence. *JAMA Internal Medicine* 178(8): 1103–1105.

Harvard, T. H. Chan School of Public Health. 2015. *Toxic Food Environment: How Our Surroundings Influence What We Eat* (http://www.hsph.harvard.edu/obesity-prevention -source/obesity-causes/food-environment-and-obesity/).

Karl, J. P., et al. 2015. Effects of carbohydrate quantity and glycemic index on resting metabolic rate and body composition during weight loss. *Obesity* 23(11): 2190–2198.

Kaur, J., et al. 2015. The association between food insecurity and obesity in children— the National and Nutrition Examination Survey. *Journal of the Academy of Nutrition and Dietetics* 115: 751–758.

Kenney, E. L., and S. L. Gortmaker. 2016. United States adolescents' television, computer, videogame, smartphone, and tablet use: Associations with sugary drinks, sleep, physical activity, and obesity. *Journal of Pediatrics* S0022-3476(16): 31243–31244.

Kerns, J. C., et al. 2017. Increased physical activity associated with less weight regain six years after "The Biggest Loser" competition. *Obesity* 25(11): 1838–1843.

Khera, R., et al. 2016. Association of pharmacological treatments for obesity with weight loss and adverse events: A systematic review and meta-analysis. *Journal of the American Medical Association* 315(22): 2424–2434.

Kiviruusu, O., et al. 2016. Self-esteem and body mass index from adolescence to midadulthood. A 26-year follow-up. *International Journal of Behavioral Medicine* 23(3): 355–363.

Knab, A. M., et al. 2011. A 45-minute vigorous exercise bout increases metabolic rate for 14 hours. *Medicine and Science in Sports and Exercise* 43(9): 1643–1648.

Lasikiewicz, N., et al. 2014. Psychological benefits of weight loss following behavioural and/or dietary weight loss interventions. A systematic research review. *Appetite* 72: 123–137.

Levis, L. 2016. Are all calories equal? *Harvard Magazine* (https://harvardmagazine .com/2016/05/are-all-calories-equal).

Ludwig, D. 2016. Lifespan weighed down by diet. *Journal of the American Medical Association* 315(21): 2269–2270.

Ludwig, D. S., and C. B. Ebbeling. 2018. The carbohydrate-insulin model of obesity beyond "calories in, calories out." *JAMA Internal Medicine* 178(8): 1098–1103.

Mayo Clinic. 2018. *Bariatric Surgery* (https://www.mayoclinic.org/tests-procedures /bariatric-surgery/about/pac-20394258).

Mayo Clinic. 2019. *Nuts and Your Heart: Eating Nuts for Heart Health* (https://www .mayoclinic.org/diseases-conditions/heart-disease/in-depth/nuts/art-20046635).

Mazidi, M., et al. 2016. Gut microbiome and metabolic syndrome. *Diabetes and Metabolic Syndrome* 10 (2 Suppl 1): S150–S157.

Mozzafarian, D. 2016. Dietary and policy priorities for cardiovascular disease, diabetes, and obesity: A comprehensive review. *Circulation* 133(2): 187–225.

National Institute of Diabetes and Digestive Kidney Diseases. 2017. *Overweight & Obesity Statistics* (https://www.niddk.nih.gov/health-information/health-statistics /overweight-obesity).

NCD Risk Factor Collaboration. 2016. Trends in adult body-mass index in 200 countries from 1975 to 2014: A pooled analysis of 1698 population-based measurement studies with 19.2 million participants. *The Lancet* 387(10026): 1377–1396.

Nunez, C., et al. 2017. Obesity, physical activity and cancer risks: Results from the Cancer, Lifestyle and Evaluation of Risk Study (CLEAR). *Cancer Epidemiology* 47: 56–63.

Ogilvie, R. P., et al. 2016. Actigraphy measured sleep indices and adiposity: The Multi-Ethnic Study of Atherosclerosis (MESA). *Sleep* 39(9): 1701–1708.

Ostendorf, D. M., et al. 2019. Physical activity energy expenditure and total daily energy expenditure in successful weight loss maintainers. *Obesity* 27(3): 496–504.

Postrach, E., et al. 2013. Determinants of successful weight loss after using a commercial web-based weight reduction program for six months: Cohort study. *Journal of Medical Internet Research* 15(10): E219.

Romieu, I., et al. Energy balance and obesity: What are the main drivers? *Cancer Causes and Control* 28(3): 247–258.

Rouhani, M. H., et al. 2016. Associations between dietary energy density and obesity: A systematic review and meta-analysis of observational studies. *Nutrition* 32(10): 1037–1047.

Sheikh, V. K., and H. A. Raynor. 2016. Decreases in high-fat and/or high added-sugar food group intake occur when a hypocaloric, low-fat diet is prescribed within a lifestyle intervention: a secondary cohort analysis. *Journal of the Academy of Nutrition and Dietetics* 116(10): 1599–1605.

Siegel, K. R., et al. 2016. Association of higher consumption of foods derived from subsidized commodities with adverse cardiometabolic risk among US adults. *JAMA Internal Medicine* 176(8): 1124–1132.

Stanhope, K. L., et al. 2018. Pathways and mechanisms linking dietary components to cardiometabolic disease: Thinking beyond calories. *Obesity Reviews* 19(9): 1205–1235.

U.S. Department of Health and Human Services and U.S. Department of Agriculture. 2015. *2015-2020 Dietary Guidelines for Americans* (8th ed.) (https://health.gov /dietaryguidelines /2015/guidelines/).

U.S. Food and Drug Administration. 2018. *Tainted Weight Loss Products* (https://www .fda.gov/Drugs/ResourcesForYou/Consumers/BuyingUsingMedicineSafely /MedicationHealthFraud/ucm234592.htm).

Weiss, E. P., et al. 2017. Effects of weight loss on lean mass, strength, bone, and aerobic capacity. *Medicine and Science in Sports and Exercise* 49(1): 206–217.

Wilson, P. 2016. Physical activity and dietary determinants of weight loss success in the U.S. general population. *American Journal of Public Health* 106(2): 321–326.

Wong, J. C., et al. 2016. A glucocorticoid- and diet-responsive pathway toggles adipocyte precursor cell activity in vivo. *Science Signaling* 9(451): ra103.

Yanovski, S. Z., and J. A. Yanovski. 2014. Long-term drug treatment for obesity: A systematic and clinical review. *Journal of the American Medical Association* 311(1): 74–86.

Yu, E., et al. 2017. Weight history and all-cause and cause-specific mortality in three prospective cohort studies. *Annals of Internal Medicine* 166(9): 613–620.

Name _____ Section _____ Date _____

LAB 9.1 Calculating Daily Energy Needs

Part I Estimating Current Energy Intake from a Food Record

If your weight is stable, your current daily energy intake is the number of calories you need to consume to maintain your weight at your current activity level. For women, average calorie requirements are 1,600–2,400 calories per day; for men, 2,000–3,000. The low end of the range is for sedentary individuals, the high end for active individuals. In addition, caloric needs tend to decrease with age.

If you completed Lab 8.2, you should have a record of your current energy intake; if you didn't complete the lab, keep a careful and complete record of everything you eat for one day, and then total the calories in all the foods and beverages you consumed. Record your total energy intake here:

Current energy intake (from food record): _____ **calories per day**

Part II Estimating Daily Energy Requirements Using Food and Nutrition Board Formulas

Many people underestimate the size of their food portions, and so energy goals based on estimates of current calorie intake from food records can be inaccurate. You can estimate your daily energy needs using the following formulas. To use the appropriate formula for your sex, you'll need to plug in the following:

- Age (in years)
- Height (in inches)

- Weight (in pounds)
- Physical activity coefficient (PA) from the following table.

To help estimate your physical activity level, consider the following guidelines: Someone who typically engages in 30 minutes of moderate-intensity activity, equivalent to walking two miles in 30 minutes, in addition to the activities involved in maintaining a sedentary lifestyle, is considered "low active"; someone who typically engages in the equivalent of 90 minutes of moderate-intensity activity is rated as "active." You might find it helpful to refer back to Lab 2.3 to estimate your physical activity level. (Note: These formulas from the Dietary Reference Intakes are appropriate for normal-weight, overweight, and obese adults ages 19 years and older. They may be less accurate for people with a history of substantial weight loss.)

Physical Activity Level	Physical Activity Coefficient (PA)	
	Men	*Women*
Sedentary	1.00	1.00
Low active	1.12	1.14
Active	1.27	1.27
Very active	1.54	1.45

Estimated Daily Energy Requirement for Weight Maintenance in Men

$$864 - (9.72 \times age) + (PA \times [(6.39 \times weight) + (12.78 \times height)])$$

1. $9.72 \times$ _____ age (years) = _____
2. $864 -$ _____ result from step 1 = _____ [*result may be a negative number*]
3. $6.39 \times$ _____ weight (pounds) = _____
4. $12.78 \times$ _____ height (inches) = _____
5. _____ result from step 3 + _____ result from step 4 = _____
6. _____ PA (from table) × _____ result from step 5 = _____
7. _____ result from step 2 + _____ result from step 6 = _____ calories per day

LABORATORY ACTIVITIES

Estimated Daily Energy Requirement for Weight Maintenance in Women

$$387 - (7.31 \times age) + (PA \times [(4.91 \times weight) + (16.78 \times height)])$$

1. 7.31 × _____ age (years) = _____

2. 387 − _____ result from step 1 = _____ [*result may be a negative number*]

3. 4.91 × _____ weight (pounds) = _____

4. 16.78 × _____ height (inches) = _____

5. _____ result from step 3 + _____ result from step 4 = _____

6. _____ PA (from table) × _____ result from step 5 = _____

7. _____ result from step 2 + _____ result from step 6 = _____ calories per day

Daily energy needs for weight maintenance (from formula): _____ **calories/day**

Part III Determining an Individual Daily Energy Goal for Weight Maintenance

If you calculated values for daily energy needs based on both methods, examine the two values. Some difference is likely—people tend to underestimate their food intake and overestimate their level of physical activity—but if the two values are very far off, check your food record and your physical activity estimate for accuracy, and make any necessary adjustments. For an individualized estimate of daily calorie needs, average the two values:

Daily energy needs = (food record result _____ **calories/day + formula result** _____ **calories/day) ÷ 2 =** _____ **calories/day**

Using Your Results

How did you score? Are you surprised by the value you calculated for your approximate daily energy needs? If so, is the value higher or lower than you expected?

What should you do next? Enter the results of this lab in the Preprogram Assessment column in Appendix B. If you want to change your energy balance to lose weight, complete Lab 9.2 to set goals and develop specific strategies for change. (If your goal is weight gain, see the section on healthy weight gain in the chapter for basic guidelines.) One of the best ways to increase energy expenditure to help avoid slow weight gain over time is to make modest increases in your daily physical activity. If you include increases in activity as part of your program, then you can use the results of this lab to chart changes in your daily energy expenditure (and needs). Look for ways to increase the amount of time you spend in physical activity, thus increasing your physical activity coefficient. After several weeks of your program, complete this lab again, and enter the results in the Postprogram Assessment column of Appendix B. How do the results compare? Did your program for increasing physical activity show up as an increase in your daily energy expenditure and need?

SOURCE: Estimating Daily Energy Requirements Using Food and Nutrition Board Formulas Part II: Reprinted with permission from Dietary Reference Intakes for Energy, Carbohydrate, Fiber, Fat, Fatty Acids, Cholesterol, Protein, and Amino Acids (Macronutrients). Reprinted with permission from the National Academies Press, Copyright 2005, National Academy of Sciences.

Name _____   Section _____   Date _____

LAB 9.2   Identifying Weight-Loss Goals

Negative Calorie Balance

Complete the following calculations to determine your daily negative calorie balance goal.

Your current weight: _____ lb

Total pounds to lose: _____ lb

Your target weight (from Lab 6.2): _____ lb

Your target date for achieving your target weight: _____

Enter your personal data (age, sex, activity level) along with your current and target weight in the National Institute of Health's Body Weight Planner (https://www.niddk.nih.gov/bwp) to provide an estimate of the calorie level you'll need to achieve to meet your weight loss goal. Don't enter any changes in activity level at this point (leave the changes in activity level at 0%). Enter your results from the tool in the space provided; if the calorie level is not realistic, adjust your target weight and/or your target date. Also consider the calculated calorie requirement for weight maintenance; you need to choose a goal body weight that you can not only reach but also maintain over the long term.

Results from the Body Weight Planner:

(1) Calories to maintain current weight: _____ calories/day

(2) Calories to reach goal by target date: _____ calories/day

Subtract value 2 from value 1 to obtain your daily negative calorie balance: _____ **calories per day**

Also note the Body Weight Planner's calculation for maintaining your goal weight: _____ calories/day

To keep your weight-loss program on schedule, you must achieve the daily negative calorie balance by either decreasing your calorie consumption (eating less) or increasing your calorie expenditure (being more active). Combining the two strategies may be most successful. Following, make a plan for changes in activity and diet that will allow you to achieve your daily negative calorie balance.

Changes in Activity Level

Adding a few minutes of exercise every day is a good way to expend calories. Use the calorie costs for different activities listed in the following table.

Activity	Cal/lb/min	×	Body weight	×	min	=	Total calories
Aerobic dance	.046		_____		_____		_____
Basketball (half court)	.045		_____		_____		_____
Bicycling (casual)	.049		_____		_____		_____
Bicycling (13 mph)	.071		_____		_____		_____
Elliptical exercise	.049		_____		_____		_____
Football (touch)	.049		_____		_____		_____
Hiking	.051		_____		_____		_____
Housework	.029		_____		_____		_____
Jogging	.060		_____		_____		_____
Rope skipping	.071		_____		_____		_____
Rowing	.032		_____		_____		_____
Skating	.049		_____		_____		_____
Soccer	.052		_____		_____		_____
Swimming	.032		_____		_____		_____
Walking (normal pace)	.029		_____		_____		_____
Walking (briskly)	.048		_____		_____		_____

Activity	Duration	Calories Used
_____	_____	_____
_____	_____	_____
_____	_____	_____

Total calories expended: _____

LABORATORY ACTIVITIES

Changes in Diet

Look closely at your diet from one day, as recorded in Lab 8.2. Identify ways to cut calorie consumption by eliminating certain items or substituting lower-calorie choices. Be realistic in your cuts and substitutions; you need to develop a plan you can live with. For your substitute foods items, consider not only calories but how the food might affect your appetite; unprocessed foods high in fiber help you feel full.

Food Item	Substitute Food Item	Calorie Savings
_____	_____	_____
_____	_____	_____
_____	_____	_____

Total calories cut: _____

Total calories expended _____ **+ total calories cut** _____ **= total negative calorie balance** _____

Common Problem Eating Behaviors

For each group of statements, check those that are true for you. If you check several statements for a given pattern or problem, it will probably be a significant factor in your weight-management program. One possible strategy for dealing with each type of problem is given. For those eating problems you identify as important, add your own ideas to the strategies listed.

1. _____ I often skip meals.

   _____ I often eat a number of snacks in place of a meal.

   _____ I don't have a regular schedule of meal and snack times.

   _____ I make up for missed meals and snacks by eating more at the next meal.

Problem: Irregular eating habits

Possible solutions:

• Write out a plan for each day's meals in advance. Carry it with you and stick to it.

• _____

• _____

2. _____ I eat more than one sweet dessert or snack each day.

   _____ I usually snack on processed foods.

   _____ I drink regular (not sugar-free) soft drinks.

   _____ I choose types of meat that are high in fat.

   _____ I consume more than one alcoholic beverage a day.

Problem: Poor food choices

Possible solutions:

• Keep a supply of raw fruits and vegetables handy for snacks.

• _____

• _____

3. _____ I always eat everything on my plate.

   _____ I often go back for seconds and thirds.

   _____ I take larger helpings than most people.

   _____ I eat leftovers instead of putting them away.

Problem: Portion sizes too large

Possible solutions:

• Measure all portions with a scale or measuring cup.

• _____

• _____

Name _____ Section _____ Date _____

LAB 9.3 Checking for Body Image Problems and Eating Disorders

Assessing Your Body Image

	Never	Sometimes	Often	Always
1. I dislike seeing myself in mirrors.	0	1	2	3
2. When I shop for clothing, I am more aware of my weight problem, and consequently I find shopping for clothes somewhat unpleasant.	0	1	2	3
3. I'm ashamed to be seen in public.	0	1	2	3
4. I prefer to avoid engaging in sports or public exercise because of my appearance.	0	1	2	3
5. I feel somewhat embarrassed about my body in the presence of someone of the other sex.	0	1	2	3
6. I think my body is ugly.	0	1	2	3
7. I feel that other people must think my body is unattractive.	0	1	2	3
8. I feel that my family or friends may be embarrassed to be seen with me.	0	1	2	3
9. I find myself comparing myself with other people to see if they are heavier than I am.	0	1	2	3
10. I find it difficult to enjoy activities because I am self-conscious about my physical appearance.	0	1	2	3
11. Feeling guilty about my weight problem occupies most of my thinking.	0	1	2	3
12. My thoughts about my body and physical appearance are negative and self-critical.	0	1	2	3
Now add up the number of points you have circled in each column: _____	0	+ _____	+ _____	+ _____

Score Interpretation

The lowest possible score is 0, and this indicates a positive body image. The highest possible score is 36, and this indicates an unhealthy body image. A score higher than 14 suggests a need to develop a healthier body image.

SOURCE: Nash, J. D. *The New Maximize Your Body Potential*. Palo Alto, CA: Bull Publishing. Reprinted with permission from Bull Publishing. All rights reserved.

Eating Attitudes Test to Evaluate Eating Disorder Risk

To help determine whether you might have an eating disorder that needs professional attention, answer the questions as accurately, honestly, and completely as possible; there are no right or wrong answers.

Part 1. Eating Attitudes Test (EAT-26)

Circle a response for each of the following statements.

	Always	Usually	Often	Sometimes	Rarely	Never
1. Am terrified about being overweight.	3	2	1	0	0	0
2. Avoid eating when I am hungry.	3	2	1	0	0	0
3. Find myself preoccupied with food.	3	2	1	0	0	0
4. Have gone on eating binges where I feel that I may not be able to stop.	3	2	1	0	0	0
5. Cut my food into small pieces.	3	2	1	0	0	0
6. Aware of the calorie content of foods that I eat.	3	2	1	0	0	0
7. Particularly avoid food with a high carbohydrate content (i.e., bread, rice, potatoes, etc.).	3	2	1	0	0	0
8. Feel that others would prefer if I ate more.	3	2	1	0	0	0

	Always	Usually	Often	Sometimes	Rarely	Never
9. Vomit after I have eaten.	3	2	1	0	0	0
10. Feel extremely guilty after eating.	3	2	1	0	0	0
11. Am preoccupied with a desire to be thinner.	3	2	1	0	0	0
12. Think about burning up calories when I exercise.	3	2	1	0	0	0
13. Other people think that I am too thin.	3	2	1	0	0	0
14. Am preoccupied with the thought of having fat on my body.	3	2	1	0	0	0
15. Take longer than others to eat my meals.	3	2	1	0	0	0
16. Avoid foods with sugar in them.	3	2	1	0	0	0
17. Eat diet foods.	3	2	1	0	0	0
18. Feel that food controls my life.	3	2	1	0	0	0
19. Display self-control around food.	3	2	1	0	0	0
20. Feel that others pressure me to eat.	3	2	1	0	0	0
21. Give too much time and thought to food.	3	2	1	0	0	0
22. Feel uncomfortable after eating sweets.	3	2	1	0	0	0
23. Engage in dieting behavior.	3	2	1	0	0	0
24. Like my stomach to be empty.	3	2	1	0	0	0
25. Have the impulse to vomit after meals.	3	2	1	0	0	0
26. Enjoy trying new rich foods.	0	0	0	1	2	3

Total the points for your responses to determine your EAT-26 score: _____

Part 2. Behavioral Questions

Answer the following questions according to your behavior in the past 6 months. Check the boxes with the most appropriate responses.

In the past 6 months have you:	Never	Once a month or less	2–3 times a month	Once a week	2–6 times a week	Once a day or more
A Gone on eating binges where you feel that you may not be able to stop?						
B Ever made yourself sick (vomited) to control your weight or shape?						
C Ever used laxatives, diet pills, or diuretics (water pills) to control your weight or shape?						
D Exercised more than 60 minutes a day to lose or to control your weight?						
E Lost 20 pounds or more in the past 6 months	Yes		No			

Interpreting Your Results

If you meet one or more of the following criteria, evaluation by a qualified professional is recommended:

- A score of 20 or higher on EAT-26,
- A check in any of the gray boxes in the Behavioral Questions section, or
- A body mass index (BMI) that classifies you as underweight or very underweight using norms for sex and age (see the following table).

This screening is not designed to make a diagnosis of an eating disorder or take the place of a professional consultation. A high score on the EAT-26 assessment does not mean that you have an eating disorder, but it does indicate that you should seek the advice of a qualified mental health professional who has experience with treating eating disorders. If you have a low score on the EAT-26, you still could have problems with eating behavior or body image; if you are suffering from feelings that are causing you concern or interfering with your daily functioning, seek help.

Body Mass Index (BMI) Cutoffs for Classification of Underweight

Age (years)	Females					Males			
	18	19	20	20+		18	19	20	20+
Very underweight	≤17.5	≤17.5	≤17.5	≤18.5		≤18.0	≤18.5	≤19.0	≤19.5
Underweight	17.6–18.0	17.6–18.0	17.6–18.5	18.6–19.0		18.1–18.5	18.6–19.0	19.1–19.5	19.6–20.0

SOURCE: Garner, D. M., et al. 1982. "The eating attitudes test: Psychometric features and clinical correlates," *Psychological Medicine* 12, no. 4: 871–878.

Using Your Results

How did you score? Are you surprised by your scores? Do the results of either assessment indicate that you may have a problem with body image or disordered eating?

What should you do next? If your results are borderline, consider trying some of the self-help strategies suggested in the chapter. If body image or disordered eating is a significant problem for you, get professional advice; a physician, therapist, and/or registered dietitian can help. Make an appointment today.

Stress Management and Sleep

LOOKING AHEAD...

After reading this chapter, you should be able to

- Explain what stress is and how people react to it.

- Describe the relationship between stress and disease.

- List common sources of stress.

- Describe techniques for preventing and managing stress.

- Put together a plan for managing the stress in your life.

- Explain the consequences of disrupted sleep and strategies for improving sleep.

TEST YOUR KNOWLEDGE

1. Which of the following events can cause stress?
   a. taking out a loan
   b. failing a test
   c. graduating from college

2. Exercise stimulates which of the following?
   a. analgesia (pain relief)
   b. birth of new brain cells
   c. relaxation

3. Which of the following can be a result of chronic stress?
   a. violence
   b. heart attack
   c. stroke

See answers on the next page.

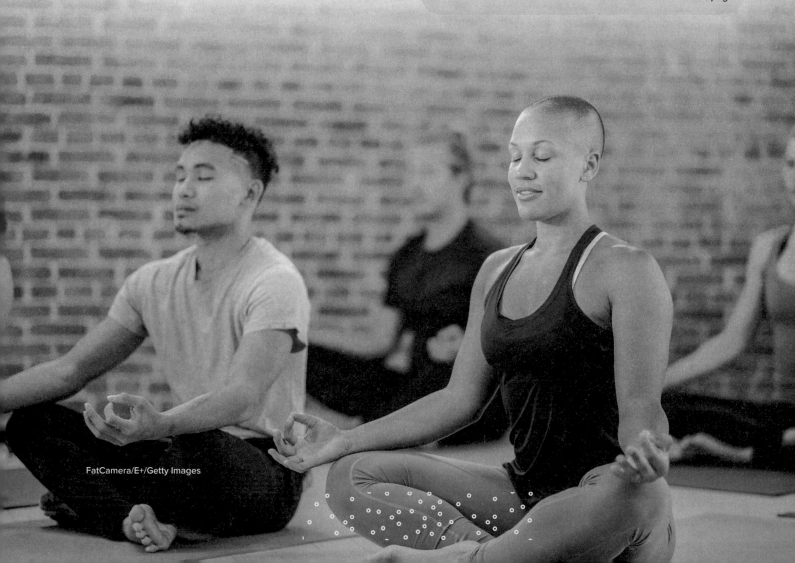

FatCamera/E+/Getty Images

Like the term *fitness, stress* is a word many people use without understanding its precise meaning. Stress is popularly viewed as an uncomfortable response to a negative event, which probably describes *nervous tension* more than the cluster of physical and psychological responses that actually constitutes stress. In fact, stress is not limited to negative situations: It is also a response to pleasurable physical challenges and the achievement of personal goals. Whether stress is experienced as pleasant or unpleasant depends largely on the situation and the individual.

Because learning effective responses to stress can enhance psychological health and help prevent a number of serious diseases, stress management can be an important part of daily life. In this chapter we explain the physiological and psychological reactions that make up the stress response and how these reactions can be risks to good health. We also present a variety of methods of managing stress and establishing healthy sleep patterns.

WHAT IS STRESS?

In common usage, the term *stress* refers to two things: the mental states or events that trigger physical and psychological reactions *and* the reactions themselves. We use the more precise term **stressor** for a situation that triggers physical and emotional reactions and the term **stress response** for those reactions. We use the term **stress** to describe the general physical and emotional state that accompanies the stress response.

Each person's experience of stress depends on many factors, including the nature of the stressor and how the person perceives it. Thoughts or feelings about an approaching event—a first date or a final exam—can be just as stressful as the event itself, or more so. Stressors take many forms. Like a fire in your home, some occur suddenly and neither last long nor repeat. Others, like air pollution or quarreling parents, can continue for a long time. The memory of a stressful occurrence, such as the loss of a loved one, can itself be a stressor years after the event. Responses to stressors can include a wide variety of physical, emotional, and behavioral changes. A short-term response might be an upset stomach or insomnia, whereas a long-term response might be a change in your personality or social relationships.

Physical Responses to Stressors

Imagine that you are crossing the street when suddenly a car comes racing around the corner, straight toward you. With a fraction of a second to spare, you leap out of harm's way. In that split second of danger and the moments that followed, you experienced a predictable series of physical reactions. Your body went from a relaxed state to one prepared for physical action to cope with a threat to your life.

Two systems in your body are responsible for your physical response to stressors: the nervous system and the endocrine system. Through rapid chemical reactions affecting almost every part of your body, these systems allow you to act quickly and appropriately.

The Nervous System The nervous system consists of the brain, spinal cord, and nerves. Part of the nervous system is under voluntary control, as when you tell your arm to reach for an orange. What is not under conscious supervision—for example, the part that controls the digestion of the orange—is the **autonomic nervous system**. In addition to digestion, it controls your heart rate, breathing, blood pressure, and hundreds of other involuntary functions.

The autonomic nervous system consists of two divisions:

- The **parasympathetic division** is in control when you are relaxed. It aids in digesting food, storing energy, and promoting growth.
- The **sympathetic division** is activated during times of arousal, including exercise, and when you face an emergency or experience severe pain, anger, or fear.

Sympathetic nerves use the neurotransmitter **norepinephrine** (or *noradrenaline*) to affect nearly every organ, sweat gland, blood vessel, and muscle to enable your body to handle an emergency. In general, the sympathetic division commands your body to stop storing energy and to use it in response to a crisis.

The Endocrine System During stress, the sympathetic nervous system triggers the **endocrine system**. This system of glands,

TERMS

stressor Any physical or psychological event or condition that produces physical and psychological reactions.

stress response The physical and emotional reactions to a stressor.

stress The general physical and emotional state that accompanies the stress response.

autonomic nervous system The branch of the nervous system that controls basic body processes; consists of the sympathetic and parasympathetic divisions.

parasympathetic division A division of the autonomic nervous system that moderates the excitatory effect of the sympathetic division, slowing metabolism and restoring energy supplies.

sympathetic division A division of the autonomic nervous system that reacts to danger or other challenges by almost instantly accelerating body processes.

norepinephrine A neurotransmitter in the central nervous system that increases alertness and arousal, and speeds reaction time; also called *noradrenaline*.

endocrine system The system of glands, tissues, and cells that secretes hormones into the bloodstream to influence metabolism and other body processes.

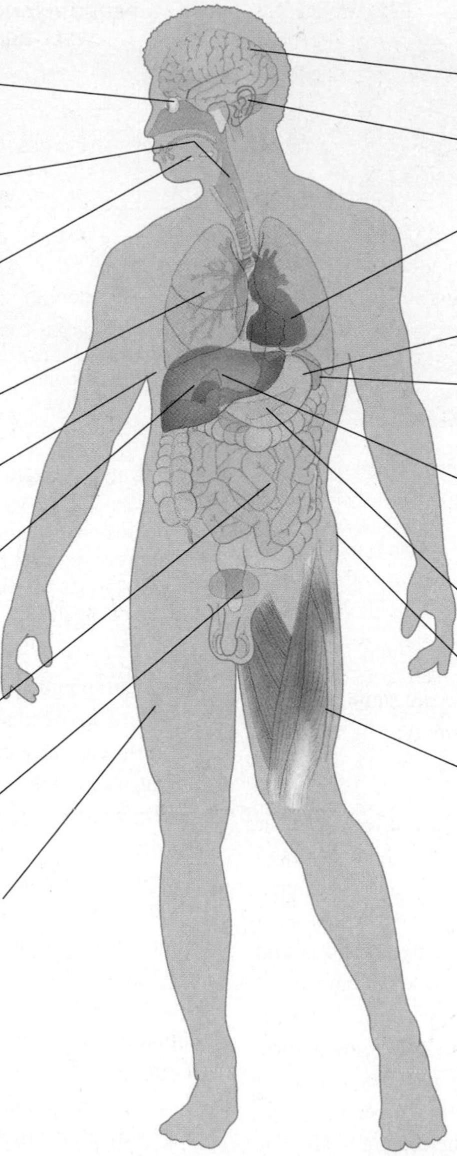

Pupils dilate to admit extra light for more sensitive vision.

Mucous membranes of nose and throat shrink, while muscles force a wider opening of passages to allow easier airflow.

Secretion of saliva and mucus decreases; digestive activities halt in an emergency.

Bronchi dilate to allow more air into lungs.

Perspiration increases, especially in armpits, groin, hands, and feet, to flush out waste and cool overheating system by evaporation.

Liver releases sugar into bloodstream to provide energy for muscles and brain.

Muscles of intestines stop contracting because digestion has halted.

Bladder relaxes. Emptying of bladder contents releases excess weight, making it easier to flee.

Blood vessels in skin and viscera contract; those in skeletal muscles dilate. This increases blood pressure and delivery of blood to where it is most needed.

Endorphins are released to block any distracting pain.

Hearing becomes more acute.

Heart rate accelerates and strength of contraction increases to allow more blood flow where it is needed.

Digestion, an unnecessary activity during an emergency, halts.

Spleen releases more red blood cells to meet an increased demand for oxygen and to replace any blood lost from injuries.

Adrenal glands stimulate secretion of epinephrine, increasing blood sugar, blood pressure, and heart rate; also spur increase in amount of fat in blood. These changes provide an energy boost.

Pancreas decreases secretions because digestion has halted.

Fat is removed from storage and broken down to supply extra energy.

Voluntary (skeletal) muscles contract throughout the body, readying them for action.

Figure 10.1   The fight-or-flight reaction.

tissues, and cells helps control body functions by releasing **hormones** and other chemical messengers into the bloodstream to influence metabolism and other body processes.

The Two Systems Together How do both systems work together in an emergency? Let's go back to your near-collision with a car. Reflexes as well as higher cognitive (thinking) areas in your brain quickly determine that you are facing a threat, and your body prepares to meet the danger. The two systems activate the adrenal glands, causing the release of the hormones **cortisol** and **epinephrine** (also called *adrenaline*). These hormones trigger the physiological changes shown in Figure 10.1. These changes, which include increases in heart and breathing rates and in the energy available to muscles, prepare your body for action. In addition, the brain releases **endorphins**—chemicals that can inhibit or block sensations of pain—in case you are injured.

Taken together, these almost-instantaneous physical changes are called the **fight-or-flight reaction**. They give you the heightened reflexes and strength you need to dodge the car or respond appropriately in the face of other stressors. Although

TERMS

hormone   A chemical messenger produced in the body and transported in the bloodstream to targeted cells or organs for specific regulation of their activities.

cortisol   A hormone secreted by the cortex (outer layer) of the adrenal gland; also called *hydrocortisone*.

epinephrine   A hormone secreted by the medulla (inner core) of the adrenal gland that affects the functioning of organs involved in responding to a stressor; also called *adrenaline*.

endorphins   Brain secretions that have pain-inhibiting effects.

fight-or-flight reaction   A defense reaction that prepares a person for conflict or escape by triggering hormonal, cardiovascular, metabolic, and other changes.

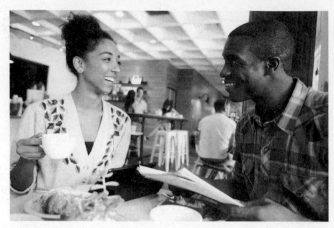

Wellness Tip Many people experience the set of almost-instantaneous physical changes that make up the stress response, such as increased heart rate and sweaty hands and feet, in reaction to positive stressors, such as a first date. Recognize the symptoms for what they are. If the physical stress response isn't appropriate for the situation, try a quick relaxation technique such as deep breathing.

monkeybusinessimages/Getty Images

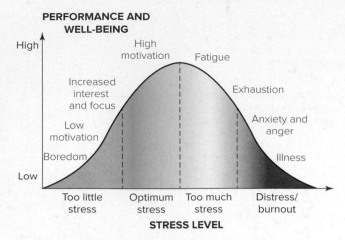

Figure 10.2 Stress level, performance, and well-being. A moderate level of stress challenges individuals in a way that promotes optimal performance and well-being. Too little stress, and people are not challenged enough to improve; too much stress, and the challenges become stressors that can impair physical and emotional health.

these physical changes may vary in intensity, the same basic set of physical reactions occurs in response to any type of stressor—positive or negative, physical or psychological.

The Return to Homeostasis A short time after your near miss with the car, you begin to feel normal again. When a stressful situation ends, the parasympathetic division of your autonomic nervous system takes command and halts the stress response. It restores **homeostasis**, a state in which your body stabilizes and maintains blood pressure, heart rate, hormone levels, and other vital functions. The parasympathetic nervous system calms your body by slowing a rapid heartbeat, drying sweaty palms, and returning breathing to normal. Gradually, your body resumes its normal "housekeeping" functions, such as digestion and temperature regulation. Ill effects of the stress response can be repaired. The day after you narrowly dodge the car, you wake up feeling fine. In this way, your body can grow, repair itself, and build energy reserves. When the next crisis comes, you'll be ready to respond again.

The Fight-or-Flight Reaction in Modern Life The fight-or-flight reaction is a part of our biological heritage, a survival mechanism that has served us well. In modern life, however, it is often absurdly inappropriate. Many stressors we face in everyday life—such as an exam, a mess left by a roommate, or a stop light—do not require a physical response. The fight-or-flight reaction prepares the body for physical action regardless of whether such action is a necessary or appropriate response to a particular stressor.

Cognitive and Psychological Responses to Stressors

We all experience a similar set of physical responses to stressors (the fight-or-flight reaction). People's perceptions of potential stressors, however—and their responses to them—can vary greatly, depending on our cognitive and psychological framework. You may feel confident about taking exams but nervous about

talking to people you don't know, while your roommate may love challenging social situations but dread taking tests.

Your cognitive appraisal of a potential stressor—how you think about it—strongly influences how you respond to it. Two factors that can reduce the magnitude of the stress response are successful prediction and the perception of control. For instance, receiving course syllabi at the beginning of the term allows you to predict the timing of major deadlines and exams. This gives you control over your study plans and can help reduce the stress caused by exams.

The way we appraise potentially stressful situations is highly individual and strongly related to emotions. The facts of a situation—Who? What? Where? When?—typically are evaluated fairly consistently from person to person. But evaluation with respect to personal outcome can vary: What does this mean for me? Can I do anything about it? Will it get better or worse? If you think you can't cope with a situation, you may respond negatively and with an inappropriate stress response. On the other hand, if you approach a situation as a challenge you can manage, you are likely to have a more positive and appropriate response. A moderate level of stress, if handled appropriately, can actually promote optimal performance (Figure 10.2).

Effective and Ineffective Responses Psychological responses to stressors include cognitive responses, which generally imply more emotion. Common psychological responses to stressors include anxiety, depression, and fear. Although emotional responses are determined in part by personality or temperament, we often moderate or learn to control them. Effective behavioral responses such as talking, laughing, exercising, meditating, learning time-management skills, and becoming more assertive can promote wellness and enable us to function at our best. Ineffective

homeostasis A state of stability and consistency in a person's physiological functioning. **TERMS**

behavioral responses to stressors include overeating; expressing hostility; and using tobacco, alcohol, or other drugs.

Personality and Stress You probably know some people who are nervous, irritable, and easily upset by minor annoyances, and other people who are calm and composed even in difficult situations. **Personality**—the sum of behavioral, cognitive, and emotional tendencies—clearly affects how people perceive and react to stressors. To investigate the links among personality, stress, and wellness, researchers have looked at characteristics such as "personality traits."

Some personality traits enable people to deal more successfully with stress. One such trait is *hardiness,* a form of optimism. People with a hardy personality view potential stressors as challenges and opportunities for growth and learning, rather than as burdens. Hardy people perceive fewer situations as stressful, and their reaction to stressors tends to be less intense. They are committed to their activities, have a sense of inner purpose and an inner locus of control, and feel at least partly in control of their lives.

Another important personality trait—*resilience*—is especially associated with social and academic success in groups at risk for stress, such as people from low-income families and those with mental or physical disabilities. Resilient people tend to face adversity by accepting the reality of their situation, holding on to a belief that life is meaningful, and possessing a great ability to improvise.

Academic resilience helps college students flourish. Whether they need to bounce back from a poor grade or negative feedback, or master the art of juggling multiple academic pressures, students can learn techniques to stay or become resilient. One technique is to identify resources such as peers and counselors to lean on in times of crisis.

Contemporary research is repeatedly demonstrating that you can change some basic elements of your personality as well as your typical behaviors and patterns of thinking by using positive stress-management techniques like those described later in the chapter.

Generation Z If you're reading this textbook in a college class, there's a good chance you belong to Generation Z, those born between 1997 and 2015. Gen Z was the focus of the American Psychological Association (APA) 2018 report, "Stress in America." Compared with other generations, Gen Zers report more stress over current issues dominating the news headlines—mass shootings, rising suicide rates, climate change and global warming, separation and deportation of immigrant and migrant families, and reports of sexual harassment and assault. Gen Zers are also the least likely to vote in elections.

Gen Zers also have a greater response to common stressors such as work, money, and health. They are the most likely of all generations to report poor mental health, especially young women. They also seek more professional help for mental health issues and are most likely to have been diagnosed with depression. Over half of Gen Zers find support by using social media—but 45% said social media makes them feel judged, and 38% said they feel bad about themselves because of using it.

Gender and Stress Your gender role—the activities, abilities, and behaviors your culture expects based on your sex—can affect your experience of stress. Some behavioral responses to stressors, such as crying or openly expressing anger, may be deemed more appropriate for one gender than another.

Strict adherence to gender roles, however, can limit your response to stress and can itself become a source of stress. Gender roles can also affect your perception of a stressor. For example, some medical situations may be more stressful for gay or bisexual men because they are often stereotyped as being HIV positive.

Since the APA began its yearly "Stress in America" survey in 2007, women have reported a higher level of stress than men. In her book *Overwhelmed,* Brigid Schulte describes a continuing unequal gendered division of labor: Families are working more hours than they used to, but American women spend even more time with their children than they did in the 1960s. How is this possible? Mothers tend to choose jobs that are flexible rather than high powered, and they spend less time cleaning (either hiring someone else or leaving their houses dirtier), sleep less, and take less time for themselves.

Cultural Background Because young adults from around the world come to the United States for a higher education, most students finish college with a greater appreciation for other cultures and worldviews. The clash of cultures, however, can be a big source of stress for many students—especially when it leads to disrespectful treatment, harassment, or violence. Everyone's reaction to stress is influenced by their upbringing and cultural background. Learning to accept and appreciate the cultural backgrounds of other people is both a mind-opening experience and a way to avoid stress over cultural differences.

Experience Past experiences can profoundly influence the way you evaluate a potential stressor. If you had a bad experience giving a speech in the past, you are much more likely to perceive an upcoming speech as stressful than someone who has had positive public-speaking experiences. Effective behavioral responses, such as preparing carefully and visualizing success, can help overcome the effects of negative past experiences.

? Ask Yourself

QUESTIONS FOR CRITICAL THINKING AND REFLECTION

Think of the last time you faced a significant stressor. How did you react? List the physical, cognitive, behavioral, and emotional reactions you experienced. Were the reactions appropriate to the circumstances? Did these reactions help you better deal with the stress, or did they interfere with your efforts to handle it?

personality The sum of behavioral, cognitive, and emotional tendencies. **TERMS**

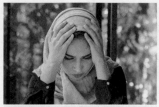
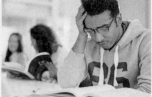

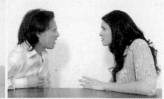

PHYSICAL SYMPTOMS	COGNITIVE SYMPTOMS	EMOTIONAL SYMPTOMS	BEHAVIORAL SYMPTOMS
Dry mouth	Confusion	Anxiety	Crying
Fatigue	Inability to concentrate	Depression	Disrupted eating habits
Frequent illnesses	Negative thinking	Edginess	Disrupted sleep
Gastrointestinal problems	Poor judgment	Hypervigilance	Problems communicating
Headaches	Worrying	Impulsiveness	Sexual problems
High blood pressure		Irritability	Social isolation
Pounding heart			Increased use of tobacco, alcohol, or other drugs
Sweating			

Figure 10.3 **Physical, cognitive, emotional, and behavioral symptoms of excessive stress.**

(left to right): Kdonmuang/Shutterstock; Tom Merton/Caia Images/Glow Images; fatchoi/iStock/Getty Images; Latinstock/Latin Stock Collection/Corbis

The Stress Experience as a Whole

As Figure 10.3 shows, the physical, emotional, cognitive, and behavioral symptoms of excess negative stress are distinct, but you might guess that they are also intimately interrelated. The more intense the emotional response, the stronger the physical response. Sometimes people have such intense responses to stressors or such ineffective coping techniques that they need professional help. More often, however, people can learn to handle stressors on their own (see the section "Managing Stress" later in the chapter).

STRESS AND WELLNESS

According to the APA "Stress in America" survey, the average overall stress level among Americans rose between 2016 and 2017, the first significant increase since the survey began in 2007. Increased stress rates corresponded to higher levels of physical and emotional stress symptoms: 80% of respondents reported having at least one symptom of stress in the past month. The role of stress in health is complex, but evidence suggests that stress can increase our vulnerability to many ailments. Several theories have been proposed to explain the relationship between stress and disease.

The General Adaptation Syndrome

The concepts of homeostasis (inner balance) and adaptations to stressors came from the work of several scientists across the 20th century. The **general adaptation syndrome (GAS)**, developed by biologist Hans Selye beginning in the 1930s and 1940s, is a theory that describes a universal and predictable response pattern to all stressors. It identifies an automatic self-regulation system of the mind and body that attempts to return the body to a state of homeostasis after being subjected to stress.

Some stressors are viewed as pleasant, such as attending a party, while others are viewed as unpleasant, such as getting a bad grade. In the GAS theory, stress triggered by a positive stressor is called **eustress**; stress triggered by a negative stressor is called **distress**. The sequence of physical responses associated with GAS (Figure 10.4) is the same for both eustress and distress and occurs in three stages:

- *Alarm.* The alarm stage includes the complex sequence of events brought on by the fight-or-flight reaction. At this stage, the body is more susceptible to disease or injury because it is geared up to deal with a crisis. Someone in this phase may experience headaches, indigestion, anxiety, and disrupted sleeping and eating patterns.

- *Resistance.* With continued stress, the body develops a new level of homeostasis in which it is more resistant to disease and injury than normal. In this stage, a person can cope with normal life and added stress.

- *Exhaustion.* The first two stages of GAS require a great deal of energy. If a stressor persists, or if several stressors occur in succession, general exhaustion results. This is not the sort of exhaustion you feel after a long, busy day. Rather, it's a life-threatening type of physiological exhaustion.

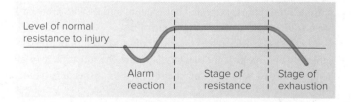

Level of normal resistance to injury

Alarm reaction | Stage of resistance | Stage of exhaustion

Figure 10.4 **The general adaptation syndrome.** During the alarm stage, a lower resistance to injury is evident. With continued stress, resistance to injury is actually enhanced. With prolonged exposure to repeated stressors, exhaustion sets in, with a return of low resistance levels seen during acute stress.

Stress research further advanced in the 1970s and 1980s with the advent of *biofeedback techniques.* Researchers developed instruments to measure brain waves, skin conduction, heart rates, and muscle tone (see discussion of biofeedback in the section "Managing Stress"). These tools allow the study of specific immediate and long-term impacts of the stress response.

Allostatic Load

The wear and tear on the body that results from long-term exposure to repeated or chronic stress is called the **allostatic load**. A person's allostatic load depends on many factors, including genetics, life experiences, and emotional and behavioral responses to stressors. The concept of allostatic load explains how frequent activation of the body's stress response, although essential for managing acute threats, can damage the body in the long run. For example, a student who suffers from test anxiety manages a week of exams but collapses on the weekend with a severe cold. Over time, the student's allostatic load, along with susceptibility to disease, can increase.

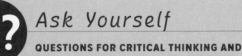

Ask Yourself

QUESTIONS FOR CRITICAL THINKING AND REFLECTION

Have you ever been so stressed that you felt ill in some way? If so, what were your symptoms? How did you handle them? Did the experience affect the way you reacted to other stressful events?

Stress and Specific Conditions

Although much remains to be learned, it is clear that people who have unresolved chronic (ongoing) stress in their lives or who handle stressors poorly are at risk for a wide range of health problems. In the short term, the problem might be a cold or a stomachache. Over the long term, the problems can be more severe, such as reduced functioning of the immune system and cardiovascular disease.

Stress and the Immune System Studies of the stress hormones cortisol and epinephrine have provided a physical link between emotions and immune function. In general, increased levels of stress hormones are linked to a decrease in the number or functioning of immune system cells. Some of the health problems linked to stress-related changes in immune function include vulnerability to colds and other infections, asthma and allergy attacks, and flare-ups of chronic diseases such as genital herpes.

Chronic stressors such as unemployment have negative effects on almost all functional measures of immunity. *Chronic stress* may cause prolonged secretion of cortisol (sometimes called the "antistress hormone" because it seeks to return the nervous system to homeostasis after a stress reaction) and may accelerate the course of diseases that involve inflammation, including multiple sclerosis, heart disease, type 2 diabetes, and clinical depression.

Mood, personality, behavior, and immune functioning are intertwined. For example, people who are generally pessimistic may neglect the basics of health care, become passive when ill, and fail to engage in health-promoting behaviors. People who are depressed may reduce physical activity and social interaction, which may in turn affect the immune system and their cognitive appraisal of stressors. Optimism, successful coping, and problem solving, by contrast, may positively influence immunity.

Cardiovascular Disease The stress response profoundly affects the cardiovascular system. During the stress response, heart rate increases, blood vessels constrict, and blood pressure rises. Chronic high blood pressure is a major cause of strokes and heart attacks (Chapter 11). As a related matter, people who react to situations with anger and hostility are more likely to have heart attacks than are people with less explosive, more relaxed personalities.

Other Health Problems Many other health problems may be caused or worsened by excessive stress, including the following:

- Digestive problems such as stomachaches, diarrhea, constipation, irritable bowel syndrome, and ulcers

- Tension headaches and migraines

- Insomnia and fatigue

- Injuries, including on-the-job injuries caused by repetitive strain

- Menstrual irregularities, impotence, and pregnancy complications

- Psychological problems, including depression, anxiety, panic attacks, eating disorders, and posttraumatic stress disorder (PTSD), which afflicts people who have suffered or witnessed severe trauma

COMMON SOURCES OF STRESS

Recognizing potential sources of stress is an important step in successfully managing the stress in your life.

Major Life Changes

Any major change in your life that requires adjustment and accommodation can be a source of stress. Early adulthood and the college years are associated with many significant changes, such as moving out of the family home and into a new, unfamiliar environment. Even changes typically thought of as positive— graduation, job promotion, marriage—can be stressful.

allostatic load The long-term negative impact of the stress response on the body.

Life changes that are traumatic, such as getting fired or divorced or experiencing the death of a loved one, may be linked to subsequent health problems in some people. Personality and coping skills, however, are important moderating influences. People with a strong support network and a stress-resistant personality are less likely to become ill in response to life changes than are people with fewer resources.

Daily Hassles

Although major life changes are undoubtedly stressful, they seldom occur regularly. Researchers have proposed that minor problems—life's daily hassles, such as losing your keys or sitting in traffic—can be an even greater source of stress because they occur much more often.

People who perceive hassles negatively are likely to experience a moderate stress response every time they are faced with one. Over time, this can take a significant toll on health. Studies indicate that for some people, daily hassles contribute to a general decrease in overall wellness.

College Stressors

College is a time of major changes and minor hassles. For many students, college means being away from home and family for the first time. Nearly all students share stresses like the following:

- *Academic stress.* Exams, grades, and heavy workloads await every college student but can be especially troublesome for young students just out of high school.

- *Interpersonal stress.* All students are more than just students; they are also friends, sons and daughters, employees, spouses, parents, and so on. Managing relationships while juggling the rigors of college life can be daunting.

- *Time pressures.* Class schedules, assignments, and deadlines are an inescapable part of college life. But these time pressures can be compounded dramatically for students who also have a job or family responsibilities.

- *Financial concerns.* The majority of college students need financial aid not just to cover the cost of tuition but also to survive from day to day while in school. For many, college life isn't possible without a job, and the pressure to stay afloat financially competes with academic and other stressors.

- *Worries about the future.* As college life comes to an end, students face the reality of life after college. This means thinking about a career, choosing a place to live, and leaving behind the friends and routines of school.

Job-Related Stressors

Worries about job performance, salary, job security, and interactions with others can contribute to stress. Tight schedules and overtime leave less time for exercising, socializing, and other stress-proofing activities. High levels of job stress are also common for people who are left out of important decisions relating

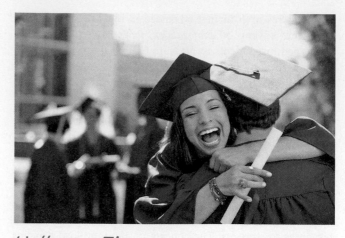

Wellness Tip Even a joyful occasion can be a source of stress, especially if it involves a major life change. To combat the stress of major life changes, develop a strong social support network and focus on the positive opportunities presented by the changes.

Paul Bradbury/OJO Images/age fotostock

to their jobs. When workers are given the opportunity to shape their job descriptions and responsibilities, job satisfaction goes up and stress levels go down.

If job-related (or college-related) stress is severe or chronic, the result can be *burnout,* a state of physical, mental, and emotional exhaustion. Burnout occurs most often in highly motivated and driven individuals who come to feel that their work is not recognized or that they are not accomplishing their goals. People in the helping professions—teachers, social workers, caregivers, police officers, and so on—are also prone to burnout. For some people who suffer from burnout, a vacation or leave of absence may be appropriate. For others, a reduced work schedule, better communication with superiors, or a change in job goals may be necessary. Improving time-management skills can also help.

Relationships and Stress

Human beings need social relationships; we cannot thrive as solitary creatures. Simply put, people need people. Even so, our interpersonal relationships—even our deepest, most intimate ones—can be one of the most significant sources of stress in our life.

The first relationships we form outside the family are friendships. Friendships give people the opportunity to share themselves and discover others. Friendships are often more stable and longer lasting than intimate partnerships. Because expectations surrounding friends differ from those surrounding romantic partners, friends are often more accepting and less critical than lovers. During times of stress, in fact, many people initially turn to their friends for comfort, rather than family members or lovers.

Intimate love relationships are among the most profound human experiences. When two people fall in love, their relationship at first is likely to be characterized by high levels of passion and rapidly increasing intimacy. In time, passion decreases as the partners become more familiar. The diminishing passion can

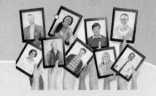

Stress is universal, but an individual's response to stress can vary depending on gender, cultural background, prior experience, and genetic factors. In diverse multiethnic and multicultural nations such as the United States, some groups face special stressors and have higher-than-average rates of stress-related physical and emotional problems. These groups include ethnic and sexual minorities, the poor, and those with physical or mental disabilities.

Discrimination occurs when people speak or act according to their prejudices—biased, negative beliefs or attitudes toward a group. Rising to the level of hate speech and criminal activity would be painting a swastika on a Jewish community center or vandalizing a mosque. A more subtle example would be when Middle Eastern American or African American students notice that shopkeepers tend to monitor them more closely. More than 60% of U.S. adults report experiencing day-to-day discrimination, such as being treated with less courtesy or respect, receiving poorer service than others, or being harassed or threatened.

Immigrants to the United States have to learn to live in a new society. Doing so requires a balance between assimilating to fit in with the majority culture and maintaining a connection to their own culture, language, and religion. The process of acculturation is generally stressful, especially when the person's background is radically different from that of the people he or she is now living among, or when people in the new community are suspicious or unwelcoming, as has recently been the case with immigrants from war-torn regions of the Middle East.

One study using 20 years of data found that the more racial discrimination participants reported experiencing or perceiving, the more dysfunctional their cortisol rhythms were. Cortisol levels normally start high in the morning, decrease throughout the day, and lower in the evening. But constant stress can alter this rhythm, keeping cortisol levels flat during the day and high at night. Irregular cortisol rhythms are linked with weakened immunity, cardiovascular disease, mental health and cognitive problems such as impaired memory, as well as fatigue and disrupted sleep. Another study showed

that while perceived discrimination produces stress in both blacks and whites, its impact on cortisol rhythms was greater for the black participants.

Many people who experience hardship and prejudice develop effective goal-directed coping skills. Some of these skills include building support networks where people share experiences; discovering and maintaining a strong cultural identity (for example, taking a class on the history of one's own cultural background, or joining campus cultural groups); and joining groups working for social action and equality.

SOURCES: Adam, E. K., et al. 2015. "Developmental histories of perceived racial discrimination and diurnal cortisol profiles in adulthood," *Psychoneuroendocrinology* 62: 279–91; American Psychological Association. 2016. *Stress in America: The Impact of Discrimination.* Washington, DC: American Psychological Association; Anderson, K. F. 2013. "Diagnosing discrimination: Stress from perceived racism and the mental and physical health effects," *Sociological Inquiry* 83: 55–81; Cook, S. H., et al. 2017. "Cortisol profiles differ by race/ethnicity among young sexual minority men," *Psychoneuroendocrinology* 75: 1–4.

create stress (usually affecting one partner more than the other) and can be experienced as a crisis in the relationship. If a quieter, more lasting love fails to emerge, the relationship will likely break up, and each person will search for another who will once again ignite his or her passion.

The key to developing and maintaining any type of friendship or intimate relationship is good communication. Miscommunication creates frustration and distances us from our friends and partners. (For more information, see the section "Communication" later in this chapter.)

Social Stressors

Social networks can be real or virtual. Both types can improve your ability to deal with stress, but they can also become stressors.

Real Social Networks The college years can be a time of great change in interpersonal relationships—becoming part of a new community, meeting people from different backgrounds, leaving old relationships behind. You may feel stress as you meet people of other ethnic, racial, or socioeconomic groups. You may feel torn between sticking with people who share your

background versus connecting with individuals and groups you've not encountered before. If English is not your first language, you may face the added burden of interacting in a language with which you are not completely comfortable. All these pressures can become significant sources of stress. (See the box "Diverse Populations, Discrimination, and Stress.")

Virtual Social Networks Technology can connect you with people all over the world and make many tasks easier, but it can also increase stress. Being electronically connected to work, family, and friends all the time can impinge on your personal space, waste time, and distract you. The 2017 "Stress in America" survey looked at "constant checkers"—the 43% of Americans who report continually checking their e-mails, texts, or social media accounts. These constant checkers report higher levels of overall stress than those who do not engage with technology as frequently. They are also more likely to report feeling disconnected from their family as a result of technology and to being stressed by political and cultural discussions on social media. Many Americans feel that taking breaks from technology is important for mental health, but fewer than 30% of them actually do so.

The overall conclusion from many published studies is that exercise—even modest activity such as taking a daily walk—can combat a variety of mental health problems. Overall, physically active people who exercise 2.5–7.5 hours per week are about 25–30% less likely to feel anxious or stressed than inactive people. Regardless of the number, age, or health status of the people being studied, those who were active managed stress better than their inactive counterparts. Among athletic teenagers, there is a correlation between exercise and improved social interaction, as well as between exercise and improved body image, two factors that contribute to good mental health. Physical activity has also been shown to improve conditions for people with anxiety; with affective, eating, and substance use disorders; and with schizophrenia and dementia.

A simple walk can be very effective: One study found that taking a long walk can reduce anxiety and blood pressure. Another showed that a brisk walk of as little as 10 minutes' duration can leave people feeling more relaxed and energetic for up to two hours. People who took three brisk 45-minute walks each week for three months reported that they perceived fewer daily hassles and had a greater sense of general wellness.

These findings are not surprising. The stress response mobilizes energy resources and readies the body for physical emergencies. If you experience stress and do not exert yourself physically, you are not completing the energy cycle. You may not be able to exercise while your daily stressors are occurring, but you can be active later in the day. Such activity allows you to expend the nervous energy you have built up and trains your body to return more readily to homeostasis after stressful situations. Physical activity also helps you sleep better, which is in turn critical to managing stress (see the section "Sleep" later in the chapter). Regular activity promotes better sleep and provides some protection against sleep interruptions such as insomnia and sleep apnea. Consistent, restful sleep is now regarded as a protective factor in disorders such as depression, anxiety, obesity, and heart disease.

SOURCES: Stubs, B., et al. 2017. "An examination of the anxiolytic effects of exercise for people with anxiety and stress-related disorders: A meta-analysis," *Psychiatry Research* 249: 102–108; Kim, Y. S., et al. 2012. "Relationship between physical activity and general mental health," *Preventive Medicine* 55(5): 458–463; Zschucke, E., et al. 2013. "Exercise and physical activity in mental disorders: Clinical and experimental evidence," *Journal of Preventive Medicine and Public Health* J46 (Suppl. 1): S12–S21; Eime, R. M., et al. 2013. "A systematic review of the psychological and social benefits of participation in sport for children and adolescents: Informing development of a conceptual model of health through sport," *International Journal of Behavioral Nutrition and Physical Activity* 10: 98.

Other Stressors

Environmental stressors are external conditions or events that cause stress and include a noisy atmosphere, unpleasant odors, pollen, industrial accidents, violence, and natural disasters. (See Appendix A for preparation and coping strategies for large-scale disasters.) Internal stressors are the pressures we put on ourselves to reach personal goals. Striving to reach goals can enhance self-esteem if the goals are reasonable, but unrealistic expectations can damage self-esteem and become a significant source of stress. Physical states such as illness and exhaustion, and emotional states such as despair or hostility, are also internal stressors.

MANAGING STRESS

Can you do anything about all this stress? A great deal.

- Develop healthy exercise and eating habits.
- Shore up your support system.
- Improve your communication skills.
- Identify and moderate individual stressors.
- Practice relaxation and mindfulness techniques.

Adequate sleep is another key strategy for managing stress and for improving your overall wellness. See the section "Sleep" later in the chapter.

Exercise

Researchers have found that people who exercise regularly react with milder physical stress responses before, during, and after exposure to stressors. Exercisers' overall sense of well-being increases as well (see the box "Does Exercise Improve Mental Health?"). Although even light exercise can have a beneficial effect, an integrated fitness program can have a significant impact on stress.

For some people, however, exercise can become just one more stressor in an already stressful life. People who exercise compulsively risk overtraining, a condition characterized by fatigue, irritability, depression, and diminished athletic performance. An overly strenuous exercise program can even make a person sick by compromising immune function. (For information on creating a safe and effective exercise program, refer to Chapter 7.)

Nutrition

A healthy, balanced diet can help you cope with stress. Eating wisely enhances your feelings of self-control and self-esteem. Avoiding or limiting caffeine may also be important in stress management. Caffeine, a mildly addictive stimulant, leaves some people jittery, irritable, and unable to sleep. Consuming caffeine during stressful situations can raise blood pressure and increase levels of cortisol. (For more on sound nutrition and for advice on evaluating dietary supplements, many of which are marketed for stress management, see Chapter 8.)

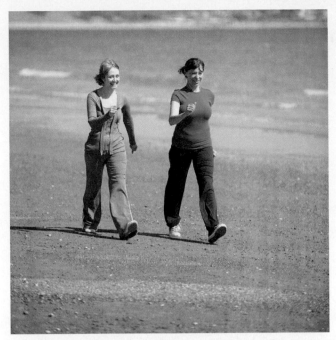

Fitness Tip Stressed out? Then walk away—literally. Walking is a proven countermeasure against stress. A brisk, 10-minute walk may be enough to help you put things in perspective and get back to your normal routine. If not, just keep walking until you feel better. As you walk, try not to think too much about anything specific; the idea is to clear your head!

Pamplemousse/OJO Images/Getty Images

Social Support

Meaningful connections with others can play a key role in stress management and overall wellness. One study of college students living in overcrowded apartments, for example, found that those with a strong social support system were less distressed by their cramped quarters than those who navigated life's challenges on their own. Other studies have shown that married people live longer than single people and have lower death rates from a wide range of conditions, although some studies suggest that marriage benefits men more than women. A sense of isolation can lead to chronic stress, which in turn can increase one's susceptibility to illnesses like colds and to chronic illnesses, such as heart disease. Although the mechanism isn't clear, social isolation can be as significant to mortality rates as factors like smoking, high blood pressure, and obesity.

Maintaining Social Ties Here are some tips for strengthening your social ties:

- *Foster friendships.* Keep in regular contact with your friends. Offer respect, trust, and acceptance, and provide help and support in times of need. Build your communication skills, and express appreciation for your friends.

- *Keep your family ties strong.* Stay in touch with the family members you feel close to. If your family doesn't function well as a support system for its members, create a second "family" of people with whom you have built meaningful ties.

- *Get involved with a group.* Do volunteer work, take a class, attend a lecture series, or join a religious group. These types of activities can give you a sense of security, a place to talk about your feelings or concerns, and a way to build new friendships. Choose activities that are meaningful to you and that include direct involvement with other people.

Combating Loneliness More than 25% of college students report stress because they are lonely. Studies show that these are mostly first-year students who are away from their friends and family and feel uncomfortable in social situations. Here are some tips toward solving this problem:

1. Start by writing down what is making you feel lonely. Validate your feelings by knowing that most people have moments of loneliness.

2. If you meet someone you like, invite him or her to lunch, coffee, or some area of the campus you like to visit. Don't be put off by one or more rejections. Keep trying.

3. Talk on the phone to friends or family. Just the sound of their voice has been shown to reduce the feeling of loneliness.

4. Find out a schedule of events on campus. Choose ones you may have a minor interest in. You are likely to meet someone like yourself.

5. If you feel uncomfortable initiating a conversation, start by making eye contact with people. This can become a lead-in to starting a conversation.

6. Volunteer for projects on campus or local nonprofit organizations. This leads to more interactions with people.

7. Speak to someone sitting near you in class. Ask him or her something about the lecture or the textbook or how to handle specific assignments.

8. Organize a group visit to a museum or nearby attraction.

9. Don't minimize what you are feeling. Ask family or a friend, "Do you ever feel lonely?" This will potentially lead to further exploration about solving this problem.

10. If you just feel stymied by this problem, ask people at the counseling center to help you.

Communication

Good communication skills can help everyone form and maintain healthy relationships. Communicating in an assertive, confident way that respects the rights of others—as well as your own—can prevent potentially stressful situations from getting out of control. When friends or partners communicate effectively, they can reduce the stresses in their relationship and spend more time focusing on the positive aspects of being together.

Three keys to good communication in relationships are self-disclosure, listening, and feedback:

- *Self-disclosure* involves revealing personal information that we ordinarily wouldn't reveal because of the risk involved. It usually increases feelings of closeness and moves the relationship to a deeper level of intimacy.

TAKE CHARGE
Guidelines for Effective Communication

Getting Started

- When you want to have a serious discussion with your partner, choose an appropriate time and place. Find a private place and a time when you will not be interrupted. Avoid having important conversations via text or other media.

- Face your partner and maintain eye contact. Use nonverbal feedback (gestures and facial expressions) to show you are interested and involved in the communication process.

Managing Conflicts

- State your concern or issue as clearly as you can.

- Use "I" statements—statements about how *you* feel—rather than statements beginning with "You," which tell another person how you think he or she feels. When you use "I" statements, you are taking responsibility for your feelings. "You" statements are often blaming or accusatory and may get a defensive or resentful response. "I feel unloved," sends a clearer, less blaming message than "You don't love me."

- Focus on a specific behavior rather than on the whole person. Be specific about the behavior you like or don't like. Avoid generalizations beginning with "You always" or "You never." Such statements make people feel defensive.

- Make constructive requests. Opening your request with "I would like" keeps the focus on your needs rather than on your partner's deficiencies.

- Avoid blaming, accusing, and belittling. Even if you are right, you have little to gain by putting people down. Studies have shown that when people feel criticized or attacked, they are less able to think rationally or solve problems constructively.

- Set your partner up for success. Tell your partner what you would like to have happen in the future; don't wait for him or her to blow it and then express anger or disappointment.

Being an Effective Listener

- Provide appropriate nonverbal feedback.

- Don't interrupt.

- Develop the skill of reflective listening. Don't judge, evaluate, analyze, or offer solutions (unless asked to do so). Your partner may just need to have you there in order to sort out feelings. By jumping in right away to "fix" the problem, you may be cutting off communication.

- Don't offer unsolicited advice. Giving advice implies that you know more about what a person needs to do than he or she does; therefore, it often evokes anger or resentment.

- Clarify your understanding of what your partner is saying by restating it in your own words and asking if your understanding is correct.

- Be sure you are really listening, not off somewhere in your mind rehearsing your reply. Tune in to your partner's feelings and needs as well as the words. Accurately reflecting the other person's feelings and needs is often a more powerful way of connecting than just reframing his or her thoughts.

- Let your partner know that you value what she or he is saying and want to understand. Respect for the other person is the cornerstone of effective communication.

- *Listening* is a rare skill. Those with good listening skills focus their time and energy on fully understanding another person's "story" rather than on judging, evaluating, blaming, advising, analyzing, or trying to control. Empathy, warmth, respect, and genuineness are qualities of skillful listeners. Attentive listening encourages friends or partners to share more and, in turn, to be attentive listeners. To connect with other people and develop real emotional intimacy, listening is essential.

- *Feedback,* a constructive response to another's self-disclosure, is the third key to good communication. Giving positive feedback means acknowledging that the friend's or partner's feelings are valid—no matter how upsetting or troubling—and offering self-disclosure in response. Self-disclosure and feedback can open the door to change.

For tips on improving your communication skills, see the box "Guidelines for Effective Communication."

Some people have trouble telling others what they need or saying no to the needs of others. They may suppress their

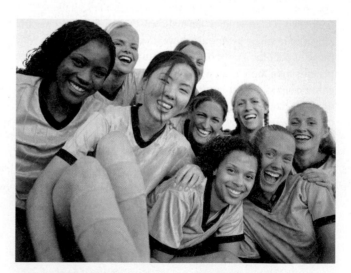

Wellness Tip Social support can be a key means of reducing stress. College offers many antidotes to loneliness in the forms of clubs, organized activities, sports, and just hanging out with friends.

Lori Adamski Peek/Getty Images

feelings of anger, frustration, and resentment, and they may end up feeling taken advantage of or suffering in unhealthy relationships. At the other extreme are people who express anger openly and directly by being verbally or physically aggressive or indirectly by making critical, hurtful comments to others. Their abusive behavior pushes other people away, so they also have problems with relationships.

If you typically suppress your feelings, you might want to take an assertiveness training course that can help you identify and change your patterns of communication. If you have trouble controlling your anger, you can benefit from learning anger-management strategies; see the box "Dealing with Anger."

Conflict Resolution

Conflict is natural in any relationship, and it can become a key source of stress for friends, coworkers, family members, and intimate partners. No matter how close two people become, they still remain separate individuals with their own needs, desires, past experiences, and ways of seeing the world. Conflict itself isn't dangerous to a relationship; it may simply indicate that the relationship is growing. But if it isn't handled in a constructive way, conflict can damage—and ultimately destroy—a relationship.

Conflict is often accompanied by anger—a universal emotion, but one that can be difficult to handle. When angry, both parties should back off, calm down, and then come back to the issue later to try to resolve it rationally.

Negotiation helps dissipate anger so the conflict can be resolved. Some basic strategies are useful in successfully negotiating with a friend, family member, colleague, or intimate partner:

1. *Clarify the issue.* Take responsibility for thinking through your feelings and discovering what's really bothering you. Agree that one of you will speak first and have the chance to speak fully while the other listens. Then reverse the roles. Try to understand the other person's position fully by repeating what you've heard and asking questions to clarify or elicit more information.

2. *Find out what each person wants.* Ask the other person to express her or his desires. Don't assume you already know what those desires are, and don't try to speak for your friend or partner.

3. *Determine how both of you can get what you want.* Brainstorm to generate a variety of options.

4. *Work out a plan for change.* For example, agree that one of you will do one task and the other will do another task or that one of you will do a task in exchange for something she or he wants.

5. *Solidify the agreements.* Go over the plan verbally and write it down, if necessary, to ensure that both of you understand and agree to it.

6. *Review and renegotiate.* Decide on a time frame for trying out the new plan and set a time to discuss how it's working. Make adjustments as needed.

Striving for Spiritual Wellness

Spiritual wellness is associated with more effective coping skills and higher levels of overall wellness. Researchers have linked spiritual wellness to longer life expectancy, reduced risk of disease, faster recovery, and improved emotional health. Although spirituality is difficult to define and study, and exactly how spirituality seems to improve health is unclear, researchers have linked spiritual wellness to longer life expectancy, reduced risk of disease, faster recovery, and improved emotional health. To develop spiritual wellness, choose activities that are meaningful to you, such as the following:

Look inward. Spend quiet time alone with your thoughts and feelings:

- Spend time in nature, experiencing continuity with the natural world.
- Notice art, architecture, or music.
- Engage in a favorite activity that allows you to express your creative side.
- Engage in a personal spiritual practice, such as prayer, meditation, or yoga.

Reach out to others:

- Share writings that inspire you.
- Practice small acts of personal kindness for people you know as well as for strangers.
- Perform community service.

Confiding in Yourself through Writing

Keeping a diary is like confiding in someone else, except that you are confiding in and becoming more attuned to yourself. This form of coping with severe stress may be especially helpful for those who find it difficult to open up to others. Although writing about traumatic and stressful events may have a short-term negative effect on mood, over the long term, stress is reduced and positive changes in health occur. A key to promoting health and well-being through journaling is to write about your emotional responses to stressful events. Set aside a special time each day or week to write down your feelings about stressful events in your life.

Time Management

Learning to manage your time can be crucial to coping with everyday stressors. Over commitment, procrastination, and even boredom are significant stressors for many people. Try these strategies for improving your time-management skills:

- *Set priorities.* Divide your tasks into three groups: essential, important, and trivial. Focus on the first two, and ignore the third.
- *Schedule tasks for peak efficiency.* You probably know that you're most productive at certain times of the day (or night). Schedule as many of your tasks for those hours as you can, and stick to your schedule.

Anger is a universal response to something we perceive as injustice, betrayal, insult, or some other wrong—whether real or imagined. We often respond physically with faster heart and breathing rates, muscle tension, trembling, a knot in the stomach, or a red face. When anger alerts us that something is wrong, it is a useful emotion that can lead to constructive change. When anger leads to loss of control and to aggression, it causes problems.

According to current popular wisdom, it's healthy to express your feelings, including anger. However, research has shown that people who are overtly hostile are at higher risk for heart disease and heart attacks than calmer people. In addition, expressing anger in thoughtless or out-of-control ways can damage personal and professional relationships.

Some people who experience rage or explosive anger may have *intermittent explosive disorder,* characterized by aggressiveness that is impulsive and out of proportion to the stimulus. Explosive anger renders people temporarily unable to think straight or act in their own best interests. Counseling can help very angry people learn how to manage their anger.

In dealing with anger, distinguish between self-assertiveness and aggression. When you are *assertive,* you stand up for your own rights at the same time that you respect the rights of others. When you are *aggressive,* you may violate the rights of others.

Managing Your Own Anger

What are the best ways to handle anger? If you find yourself in a situation where you are getting angry, answer these questions:

- Is the situation important enough to get angry about?
- Are you truly justified in getting angry?
- Is expressing your anger going to make a positive difference?

If the answer to all these questions is yes, then calm, assertive communication may be appropriate. Use "I" statements to express your feelings ("I would like . . ." "I feel . . ."), and listen respectfully to the other person's point of view. Don't attack verbally or make demands; try to negotiate a constructive, mutually satisfying solution.

If you answer no to any of the questions, try to calm yourself. First, reframe the situation by thinking about it differently. Try these strategies:

- Don't take it personally. Maybe the driver who cut you off simply didn't see you.
- Look for mitigating factors. Maybe the classmate who didn't say hello was preoccupied.
- Practice empathy. See the situation from the other person's point of view.
- Ask questions. Clarify the situation by asking what the other person meant. Avoid defensiveness.
- Focus on the present. Don't let this situation trigger thoughts of past incidents that you perceive as similar.

Second, calm your body.

- Use the old trick of counting to 10 before you respond.
- Concentrate on your breathing, taking long, slow breaths.
- Imagine yourself in a beautiful, peaceful place.
- If needed, take a longer cooling-off period by leaving the situation until your anger has subsided.

Dealing with Other People's Anger

If someone you are with becomes very angry, try these strategies:

- Respond "asymmetrically" by reacting not with anger but with calm.
- Apologize if you think you are to blame. (Don't apologize if you don't think you are to blame.)
- Validate the other person by acknowledging that he or she has some reason to be angry. However, don't accept verbal abuse.
- Focus on the problem and ask what can be done to alleviate the situation.
- If the person cannot be calmed, disengage from the situation, at least temporarily. After a time-out, attempts at rational problem solving may be more successful.

Warning Signs of Violence

Violence is never acceptable. The following behaviors, feelings, or circumstances over a period of time suggest the potential for violence:

- A history of making threats and engaging in aggressive behavior
- Drug or alcohol abuse
- Gang membership
- Access to or fascination with weapons
- Expression of feelings of rejection or aloneness, of constantly being disrespected or of victimization by bullies
- Withdrawal from usual activities and friends; poor school performance
- Failure to acknowledge the rights of others

The following are immediate warning signs of violence:

- Daily loss of temper or frequent physical fighting
- Significant vandalism or property damage
- Increased risk-taking behavior; increased drug or alcohol abuse
- Threats or detailed plans to commit acts of violence
- Pleasure in hurting animals
- The presence of weapons

Avoid people who shows these warning signs of violence. Don't carry a weapon or resort to violence to protect yourself. Ask someone in authority or an experienced professional for help.

- *Set realistic goals and write them down.* Attainable goals spur you on. Impossible goals, by definition, cause frustration and failure. Fully commit yourself to achieving your goals by putting them in writing.

- *Budget enough time.* For each project you undertake, calculate how much time you will need to finish it. Then tack on another 10–15%, or even 25%, as a buffer.

- *Break up long-term goals into short-term ones.* Instead of waiting for large blocks of time, use short amounts of time to start a project or keep it moving.

- *Visualize achieving your goal.* By mentally rehearsing a task, you will be able to do it more smoothly.

- *Keep track of the tasks you put off.* Analyze the reasons you procrastinate. If the task is difficult or unpleasant, look for ways to make it easier or more fun. For example, if you find the readings for one of your classes particularly difficult, choose an especially nice setting for your reading, and then reward yourself each time you complete a section or chapter.

- *Consider doing your least favorite tasks first.* Once you have the most unpleasant ones out of the way, you can work on the tasks you enjoy more.

- *Consolidate tasks when possible.* For example, try walking to the store so that you run your errands and exercise in the same block of time.

- *Identify quick transitional tasks.* Keep a list of 5- to 10-minute tasks you can do while waiting or between other tasks, such as watering your plants, doing the dishes, or checking a homework assignment.

- *Delegate responsibility.* Asking for help when you have too much to do is no cop-out; it's good time management. Just don't delegate the jobs you know you should do yourself.

- *Say no when necessary.* If the demands made on you don't seem reasonable, say no—tactfully but without guilt or apology.

- *Give yourself a break.* Allow time for play—free, unstructured time when you can ignore the clock. Don't consider this a waste of time. Play renews you and enables you to work more efficiently.

- *Avoid your personal "time sinks."* You can probably identify your own time sinks—activities like watching television, surfing the internet, or talking on the phone—that consistently use up more time than you anticipate and put you behind schedule. On particularly busy days, avoid these problematic activities altogether; for example, if you have a big paper due, don't sit down for a five-minute TV break if it is likely to turn into a two-hour break. Try a five-minute walk instead.

- *Stop thinking or talking about what you're going to do, and just do it!* Sometimes the best solution for procrastination is to stop waiting for the right moment and just get started. You will probably find that things are not as bad as you feared, and your momentum will keep you going.

For more help with time management, complete Activity 10 in the Behavior Change Workbook.

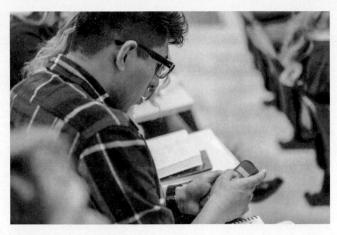

Wellness Tip Managing the many commitments of adult life—including work, school, and parenthood—can sometimes feel overwhelming and produce a great deal of stress. Time-management and problem-solving skills, including careful scheduling with a date book, smartphone, or tablet, can help you cope with busy days.
Hill Street Studios/Tobin Rogers/Getty Images

Cognitive Techniques

Certain thought patterns and ways of thinking, including ideas, beliefs, and perceptions, can contribute to stress and have a negative impact on health. But other habits of mind, if practiced with patience and consistency, can help break unhealthy thought patterns. An important skill is to distinguish between types of stressors: *eustress* or "challenge stressors" create positive experiences and opportunities for growth, versus *distress* or "hindrance stressors," which can impede growth and life satisfaction levels.

Practice Affirmations and Avoid Negative Self-Talk If you tend to beat up on yourself—"Late for class again! You can't even cope with college! How do you expect to ever hold down a real job?"—try being kind to yourself instead. Monitor your self-talk and try to minimize hostile, critical, suspicious, and self-deprecating thoughts. Substituting positive self-talk for negative self-talk can help you build and maintain self-esteem and cope better with the challenges in your life (Table 10.1).

Act Constructively and Problem Solve Focus on things you can control. Accept what you can't change, forgive others for their faults, and be flexible. Identify key stressors that you can address, and take a constructive approach to dealing with them. If you find yourself stewing over a problem, try this approach:

1. Define the problem in one or two sentences.

2. Identify the causes of the problem.

3. Consider several alternative solutions. Don't stop with the most obvious one.

4. Weigh positive and negative consequences for each alternative.

Table 10.1	Avoiding Negative Self-Talk	
COGNITIVE DISTORTION	NEGATIVE SELF-TALK	POSITIVE SELF-TALK
Focusing on negatives	School is so discouraging—nothing but one hassle after another.	School is pretty challenging and has its difficulties, but there certainly are rewards. It's really a mixture of good and bad.
Expecting the worst	Why would my boss want to meet with me this afternoon if not to fire me?	I wonder why my boss wants to meet with me. I guess I'll just have to wait and see.
Overgeneralizing	[After getting a poor grade on a paper] Just as I thought—I'm incompetent at everything.	I'll start working on the next paper earlier. That way, if I run into problems I'll have time to talk to the TA.
Minimizing	I won the speech contest, but none of the other speakers was very good. I wouldn't have done as well against stiffer competition.	It may not have been the best speech I'll ever give, but it was good enough to win the contest.
Blaming others	I wouldn't have eaten so much last night if my friends hadn't insisted on going to that restaurant.	I overdid it last night. Next time I'll make different choices.
Expecting perfection	I should have scored 100% on this test. I can't believe I missed that one problem through a careless mistake.	Too bad I missed one problem through carelessness, but overall I did very well on this test. Next time I'll be more careful.

5. Make a decision—that is, choose a solution.

6. Make a list of things you must do to act on your decision.

7. Do them.

8. Evaluate the outcome and revise your approach if necessary.

Modify Your Expectations and Live in the Present

The fewer expectations you have, the more you can live spontaneously and joyfully in the present. Try to accept life as it comes. The more you expect from others, the more often you will feel let down. And trying to meet the expectations others have of you is often futile.

Cultivate Your Sense of Humor

Even a fleeting smile produces changes in your autonomic nervous system that can lift your spirits. Hearty laughter triggers the release of endorphins, and after a good laugh, your muscles go slack and your pulse and blood pressure dip below normal; you are relaxed.

Relaxation and Body Awareness Techniques

The **relaxation response** is a physiological state characterized by a feeling of warmth and quiet mental alertness. This state is the opposite of the fight-or-flight response. When you induce the relaxation response by using a relaxation technique, your heart rate, breathing, and metabolism slow down. Blood pressure and oxygen consumption decrease. At the same time, blood flow to the brain and skin increases, and brain waves shift from an alert beta rhythm to a relaxed alpha rhythm.

relaxation response A physiological state characterized by a feeling of warmth and quiet mental alertness.

TERMS

The techniques described in this section are among the most popular and easiest to learn. All of them take practice, so it may be several weeks before the benefits become noticeable in everyday life.

Progressive Muscle Relaxation In this simple relaxation technique, you tense and then relax the muscles of the body one group at a time. Also known as deep muscle relaxation, this technique addresses the muscle tension that occurs when the body is experiencing stress. Consciously relaxing tensed muscles sends a message to other body systems to reduce the stress response.

To practice progressive relaxation, begin by inhaling as you contract your right fist. Then exhale as you release your fist. Repeat. Contract and relax your right bicep. Repeat. Do the same using your left arm. Then, working from forehead to feet, contract and relax other muscles. Repeat each contraction at least once, inhaling as you tense and exhaling as you relax. To speed up the process, tense and relax more muscles at one time—for example, both arms simultaneously. With practice, you'll be able to relax quickly just by clenching and releasing only your fists.

Visualization Also known as imagery, visualization is so effective in enhancing sports performance that it has become part of the curriculum at training camps for U.S. Olympic athletes. This same technique can be used to improve performance on an exam, on stage, or on a playing field. Imagery can also help change habits and induce relaxation.

To practice visualization, imagine yourself floating on a cloud, sitting on a mountaintop, or lying in a meadow. Try to identify all the perceptible qualities of the environment—sight, sound, temperature, smell, and so on. Your body will respond as if your imagery were real.

An alternative is to close your eyes and imagine a deep purple light filling your body. Then change the color to a soothing gold. As the color lightens, so should your distress.

Deep Breathing Your breathing pattern is closely tied to your stress level. Deep, slow breathing is associated with relaxation. Rapid, shallow, often irregular breathing occurs during the stress response. With practice, you can learn to slow and quiet your breathing pattern, thereby also quieting your mind and relaxing your body. Try one of the breathing techniques described here for on-the-spot tension relief, as well as for long-term stress reduction.

BELLY BREATHING:

1. Lie on your back and relax.
2. Place one hand on your chest and the other on your abdomen. Your hands will help you gauge your breathing.
3. Take in a slow, deep breath through your nose and into your belly. Your abdomen should rise significantly (check with your hand); your chest should rise only slightly. Focus on filling your abdomen with air.
4. Exhale through your mouth, gently pushing out the air from your abdomen.

TENSION-RELEASE BREATHING:

1. Lie down or sit in a chair and get comfortable.
2. Take a slow, deep breath into your abdomen. Inhale through your nose. Try to visualize the air moving to every part of your body. As you breathe in, say to yourself, "Breathe in relaxation."
3. Exhale through your mouth. Visualize tension leaving your body. Say to yourself, "Breathe out tension."

These techniques have many variations. For example, sit in a chair and raise your arms, shoulders, and chin as you inhale; lower them as you exhale. Or slowly count to four as you inhale, then again as you exhale. Breathing in time to soothing music can work well, too. Experts suggest inhaling through the nose and exhaling through the mouth. Breathe slowly, deeply, and gently. To focus on breathing gently, imagine a candle burning a few inches in front of you. Try to exhale softly enough to make the candle's flame flicker, not hard enough to blow it out. Practice is important, too. Perform your chosen breathing exercise two or more times daily, for 5–10 minutes per session.

Body Awareness Techniques and Mindfulness
Mindfulness is both a mental state and the practices that cultivate this mental state. We cultivate mindfulness by paying attention to our mental states, physical activities, and behaviors as they happen. Practicing mindfulness promotes stronger connections between the brain's prefrontal cortex and amygdala. These connections have been demonstrated to facilitate improved problem-solving skills, emotional self-regulation, and resilience.

> **mindfulness** The intentional cultivation of attention in a way that is nonjudging and nonstriving. **TERMS**

Techniques for practicing mindfulness include forms of meditation (see the box "Mindfulness Meditation") as well as more familiar forms of neuromuscular activities.

YOGA Hatha yoga, the most common yoga style practiced in the United States, emphasizes physical balance and breath control. It integrates components of flexibility, muscular strength, endurance, and muscle relaxation. A session of yoga typically involves a series of postures, each held for a few seconds to several minutes. With yoga, you can cultivate body awareness, ease, and flexibility. If you are interested in trying yoga, take a class with an experienced instructor.

TAI CHI This martial art (in Chinese, *taijiquan*) is a system of self-defense that incorporates philosophical concepts from Taoism and Confucianism. Tai chi aims to bring the body into balance and harmony to promote health and spiritual growth. It teaches practitioners to remain calm and centered, to conserve and concentrate energy, and to manipulate force by becoming part of it—by "going with the flow." Tai chi consists of a series of slow, fluid, elegant movements that reinforce the idea of moving *with* rather than against the stressors of everyday life. As with yoga, it's best to start tai chi with a class led by an experienced instructor.

Listening to Music Music can relax us. It influences pulse, blood pressure, and the electrical activity of muscles. Listening to soothing music can lessen depression, anxiety, and stress levels. To experience the stress-management benefits of music, set aside a period of at least 15 minutes to listen quietly. Choose music you enjoy and selections that make you feel relaxed.

Other Stress-Management Techniques

Techniques such as biofeedback, hypnosis and self-hypnosis, and massage require a partner or professional training or assistance. As with the relaxation techniques presented, all take practice, and it may be several weeks before the benefits are noticeable.

Biofeedback helps people reduce their response to stress by enabling them to become more aware of their level of physiological arousal. In biofeedback, some measure of stress—perspiration, heart rate, skin temperature, or muscle tension—is electronically monitored, and feedback is given using sound (a tone or music), light, or a meter or dial. With practice, people begin to exercise conscious control over their physiological stress responses. The point of biofeedback training is to develop the ability to transfer the skill to daily life without the use of electronic equipment.

Counterproductive Strategies for Coping with Stress

As we've seen, there are many effective coping techniques for dealing with stress. However, college students sometimes develop habits in response to stress that are ineffective and

Mindfulness Meditation

Mindful Breathing

You are always breathing, so this is a powerful and convenient way to become present wherever you go and whatever you do. After you read these instructions, close your eyes and invest 5–15 minutes in being present with your breath. Sitting comfortably where you are right now, bring your body into a posture that is upright and supported, with a sense of balance and dignity. See if you can align your head, neck, and body in a way that is neither too rigid nor too relaxed, but somewhere in between. The intention is to be wakeful and alert, yet not tense; at ease, but not sleeping.

Bring attention to your breathing, wherever you feel it most prominently and notice the sensations of your breath coming and going as it will, in its own way and with its own pace. If your mind wanders from your breath, return to it by feeling the sensations of the breath as they come and go. Use these sensations as your way to be present, here and now, in each successive moment for the time you have set aside. Research has repeatedly demonstrated that extending this practice to 30 or 45 minutes on a regular basis significantly reduces stress and stress-related illnesses and conditions.

Many cultures have developed ways of quieting the mind over the centuries. Qigong, yoga, tai chi, and meditation can all complement or supplement other stress therapies.

At its most basic level, meditation involves quieting or emptying the mind to achieve deep relaxation. Some practitioners of meditation view it on a deeper level as a means of focusing concentration, increasing self-awareness, and bringing enlightenment to their lives. Meditation has been integrated into the practices of several religions—Buddhism, Hinduism, Confucianism, Taoism—but it is not a religion itself, nor does its practice require any special knowledge, belief, or background.

Walking Meditation

Find a place where you can walk and be uninterrupted by other people or traffic—if possible, in natural surroundings. You can adapt this practice to fit yourself, whatever your circumstances are with mobility—for example, it can become a mindful-rolling practice if you use a wheelchair. Once you're ready, begin walking—slowly at first (as slowly as possible for about 10 minutes)—paying close attention to each step and using the sensations of each foot touching the ground as your way to be present. When you are ready, accelerate your pace, broadening your attention to take in more of your experience as you walk. In this mindful-movement practice, you may walk any distance, anywhere, at any speed that feels right for you. In the beginning, however, give yourself about 30 minutes.

The key instruction is to be fully present in each moment you are walking rather than consumed with mind chatter or destination. Be open to the experience of your environment and notice, for example, the way clouds move or how the sunlight glistens in the trees and foliage around you. Turn toward whatever calls your attention and be with it as long as you like, stopping if you want to take a close look at a bug or flowers or to listen to the rustling of leaves.

As you become more skilled in mindful awareness practice, you will be able to do this anywhere, even on a bustling college campus. If you want to pick up the speed or duration of your walk, you can make this walking practice part of a regular exercise program, and you will grow in strength and cardiovascular health as well as mindfulness.

---

even unhealthy. Here are a few unhealthy coping techniques to avoid:

- *Alcohol.* A few drinks might make you feel at ease, and getting drunk may help you forget the stress in your life—but any relief alcohol provides is temporary. Binge drinking and excessive alcohol consumption are not effective ways to handle stress, and using alcohol to deal with stress puts you at risk for all the short- and long-term problems associated with alcohol abuse.

- *Tobacco.* The nicotine in cigarettes and other tobacco products can make you feel relaxed and may even increase your ability to concentrate. Tobacco, however, is highly addictive, and smoking causes cancer, heart disease, sexual problems, and many other health problems. Tobacco use is the leading preventable cause of death in the United States.

- *Other drugs.* Altering your body chemistry to cope with stress is a strategy with many pitfalls. Stimulants, such as amphetamines, can activate the stress response; they also affect the same areas of the brain that are involved in regulating the stress response. Repeated use of marijuana can elicit panic attacks. Opioids such as morphine and heroin can mimic the effects of your body's natural pain-killers and reduce anxiety; however, tolerance develops quickly, and many users become dependent.

- *Binge eating.* Eating can induce relaxation, which reduces stress. Eating as a means of coping with stress, however, may lead to weight gain and eating disorders.

There is one other problem with these methods of fighting stress: None of them addresses the actual cause of the stress in your life. To combat stress in a healthy way, learn some of the stress-management techniques described in this chapter.

GETTING HELP

You can use the principles of behavioral self-management described in Chapter 1 to create a stress-management program tailored specifically to your needs. The starting point of a successful program is to listen to your body. When you learn to

Choosing and Evaluating Mental Health Professionals

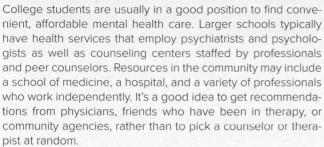

College students are usually in a good position to find convenient, affordable mental health care. Larger schools typically have health services that employ psychiatrists and psychologists as well as counseling centers staffed by professionals and peer counselors. Resources in the community may include a school of medicine, a hospital, and a variety of professionals who work independently. It's a good idea to get recommendations from physicians, friends who have been in therapy, or community agencies, rather than to pick a counselor or therapist at random.

In choosing a mental health professional, financial considerations are also important. Find out the costs and what your health insurance will cover. If you're not adequately covered by a health plan, don't let that stop you from getting help; investigate low-cost alternatives on campus and in your community. The cost of treatment is linked to how many therapy sessions will be needed, which in turn depends on the type of therapy and the nature of the problem. Psychological therapies focusing on specific problems may require 8–24 sessions at weekly intervals. Therapies aiming for psychological awareness and personality change can last months or years.

Deciding whether a therapist is right for you requires meeting the therapist in person. Before or during your first meeting, find out about the therapist's background and training:

- Does the therapist have a degree from an appropriate professional school and a state license to practice?

- Has the therapist had experience treating people with problems similar to yours?

- How much will therapy cost?

You have a right to know the answers to these questions and should not hesitate to ask them. After your initial meeting, evaluate your impressions:

- Does the therapist seem like a warm, intelligent person who would be able to help you and is interested in doing so?

- Are you comfortable with the personality, values, and beliefs of the therapist?

- Is the therapist willing to talk about the techniques he or she will use? Do these techniques make sense to you?

If you answer yes to these questions, this therapist may be satisfactory for you. If you feel uncomfortable—and if you are not in need of emergency care—it's worthwhile to set up one-time consultations with one or two others before you make up your mind. Take the time to find someone who feels right for you.

Later in your treatment, evaluate your progress:

- Are you being helped by the treatment?

- If you are displeased, is it because you aren't making progress or because therapy is raising difficult, painful issues you don't want to deal with?

- Can you express dissatisfaction to your therapist? Such feedback can improve your treatment.

If you're convinced your therapy isn't working or is harmful, thank your therapist for her or his efforts and find another.

---

recognize the stress response and the emotions and thoughts that accompany it, you'll be in a position to begin handling stress. Labs 10.1 and 10.2 can guide you in identifying and finding ways to cope with stress-inducing situations.

If you feel you need guidance beyond the information in this text, excellent self-help guides can be found in bookstores or the library; helpful websites are listed in "For Further Exploration" at the end of the chapter. Some people also find it helpful to express their feelings in a journal. Grappling with a painful experience in this way provides an emotional release and can help you develop more constructive ways of dealing with similar situations in the future.

Peer Counseling and Support Groups

If you still feel overwhelmed despite efforts to manage your stress, you may want to seek outside help. Peer counseling, often available through the student health center or counseling center, is usually staffed by volunteer students with special training that emphasizes maintaining confidentiality. Peer counselors can steer those seeking help to appropriate campus and community resources or just offer sympathetic listening.

Support groups are typically organized around a particular issue or problem: All group members might be entering a new school, reentering school after an interruption, struggling with

single parenting, experiencing eating disorders, or coping with particular kinds of trauma. Simply voicing concerns that others share can relieve stress.

Professional Help

Psychotherapy, especially a short-term course of sessions, can also be tremendously helpful in dealing with stress-related problems. Not all therapists are right for all people, so it's a good idea to shop around for a compatible psychotherapist who has reasonable fees. (See the box "Choosing and Evaluating Mental Health Professionals.")

Is It Stress or Something More Serious?

Most of us have periods of feeling down when we become pessimistic, anxious, less energetic, and less able to enjoy life. Such feelings and thoughts can be normal responses to the ordinary challenges of life. Symptoms that may indicate a more serious problem include the following:

- Depression, anxiety, or other emotional problems that interfere seriously with school or work performance or in getting along with others

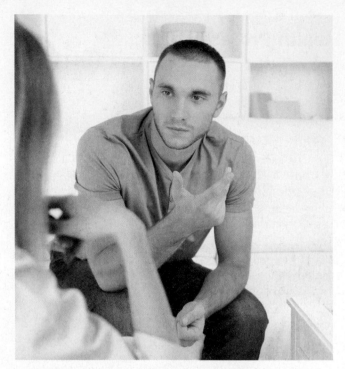

Wellness Tip The most important predictor of whether therapy will be helpful is how much rapport you feel with your therapist at the first session. You have to like your therapist and feel that she or he will be able to help you. If you do, there's a good chance that therapy will be helpful. If you seek professional help for stress-related problems, take the time to find someone who feels right for you.

Africa Studio/Shutterstock

- Attempted or serious consideration of suicide
- Symptoms such as hallucinations, delusions, incoherent speech, or loss of memory
- Alcohol or drug use to the extent that they impair normal functioning, occupy much of the week, or result in psychological or physical withdrawal symptoms when a dosage is reduced

Depression is of particular concern because severe depression is linked to suicide, one of the leading causes of death among college students, and the second leading cause of death for people age 10–34 years. In some cases, depression, like severe stress, is a clear-cut reaction to a specific event, such as losing a loved one or failing in school or work. In other cases, no trigger event is obvious. Depression differs from person to person but includes the following symptoms that persist most of the day and last more than two consecutive weeks:

- A feeling of sadness and hopelessness or loss of pleasure in doing usual activities (anhedonia)

depression A mood disorder characterized by loss of interest, sadness, hopelessness, loss of appetite, disturbed sleep, and other physical symptoms.

TERMS

- Poor appetite and weight loss, or alternatively, increased eating compared to usual
- Insomnia or disturbed sleep, including waking up and being unable to fall back to sleep or sleeping more than normal
- Decreased energy
- Restlessness or, alternatively, slowed thinking or activity
- Thoughts of worthlessness and guilt
- Trouble concentrating or making decisions
- Thoughts of death or suicide

Not everyone who is depressed has all these symptoms, but most have depressed mood or anhedonia and at least four other symptoms. Someone who has symptoms of major depression for more than two weeks, even if it is in reaction to a specific event, should consider treatment. About 60% of people who commit suicide are depressed. The more symptoms of depression a person has, the greater the risk. Warning signs of suicide include expressing the wish to be dead, revealing contemplated suicide methods, increasing social withdrawal and isolation, and exhibiting a sudden, inexplicable lightening of mood (which can indicate the person has finally decided to commit suicide).

If you are severely depressed or know someone who is, expert help from a mental health professional is essential. Most communities and many colleges have hotlines and/or health services and counseling centers that can provide help. The National Suicide Prevention Lifeline can be reached at 1-800-273-TALK. Treatments for depression and many other psychological disorders are highly effective.

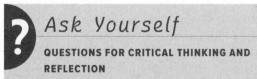

? *Ask Yourself*

QUESTIONS FOR CRITICAL THINKING AND REFLECTION

Have you ever felt depressed? If you have had symptoms of depression, did you do anything to relieve them? Have you considered seeking professional help?

SLEEP

The benefits of adequate sleep can hardly be overstated: Sleep is as important to healthy living as are healthful diet and exercise. To say that sleep has magical qualities is not an exaggeration. Adequate sleep improves memory, creativity, and mood; fosters feelings of competence and self-worth; and works against depression and anxiety. It lowers food craving and maintains a healthier immune system. New evidence continues to show that sleep helps prevent cardiovascular disease, diabetes, weight gain, certain cancers, and neurodegenerative diseases. The list goes on.

How Sleep Works: The Physiology of Sleep

During wakefulness the brain works with fast-frequency chaotic brain wave activity as it learns and takes in new experiences. Sleep then occurs in two phases with dramatically different purposes, characteristics, and brain wave patterns: non-rapid eye movement sleep (NREM) and rapid eye movement sleep (REM).

NREM Sleep NREM sleep includes stages of successively deeper sleep (N1, N2, N3). As you move through these stages, a variety of physiological changes occur: Your blood pressure drops, respiration and heart rates slow, body temperature declines, and growth hormone is released. Each state of sleep is characterized by a different pattern of electrical brain activity. Brain waves become slow and even in NREM sleep. Parts of the brain associated with memory, learning, and other cognitive functions can become active during stages N2 and N3. People in the deepest NREM stage are difficult to arouse quickly, and when awakened, they may be confused. For feeling rested, this stage is the most necessary.

REM Sleep The second phase of one sleep cycle, during which dreams occur. REM sleep is characterized by rapid movement of the eyes under closed eyelids, similar to when people move their eyes while awake. REM sleep waves closely resemble brain waves of alert wakefulness. Blood pressure and respiration and heart rates rise, protein synthesis peaks, and brain activity increases to levels equal to or greater than those during waking hours. In contrast, muscles in the limbs relax completely because the body is prevented from moving during dreaming, a form of paralysis.

Sleep Cycles When people fall asleep, they cycle through the stages of NREM and then REM sleep (Figure 10.5). The sequence lasts about 90 minutes, and then the ratios of NREM to REM repeats. During one night of sleep, a person is likely to go through four or five cycles, but the ratios of NREM to REM differ throughout the night: NREM periods are longer in the first part, and REM periods are longer in the last part. Because of this pattern, confusional awakening and sleepwalking are more likely to occur in the earlier part of the night, whereas dreaming is more likely to occur in the last part of the night.

Natural Sleep Drives

Two main forces drive us toward sleep—the homeostatic sleep drive and the circadian rhythm. Understanding how these work and learning how to strengthen them can have a big impact on sleep.

Homeostatic Sleep Drive The homeostatic sleep drive is the drive for sleep that builds up the longer you are awake. If you do not sleep all night, and you stay up the next day, you will feel an ever-increasing need to sleep. During daytime wakefulness, a neurochemical called adenosine accumulates in the brain. This is a by-product of energy used by the brain, and it promotes sleep onset. The homeostatic drive is strengthened if you get up at a reasonably early time in the morning and then remain awake until your intended bedtime at night. Naps or dozing in the afternoon will strongly reduce this sleep drive at night, as will sleeping late in the morning. People who have problems falling asleep or staying asleep can strengthen the sleep drive by avoiding naps and setting a reasonably early wake time goal every day. This allows for enough wake time during the day for the sleep drive to accumulate. Caffeine blocks the homeostatic sleep drive by blocking adenosine receptors in the brain. If a person has problems falling asleep, reducing caffeine intake can be very important.

Circadian Rhythm The circadian rhythm is the sleep and wake pattern coordinated by the brain's master internal clock, which sends signals throughout the body. You may be familiar with the sensation of jet lag—when a change of time zone causes the internal body clock to be out of sync with the new environment—but travel between time zones is not the only disrupter of circadian rhythm. Some people have habits that cause their internal body clocks to be set at a time that differs from the time zone where they live. An example is a person who stays up regularly until four in the morning and then sleeps until noon, a pattern called delayed sleep phase. When this person has to wake up earlier, the change can be difficult, and the person will feel poorly, just like a person with jet lag.

The master clock can be reset by "time-givers," or *zeitgebers*. Although there are many zeitgebers, including activity, exercise, and eating, the strongest is light. If a person is exposed to light in the morning at a certain time on a regular basis, it will indicate to the brain that it should set the internal clock to wake around that time. When light is reduced at night, as when natural dusk occurs, the internal clock triggers the production of melatonin. Melatonin signals

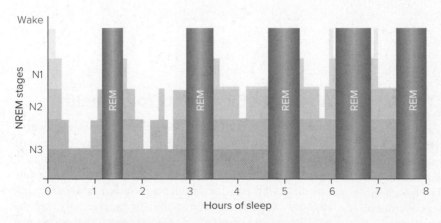

Figure 10.5 **Sleep stages and cycles.** During one night of sleep, we typically go through cycles of progressively deeper sleep stages followed by REM sleep.

SOURCES: Adapted from Krejcar, O., J. Jirka, and D. Janckulik. 2011. "Use of mobile phones as intelligent sensors for sound input analysis and sleep state detection," *Sensors* 11(6): 6037–6055.

Many apps are promoted as sleep aids and trackers. Can they really improve sleep? Or can using digital devices hurt the body's natural sleep cycles?

Digital Devices and Sleep

Before we look at sleep apps, let's consider how use of your digital devices can negatively affect your sleep. Tablets, smartphones, and computers emit blue light, which impedes the release of melatonin, a hormone that affects sleep and wake cycles. In one study, researchers compared the sleep of people who read an e-book on a digital device in the hours before bedtime with people who did so with a print book. Those who read the digital book took longer to fall asleep, had reduced melatonin release, and were less alert the next morning. In another study that compared the impact of playing smartphone games with either a standard or suppressed blue light phone, use of the blue light phone was associated with decreased sleepiness and worsened mood as well as a decline in memory performance.

Does heavy texting affect sleep? Psychologist Karla Murdock reported that texting was a direct predictor of sleep problems among first-year students in a study that examined links among interpersonal stress, text-messaging behavior, and three indicators of college students' health: burnout, sleep problems, and emotional well-being.

Murdock and other sleep experts suggest turning off your screens. Use them less during the day and also when preparing to sleep at night. If you have trouble relaxing and transitioning to sleep in the evenings, shut down all your devices an hour or more before you intend to sleep. Now that you are resting in the dark, why would you consider using a sleep app or digital tracker? Ironically, a smartphone may help you get to sleep—if you tuck it into the corner of your bed.

Digital Aids for Relaxation

Many free and low-cost apps provide aids to assist with relaxation and improve sleep. Some include music, white noise, or sounds of nature (e.g., wind, rain, waves, or songbirds). Others offer specific techniques, such as guided meditation or breathing exercises, to promote relaxation and sleep. Experiment to find the aids that work best for you.

Digital Sleep Trackers

More complicated technologies attempt to track and analyze sleep. Many are based on movement detectors in smartphones. These apps estimate the amount and type of sleep you get based on your movements during the night; they may generate detailed graphs of your sleep quality and then time your wake-up alarm to a specific sleep cycle. Some apps also include a sound recorder, which detects sleep talking, snoring, and other night noises, providing further information.

In addition to smartphone apps, specialized fitness wristbands such as those by Fitbit and Garmin include sleep trackers. Many of these are also based on movement detectors, but some incorporate heart-rate data as well; preliminary research indicates that adding heart-rate data to movement tracking may improve the accuracy of the results. Fitbit and other wearables, along with some apps, may combine sleep and fitness data into an overall picture of an individual's activity over the course of a day.

Apps and devices may be popular, but no consumer technology yet developed can equal the capability of a sleep lab at detecting sleep stages or diagnosing specific sleep disorders. If you enjoy the features of an app or wearable tracker, go ahead and use them, but don't rely on an app to diagnose the presence or absence of a serious sleep problem. One good effect of using a sleep tracker is simply the greater focus it places on sleep.

SOURCES: Heo, J. Y., et al. 2016. "Effects of smartphone use with and without blue light at night in healthy adults: A randomized, double-blind, cross-over, placebo-controlled comparison," *Journal of Psychiatric Research* 87: 61–70; Chang, A. M., et al. 2015. "Evening use of light-emitting eReaders negatively affects sleep, circadian timing, and next-morning alertness," *Proceedings of the National Academy of Sciences* 112(4): 1232–1237; Bhat, S., et al. 2015. "Is there a clinical role for smartphone sleep apps? Comparison of sleep cycle detection by a smartphone application to polysomnography," *Journal of Clinical Sleep Medicine,* February 3; Behar, J., et al. 2013. "A review of current sleep screening applications for smartphones," *Physiological Measurement* 34(7): R29–R46; Lewis, J. G. 2013. *Sleep cycle app: Precise, or placebo? Mind Read: Connecting Brain and Behavior* (http://www.nature.com/scitable/blog/mind-read/sleep_cycle_app_precise_or); Murdock, K. K. 2013. "Texting while stressed: Implications for students' burnout, sleep, and well-being," *Psychology of Popular Media Culture* 2(4): 207–221.

systems involved in preparation for sleep. People who are blind often have problems with sleep because they do not have the usual light signals to help synchronize their circadian rhythms.

The breakdown of circadian rhythm increases risk for illnesses such as diabetes, heart disease, and dementia. To strengthen the circadian rhythm, get good light exposure in the morning and daytime and reduce exposure to light at night. The challenge in the modern age is that we live with abundant sources of artificial light, which can insulate us from the natural 24-hour rhythm of the sun. For information on personal electronic devices and sleep, see the box "Digital Devices: Help or Harm for a Good Night's Sleep?"

Adequate Sleep and Your Health

Poor-quality or insufficient sleep has been associated with a number of health problems and impairments, including heart disease, high blood pressure, depression, stress, earlier death, increased risk for dementia, weight gain, poorer glucose control, increased risk for accidents, reduced motivation and attention, and increased irritability or hyperactivity (see the box "Sleep and Learning"). The good news is that people can improve their sleep and, in turn, their health. Along with exercise and good nutrition, good sleep is a critical pillar of good health.

Important learning occurs during sleep. Recent memories are reinforced, and some of them become permanent when awake. The connection of sleep to memory and learning is a relatively recent area of sleep science research. Around 100 years ago, the first sleep-memory experiments asked their subjects to learn a list of nonsense syllables. When subjects slept directly after learning the list, they could recall more syllables than if they had stayed awake. In a recent Harvard study, students learned to navigate a complex maze. Some then napped 90 minutes; others stayed awake. When the students tried to solve the maze again, only the few who dreamed about it during their naps did better. These results suggest that dreaming may reactivate and reorganize recently learned material, which would facilitate memorizing and boost performance.

How does sleeping help us learn? Our memories develop in three stages: encoding, consolidating, and retrieving. When we first register information, it is encoded, or converted from sensory stimuli into a representation stored in the area of the brain called the hippocampus. While we then sleep, some newly encoded memories are consolidated, or stabilized in the cerebral cortex, where they become more permanent. The recently learned information is selected to be rehearsed and becomes ingrained and available for later retrieval, or reactivation.

Some studies indicate that NREM sleep is especially important for specific types of learning, such as learning a new motor sequencing task or new word associations. But REM sleep might be better for learning consolidation and problem solving. Researchers gave 77 participants a list of creative problems in the morning. Everyone was asked to think about solutions, and half the participants napped before being tested. All the nappers were monitored during sleep. Only those who took longer naps entered REM sleep, which occupied about 14 minutes of the 73-minute naps. NREM napping did not boost creative problem solving, but people who entered REM sleep enhanced their performance by nearly 40%, as compared with non-nappers and NREM nappers. The improvement was specific for problems that were introduced before napping: Rather than simply boosting alertness and attention, REM sleep allowed the brain to work creatively on problems posed before sleep.

When sleep is disrupted, we can develop problems with attention, which can interfere with learning. Children and young adults who have trouble sleeping at night are especially prone to developing problems during the day—not so much that they become sleepy, but that they have trouble focusing their attention. One study looked at sleep apnea in first-graders who were performing at or below the 10th percentile. Among the group who screened positive for sleep apnea, some followed a treatment plan. In the next grade, those children who were treated increased their performance to the 50th percentile; those who did not receive treatment remained at or below the 10th percentile.

Pulling all-nighters does not help grades and learning. In one study, subjects who stayed awake 35 hours managed performances on memory tests that would earn them the equivalent of two letter grades lower than subjects who had slept.

The bottom line is that sleep, both before and after learning new material, plays a critical role in the consolidation of memories. To enhance memory and learning, prioritize healthy sleep habits.

SOURCES: Puller, K. A., and D. Oudielle. 2018. "Sleep learning gets real," *Scientific American* 319(5): 27–31; Vorster, A. P., and J. Borna. 2015. "Sleep and memory in mammals, birds and invertebrates," *Neuroscience & Biobehavioral Reviews* 50: 103–119; Hershner, S. D., and R. D. Chervin. 2014. "Causes and consequences of sleepiness among college students," *Nature and Science of Sleep* 6: 73–84; Harvard Men's Health Watch. 2012. *Learning While You Sleep: Dream or Reality*. Harvard Health Publishing, Harvard Medical School (https://www.health.harvard.edu/staying-healthy/learning-while-you-sleep-dream-or-reality).

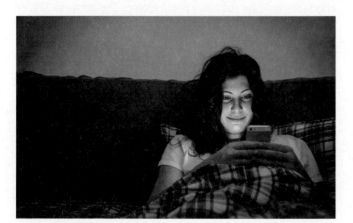

Wellness Tip Don't use electronic devices, especially those that emit blue light, in the hour before bed. Use of blue-light-emitting devices affects melatonin levels and is associated with problems falling asleep and greater sleepiness the following day. Take a break from your devices.

acinquantadue/Shutterstock

Sleep and Stress Hormones Stress-hormone—cortisol—levels in the bloodstream vary throughout the day and are related to sleep patterns. Stress-hormone levels are low during NREM sleep and increase during REM sleep. Peak concentrations occur in the early morning, followed by a slow decline during the day and evening.

Even though cortisol is released during sleep, it is the lack of sleep that has the greatest impact on stress. In someone who is suffering from sleep deprivation (not getting enough sleep over time), mental and physical processes deteriorate steadily. A sleep-deprived person experiences headaches, feels irritable, cannot concentrate, and is prone to forgetfulness. Acute sleep deprivation slows the daytime decline in stress hormones, so evening levels are higher than normal. A decrease in total sleep time also causes an increase in the level of stress hormones. Together these changes may increase stress-hormone levels throughout the day and contribute to physical and mental exhaustion. Extreme sleep deprivation can lead to hallucinations and other psychotic symptoms, as well as to a significant increase in heart attack risk.

Most people can overcome insomnia by discovering the cause of poor sleep and taking steps to remedy it. If you're bothered by insomnia, try the following:

- Determine how much sleep you need to feel refreshed the next day.

- Go to bed at the same time every night and, more important, get up at the same time every morning, seven days a week, regardless of how much sleep you got. Adjust your sleep schedule to keep your wake time consistent and early enough for the sleep drive to accumulate.

- Anchor your circadian rhythm with more light in the morning.

- Don't nap during the day if you can help it. If you fall asleep in the afternoon, make the nap short—less than 30 minutes.

- Exercise every day, but not too close to bedtime. Your metabolism takes up to six hours to slow down after exercise.

- Avoid caffeine late in the day and alcohol before bedtime (it causes disturbed, fragmented sleep). If you take any medications (prescription or not), ask your doctor or pharmacist if they are known to interfere with sleep.

- Do what you can to make your sleeping environment quiet, dark, and a comfortable temperature. Overhearing music or talking can make it hard to sleep.

- Have a light snack before bedtime; you'll sleep better if you're not hungry.

- Use your bed only for sleep. Don't eat, read, study, or watch television in bed.

- Relax before bedtime with a bath, a book, music, or relaxation exercises. Avoid bright lights and electronic activities in the hour prior to bedtime.

- If you don't fall asleep in 15–20 minutes, or if you wake up and can't fall asleep again, turn on your back and engage in a mindful breathing exercise.

If sleep problems last more than six months and interfere with daytime functioning, ask your physician for a referral to a sleep specialist. You may be a candidate for a sleep study—an overnight evaluation of your sleep pattern that can uncover many sleep-related disorders. Sleeping pills are not recommended for chronic insomnia because they can be habit-forming; they often lose their effectiveness over time.

Sleep and Driving Drowsy driving is responsible for more than 109,000 injuries and 6,400 deaths each year. Even if you don't fall asleep completely, drowsiness slows your reaction time and lessens your ability to pay attention and make good decisions. Going 24 hours without sleep can impair a driver to the same extent as a blood alcohol level of 0.10%, which is above the legal limit.

People who are most at risk for falling asleep while driving include young adults aged 18–29, with men at slightly greater risk than women; parents with small children; shift workers; people who have accumulated sleep debt; and those who have other untreated sleep disorders such as sleep apnea or insomnia. Sleepiness is worsened when people take substances such as muscle relaxants, antihistamines, cold medicines, or alcohol.

The good news is that accidents due to sleepiness are preventable. First and foremost, if you find yourself drowsy while driving, pull over. Taking a nap or short rest can help, but if drowsiness persists, let someone else do the driving.

Sleep Disorders

Although many of us can attribute the lack of sleep to long workdays and family responsibilities, as many as 70 million Americans suffer from chronic sleep disorders—medical conditions that prevent them from sleeping well. Some of the most common ones are described in the sections that follow.

Chronic Insomnia Many people have trouble falling asleep or staying asleep—a condition called insomnia. For most people, insomnia is brief and due to life circumstances, such as worrying about an upcoming deadline or consuming too much caffeine or alcohol on a particular day. A person is considered to have chronic insomnia if sleep disruption occurs at least three nights per week and lasts at least three months. If you experience insomnia, try the strategies described in this chapter for promoting healthy sleep patterns and in the box "Overcoming Insomnia."

Restless Leg Syndrome Restless leg syndrome (RLS) affects about 5% of the adult population and as many as 25% of pregnant women. RLS is characterized by muscle throbbing or creeping or other uncomfortable sensations in the legs, which create an uncontrollable urge to move them. Symptoms occur primarily at night or while resting.

RLS can be associated with small kicking movements during the night, can interfere with falling asleep, and can make falling back to sleep more difficult. Simple measures that help RLS include getting more exercise during the day; avoiding all caffeine, tobacco, and alcohol; massaging the legs or using heating pads or a warm bath; maintaining a regular sleep pattern; and correcting any deficiencies in iron, folate, or magnesium. Medications are also available, but certain substances should be avoided: Diphenhydramine (Benadryl), which is a common ingredient in over-the-counter sleeping pills, paradoxically worsens RLS symptoms and can worsen sleep.

Sleep Apnea Sleep apnea occurs when a person repeatedly stops breathing for short periods while asleep. Apnea is caused by a number of factors, but typically results when soft tissue at the

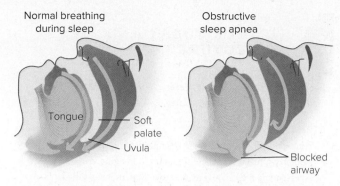

Normal breathing during sleep

Obstructive sleep apnea

Tongue

Soft palate

Uvula

Blocked airway

Figure 10.6 Sleep apnea. Sleep apnea occurs when soft tissues surrounding the airway relax, "collapsing" the airway and restricting airflow.

back of the mouth (such as the tongue or soft palate) "collapses" during sleep, blocking the airway (Figure 10.6). Interrupted breathing normally awakens a sleeper, and usually without the sleeper's awareness. However, the disruption to sleep can be significant, and over time, acute sleep deprivation can result.

Apnea is hard to detect: Its main symptom is excessive daytime sleepiness, and it doesn't hurt. For these reasons the American Sleep Apnea Organization estimates that 22 million Americans suffer from sleep apnea, and 80% of cases of moderate and severe obstructive sleep apnea go undiagnosed.

Sleep apnea is more common among people who are overweight, but it can occur in people at normal weight. Risk increases with age, and up to 50% of adults over age 65 may have some degree of sleep apnea. Untreated, sleep apnea increases the risk of high blood pressure, heart attack, stroke, obesity, and diabetes. It also increases the risk of work-related or driving accidents. Treatments for sleep apnea include the following:

- Lifestyle changes, including weight loss, sleeping on your side, quitting smoking, and using nasal sprays or allergy medicines to keep nasal passages open at night.

- Mouthpieces (oral appliances) that are worn at night and adjust the position of the lower jaw to help keep airways open.

- Breathing devices such as the continuous positive airway pressure (CPAP) machine, which uses a mask over the mouth and/or nose to blow air into the throat, adjusting the force to keep airways open.

Improving Sleep

If you're like the average American, you get less than the recommended amount of sleep each night (see Figure 10.7). The Centers for Disease Control and Prevention calls sleep deprivation a national public epidemic. In adults, between seven and nine hours of sleep is generally sufficient, but sleep needs vary from person to person; some people need only six hours, while others need more than nine. Complete Lab 10.3 to learn more about your current sleep.

Support Natural Sleep Rhythms and Drives Sleep is a natural physiological process, so you can't "will" yourself to sleep—meaning, don't get frustrated if you don't fall asleep. As

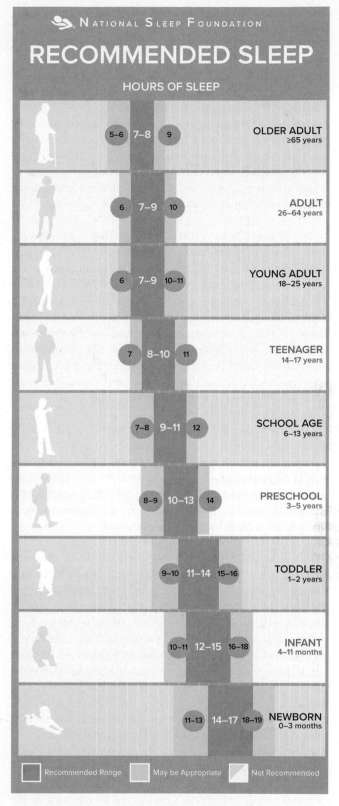

RECOMMENDED SLEEP

HOURS OF SLEEP

OLDER ADULT ≥65 years	5–6 7–8 9	
ADULT 26–64 years	6 7–9 10	
YOUNG ADULT 18–25 years	6 7–9 10–11	
TEENAGER 14–17 years	7 8–10 11	
SCHOOL AGE 6–13 years	7–8 9–11 12	
PRESCHOOL 3–5 years	8–9 10–13 14	
TODDLER 1–2 years	9–10 11–14 15–16	
INFANT 4–11 months	10–11 12–15 16–18	
NEWBORN 0–3 months	11–13 14–17 18–19	

Recommended Range   May be Appropriate   Not Recommended

Figure 10.7 Sleep needs change over the source of the life span.
SOURCE: National Sleep Foundation. "How much sleep do we really need?" n.d. (https://www.sleepfoundation.org/excessive-sleepiness/support/how-much-sleep-do-we-really-need).

noted, to strengthen physiological sleep drives, keep a consistent sleep schedule throughout the week, including the weekends. To support circadian rhythm, set a target wake time with good light exposure, and avoid bright lights and electronic devices at night. To enhance the homeostatic drive, make your wake time sufficiently early, avoid naps, and minimize caffeine.

Create a Good Sleep Environment Your bedroom should be cool, dark, and quiet, ideally without pets. Although you'll want to be warm when you get into bed, sleep comes more easily in cool temperatures. Therefore, you may want to take a warm shower or bath before bed, to warm the body, and wear socks if you tend to have cold extremities at night. But after that, fewer blankets and a cooler temperature setting are beneficial. Generally if you tend to awaken at night, avoid activities in the bedroom that might be stimulating, such as watching television or using electronic devices.

Avoid Substances That Disrupt Sleep People vary greatly in how they are affected by caffeine, but those with poor-quality sleep, difficulty falling asleep, or nighttime awakenings need to be especially careful. Caffeine can have physiological effects for over 24 hours in susceptible people, and even caffeine consumed in the morning can affect sleep throughout the night. Alcohol is another substance that can affect sleep. Some people think that alcohol improves sleep, but it can cause poorer sleep in the second part of the night when the effects wear off, leading to increased activation and arousal. For people with poor sleep, reducing alcohol consumption can be beneficial.

Treat Conditions That Interfere with Sleep A number of readily treated medical conditions, including nasal congestion and acid reflux, can disrupt sleep. Simple interventions, such as using medications or saline spray to treat allergies or limiting foods and fluids for several hours before bedtime, can help in some cases. If symptoms are severe and continue to interfere with sleep, consult a health care provider.

Don't Equate Sleeplessness with Job or School Performance We live in a society where people work long hours, and our culture can seem to reward people who sleep less and work more. But establishing balance between sleep and life activities is important. "Cramming" all night before an exam, or staying up all night to write a paper, is something most college students have been tempted to do, but all-nighters can interfere with learning and memory. Having a full night's sleep after studying promotes long-term memory formation (see the box "Can We Learn While Sleeping?").

Similarly, some job environments encourage longer working hours. But equating work ethic with long work hours and less sleep can lead to burnout and lower productivity. People who work the night shift must try especially hard to protect downtime and sleep periods and refrain from adding other daytime commitments that interfere with sleep. It can be tempting in the short term to cut back on sleep, but in the longer term this is likely to backfire, resulting in increased mood problems and the health-related issues associated with sleep loss.

Avoid Sleep Pitfalls Don't be concerned with a bout of sleeplessness. Worry can worsen sleep, and when you are having trouble sleeping, it can be easy to start worrying about the

TIPS FOR TODAY AND THE FUTURE

For the stress you can't avoid, develop a range of stress-management techniques and strategies.

RIGHT NOW YOU CAN

- Practice deep breathing for 5–10 minutes.
- Visualize a relaxing, peaceful place and imagine yourself experiencing it as vividly as possible. Stay there as long as you can.
- Do some stretching exercises.
- Get out your datebook and schedule what you'll be doing the rest of today and tomorrow. Plan a short walk and a conversation with a friend. Schedule a reasonable bedtime to ensure adequate sleep.

IN THE FUTURE YOU CAN

- Take a class or workshop, such as one in assertiveness training or time management, that can help you overcome a source of stress.
- Find a way to build relaxing time into every day. Just 15 minutes of meditation, stretching, or deep breathing can induce the relaxation response.
- Evaluate your sleep patterns and gradually make changes that will help you get the sleep you need to feel and do your best.

consequences for the next day. Most of the time, even if you sleep poorly, the next day's activities will be fine. The ups and down of mental and physical performance are not always correlated to the prior night's sleep. In addition, remember the value of relaxation. Quiet relaxation has restorative value. You don't have to be sound asleep to benefit from quiet time during the night; resting, relaxing, and dozing can also be beneficial. Consider the relaxation techniques presented earlier in this chapter. If you find that despite everything, you feel anxious or frustrated during the night when awake, leave the bedroom and engage in a quiet activity like reading until you feel more relaxed and sleepy again.

SUMMARY

- Stress is the collective physiological and emotional response to any stressor. Physiological responses to stressors are the same for everyone.

- The autonomic nervous system and the endocrine system are responsible for the body's physical response to stressors. The sympathetic nervous system mobilizes the body and activates key hormones of the endocrine system, causing the fight-or-flight reaction. The parasympathetic system returns the body to homeostasis.

- Behavioral responses to stress are controlled by the somatic nervous system and fall under a person's conscious control, though personality, gender, culture, and experience affect one's response to stress.

COMMON QUESTIONS ANSWERED

Q **Are there any relaxation techniques I can use in response to an immediate stressor?**

A Yes. Try the deep breathing techniques described in the chapter, and try some of the following to see which work best for you:

• Do a full-body stretch while standing or sitting. Stretch your arms out to the sides and then reach them as far as possible over your head. Rotate your body from the waist. Bend over as far as is comfortable for you.

• Do a partial session of progressive muscle relaxation. Tense and then relax some of the muscles in your body. Focus on the muscles that are stiff or tense. Shake out your arms and legs.

• Take a short, brisk walk (three to five minutes). Breathe deeply.

• Engage in realistic self-talk about the stressor. Mentally rehearse dealing successfully with the stressor. As an alternative, focus your mind on some other activity.

• Briefly reflect on something personally meaningful. In one study of college students, researchers found that self-reflection on important personal values prior to a stressful task reduces the hormonal response to the stressor.

Q **Can stress cause headaches?**

A Stress is one possible cause of the most common type of headache, the tension headache. About 90% of headaches are tension headaches, characterized by a dull, steady pain, usually on both sides of the head. It may feel as though a band of pressure is tightening around the head, and the pain may extend to the neck and shoulders. Acute tension headaches may last from hours to days, while chronic tension headaches may occur almost every day for months or even years. Ineffective stress-management skills, poor posture, and immobility are leading causes of tension headaches. There is no cure, but the pain can sometimes be avoided and relieved with mindfulness skills and over-the-counter painkillers; many people also try therapies such as massage, relaxation, hot or cold showers, and rest. Stress is also one possible trigger of migraine headaches, which are typically characterized by throbbing pain (often on one side of the head), heightened sensitivity to light and noise, visual disturbances such as flashing lights, nausea, and fatigue.

If your headaches are frequent, keep a journal with details about the events surrounding each one. Are your tension headaches associated with late nights, academic deadlines, or long periods spent sitting at a computer? Are migraines associated with certain foods, stress, fatigue, specific sounds or odors, or (in women) menstruation? If you can identify the stressors or other factors that are consistently associated with your headaches, you can begin to gain more control over the situation. If you suffer persistent tension or migraine headaches, consult your physician.

• The general adaptation syndrome model contributes to our understanding of the links between stress and disease. People who have many stressors in their lives or who handle stress poorly are at risk for cardiovascular disease, impairment of the immune system, and many other problems.

• Potential sources of stress include major life changes, daily hassles, college- and job-related stressors, and interpersonal and social stressors, both real and virtual.

• Positive ways of managing stress include regular exercise; good nutrition; support from other people; clear communication; conflict resolution; spiritual wellness; effective time management; cognitive techniques; and techniques for relaxation, body awareness, and mindfulness.

• If a personal program for stress management doesn't work, peer counseling, support groups, and psychotherapy are available.

• Adequate sleep improves memory, creativity, and mood; fosters feelings of competence and self-worth; and works against stress, depression, and anxiety. It lowers food craving and maintains a healthier immune system, and helps prevent cardiovascular disease, diabetes, weight gain, certain cancers, and neurodegenerative diseases.

• Two phases of sleep patterns—non-rapid eye movement sleep (NREM) and rapid eye movement (REM)—are characterized by a different pattern of electrical brain activity. Brain waves become slow and even in NREM sleep. REM sleep waves closely resemble those of alert wakefulness.

• The body's master clock can be set backward or forward by light. To strengthen your circadian rhythm, get good light exposure in the morning and daytime, and reduce exposure to light at night.

FOR FURTHER EXPLORATION

American Academy of Sleep Medicine. Advocates research and advocacy to improve sleep health.

https://aasm.org/

American Headache Society. Provides information for consumers and clinicians about different types of headaches, their causes, and their treatment.

http://www.americanheadachesociety.org/

American Sleep Association. Advances the medical specialty of sleep medicine.

http://www.sleepassociation.org

American Institute of Stress. A resource of in-depth information on stress, its causes, and its treatments.

http://www.stress.org

American Psychiatric Association: Blogs. Provides information on topics related to mental health and well-being, including stress, anxiety, and depression.

https://www.psychiatry.org/news-room/apa-blogs

American Psychological Association. Provides information on stress management and psychological disorders.

http://www.apa.org

http://www.apa.org/helpcenter/index.aspx

Association for Applied Psychophysiology and Biofeedback. Provides information about biofeedback and referrals to certified biofeedback practitioners.

http://www.aapb.org

Benson-Henry Institute for Mind Body Medicine. Provides information about stress management and relaxation techniques.

http://www.massgeneral.org/bhi

Choose Sleep. Aims to increase awareness about the risks of sleep disorders and the importance of sleep.

http://www.choosesleep.org

Harvard Medical School Division of Sleep Medicine: Sleep and Health Education Program. Provides information about the importance of sleep, improving sleep, and sleep disorders.

http://healthysleep.med.harvard.edu/portal/

National Institute of Mental Health (NIMH). Publishes informative brochures about stress and stress management as well as other aspects of mental health.

http://www.nimh.nih.gov

National Sleep Foundation. Provides information about sleep and how to overcome sleep problems such as insomnia, apnea, and jet lag.

http://www.sleepfoundation.org

WebMD Stress Management Health Center. Offers a range of digestible subtopics of stress.

http://www.webmd.com/balance/stress-management/default.htm

SELECTED BIBLIOGRAPHY

AAA Foundation for Traffic Safety. 2018. *Prevalence of Drowsy Driving Crashes: Estimates from a Large-Scale Naturalistic Driving Study.* AAA Foundation for Traffic Safety.

American College Health Association. 2017. *American College Health Association-National College Health Assessment II Reference Group Executive Summary, Fall 2017.* Hanover, MD: American College Health Association.

American Psychological Association. 2017. *Stress in America 2017 Part 1: Coping with Change.* Washington, DC: American Psychological Association.

American Psychological Association. 2017. *Stress in America 2017 Part 2: Technology and Social Media.* Washington, DC: American Psychological Association.

American Psychological Association. 2018. *Stress in America: Generation Z.* Stress in America™ Survey.

Cassidy, S. 2016. The Academic Resilience Scale (ARS-30): A new multidimensional construct measure. *Frontiers in Psychology* 7: 1787.

Dyar, C., et al. 2016. The mediating roles of rejection sensitivity and proximal stress in the association between discrimination and internalizing symptoms among sexual minority women. *Archives of Sexual Behavior.* doi:10.1007/s10508-016-0869-1.

Edes, A. N., and D. E. Crews. 2017. Allostatic load and biological anthropology. *American Journal of Physical Anthropology* 162(S63): 44–70.

Flinchbaugh, C., et al. 2015. A challenge or a hindrance? Understanding the effects of stressors and thriving on life satisfaction. *International Journal of Stress Management* 22(4): 323.

Greenberg, J. 2016. *Comprehensive Stress Management* (14th ed.). New York: McGraw-Hill.

Kabat-Zinn, J. 2011. *Mindfulness for Beginners: Reclaiming the Present Moment—and Your Life.* Louisville, CO: Sounds True.

Kurek Jr., S. J. 2016. EAST 2016 presidential address: Resilience. *Journal of Trauma and Acute Care Surgery* 81(1): 1–87.

Leppink, E. W., et al. 2016. The young and the stressed: Stress, impulse control, and health in college students. *Journal of Nervous and Mental Disease* 204(12):931–938.

Manzoni, G. C., et al. 2016. Age of onset of episodic and chronic cluster headache—a review of a large case series from a single headache centre. *Journal of Headache Pain* 17: 44.

Mayo Foundation for Medical Education and Research. 2016. *Stress: Constant Stress Puts You Health at Risk* (http://www.mayoclinic.com/health/stress/SR00001).

McGonigal, K. 2015. *The Upside of Stress: Why Stress Is Good for You, and How to Get Good at It.* New York: Avery.

National Institute of Neurological Disorders and Stroke. 2018. *Restless Legs Syndrome Fact Sheet* (http://www.ninds.nih.gov/disorders/restless_egs/detail_restless_legs.htm).

O'Driscoll, M., et al. 2017. The effects of mindfulness-based interventions for health and social care undergraduate students: A systematic review of the literature. *Psychology, Health, and Medicine.* doi:10.1080/13548506.2017.1280178.

Pascoe, M. C., and I. E. Bauer. 2015. A systematic review of randomised control trials on the effects of yoga on stress measures and mood. *Journal of Psychiatric Research* 68: 270–282.

Pennebaker, J. W., and J. Evans. 2014. *Expressive Writing: Words That Heal.* Enumclaw, WA: Idyll Arbor.

Pew Research Center. 2013. *Modern Parenthood: How Mothers and Fathers Spend Their Time* (http://www.pewsocialtrends.org/2013/03/14/chapter-4-how-mothers-and-fathers-spend-their-time/).

Ramikie, T. S., et al. 2014. Multiple mechanistically distinct modes of endocannabinoid mobilization at central amygdala glutamatergic synapses. *Neuron* 81(5): 1111–1125.

Schulte, B. 2014. *Overwhelmed.* New York: Sarah Crichton Books.

Seaward, B. L. 2015. *Managing Stress: Principles and Strategies for Health and Well-Being* (8th ed.). Boston: Jones and Bartlett.

Turner, J. B., and R. J. Turner. 2013. Social relations, social integration, and social support. In *Handbook of the Sociology of Mental Health* (pp. 341–456), ed. C. S. Aneshensel, J. C. Phelan, and A. Bierman. Dordrecht, Netherlands: Springer.

U.S. Department of Health and Human Services, National Institutes of Health. 2015. *Stress* (http://www.nlm.nih.gov/medlineplus/stress.html).

Vaccarino, V., et al. 2016. Sex differences in mental stress-induced myocardial ischemia in patients with coronary heart disease. *Journal of the American Heart Association* 5(9): e003630.

Van der Zwan, J. E., et al. 2015. Physical activity, mindfulness meditation, or heart rate variability biofeedback for stress reduction: A randomized controlled trial. *Applied Psychophysiology and Biofeedback* 40(4): 257–268.

Wang C.-W., et al. 2014. Managing stress and anxiety through qigong exercise in healthy adults: A systematic review and meta-analysis of randomized controlled trials. *BMC Complementary and Alternative Medicine* 14: 8.

White, R. L., et al. 2017. Domain-specific physical activity and mental health: A meta-analysis. *American Journal of Preventive Medicine.* doi:10.1016/j.amepre.2016.12.008.

Yano, Y., et al. 2016. Blood pressure reactivity to psychological stress in young adults and cognition in midlife: The Coronary Artery Risk Development in Young Adults (CARDIA) study. *Journal of the American Heart Association* 5(1): e002718.

Name _____ Section _____ Date _____

LAB 10.1 Identifying Your Stress Level and Key Stressors

How Stressed Are You?

To help determine how much stress you experience on a daily basis, answer the following questions.
How many of the symptoms of excessive stress in the list do you experience frequently?

Symptoms of Excessive Stress

Physical Symptoms	*Cognitive Symptoms*	*Emotional Symptoms*	*Behavioral Symptoms*
Dry mouth	Confusion	Anxiety	Crying
Fatigue	Inability to concentrate	Depression	Disrupted eating habits
Frequent illnesses	Negative thinking	Edginess	Disrupted sleep
Gastrointestinal problems	Poor judgment	Hypervigilance	Increased use of tobacco, alcohol, or other drugs
Headaches	Worrying	Impulsiveness	Problems communicating
High blood pressure		Irritability	Sexual problems
Pounding heart			Social isolation
Sweating			

Yes	No	
_____	_____	1. Are you easily startled or irritated?
_____	_____	2. Are you increasingly forgetful?
_____	_____	3. Do you have trouble falling or staying asleep?
_____	_____	4. Do you continually worry about events in your future?
_____	_____	5. Do you feel as if you are constantly under pressure to produce?
_____	_____	6. Do you frequently use tobacco, alcohol, or other drugs to help you relax?
_____	_____	7. Do you often feel as if you have less energy than you need to finish the day?
_____	_____	8. Do you have recurrent stomachaches or headaches?
_____	_____	9. Is it difficult for you to find satisfaction in simple life pleasures?
_____	_____	10. Are you often disappointed in yourself and others?
_____	_____	11. Are you overly concerned with being liked or accepted by others?
_____	_____	12. Have you lost interest in intimacy or sex?
_____	_____	13. Are you concerned that you do not have enough money?

Experiencing some stress-related symptoms or answering yes to a few questions is normal. However, if you experience a large number of stress symptoms or you answered yes to a majority of the questions, you may be experiencing a high level of stress. Take time out to develop effective stress-management techniques. Many coping strategies that can aid you in dealing with college stressors are described in this chapter. In addition, your school's counseling center can provide valuable support.

LABORATORY ACTIVITIES

Weekly Stress Log

Now that you are familiar with the signals of stress, complete the weekly stress log to map patterns in your stress levels and identify sources of stress. Enter a score for each hour of each day according to the ratings listed here.

	A.M.							P.M.												Average
	6	7	8	9	10	11	12	1	2	3	4	5	6	7	8	9	10	11	12	*Average*
Monday																				
Tuesday																				
Wednesday																				
Thursday																				
Friday																				
Saturday																				
Sunday																				
Average																				

Ratings:
- 0 = Asleep
- 1 = No anxiety; general feeling of well-being
- 2 = Mild anxiety; no interference with activity
- 3 = Moderate anxiety; specific signal(s) of stress present
- 4 = High anxiety; interference with activity
- 5 = Very high anxiety and panic reactions; general inability to engage in activity

To identify daily or weekly patterns in your stress level, average your stress rating for each hour and each day. For example, if your scores for 10:00 a.m. are 4, 3, 4, 3, 4, 3, and 4, your 10:00 a.m. rating would be 25 ÷ 7 , or 3.6 (moderate to high anxiety). Then calculate an average weekly stress score by averaging your daily average stress scores. Your weekly average will give you a sense of your overall level of stress.

Using Your Results

How did you score? How high are your daily and weekly stress scores? Are you satisfied with your stress rating? If not, set a specific goal:

What should you do next? Enter the results of this lab in the Preprogram Assessment column in Appendix B. If you've set a goal for improvement, begin by using your log to look for patterns and significant time periods in order to identify key stressors in your life. Here, list any stressors that caused you a significant amount of discomfort this week; these can be people, places, events, or recurring thoughts or worries. For each, enter one strategy that would help you deal more successfully with the stressor. Examples of strategies might include practicing an oral presentation in front of a friend or engaging in positive self-talk.

Next, begin to put your strategies into action. In addition, complete Lab 10.2 to help you incorporate lifestyle stress-management techniques into your daily routine.

Name _____ **Section** _____ **Date** _____

LAB 10.2 Stress-Management Techniques

Part I Lifestyle Stress Management

For each of the areas listed in the following table, describe your current lifestyle as it relates to stress management. For example, do you have enough social support? How are your exercise and nutrition habits? Is time management a problem for you? For each area, list two ways that you could change your current habits to help you manage your stress. Sample strategies might include calling a friend before a challenging class, taking a walk before lunch, and using a datebook to track your time.

	CURRENT LIFESTYLE	LIFESTYLE CHANGE #1	LIFESTYLE CHANGE #2
Social support system			
Exercise habits			
Nutrition habits			
Time-management techniques			
Self-talk patterns			
Sleep habits			

LABORATORY ACTIVITIES

Part II Relaxation Techniques

Choose two relaxation techniques described in this chapter (progressive relaxation, visualization, deep breathing, meditation, listening to music). If a recording is available for progressive relaxation or visualization, these techniques can be performed by your entire class as a group.

List the techniques you tried.

1. _____

2. _____

How did you feel before you tried these techniques?

_____

_____

_____

What did you think or how did you feel during each of the techniques you tried?

1. _____

_____

_____

2. _____

_____

_____

How did you feel after you tried these techniques?

_____

_____

_____

Name _____ **Section** _____ **Date** _____

LAB 10.3   Evaluating and Improving Sleep

Adequate sleep helps you stay healthy and function at your best. However, chronic sleep loss and sleep disorders affect many Americans and contribute to lost productivity as well as health care expenses. Complete the following checklists, log, and analysis to evaluate and improve your sleep habits.

Do You Get Enough Sleep?

To determine whether you get enough high-quality sleep, review the following list of statements and check any that are true for you.

_____ 1. I feel very tired during the day.

_____ 2. I do not feel refreshed and alert when I wake up.

_____ 3. I often feel I could doze off while

_____ sitting and reading or watching media.

_____ sitting in a public place, such as a classroom, meeting, or movie theater.

_____ riding in a car for an hour without stopping.

_____ sitting and talking to someone.

_____ sitting quietly after lunch.

_____ sitting in traffic for a few minutes.

_____ 4. I often have trouble focusing, making decisions, solving problems, remembering things, and coping with change.

The more items you check, the more likely it is that you are not getting enough sleep. Insufficient or poor sleep can be due to a sleep disorder (see next section) or to not allotting enough time for sleep.

Do You Have Signs of a Sleep Disorder?

Review this list of common signs of a sleep disorder and check any that are true for you on three or more nights per week.

_____ 1. It takes me more than 30 minutes to fall asleep at night.

_____ 2. I awaken frequently in the night and then have trouble falling back to sleep again.

_____ 3. I awaken too early in the morning.

_____ 4. I often don't feel well rested despite spending seven to eight hours or more asleep at night.

_____ 5. I feel sleepy during the day and fall asleep within five minutes if I have an opportunity to nap, or I fall asleep unexpectedly or at inappropriate times during the day.

_____ 6. My bed partner claims that I snore loudly, snort, gasp, or make choking sounds while I sleep, or that my breathing stops for short periods.

_____ 7. I have creeping, tingling, or crawling feelings in my legs that are relieved by moving or massaging them, especially in the evening and when I try to fall asleep.

_____ 8. I have vivid, dreamlike experiences while falling asleep or dozing.

_____ 9. I have episodes of sudden muscle weakness when I am angry or fearful, or when I laugh.

_____ 10. I feel as though I cannot move when I first wake up.

_____ 11. My bed partner notes that my legs or arms jerk often during sleep.

_____ 12. I regularly need to use stimulants to stay awake during the day.

LABORATORY ACTIVITIES

If you checked any of these items, get an evaluation by a health care provider. Some items on the list can be symptoms of multiple types of sleep disorders, but some are characteristic of specific disorders:

- *Chronic insomnia:* Difficulty falling asleep or staying asleep on at least three nights per week for more than one month

- *Sleep apnea:* Intermittent blocking of the upper airway, causing pauses in breathing and sleep; often characterized by loud and frequent snoring, with periodic gasping or snorting noises

- *Restless leg syndrome:* Unpleasant prickling or tingling in the legs that is relieved by moving or massaging them; may also be characterized by brief and abrupt limb movements during sleep that can awaken the sleeper

- *Narcolepsy:* Overwhelming daytime sleepiness, sudden muscle weakness, sleep paralysis, and vivid dreams

Tracking Your Sleep

One of the best ways to determine if you are getting enough high-quality sleep, or if you have signs of a sleep disorder, is to keep a sleep log. Your log will give you an idea of how much uninterrupted sleep you need to avoid daytime sleepiness. You can also use the log to identify patterns or practices that may keep you from getting a good night's sleep.

Complete the log for at least a week to capture your typical pattern, which may vary between weekdays and weekends. You don't need to be exact; your best estimate is good enough. You may use a sleep app to inform your estimates, but don't keep checking the time, as that may negatively affect your sleep.

Date							
Complete in the morning:							
Time I went to bed last night							
Time I got up this morning							
How long I took to fall asleep last night							
Number of awakenings							
Total time awake last night							
Number of hours of sleep last night							
Medications taken last night							
How awake did I feel this morning 1 = wide awake 2 = awake but a little tired 3 = sleepy							
Complete in the evening:							
Number of caffeinated drinks and time when I had them today							
Number of alcoholic drinks and time when I had them today							
Naptimes and lengths today							
Exercise times and lengths today							
How sleepy did I feel today? 1 = so sleepy I had to struggle to stay awake 2 = somewhat tired 3 = fairly alert 4 = wide awake							

Analyzing Your Sleep Log

What is your current sleep schedule during the week? On the weekends?

How many hours of sleep do you currently average per night? How much sleep do you need to function well? How do the numbers compare? Remember, the amount of sleep time varies by individual; if you get eight hours of sleep a night and are still sleepy during the day, you may naturally require more sleep and should plan accordingly.

What would be your ideal sleep period if you could sleep anytime you wanted? What would be the best sleep period for you to get adequate sleep, considering your obligations and preferences? Why?

Could your consumption of caffeine or alcohol be affecting your sleep? What about your pattern of exercise? Do you have any medical conditions like nasal allergies or acid reflux that could interfere with sleep? Do you take any medications that can affect sleep?

Using Your Results

How did you score? Do you have signs of insufficient sleep or a sleep disorder? What did you learn from your sleep log?

What should you do next? Based on your analysis, identify at least one problem with your sleep pattern or with possible blockers of quality sleep. Set an appropriate SMART goal to address the problem, and then identify at least two concrete strategies to try. Your goal and strategies can focus on a specific sleep problem or on a time-management issue that limits your ability to schedule enough time for sleep.

SOURCES: Centers for Disease Control and Prevention. 2014. *Key Sleep Disorders* (https://www.cdc.gov/sleep/about_sleep/key_disorders.html); U.S. Department of Health and Human Services, National Institutes of Health, National Heart Lung and Blood Institute. 2011. *Your Guide to Healthy Sleep.* NIH Publication No. 11-5271.

Cardiovascular Health and Diabetes

LOOKING AHEAD...

After reading this chapter, you should be able to

- Summarize the major forms of cardiovascular disease and how they develop.

- Describe the risk factors associated with cardiovascular disease.

- List the steps you can take to protect yourself against cardiovascular disease.

- Describe types, risk factors, and prevention strategies for diabetes.

TEST YOUR KNOWLEDGE

1. Women are less likely to die of cardiovascular disease than they are to die of breast cancer. True or false?

2. On average, how much earlier does heart disease develop in people who don't exercise regularly than in people who do?
   a. 6 months
   b. 2 years
   c. 6 years

3. Which of the following foods would be a good choice for promoting heart health?
   a. whole grains
   b. salmon
   c. bananas

See answers on the next page.

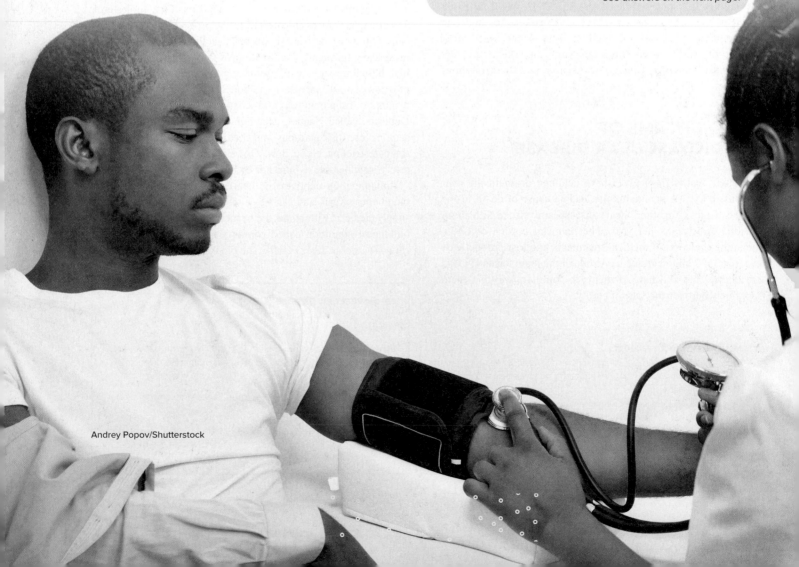

Andrey Popov/Shutterstock

Cardiovascular disease (CVD) includes the diseases that affect the heart and blood vessels: heart disease, heart attack, stroke, and angina (chest pain), as well as blood vessel diseases, arrhythmias (heart rhythm problems), congenital heart defects, and other conditions affecting the heart's muscle, valves, or rhythms.

As the country's leading cause of death, CVD claims more than 2,300 American lives every day. Nearly half (48%) of American adults have one or more types of CVD. Heart disease, one form of CVD, is the leading cause of death for both U.S. men and women; strokes rank fifth. High blood pressure, which is both a form of CVD and a risk factor for other types of disease, affects nearly half of all American adults, including 26% of those ages 20 to 44. Although CVD may seem like a disease that affects only older adults, evidence has been mounting that atherosclerosis, the underlying cause of CVD, begins in childhood.

CVD is largely due to our way of life. Millions of Americans are overweight and sedentary; we smoke, manage stress ineffectively, have uncontrolled high blood pressure or high cholesterol levels, and don't know the signs of CVD. Not all risk factors for CVD are controllable—for example, some people have an inherited tendency toward high cholesterol levels—but many risk factors are within your control.

In this chapter you'll learn about the major forms of CVD, including hypertension, atherosclerosis, and stroke, and also the factors that put people at risk for CVD. We'll also talk about diabetes because it is a key CVD risk factor and one of the leading causes of death among Americans. Most important, you'll learn the steps you can take to protect your heart and promote cardiovascular health throughout your life.

MAJOR FORMS OF CARDIOVASCULAR DISEASE

Although deaths from CVD have declined dramatically over the past 60 years, it remains the leading cause of death in the United States. Together, heart disease and stroke kill about 775,000 Americans per year. The financial burden of CVD, including the costs of medical treatments and lost productivity, exceeds $320 billion annually. Although the main forms of CVD are interrelated and have elements in common, we treat them separately here for the sake of clarity.

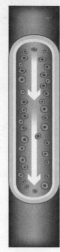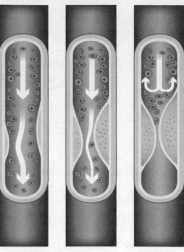

A healthy artery allows blood to flow freely.

As plaque builds up in the arteries, the inside of the arteries begins to narrow, which lessens or blocks the flow of blood. Plaques can also rupture, causing a blood clot to form on the plaque and blocking the flow of blood.

Figure 11.1 Atherosclerosis: The process of cardiovascular disease.
SOURCE: Centers for Disease Control and Prevention. (n.d.) Heart Disease Facts. (https://www.cdc.gov/heartdisease/facts.htm)

Atherosclerosis

Atherosclerosis is a thickening and hardening of the arteries. In atherosclerosis, arteries narrow from deposits of fat, cholesterol, and other substances (Figure 11.1). The process begins when the cells lining the arteries (endothelial cells) become damaged, most likely through a combination of factors such as smoking, high blood pressure, high insulin or glucose levels, and deposits of oxidized LDL particles. The body's response to this damage results in inflammation and changes in the artery lining. Deposits, called **plaques**, accumulate on artery walls, and the arteries lose their elasticity and their ability to expand and contract, restricting blood flow. Once narrowed by a plaque, an artery is vulnerable to blockage by blood clots.

Inflammation deprives the heart, brain, or other organs of blood and oxygen, and can be deadly. Coronary arteries, which supply the heart with blood, are particularly susceptible to plaque buildup, a condition called **coronary heart disease (CHD)**, or *coronary artery disease* (*CAD*). The blockage of a coronary artery

> **cardiovascular disease (CVD)** A collective term for various diseases of the heart and blood vessels.
>
> **TERMS**
>
> **atherosclerosis** A form of CVD in which the inner layers of artery walls are made thick and irregular by plaque deposits; arteries become narrowed, and blood supply is reduced.
>
> **plaque** A deposit of fatty (and other) substances on the inner wall of an artery.
>
> **coronary heart disease (CHD)** Heart disease caused by atherosclerosis in the arteries that supply blood to the heart muscle; also called *coronary artery disease (CAD)*.

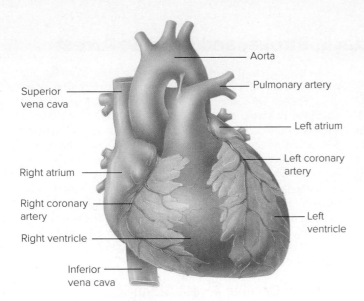

Figure 11.2   Blood supply to the heart. Blood is supplied to the heart from the right and left coronary arteries, which branch off the aorta. If a coronary artery becomes blocked by plaque buildup or a blood clot, a heart attack occurs; part of the heart muscle may die due to lack of oxygen.

causes a heart attack. If a cerebral artery (leading to the brain) is blocked, the result is a stroke. The main risk factors for atherosclerosis are cigarette smoking, physical inactivity, high levels of blood cholesterol, high blood pressure, and diabetes.

Heart Disease and Heart Attacks

The American Heart Association estimates that 800,000 people in the United States have heart attacks each year. Of those, about 112,000 will die. Although a **heart attack**, also called *myocardial infarction (MI)*, may come without warning, it is usually the end result of a long-term disease process. The heart requires a steady supply of oxygen-rich blood to function properly (Figure 11.2). If one coronary artery that supplies blood to the heart becomes blocked, a heart attack results. A heart attack caused by a blood clot is called *coronary thrombosis*. During a heart attack, part of the heart muscle (myocardium) may die from lack of blood flow.

Chest pain, called **angina pectoris**, is a signal that the heart isn't getting enough oxygen to supply its needs. Although not actually a heart attack, angina—felt as an extreme tightness in the chest and heavy pressure behind the breastbone or in the shoulder, neck, arm, hand, or back—is a warning that the heart is overloaded.

If the electrical impulses that control heartbeat are disrupted, the heart may beat too quickly, too slowly, or in an irregular fashion, a condition known as **arrhythmia**. The symptoms of arrhythmia range from imperceptible to severe and even fatal. **Sudden cardiac death**, also called *cardiac arrest,* is most often caused by an arrhythmia called *ventricular fibrillation,* a kind of "quivering" of the ventricle that makes it ineffective in pumping blood. If ventricular fibrillation continues for more than a few minutes, it is generally fatal. Cardiac defibrillation, in which an electrical shock is delivered to the heart, can jolt the heart into a more efficient rhythm. This shock can be administered with an automated external defibrillator (AED), a first-aid device that is available in many public places in case someone experiences a heart attack.

Heart attack symptoms may include pain or pressure in the chest; pain in the arm, neck, or jaw; difficulty breathing; excessive sweating; nausea and vomiting; and loss of consciousness. But not all heart attacks involve sharp chest pain. Women, in particular, are more likely to have different symptoms—shortness of breath, weakness, unusual fatigue, cold sweat, and dizziness.

If symptoms of heart trouble occur, contact an emergency medical service or go immediately to the nearest hospital or clinic (see the box "Warning Signs of Heart Attack, Stroke, and Cardiac Arrest"). Many experts also suggest that the heart attack victim chew and swallow one adult aspirin tablet (325 mg); aspirin has an immediate anticlotting effect. If someone having a heart attack gets to the emergency department quickly enough, an injection can be used to dissolve a clot in the coronary artery, reducing the amount of damage to the heart muscle.

Physicians have a variety of diagnostic tools and treatments for heart disease. Patients may undergo a stress or exercise test, in which they run on a treadmill or pedal a stationary cycle while being monitored with an electrocardiogram (ECG or EKG). Characteristic changes in the heart's electrical activity during the test can reveal particular heart problems, such as restricted blood flow to the heart muscle. Tools that allow the physician to visualize a patient's heart and arteries include a special type of X-ray known as an angiogram, magnetic resonance imaging (MRI), electron-beam computed tomography (EBCT), echocardiograms, and others.

If tests indicate a cardiovascular problem, or if a person has already had a heart attack, several treatments are possible. Along with a low-fat diet, regular exercise, and smoking cessation, many patients are also advised to take a low-dose aspirin tablet (81 mg) daily. Aspirin has an anticlotting effect, keeping platelets in the blood from sticking to arterial plaques and forming clots; it also reduces inflammation. Low-dose aspirin therapy may help prevent heart attacks and strokes. In addition to aspirin, prescription drugs can also help reduce the strain on the heart.

Several surgical treatments exist for certain forms of heart disease. *Balloon angioplasty* threads a catheter with an inflatable balloon tip through a coronary artery until it reaches the area of blockage; as the balloon is inflated, it flattens the plaque, widening the arterial opening. Many surgeons implant permanent

---

TERMS

heart attack   Damage to, or death of, heart muscle, resulting from a failure of the coronary arteries to deliver enough blood to the heart; also known as *myocardial infarction (MI).*

angina pectoris   A condition in which the heart muscle does not receive enough blood, causing severe pain in the chest and often in the arm and shoulder.

arrhythmia   A change in the normal pattern of the heartbeat.

sudden cardiac death   A nontraumatic, unexpected death from sudden cardiac arrest, most often due to arrhythmia; in most instances, victims have underlying heart disease.

Warning Signs of Heart Attack, Stroke, and Cardiac Arrest

Heart Attack Warning Signs

The most common warning symptoms of a heart attack for both men and women are the following:

- *Chest pain or discomfort* (*angina*) in the center or left side of the chest that usually lasts for more than a few minutes or goes away and comes back. It can feel like pressure, squeezing, fullness, or pain. It can also feel like heartburn or indigestion and can be mild or severe.

- *Upper body discomfort* in one or both arms, the back, shoulders, neck, jaw, or upper part of the stomach (above the navel).

- *Shortness of breath* may be the only symptom, or it may occur before or along with chest pain or discomfort. It can occur when you are resting or doing mild physical activity.

But remember these additional facts:

- Heart attacks can start slowly and cause only mild pain or discomfort. Symptoms can be mild or more intense and sudden. Symptoms also may come and go over several hours.

- People who have high blood sugar (diabetes) may have no symptoms or very mild ones. Heart attacks without symptoms or with very mild symptoms are called silent heart attacks.

- Women are somewhat more likely to have shortness of breath; nausea and vomiting; unusual tiredness (sometimes for days); and pain in the back, shoulders, and jaw.

- Other possible symptoms include breaking out in a cold sweat, light-headedness or sudden dizziness, or a change in the pattern of usual symptoms.

The signs and symptoms of a heart attack can develop suddenly or slowly—within hours, days, or weeks. If you or someone you know might be having a heart attack, don't ignore it or feel embarrassed to call for help. **Call 9-1-1 right away.** Here's why:

- Acting fast can be life saving. Every minute matters.

- An ambulance is the best and safest way to get to the hospital. Emergency medical services (EMS) personnel start lifesaving treatments right away. People who arrive by ambulance often receive faster treatment at the hospital.

- The 9-1-1 operator or EMS technician can give you advice. You might be told to crush or chew an aspirin if you're not allergic, unless there is a medical reason for you not to take one.

Stroke Warning Signs

The symptoms of stroke are distinctive because they happen quickly:

- Sudden numbness or weakness of the face, arm, or leg (especially on one side of the body)

- Sudden confusion, trouble speaking or understanding speech

- Sudden trouble seeing from one or both eyes

- Sudden trouble walking, dizziness, loss of balance or coordination

- Sudden severe headache with no known cause

An acronym to help you remember the signs of stroke and what to do is FAST. This stands for Facial drooping, Arm weakness, Speech difficulties, and Time to call 9-1-1. If you believe someone is having a stroke, call 9-1-1 immediately. Ischemic strokes, the most common type, can be treated with a drug called t-PA, which dissolves blood clots. The drug must be administered within three hours, but to be evaluated and treated in time, patients must get to the hospital within 60 minutes.

A transient ischemic attack (TIA) occurs when blood to the brain is briefly blocked. TIAs have the same signs and symptoms as a stroke but usually last less than 1–2 hours (although they may last up to 24 hours). A TIA, which may occur only once in a person's lifetime or more often, can be a warning sign for future strokes.

Sudden Cardiac Arrest Signs

In sudden cardiac arrest (SCA), the heart suddenly and unexpectedly stops beating. As a result, blood stops flowing to the brain and other vital organs. The person suddenly becomes unresponsive and stops breathing, and if not treated within minutes, death can occur. Some people may have a racing heartbeat or feel dizzy or light-headed just before they lose consciousness (faint). Within an hour before SCA, some people have chest pain, shortness of breath, nausea, or vomiting. Usually, however, the first sign of SCA is loss of consciousness. At the same time, no heartbeat (or pulse) can be felt.

If you are with someone who suddenly experiences these symptoms, begin CPR (see Appendix A) and call 9-1-1 immediately. Rapid treatment of SCA with a defibrillator can save a life. A defibrillator is a device that sends an electric shock to the heart to restore its normal rhythm. Automated external defibrillators (AEDs) can be used by bystanders to save the lives of people who are having SCA. (See how to use one at the National Heart, Blood, and Lung Institute website: https://www.nhlbi.nih.gov/health/health-topics/topics/aed/howtouse.) These portable devices are often found in public places, such as shopping malls, golf courses, businesses, airports, airplanes, convention centers, hotels, sports venues, and schools.

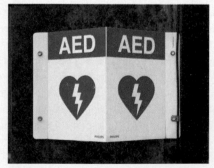

Robert Alexander/Archive Photos/Getty Images

SOURCES: National Heart, Lung, and Blood Institute. 2011. *Don't Take a Chance with a Heart Attack: Know the Facts* (https://www.nhlbi.nih.gov/files/docs/public/heart/heart_attack_fs_en.pdf); National Institute of Neurological disorders and Stroke. 2013. *Know Stroke. Know the Signs. Act in Time* (https://www.stroke.nih.gov/materials/actintime.htm); National Heart, Lung, and Blood Institute. 2016. *Sudden Cardiac Arrest* (https://www.nhlbi.nih.gov/health-topics/sudden-cardiac-arrest).

coronary *stents*—flexible stainless steel tubes—to prop open the artery and prevent reclogging after angioplasty. In coronary bypass surgery, healthy blood vessels are grafted to coronary arteries to bypass blockages.

Stroke

A **stroke**, called a *cerebrovascular accident* (*CVA*), occurs when the blood supply to the brain is cut off. If brain cells are deprived of blood for more than a few minutes, they die. About two million cells are lost every minute that blood flow is not restored. Nerve cells control sensation and most body movements; depending on the area of the brain affected, a stroke may cause paralysis, walking disability, speech impairment, memory loss, and changes in behavior. Prompt treatment of stroke can greatly decrease the risk of permanent disability. The American Heart Association estimates that 795,000 Americans suffer a stroke each year.

There are two major types of strokes: ischemic and hemorrhagic. Ischemic strokes are the more common type and account for 87% of all strokes. They are caused by a blockage in a blood vessel. There are two types of ischemic strokes:

- A *thrombotic stroke* is caused by a blood clot that forms in a cerebral or carotid artery that has been narrowed or damaged by atherosclerosis.

- An *embolic stroke* is caused by an embolus, a wandering blood clot that is carried in the bloodstream and may become wedged in a cerebral artery.

A *hemorrhagic stroke* occurs when a blood vessel in the brain bursts, spilling blood into the surrounding tissue. Cells normally nourished by the vessel are deprived of blood and cannot function. In addition, accumulated blood from the burst vessel may put pressure on surrounding brain tissue, causing damage and even death.

Hemorrhages can be caused by head injuries, by a malformed blood vessel bursting, or by an *aneurysm,* which is a blood-filled pocket that bulges out from a weak spot in the artery wall. Aneurysms in the brain may remain stable and never break, but when they do, the result is a hemorrhagic stroke. Aneurysms may be caused or worsened by hypertension.

Many people have strokes without knowing it. Because silent strokes do not cause symptoms while they are occurring, many people do not realize they need evaluation or treatment for the risk of a full-blown stroke in the future. Although they may be mild, silent strokes leave their victims at a higher risk for subsequent and more serious strokes later in life. They also contribute to loss of mental and cognitive skills.

Some stroke victims have a transient ischemic attack (TIA), or "ministroke," days, weeks, or months before they have a full-blown stroke (see the box "Warning Signs of Heart Attack, Stroke, and Cardiac Arrest"). A TIA produces temporary stroke-like symptoms, such as weakness or numbness in an arm or a leg, speech difficulty, or dizziness. These symptoms are brief, often lasting just a few minutes, and do not cause permanent damage. Still, anyone with a suspected TIA should get immediate medical attention.

Congestive Heart Failure

The heart's pumping mechanism can be damaged by a number of conditions, including high blood pressure, heart attack, atherosclerosis, viral infections, rheumatic fever, and birth defects. When the heart cannot maintain its regular pumping rate and force, fluids begin to back up. When extra fluid seeps through capillary walls, edema (swelling) results, usually in the legs and ankles. Fluid can also collect in the lungs and interfere with breathing, particularly when a person is lying down. This condition is called *pulmonary edema,* and the entire process is known as **congestive heart failure**. Treatment includes reducing the workload on the heart, modifying salt intake, and using drugs that help the body eliminate excess fluid.

RISK FACTORS FOR CARDIOVASCULAR DISEASE

Researchers have identified a variety of factors associated with an increased risk of developing CVD. They have categorized them as major risk factors and contributing risk factors. Some are linked to controllable aspects of lifestyle and can therefore be changed. Others are beyond your control. (You can evaluate your personal CVD risk factors in Part I of Lab 11.1.)

Major Risk Factors That Can Be Changed

The American Heart Association (AHA) has identified six major risk factors for CVD that can be changed: tobacco smoke, high blood pressure, unhealthy cholesterol levels, physical inactivity, obesity, and diabetes. Most Americans, including young adults, have at least one major risk factor for CVD that they can control.

Tobacco Smoke Annually, nearly 1 in 5 deaths is attributable to smoking, equivalent to 1,300 deaths per day. Smoking remains the leading preventable causes of CVD in the United States. People who smoke a pack of cigarettes a day have twice the risk of heart attack that nonsmokers do; smoking two or more packs a day triples the risk. When smokers have heart attacks, they are two to three times more likely than nonsmokers to die from them. Cigarette smoking also doubles the risk of stroke.

> **stroke** An impeded blood supply to some part of the brain, resulting in the destruction of brain cells; also called *cerebrovascular accident* (*CVA*).
>
> **congestive heart failure** A condition resulting from the heart's inability to pump out all the blood that returns to it; blood backs up in the veins leading to the heart, causing an accumulation of fluid in various parts of the body.

TERMS

Smoking harms the cardiovascular system in several ways:

- It damages the lining of arteries.
- It reduces the level of *high-density lipoproteins* (*HDL*), or "good" cholesterol.
- It raises the levels of triglycerides and *low-density lipoproteins* (*LDL*), or "bad" cholesterol.
- Nicotine increases blood pressure and heart rate.
- The carbon monoxide in cigarette smoke displaces oxygen in the blood, reducing the oxygen available to the body, and decreases exercise tolerance.
- Smoking causes **platelets** to stick together in the blood-stream, leading to clotting.
- Smoking speeds the development of fatty deposits in the arteries.

Exposure to other people's smoke also increases the risk of heart disease even for nonsmokers. You don't have to smoke to be affected. The risk of developing heart disease increases up to 30% among people exposed to environmental tobacco smoke (ETS)—also known as "secondhand smoke." Researchers estimate that about 33,950 nonsmokers die from heart disease each year as a result of exposure to ETS.

Recently, electronic cigarettes (or e-cigarettes) have become popular, especially among teenagers and young adults. As of 2018, almost one-third of 12th graders were using electronic cigarettes. Notably, e-cigarettes contain nicotine, which causes addiction, may harm brain development, affects cardiovascular function, and could lead to continued tobacco use into adulthood. The Centers for Disease Control and Prevention (CDC) has identified electronic cigarettes as an area of concern due to the potential harm to public health in the United States.

High Blood Pressure In addition to being a form of CVD in itself, high blood pressure, or **hypertension**, is a risk factor for other forms of cardiovascular disease, including heart attacks and strokes.

Created by the pumping action of the heart, blood pressure is the force exerted by the blood on the vessel walls. High blood pressure occurs when too much force is exerted against the walls of the arteries, thereby increasing the heart's workload and decreasing its efficiency. Short periods of high blood pressure—such as in response to excitement or exertion—are normal, but chronic high blood pressure is a health risk.

Blood pressure is expressed as two numbers—for example, 120 over 80—and measured in millimeters of mercury (mmHg). The first number measures systolic blood pressure, the greatest pressure your blood exerts against artery walls as your heart beats, pushing blood around the body. The second measures diastolic blood pressure, the lowest pressure, which occurs when

platelets Cell fragments in the blood that are necessary for the formation of blood clots.

hypertension Sustained abnormally high blood pressure.

Table 11.1	Blood Pressure Classification for Healthy Adults			
CATEGORY[a]	SYSTOLIC (mmHg)			DIASTOLIC (mmHg)
Normal[b]	below 120	and		below 80
Elevated	120–129	and		below 80
Hypertension[c]				
Stage 1	130–139	or		80–89
Stage 2	140 or higher	or		90 or higher

[a]When systolic and diastolic pressures fall into different categories, the higher category should be used to classify blood pressure status.

[b]The risk of death from heart attack and stroke begins to rise when blood pressure is above 115/75.

[c]Based on the average of two or more readings taken at different physician visits. In people older than 50, systolic blood pressure greater than 140 mmHg is a much more significant CVD risk factor than diastolic blood pressure.

SOURCE: Whelton, P., et al. 2017. "2017 ACC/AHA/AAPA/ABC/ACPM/AGS/APhA/ASH/ASPC/NMA/PCNA guideline for the prevention, detection, evaluation, and management of high blood pressure in adults," *Journal of the American College of Cardiology*, 1–176. (https://doi:10.1016/j.jacc.2017.11.006).

your heart relaxes between beats (see Chapter 3). A normal blood pressure reading for a healthy adult is below 120 systolic and below 80 diastolic. Blood pressure readings above this level indicate an increased risk for CVD and are classified as prehypertension or hypertension. High blood pressure (hypertension) in adults is defined as equal to or greater than 130 systolic or 80 diastolic (Table 11.1). Health care professionals measure blood pressure with a stethoscope and an instrument called a *sphygmomanometer*. Professional measurement is needed for a diagnosis of hypertension, but you can track your own blood pressure at a drugstore or at home with an inexpensive monitor, and some new technologies measure blood pressure with wearable devices.

High blood pressure results from the heart's increased output of blood or from the arteries' increased resistance to blood flow. Arterial resistance can be caused by the constriction of smooth muscle surrounding the arteries or by atherosclerosis. High blood pressure also scars and hardens arteries, making them less elastic and further increasing blood pressure. High blood pressure makes the heart work harder than normal to force blood through the narrowed and stiffened arteries, straining both the heart and the arteries. Eventually, the strained heart weakens and tends to enlarge, which weakens it even more.

High blood pressure is often called a silent killer, because it usually has no symptoms. A person may have high blood pressure for years without realizing it. But during that time, it damages vital organs and increases the risk of heart attack, congestive heart failure, stroke, kidney failure, and blindness.

Recent research has shed new light on the importance of lowering blood pressure to improve cardiovascular health. Doctors now target lower blood pressures than goals used in the past: The risk of death from heart attack or stroke begins to rise even when blood pressure is just above 120 over 80 mmHg, in the range referred to as "elevated."

Hypertension is common. Under the newly updated blood pressure guidelines, about 46% of adults have hypertension (defined as systolic pressure of 120–129 mmHg and diastolic pressure of less than 80 mmHg), with the greatest impact among younger individuals. In most cases, hypertension cannot be cured, but it can be controlled. The key to avoiding complications is to have your blood pressure tested at least once every two years (or if you have other CVD risk factors, at least once every year).

Lifestyle changes are recommended for everyone with elevated blood pressure and hypertension. These changes include weight reduction, regular physical activity, a healthy diet, and moderation of alcohol use. The DASH diet (see Chapter 8) is recommended specifically for people with high blood pressure; it emphasizes fruits, vegetables, and whole grains—foods that are rich in potassium and fiber, both of which may reduce blood pressure. Sodium restriction is also helpful. The *2015–2020 Dietary Guidelines for Americans* recommends restricting sodium consumption to less than 2,300 mg (equivalent to a teaspoon of salt) per day for adults and children age 14 and older. This recommendation applies to all people but is particularly important for those with hypertension or prehypertension, African Americans, and middle-aged and older adults. For these groups, further reduction in sodium intake to 1,500 mg per day can result in even greater blood pressure reduction. Adequate potassium intake is also important. New blood pressure drug treatments are available, as well as particular combinations for the elderly and people with diabetes, chronic kidney disease, and cardiovascular diseases. People who fall into the category of prehypertension or the high normal blood pressure range may not benefit from drug therapy.

Unhealthy Cholesterol Levels

Cholesterol is a fatty, wax-like substance that circulates through the bloodstream and is an important component of cell membranes, sex hormones, vitamin D, the fluid that coats the lungs, and the protective sheaths around nerves. Adequate cholesterol is essential for the proper functioning of the body. Excess cholesterol, however, can clog arteries and increase the risk of CVD (Figure 11.3). Your liver manufactures cholesterol; foods can also increase your cholesterol level.

GOOD VERSUS BAD CHOLESTEROL Cholesterol is carried in the blood by protein-lipid packages called **lipoproteins**. **Low-density lipoproteins (LDLs)** shuttle cholesterol from the liver to the organs and tissues that require it. LDL is known as "bad" cholesterol because if there is more than the body can use, the excess can be deposited in the blood vessels. The accumulated LDL becomes encased in artery walls and may be oxidized by free radicals, speeding inflammation and damage to artery walls and increasing the likelihood that an artery will become blocked, causing a heart attack or stroke. **High-density lipoproteins (HDLs)**, or "good" cholesterol, act as scavengers and are transported in a protein package that takes LDL cholesterol back to the liver for recycling. By removing cholesterol from blood vessels, HDLs help protect against atherosclerosis.

RECOMMENDED BLOOD CHOLESTEROL LEVELS Screening for cholesterol provides one part of the assessment of the risk of cardiovascular disease. This risk for CVD increases with higher LDL cholesterol levels. The National Cholesterol Education Program recommends testing at least once every five years for all adults, beginning at age 20. The recommended test is a fasting lipoprotein profile that measures total cholesterol, LDL cholesterol, HDL cholesterol, and triglycerides (a type of blood fat). In general, high LDL, total cholesterol, and triglyceride levels, combined with low HDL levels, are associated with a higher risk for CVD. You can reduce this risk by lowering LDL, total cholesterol, and triglycerides. Raising HDL is important because a high HDL level seems to offer some protection from CVD even in cases where total cholesterol is high. This appears to be especially true for women.

The latest American College of Cardiology (ACC) and the AHA guidelines for the treatment of elevated blood cholesterol levels focus on lifestyle change as well as therapy with *statins,* a group of medications that lower LDL. Although the previous guidelines set specific targets for LDL and HDL, the new guidelines instead focus on identifying the groups of people for whom medical treatment has the greatest chance of preventing heart attacks and strokes (Table 11.2). Experts hope that the new recommendations will mean that more people who would benefit from statin therapy will get it, while those who would not benefit will avoid unnecessary treatment.

People can review their specific risk factors and the pros and cons of therapy with their health care providers. Lifestyle choices to help improve cholesterol levels include exercising regularly, limiting saturated and trans fat intake, and choosing a healthy dietary pattern. To lower LDL, the ACC and AHA recommend a dietary pattern that is rich in fruits, vegetables, and whole grains; includes low-fat dairy, poultry, fish, legumes, nontropical vegetable oils, and nuts; and limits sweets, sugar-sweetened beverages, and red meats.

Physical Inactivity

At risk for CVD, about 1 in every 3 Americans is sedentary during leisure time. Exercise is thought to be the closest thing we have to a magic bullet against heart disease. It lowers CVD risk by helping to decrease blood pressure and resting heart rate, increase HDL levels, maintain desirable weight, improve the condition of the blood vessels, and prevent or control diabetes. One study found that women who got in at least three hours of brisk walking each week cut their risk of heart attack and stroke by more than half. (See Chapter 3 for more information on the benefits of cardiorespiratory exercise.)

---

lipoproteins Protein-and-lipid substances in the blood that carry fats and cholesterol; classified according to size, density, and chemical composition.

low-density lipoprotein (LDL) A lipoprotein containing a moderate amount of protein and a large amount of cholesterol; "bad" cholesterol.

high-density lipoprotein (HDL) A lipoprotein containing relatively little cholesterol that helps transport cholesterol out of the arteries; "good" cholesterol.

TERMS

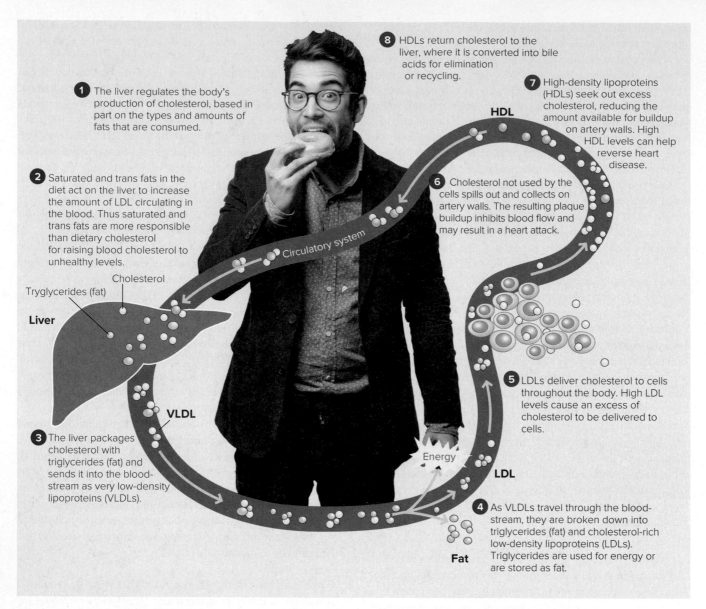

Figure 11.3 Travels with cholesterol.

Asier Romero/Shutterstock

The following labels appear in the figure:

1 The liver regulates the body's production of cholesterol, based in part on the types and amounts of fats that are consumed.

2 Saturated and trans fats in the diet act on the liver to increase the amount of LDL circulating in the blood. Thus saturated and trans fats are more responsible than dietary cholesterol for raising blood cholesterol to unhealthy levels.

Tryglycerides (fat)

Cholesterol

Liver

3 The liver packages cholesterol with triglycerides (fat) and sends it into the blood-stream as very low-density lipoproteins (VLDLs).

VLDL

Circulatory system

Energy

Fat

4 As VLDLs travel through the blood-stream, they are broken down into triglycerides (fat) and cholesterol-rich low-density lipoproteins (LDLs). Triglycerides are used for energy or are stored as fat.

LDL

5 LDLs deliver cholesterol to cells throughout the body. High LDL levels cause an excess of cholesterol to be delivered to cells.

6 Cholesterol not used by the cells spills out and collects on artery walls. The resulting plaque buildup inhibits blood flow and may result in a heart attack.

7 High-density lipoproteins (HDLs) seek out excess cholesterol, reducing the amount available for buildup on artery walls. High HDL levels can help reverse heart disease.

HDL

8 HDLs return cholesterol to the liver, where it is converted into bile acids for elimination or recycling.

Obesity The risk of death from CVD is two to three times higher in obese people (BMI ≥ 30) than it is in lean people (BMI 18.5–24.9), and for every five-unit increment of BMI, a person's risk of death from coronary heart disease increases by 30%. Excess weight increases the strain on the heart by contributing to high blood pressure and high cholesterol. It can also lead to diabetes, another CVD risk factor (see the next section). As discussed in Chapter 6, distribution of body fat is also significant: Fat that collects in the abdomen is more dangerous than fat that collects around the hips. Obesity in general, and abdominal obesity in particular, is significantly associated with narrowing of the coronary arteries, even in young adults in their 20s.

A sensible diet and regular exercise are the best ways to achieve and maintain a healthy body weight (see Chapter 9 for an extensive discussion of weight control). For someone who is overweight, even modest weight reduction can reduce CVD risk by lowering blood pressure, improving cholesterol levels, and reducing diabetes risk.

Diabetes **Diabetes mellitus** is a disorder in which the metabolism of glucose is disrupted, causing a buildup of glucose in the bloodstream. People with diabetes are at increased risk for CVD, partly because elevated blood glucose levels can damage the lining of arteries, making them more vulnerable to

diabetes mellitus A disease that disrupts normal metabolism, interfering with cells' ability to take in glucose for energy production. **TERMS**

atherosclerosis. Diabetics also often have other risk factors, including hypertension, obesity, unhealthy cholesterol and triglyceride levels, and platelet and blood coagulation abnormalities. Even people whose diabetes is under control face an increased risk of CVD. Therefore, careful control of other risk factors is critical for people with diabetes. Diabetes is described in detail later in the chapter.

Contributing Risk Factors That Can Be Changed

As with the major risk factors, some contributing CVD risk factors can be changed, including triglyceride levels, psychological and social factors, and drug use.

High Triglyceride Levels *Triglycerides* are blood fats that are absorbed from food and manufactured by the body. High triglyceride levels are a reliable predictor of heart disease, especially if associated with other risk factors, such as low HDL levels, obesity, and diabetes. Factors contributing to elevated triglyceride levels include excess body fat, physical inactivity, cigarette smoking, type 2 diabetes, excessive alcohol intake, very-high-carbohydrate diets, and certain diseases and medications. A full lipid profile should include testing and evaluation of triglyceride levels.

For people with high triglyceride levels, lifestyle changes can bring levels down into the healthy range: losing weight, reducing intake of added sugars while increasing intake of unsaturated fats, and increasing physical activity. Limiting alcohol use is also helpful. For some people with very high triglyceride levels, drug therapy may be prescribed.

Insulin Resistance and Metabolic Syndrome As people gain weight and become less active, their muscles, fat, and liver become less sensitive to the effect of insulin—a condition known as *insulin resistance* (or prediabetes). As the body becomes increasingly insulin resistant, the pancreas must secrete more and more insulin (hyperinsulinemia) to keep glucose levels within a normal range. Eventually even high levels of insulin may become insufficient, and blood glucose levels start to rise (hyperglycemia), resulting in type 2 diabetes.

Those who have insulin resistance tend to have several other related risk factors. This cluster of abnormalities is called *metabolic syndrome* or *insulin resistance syndrome* (Table 11.3). Metabolic syndrome significantly increases the risk of CVD—more so in women than in men. It is estimated that about 34% of the adult U.S. population has metabolic syndrome.

To reduce your risk of developing metabolic syndrome, choose a healthy dietary pattern and get plenty of aerobic exercise. Reducing calorie intake to prevent weight gain, or losing weight if needed, also reduces insulin resistance. Eating more protein, vegetables, and fiber while limiting fat, added sugars, and starches may be beneficial.

Inflammation Inflammation plays a key role in the development of CVD. When an artery is injured by hypertension, smoking, cholesterol, or other factors, the body's response is to produce inflammation. A substance called C-reactive protein (CRP) is released into the bloodstream during the inflammatory response, and high levels of CRP indicate a substantially elevated risk of heart attack and stroke. CRP may also be harmful to the coronary arteries themselves. Gum disease involves another type of inflammation that may moderately influence the progress of coronary heart disease.

Table 11.3	Characteristics of Metabolic Syndrome*	
FACTOR	**CRITERIA**	
Large waistline	35 or more inches for women	
	40 or more inches for men	
High triglyceride level	150 mg/dL or higher	
	Or taking medication to treat high triglycerides	
Low HDL level	Less than 50 mg/dL for women	
	Less than 40 mg/dL for men	
	Or taking medication to treat low HDL	
High blood pressure	130/85 mmHg or higher (one or both numbers)	
	Or taking medication to treat high blood pressure	
High fasting blood sugar	100 mg/dL or higher	
	Or taking medication to treat high blood sugar	

*A person having three or more factors listed here is diagnosed with metabolic syndrome.

SOURCE: Adapted from National Heart, Lung, and Blood Institute. 2011. *How Is Metabolic Syndrome Diagnosed?* (http://www.nhlbi.nih.gov/health/health-topics/topics/ms/diagnosis).

Lifestyle changes and certain drugs can reduce inflammation and CRP levels. Statin drugs, widely prescribed to lower cholesterol, also decrease inflammation; this may be one reason that statin drugs seem to lower CVD risk even in people with normal blood lipid levels.

Psychological and Social Factors Many of the psychological and social factors that influence other areas of wellness are also important risk factors for CVD. They include chronic stress, chronic hostility and anger, lack of social support, and others. The cardiovascular system is affected by both sudden, acute episodes of mental stress and the more chronic, underlying emotions of anger, anxiety, and depression. See Chapter 10 for more information on stress, its effects, and ways to combat these effects.

Alcohol and Drugs Drinking too much alcohol raises blood pressure and can increase the risk of stroke and heart failure. Stimulant drugs, particularly cocaine and methamphetamines—and stimulants such as ecstasy (MDMA)—can also cause serious cardiac problems, including heart attack, stroke, and sudden cardiac death. Injection drug use can cause heart infections and stroke.

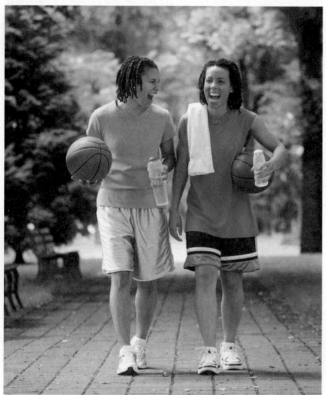

Wellness Tip Stress and social isolation increase the risk of cardiovascular disease, whereas social support buffers risk and may prevent or delay the onset of CVD. A strong social support network improves both heart health and overall wellness and can provide opportunities for exercise and relaxation. Take time out to develop and nurture friendships and family ties.

David Buffington/Blend Images/Getty Images

Major Risk Factors That Can't Be Changed

A number of major risk factors for CVD cannot be changed. They include genetics, aging, being male, and ethnicity.

Genetics Multiple genes contribute to the development of CVD and its risk factors. Having an unfavorable set of genes increases your risk, but risk is modifiable by lifestyle factors such as whether you smoke, exercise, or eat a healthy diet. People who inherit a tendency for CVD are not destined to develop it, but they may have to work harder than other people to prevent it.

Age About 70% of all heart attack victims are age 65 or older, and about 75% who suffer fatal heart attacks are over 65. For people over 55, the incidence of stroke more than doubles in each successive decade. However, even people in their 30s and 40s can have heart attacks.

Gender Although CVD is the leading killer of both men and women in the United States, men face a greater risk of heart attack than women, especially earlier in life. Until age 55, men also have a greater risk of hypertension than women. The incidence of stroke is higher for males than females until age 65. Estrogen production, which is highest during the child-bearing years, may protect premenopausal women against CVD (see the box "Gender, Race/Ethnicity, and CVD"). By age 75, the gender gap nearly disappears.

Race/Ethnicity Rates of heart disease and CVD risk factors vary among racial and ethnic groups in the United States. African Americans have much higher rates of hypertension, heart disease, and stroke than other groups do. Figure 11.4 shows how rates of CVD compare among racial and ethnic groups in the United States. American Indians and Alaska Natives have higher rates of hypertension than non-Hispanic whites; Hispanic women have higher rates of angina (a warning

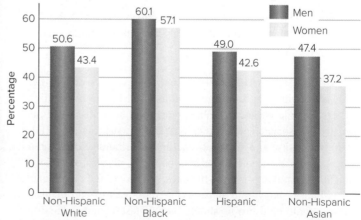

Figure 11.4 Percentage of adult Americans with cardiovascular disease.

SOURCE: Benjamin, E. J., et al. 2019. "Heart disease and stroke statistics–2019 update," *Circulation*, 139, no. 10: e56–528. (https://DOI: 10.1161 /CIR.0000000000000659).

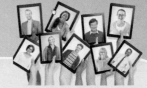

CVD is the leading cause of death for all Americans, but significant differences exist between men and women and among racial/ethnic groups in the incidence, diagnosis, and treatment of this deadly disease.

CVD in Women

CVD has been thought of as a "man's disease," but it actually kills more women than men. Polls indicate that women vastly underestimate their risk of dying of a heart attack and overestimate their risk of dying of breast cancer. In reality, women are 10 times more likely to die of heart disease than breast cancer. In the past, CVD rarely developed in women under age 50, but new research suggests that CVD deaths in women aged 35–54 is increasing. Young women receive fewer treatments and preventative medications for CVD, probably because they do not fit the typical CVD patient profile many doctors are familiar with.

The hormone estrogen, produced naturally by a woman's ovaries until menopause, improves blood lipid concentrations and reduces other CVD risk factors. For several decades, many physicians encouraged menopausal women to take hormone replacement therapy (HRT), which includes estrogen, to relieve menopause symptoms and presumably to reduce their risk of CVD. However, some studies found that HRT may actually *increase* a woman's risk for heart disease and other health problems, including breast cancer. Some newer studies have found that the increased risk of CVD in women who start HRT may be age dependent; women in the early stages of menopause or ages 50–59 did not appear to have excess risk. This suggests that outcomes may depend on several factors, including the timing of hormone use. The U.S. Preventive Services Task Force and the American Heart Association recommend that HRT not be used to protect against CVD.

When women have heart attacks, they are more likely than men to die within a year. One reason is that because they develop heart disease at older ages, women are more likely to have other health problems that complicate treatment. Women with CVD are less likely than men to report the usual symptoms of a heart attack, such as chest pain, and more likely to report less-specific symptoms; this pattern may obscure the diagnosis. These less-specific symptoms include fatigue, weakness, shortness of breath, nausea, vomiting, and pain in the abdomen, neck, jaw, and back. Women are also more likely than men to have pain at rest, during sleep, or accompanying mental stress. A woman who experiences these symptoms should be persistent in seeking accurate diagnosis and appropriate treatment.

Careful diagnosis of cardiac symptoms is also key in avoiding unnecessary invasive procedures in cases of stress cardiomyopathy ("broken heart syndrome"), which occurs much more commonly in women than in men. In this condition, hormones and neurotransmitters associated with a severe stress response stun the heart, producing heart-attack-like symptoms and decreased pumping function of the heart, but no damage to the heart muscle. Typically, the condition reverses quickly.

Women should be aware of their CVD risk factors and consult with a physician to assess their risk and determine the best way to prevent CVD.

CVD in African Americans and Other Racial/Ethnic Groups

Although cardiovascular disease is the leading cause of death for all Americans, there is a higher prevalence of CVD in adult African Americans, and a higher prevalence of many associated risk factors in Mexican Americans, than in non-Hispanic whites and Asian Americans. The reasons for these disparities likely include both genetic and environmental factors.

African Americans tend to develop hypertension at an earlier age than non-Hispanic whites, and their average blood pressures are much higher. African Americans have a higher risk of stroke and have strokes at younger ages. Survivors have more significant stroke-related disabilities. Some experts recommend that African Americans begin taking antihypertensive drugs when blood pressure reaches 130/80 rather than the typical 140/90 cutoff for hypertension.

A number of genetic and biological factors may contribute to CVD in African Americans. For instance, a higher sensitivity to dietary sodium may lead to greater blood pressure elevation in response to a given amount of sodium. African Americans may also experience less dilation of blood vessels in response to stress (see Chapter 10).

Genetics also plays a large role in the tendency to develop diabetes, another important CVD risk factor that is more common in non-Hispanic blacks and Hispanics than in non-Hispanic whites. However, the prevalence of diabetes varies among those with different Hispanic backgrounds; for example, the rate of diabetes among Mexican Americans is nearly twice that of people who trace their background to South America.

Racial and ethnic groups other than non-Hispanic whites are more likely to be poor, and low income is associated with reduced access to health care and healthy dietary options for CVD prevention. Associated with low income is low educational attainment, which often means less access to information about preventive health measures, such as diet and stress management. Populations with low incomes tend to smoke more, consume more salt, and exercise less than those with higher incomes. Residents of low-income neighborhoods also experience longer delays between the onset of heart attack symptoms and reaching a hospital.

Discrimination may also play a role in CVD. Physicians and hospitals may treat the medical problems of non-whites differently from those of whites. Discrimination, low income, and other forms of deprivation may also increase stress, which is linked to hypertension and CVD. Lack of insurance coverage and less-advanced medical technologies in hospitals that serve minority and low-income neighborhoods may also play a role.

All Americans, regardless of background, are advised to have their blood pressure checked regularly, exercise on a regular basis, eat a healthy diet, manage stress, and avoid tobacco products. Tailoring your lifestyle to any risk factors especially relevant for you can also help. Discuss your particular risk profile with your physician to help identify the lifestyle changes most appropriate for you.

sign of heart disease) than other racial/ethnic groups. Asian Americans historically have had far lower rates of CVD than white Americans.

Possible Risk Factors Currently Being Studied

In recent years, several other possible risk factors for cardiovascular disease have been identified.

Elevated blood levels of homocysteine, an amino acid that may damage the lining of blood vessels, are associated with an increased risk of CVD. Men generally have higher homocysteine levels than women, as do individuals with diets low in folic acid, vitamin B-12, and vitamin B-6. Most people can lower homocysteine levels easily by adopting a healthy diet rich in fruits, vegetables, and grains. Severe vitamin D deficiency has also been associated with heart dysfunction, independent of homocysteine levels.

Several infectious agents, including *Chlamydia pneumoniae,* cytomegalovirus, and *Helicobacter pylori,* have also been identified as possible risk factors for cardiovascular disease. *Chlamydia pneumoniae,* a common cause of flulike respiratory infections, has been found in sections of clogged, damaged arteries but not in sections of healthy arteries. This effect may be secondary to the inflammation that many infectious agents produce.

Gum disease has long been suspected to be linked to CVD. Gingivitis, the beginning stages of gum disease, occurs when bacteria accumulate on the teeth, causing inflammation of the gums. For recommendations on good dental self-care, visit the American Dental Association's consumer website: http://www.mouthhealthy.org.

? Ask Yourself

QUESTIONS FOR CRITICAL THINKING AND REFLECTION?

What risk factors do you have for cardiovascular disease? Which ones are factors you have control over, and which are factors you can't change? If you have risk factors you cannot change (such as a family history of CVD), were you aware that you can make lifestyle adjustments to reduce your risk? Do you think you will make them? Why or why not?

PROTECTING YOURSELF AGAINST CARDIOVASCULAR DISEASE

You can take several important steps right now to lower your risk of developing CVD (Figure 11.5). Reducing CVD risk factors when you are young can pay off with many extra years of life and good health. CVD can begin very early in life. For example, fatty streaks (very early atherosclerosis) can be seen on the aorta in children younger than age 10.

Eat a Heart-Healthy Diet

A dietary pattern for heart health emphasizes whole grains, a variety of fruits and vegetables, low-fat dairy products, nuts, legumes, fish, lean meats, and vegetable oils. Limit saturated and trans fats, sweets and sugar-sweetened beverages, sodium, and

Do More

- Eat a diet rich in fruits, vegetables, whole grains, and low-fat or fat-free dairy products. Eat five to nine servings of fruits and vegetables each day.

- Eat several servings of high-fiber foods each day.

- Eat two or more servings of fish per week; try a few servings of nuts and soy foods each week.

- Choose unsaturated fats rather than saturated and trans fats.

  - Be physically active; do both aerobic exercise and strength training on a regular basis.

  - Achieve and maintain a healthy weight.

- Develop effective strategies for handling stress and anger. Nurture old friendships and family ties, and make new friends; pay attention to your spiritual side.

- Obtain recommended screening tests and follow your physician's recommendations.

Do Less

- Don't use tobacco in any form: cigarettes, e-cigarettes, spit tobacco, cigars and pipes, bidis, and clove cigarettes.

- Limit consumption of trans fats and saturated fats.

- Limit consumption of salt to no more than 2,300 mg of sodium per day (1,500 mg if you have or are at high risk for hypertension).

- Avoid exposure to environmental tobacco smoke.

- Avoid excessive alcohol consumption— no more than one drink per day for women and two drinks per day for men.

- Limit consumption of added sugars and refined carbohydrates.

- Avoid excess stress, anger, and hostility.

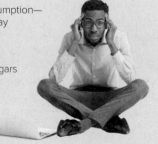

Figure 11.5   Strategies for reducing your risk of cardiovascular disease.

(left): Jessica Peterson/Rubberball/Getty Images; (right): Vladyslav Starozhylov/Alamy Stock Photo

red meat. Specific guidelines for heart health include the following:

- *Fats:* Saturated fats should be limited to 7% of total daily calories, or 5–6% for adults who have elevated LDL. Trans fats should be avoided. The majority of fats in your diet should be unsaturated, from sources such as vegetable oils, fish, and nuts.

- *Fiber:* Studies have shown that a high-fiber diet is associated with a 40–50% reduction in the risk of heart attack and stroke. To get the recommended 25–38 grams of dietary fiber a day, eat whole grains, fruits, and vegetables. Good sources of fiber include oatmeal, some breakfast cereals, barley, legumes, and most fruits and vegetables.

- *Sodium and potassium:* Reducing sodium intake to recommended levels, while also increasing potassium intake, can help reduce blood pressure for many people. Limit sodium intake to no more than 2,300 mg (about 1 teaspoon) per day for all Americans. Reducing sodium intake further, to 1,500 mg/day, is associated with even greater reductions in blood pressure.

- *Alcohol:* Moderate alcohol use may increase HDL cholesterol; it may also reduce stroke risk, possibly by dampening the inflammatory response or by affecting blood clotting. For most people under age 45, however, the risks of alcohol use probably outweigh any health benefit. Excessive alcohol consumption increases the risk of a variety of serious health problems, including hypertension, stroke, some cancers, liver disease, alcohol dependence, and injuries.

Exercise Regularly

You can significantly reduce your risk of CVD with a moderate amount of physical activity (see the box "How Does Exercise Affect CVD Risk?"). Refer to Chapters 2 through 7 to learn how to create and implement a complete exercise program.

Avoid Tobacco

The number-one risk factor for CVD that you can control is smoking. If you smoke, quit or enroll in a stop-smoking program. If you don't smoke, don't start. If you live or work with people who smoke, encourage them to quit—for their sake and yours. If you find yourself breathing in smoke, take steps to prevent or stop this exposure.

Know and Manage Your Blood Pressure

If you have no CVD risk factors, have your blood pressure measured at least once every two years; yearly tests are recommended if you have other risk factors. If your blood pressure is high, follow your physician's advice on lowering it.

Know and Manage Your Cholesterol Levels

All people age 20 and over should have their cholesterol checked at least once every five years. The National Cholesterol Education Program recommends a fasting lipoprotein profile that measures total cholesterol, HDL, LDL, and triglyceride levels. After you know your baseline numbers, you and your physician can develop a treatment and lifestyle plan.

Develop Ways to Handle Stress and Anger

To reduce the psychological and social risk factors for CVD, develop effective strategies for handling the stress in your life. Shore up your social support network, and try some techniques described in Chapter 10 for managing stress and anger.

Ask Yourself

QUESTIONS FOR CRITICAL THINKING AND REFLECTION?

Do you know what your blood pressure and cholesterol levels are? If not, is there something preventing you from getting this information about yourself? How can you motivate yourself to have these easy but important health checks?

DIABETES

As described earlier, diabetes mellitus is both a major risk factor for cardiovascular disease and a leading cause of death among Americans. In diabetes, the process of metabolism is disrupted (Figure 11.6). The pancreas normally secretes insulin, which stimulates cells to take up glucose (blood sugar) to produce energy. Diabetes interferes with this process, causing a buildup of glucose in the bloodstream.

Types of Diabetes

About 30.3 million Americans (9.3% of the population) have one of two major forms of diabetes—more than double the number of people affected in 1995. About 5–10% of people with diabetes have the more serious form, known as *type 1 diabetes*. In this type of diabetes, the body's immune system, triggered by a viral infection or some other environmental factor, destroys the insulin-producing cells in the pancreas. The pancreas produces little or no insulin, so daily doses of insulin are required; without insulin, a person will lapse into a coma. Type 1 diabetes usually begins in childhood or adolescence and is not related to obesity.

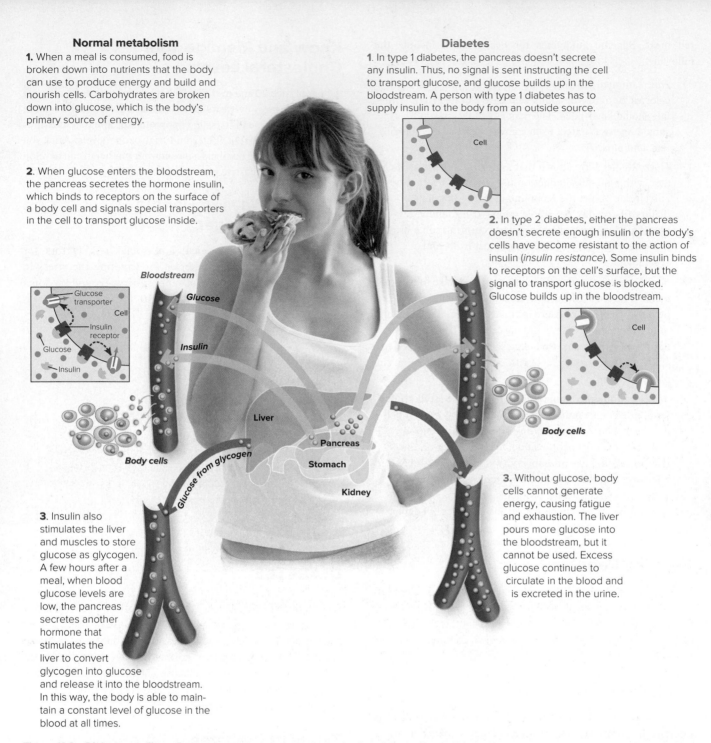

Normal metabolism

1. When a meal is consumed, food is broken down into nutrients that the body can use to produce energy and build and nourish cells. Carbohydrates are broken down into glucose, which is the body's primary source of energy.

2. When glucose enters the bloodstream, the pancreas secretes the hormone insulin, which binds to receptors on the surface of a body cell and signals special transporters in the cell to transport glucose inside.

3. Insulin also stimulates the liver and muscles to store glucose as glycogen. A few hours after a meal, when blood glucose levels are low, the pancreas secretes another hormone that stimulates the liver to convert glycogen into glucose and release it into the bloodstream. In this way, the body is able to maintain a constant level of glucose in the blood at all times.

Diabetes

1. In type 1 diabetes, the pancreas doesn't secrete any insulin. Thus, no signal is sent instructing the cell to transport glucose, and glucose builds up in the bloodstream. A person with type 1 diabetes has to supply insulin to the body from an outside source.

2. In type 2 diabetes, either the pancreas doesn't secrete enough insulin or the body's cells have become resistant to the action of insulin (*insulin resistance*). Some insulin binds to receptors on the cell's surface, but the signal to transport glucose is blocked. Glucose builds up in the bloodstream.

3. Without glucose, body cells cannot generate energy, causing fatigue and exhaustion. The liver pours more glucose into the bloodstream, but it cannot be used. Excess glucose continues to circulate in the blood and is excreted in the urine.

Bloodstream
Glucose transporter
Cell
Insulin receptor
Glucose
Insulin
Cell
Glucose
Insulin
Body cells
Liver
Glucose from glycogen
Pancreas
Stomach
Kidney
Body cells

Figure 11.6 Diabetes mellitus. During digestion, carbohydrates are broken down in the small intestine into glucose, a simple sugar that enters the bloodstream. The presence of glucose signals the pancreas to release insulin, a hormone that helps cells take up glucose; once inside a cell, glucose can be converted to energy. In diabetes, this process is disrupted, resulting in a buildup of glucose in the bloodstream.

webphotographeer/iStock/Getty Images

The remaining Americans with diabetes have *type 2 diabetes.* This condition can develop slowly, and about a quarter of affected individuals are unaware of their condition. In type 2 diabetes, the pancreas fails to produce enough insulin, cells are resistant to insulin, or both. This condition is usually diagnosed in people over age 40, although there has been a tenfold increase in type 2 diabetes in children in the past two decades. About one-third of people with type 2 diabetes must take insulin; others may take medications that increase insulin production or stimulate cells to take up glucose.

A third type of diabetes occurs in 2–10% of women during pregnancy. *Gestational diabetes* usually disappears after pregnancy. Women who had gestational diabetes during pregnancy have up to a 60% chance of developing diabetes within 10–20 years.

Regular exercise directly and indirectly benefits your cardiovascular health and can help you avoid a heart attack or stroke. The evidence comes from dozens of large-scale, population-based studies conducted over the past several decades. There is so much evidence about the cardiovascular health benefits of exercise, in fact, that physicians regard physical activity as a magic bullet against heart disease.

Physical activity has an inverse relationship with cardiovascular disease, meaning that the more exercise you get, the less likely you are to develop or die from CVD. Compared to sedentary individuals, people who engage in regular, moderate physical activity lower their risk of CVD by 20% or more. People who get regular, vigorous exercise reduce their risk of CVD by 30% or more. This positive benefit applies regardless of gender, age, race, or ethnicity.

Most studies focus on various aerobic endurance exercises, such as walking, running on a treadmill, or biking. The type of exercise performed is less important than the amount of energy expended during the activity. The greater the energy expenditure, the greater the health benefits.

Exercise affects heart health via many mechanisms, all of which are being studied. For example, exercise helps people lose weight and improve body composition. Weight loss can improve heart health by reducing the amount of stress on the heart. Changing body composition to a more positive ratio of fat to fat-free mass boosts resting metabolic rate. Exercise directly strengthens the heart muscle itself, and it improves the balance of fats in the blood by boosting HDL and reducing LDL and triglyceride levels.

Exercise improves the health and function of the endothelial cells—the inner lining of the arteries. These cells secrete nitric oxide, which regulates blood flow, improves nerve function, strengthens the immune system, enhances reproductive health, and suppresses inflammation. Exercise training also improves the function of sodium-potassium pumps, which regulate fluid and electrolyte balance and cellular communication throughout the body.

One of the clearest positive effects of exercise is on hypertension. Many studies, involving thousands of people, have shown that physical activity reduces both systolic and diastolic blood pressure. These studies showed that people who engaged in regular aerobic exercise lowered their resting blood pressure by 2–4%, on average. Lowered blood pressure itself reduces the risk of other kinds of CVD.

Even with limited evidence, there appears to be an inverse relationship between physical activity and stroke. That is, according to a handful of studies, the most physically active people reduced their risk of both ischemic and hemorrhagic strokes by up to 30%. Although this benefit appears to apply equally to men and women, there is not sufficient evidence that it applies equally across races or ethnicities.

Of course, exercise isn't possible for everyone and may actually be dangerous for some people. People with CVD or serious risk factors for heart disease should work with their physician to determine whether or how to exercise.

Keep these guidelines in mind as you strive to reduce CVD risk factors:

- **Set goals.** Target a behavior (such as exercising for 30 minutes per day).

- **Monitor yourself.** Self-monitoring increases your awareness of physical cues and behaviors and helps you identify the barriers to changing a behavior.

- **Schedule follow-up exercise sessions.** Multiple sessions are more effective than single sessions.

- **Get feedback from your health care provider.** Feedback can encourage healthy choices by giving you an external measuring stick you can use to monitor your progress.

- **Keep a positive outlook on your progress.** A feeling of accomplishment is very important in motivating you to initiate new behaviors and continue your efforts.

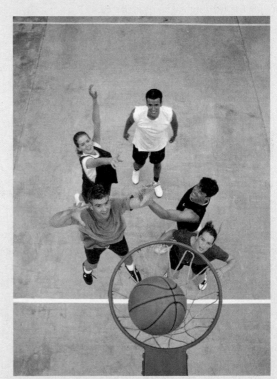

Photodisc/Getty Images

SOURCES: Brawner, C. A., et al. 2017. "Maximal exercise capacity is associated with survival in men and women," *Mayo Clinic Proceedings* 92(3): 383–390; Eckel, R. H., et al. 2014. "2013 AHA/ACC guideline on lifestyle management to reduce cardiovascular risk: A report of the American College of Cardiology/American Heart Association Task Force on Practice Guidelines," *Journal of the American College of Cardiology* 63(25_PA); Physical Activity Guidelines Advisory Committee. 2008. *Physical Activity Guidelines Advisory Committee Report, 2008.* Washington, DC: U.S. Department of Health and Human Services.

The term *prediabetes* describes blood glucose levels that are higher than normal but not high enough for a diagnosis of full-blown diabetes. The American Heart Association estimates that about 92 million Americans have prediabetes. Experts warn that most people with the condition will develop type 2 diabetes unless they adopt preventive lifestyle measures. People with prediabetes also face a significantly increased risk of CVD.

The major factors involved in the development of type 2 diabetes are age, obesity, physical inactivity, a family history of diabetes, and lifestyle. Excess body fat reduces cell sensitivity to insulin, and insulin resistance is usually a precursor of type 2 diabetes. Race and ethnicity also play a role. According to the Centers for Disease Control and Prevention, the rate of diagnosed diabetes cases is highest among Native Americans and Alaska Natives, followed by blacks, Hispanics, Asian Americans, and white Americans. About 26% of all Americans age 65 and older have diabetes, either diagnosed or undiagnosed.

Warning Signs and Testing

Be alert for the warning signs of diabetes:

- Frequent urination
- Extreme hunger or thirst
- Unexplained weight loss
- Extreme fatigue
- Blurred vision
- Frequent infections
- Cuts and bruises that are slow to heal
- Tingling or numbness in the hands or feet
- Generalized itching with no rash

The best way to avoid complications is to recognize these symptoms and get early diagnosis and treatment. Because type 2 diabetes is often asymptomatic in the early stages, major health organizations now recommend routine screening for people over age 45 and anyone younger who is at high risk, including those who are obese.

Screening involves a blood test to check glucose levels after either a period of fasting or the administration of a set dose of glucose. A fasting glucose level of 126 mg/dl or higher indicates diabetes; a level of 100–125 mg/dl indicates prediabetes. If you are concerned about your risk for diabetes, talk with your physician about being tested.

Treatment

There is no cure for diabetes, but it can be managed successfully by keeping blood sugar levels within safe limits through diet, exercise, and, if necessary, medication. Blood sugar levels can be monitored with a home test; close control of glucose levels can significantly reduce the rate of serious complications.

Nearly 88% of people with type 2 diabetes are overweight when diagnosed, including 43.5% who are obese. An important

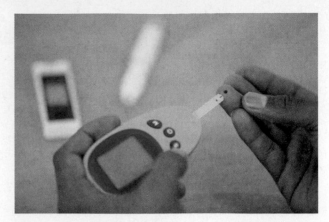

Wellness Tip Most cases of type 2 diabetes can be prevented through lifestyle measures such as regular physical activity and modest weight loss. For those who have type 2 diabetes, careful management to keep blood sugar levels within a healthy range through diet, exercise, and, if needed, medication can reduce the rate of complications from the disorder.

Sean Prior/Alamy Stock Photo

step in treatment is to lose weight. Even a small amount of exercise and weight loss can be beneficial. Regular exercise and a healthy diet are often sufficient to control type 2 diabetes.

Prevention

It is estimated that 90% of cases of type 2 diabetes could be prevented if people adopted healthy lifestyle behaviors, including regular physical activity, a moderate diet, and modest weight loss. For people with prediabetes, lifestyle measures are more effective than medication for delaying or preventing the development of diabetes. Studies of people with prediabetes show that a 5–7% weight loss can lower diabetes onset by nearly 60%. Exercise (endurance and/or strength training) makes cells more sensitive to insulin and helps stabilize blood glucose levels; it also helps keep body fat at healthy levels.

A moderate diet to control body fat is perhaps the most important dietary recommendation for the prevention of diabetes. However, the composition of the diet may also be important. Studies have linked diets low in fiber and high in sugar, refined carbohydrates, saturated fat, red meat, and high-fat dairy products to increased risk of diabetes. Specific foods linked to higher diabetes risk include soft drinks, white bread, white rice, French fries, processed meats, and sugary desserts. Diets rich in whole grains, fruits, vegetables, legumes, fish, and poultry may be protective.

Smoking contributes to insulin resistance, so not smoking—or quitting if you currently smoke—can also help prevent or delay getting type 2 diabetes. If you are at increased risk for diabetes, talk to your health care provider and consider participating in a local or online CDC-recognized lifestyle change program for diabetes prevention (https://www.cdc.gov/diabetes/prevention/lifestyle-program). These programs have been shown to reduce the risk for diabetes, heart attack, and stroke; some participants even reverse a prediabetes diagnosis.

COMMON QUESTIONS ANSWERED

Q I know what foods to avoid to prevent CVD, but are there any foods I should eat to help protect myself from CVD?

A The most important dietary change for CVD prevention is a negative one: cutting back on foods high in sugar and in saturated and trans fat. However, certain foods may be helpful. The positive effects of unsaturated fats, soluble fiber, and limited alcohol on heart health (alcohol for those over age 45) were discussed earlier in the chapter. Other potentially beneficial foods include those rich in the following:

- *Omega-3 fatty acids.* Found in fish, shellfish, and some nuts and seeds, omega-3 fatty acids reduce clotting and inflammation and may lower the risk of fatal arrhythmia.

- *Folic acid, vitamin B-6, and vitamin B-12.* These vitamins may affect CVD risk by lowering homocysteine levels; see Table 8.6 for a list of food sources.

- *Plant stanols and sterols.* Plant stanols and sterols, found in some types of trans-fat-free margarines and other products, reduce the absorption of cholesterol in the body and help lower LDL levels.

- *Soy protein.* Replacing some animal protein with soy protein can lower LDL cholesterol. Soy-based foods include tofu, tempeh, and soy-based beverages.

- *Calcium.* Diets rich in calcium may help prevent hypertension and possibly stroke by reducing insulin resistance and platelet aggregation. Low-fat and fat-free dairy products are rich in calcium; refer to Chapter 8 for other sources.

Q The advice I hear from the media about protecting myself from CVD seems to be changing all the time. What should I believe?

A Health-related research is now described in popular newspapers and magazines rather than just medical journals, meaning that more and more people have access to the information. Researchers do not deliberately set out to mislead or confuse people. However, news reports may oversimplify the results of research studies, omitting some qualifications and questions the researchers present with their findings. In addition, news reports may not differentiate between a preliminary finding and a result that has been verified by a large number of long-term studies. And researchers themselves must strike a balance between reporting promising preliminary findings to the public, thereby allowing people to act on them, and waiting 10–20 years until long-term studies confirm (or disprove) a particular theory.

Although you cannot become an expert on all subjects, there are some strategies you can use to assess the health advice that appears in the media; see the box "Evaluating Sources of Health Information" in Chapter 1.

Q What's a heart murmur, and is it dangerous?

A A heart murmur is an extra or altered heart sound detectable during a routine medical exam. The source is often a problem with one of the heart valves that separate the chambers of the heart. Congenital defects and certain infections can cause abnormalities in the valves. The most common heart valve disorder is mitral valve prolapse (MVP), which occurs in about 4% of the population. MVP is characterized by a "billowing" of the mitral valve, which separates the left ventricle and left atrium, during ventricular contraction. In some cases, blood leaks from the ventricle into the atrium. Most people with MVP have no symptoms; they have the same capability for exercising as people without MVP, and they also live as long.

Q How does stress contribute to cardiovascular disease?

A With stress, the brain tells the adrenal glands to secrete cortisol and other hormones and neurotransmitters, which in turn activate the sympathetic nervous system—causing the fight-or-flight response. This response increases heart rate and blood pressure so that more blood is distributed to the heart and other muscles in anticipation of physical activity. Blood glucose concentrations and cholesterol also increase to provide a source of energy, and the platelets become activated so that they will be more likely to clot in case of injury. Such a response can be adaptive if you're being chased by a hungry lion but may be more detrimental than useful if you're sitting at a desk taking an exam or feeling frustrated by a task given to you by your boss.

If you are healthy, you can tolerate the cardiovascular responses that take place during stress, but if you already have CVD, stress can lead to adverse outcomes such as abnormal heart rhythms, heart attacks, and sudden cardiac death. It has long been known that an increase in heart rhythm problems and deaths is associated with acute mental stress. For example, the rate of potentially life-threatening arrhythmias in patients who already had underlying heart disease doubled during the month after the September 11 terrorist attacks; this increase was not limited to people in proximity to Manhattan.

Because avoiding all stress is impossible, having healthy mechanisms to cope with it is your best defense. Instead of adopting unhealthy habits such as smoking, drinking, or overeating to deal with stress, try healthier coping techniques such as exercising, getting enough sleep, meditating, and talking to family and friends.

TIPS FOR TODAY AND THE FUTURE

Because cardiovascular disease and diabetes can develop slowly, beginning when you're young, it's important to develop healthy habits early in life.

RIGHT NOW YOU CAN

- Make an appointment to have your blood pressure, cholesterol, and glucose levels checked.
- List key stressors in your life, and decide what to do about the ones that bother you most.
- Plan to replace one high-fat, high-sugar item in your diet with one that is high in fiber. For example, replace a doughnut with a bowl of whole-grain cereal.

IN THE FUTURE YOU CAN

- Track your eating choices for one week, then compare them to the DASH eating plan. Make adjustments to bring your diet closer to the DASH recommendations.
- Sign up for a class in CPR. A CPR certification equips you with valuable lifesaving skills you can use to help someone who is choking, having a heart attack, or experiencing cardiac arrest.

SUMMARY

- The major controllable risk factors for CVD are smoking, hypertension, unhealthy cholesterol levels, inactivity, overweight and obesity, and diabetes.

- Contributing factors for CVD that can be changed include high triglyceride levels, inadequate stress management, a hostile personality, depression, anxiety, lack of social support, poverty, and alcohol and drug use.

- Major risk factors for CVD that can't be changed are heredity, aging, being male, and ethnicity.

- Hypertension weakens the heart and scars and hardens arteries, causing resistance to blood flow. It is defined as blood pressure equal to or higher than 130 over 80.

- Atherosclerosis is a progressive hardening and narrowing of arteries that can lead to restricted blood flow and even complete blockage.

- Heart attacks, strokes, and congestive heart failure are the results of a long-term disease process; hypertension and atherosclerosis are usually involved.

- Reducing heart disease risk involves eating a heart-healthy diet, exercising regularly, avoiding tobacco, managing blood pressure and cholesterol levels, and managing stress and anger.

- The most common type of diabetes, a disorder of metabolism, is linked to older age and lifestyle factors, including inactivity and obesity; treatment can help reduce the rate of serious complications.

FOR FURTHER EXPLORATION

American Diabetes Association. Provides information, a free newsletter, and referrals to local support groups; the website includes an online diabetes risk assessment.

http://www.diabetes.org

American Heart Association. Provides information on hundreds of topics relating to the prevention and control of CVD. See especially "My Life Check–Life's Simple 7" for seven factors to ideal cardiovascular health.

http://www.heart.org

Centers for Disease Control and Prevention: Preventing or Managing High Cholesterol. Gives succinct advice on diet, weight, physical activity, smoking, and drinking alcohol, as well as links to other CDC websites.

https://www.cdc.gov/cholesterol/prevention-management.htm

Franklin Institute: The Heart: The Engine of Life. An online museum exhibit containing information on the structure and function of the heart, how to monitor your heart's health, and how to maintain a healthy heart.

https://www.fi.edu/heart-engine-of-life

Mayo Clinic. Gives reader-friendly definitions and descriptions of symptoms, tests, and treatments, and prepares you to discuss your health with an expert.

https://www.mayoclinic.org/diseases-conditions/heart-disease/in-depth/heart-disease-prevention/art-20046502

MedlinePlus: Blood, Heart and Circulation Topics. Provides links to reliable sources of information on cardiovascular health.

http://www.nlm.nih.gov/medlineplus/bloodheartandcirculation.html

National Heart, Lung, and Blood Institute. Provides information on a variety of topics relating to cardiovascular health and disease, including cholesterol, smoking, obesity, hypertension, and the DASH diet.

http://www.nhlbi.nih.gov/

National Stroke Association. Provides information and referrals for stroke victims and their families; the website has a stroke risk assessment.

http://www.stroke.org/site/PageNavigator/HOME

See also the listings for Chapters 9 and 10.

SELECTED BIBLIOGRAPHY

Akesson, A., et al. 2014. Low-risk diet and lifestyle habits in the primary prevention of myocardial infarction in men: A population-based prospective cohort study. *Journal of the American College of Cardiology* 64(13): 1299–1306.

American Heart Association. 2014. *Diet and Lifestyle Recommendations* (http://www.heart.org/HEARTORG/GettingHealthy/NutritionCenter/HealthyEating/The-American-Heart-Associations-Diet-and-Lifestyle-Recommendations_ UCM_305855_Article.jsp).

American Heart Association. 2015. *Dental Health and Heart Health* (https://newsroom.heart.org/news/poor-oral-health-linked-to-higher-blood-pressure-worse-blood-pressure-control).

American Heart Association. 2016. *Understand Your Risks to Prevent Heart Attack* (http://www.heart.org/HEARTORG/Conditions/HeartAttack/UnderstandYourRiskstoPreventaHeartAttack/Understand-Your-Risks-to-Prevent-a-Heart-Attack_UCM_002040_Article.jsp).

American Heart Association. 2017. *The Facts About High Blood Pressure* (http://www.heart.org/HEARTORG/Conditions/HighBloodPressure/GettheFactsAboutHighBloodPressure/The-Facts-About-High-Blood-Pressure_UCM_002050_Article.jsp).

American Heart Association. 2017. *Heart Attack Symptoms in Women* (http://www
.heart.org/HEARTORG/Conditions/HeartAttack/WarningSignsofaHeartAttack
/Heart-Attack-Symptoms-in-Women_UCM_436448_Article.jsp).

American Lung Association. 2019. *Health Effects of Secondhand Smoke* (https://www
.lung.org/stop-smoking/smoking-facts/health-effects-of-secondhand-smoke.html).

Bavry, A. A., and M. C. Limacher. 2014. Prevention of cardiovascular disease in women.
Seminars in Reproductive Medicine 32(06): 447–453.

Benjamin, E. J., et al. 2019. Heart disease and stroke statistics—2019 update. *Circulation*
139(10): e56–e528.

Bucholz, E. M., et al. 2016. Life expectancy after myocardial infarction, according to
hospital performance. *New England Journal of Medicine* 375(14): 1332–1342.

Centers for Disease Control and Prevention. 2017. *Cholesterol* (http://www.cdc.gov
/cholesterol/treating_cholesterol.htm).

Centers for Disease Control and Prevention. 2018. *Current Cigarette Smoking among
Adults in the United States* (http://www.cdc.gov/tobacco/data_statistics/fact
_sheets/adult_data/cig_smoking/index.htm).

Centers for Disease Control and Prevention. 2017. *Heart Disease Fact Sheet* (http://
www.cdc.gov/dhdsp/data_statistics/fact_sheets/fs_heart_disease.htm).

Centers for Disease Control and Prevention. 2016. *High Blood Pressure Fact Sheet*
(http://www.cdc.gov/dhdsp/data_statistics/fact_sheets/fs_bloodpressure.htm).

Centers for Disease Control and Prevention, National Center for Health Statistics.
2018. *Underlying Cause of Death 1999–2017* on CDC WONDER Online Database.
Data are from the Multiple Cause of Death Files, 1999–2017, as compiled from
data provided by the 57 vital statistics jurisdictions through the Vital Statistics
Cooperative Program (http://wonder.cdc.gov/ucd-icd10.html).

Diabetes Prevention Program Research Group. 2015. Long-term effects of lifestyle
intervention or metformin on diabetes development and microvascular complications over 15-year follow-up: The Diabetes Prevention Program Outcomes Study.
Lancet: Diabetes & Endocrinology 3(11): 866–875.

Giedrimiene, D., and R. King. 2017. Abstract 207: Burden of cardiovascular disease
(cvd) on economic cost comparison of outcomes in US and Europe. *Circulation*
10: A2017.

Grundy, S. M., et al. 2019. 2018 AHA/ACC/AACVPR/AAPA/ABC/ACPM/ADA/AGS/
APhA/ASPC/NLA/PCNA guideline on the management of blood cholesterol. A
report of the American College of Cardiology/American Heart Association Task
Force on Clinical Practice Guidelines. *Journal of the American College of Cardiology*
73(24): e1082–e1143.

Guan, W., et al. 2015. Race is a key variable in assigning lipoprotein(a) cutoff values for
coronary heart disease risk assessment: The Multi-Ethnic Study of Atherosclerosis.
Arteriosclerosis, Thrombosis, and Vascular Biology 35(4): 996–1001.

Heinl, R. E., et al. 2016. Comprehensive cardiovascular risk reduction and cardiac
rehabilitation in diabetes and the metabolic syndrome. *Canadian Journal of
Cardiology* 32(10S2): S349–S357.

Hernandez, D. C., et al. 2014. Social support and cardiovascular risk factors among
black adults. *Ethnicity and Disease* 24(4): 444–450.

James, P. A., et al. 2014. Evidence-based guideline for the management of high blood
pressure in adults: Report from the panel members appointed to the Eighth Joint
National Committee (JNC 8). *JAMA* 311(5): 507–520.

Johnston, L. D., et al. 2018. *Monitoring the Future national survey results on drug use,
1975–2017: Overview, key findings on adolescent drug use.* Ann Arbor: Institute for
Social Research, The University of Michigan.

Kones, R., and U. Rumana. 2015. Current treatment of dyslipidemia: A new paradigm
for statin drug use and the need for additional therapies. *Drugs,* June 27.

Larsson, S. C., et al. 2015. Primary prevention of stroke by a healthy lifestyle in a high-
risk group. *Neurology* 84(22): 2224–2228.

Micha, R., et al. 2017. Association between dietary factors and mortality from heart
disease, stroke, and type 2 diabetes in the United States. *JAMA* 317(9): 912–924.

Miller, M., et al. 2011. Triglycerides and cardiovascular disease: A scientific statement
from the American Heart Association. *Circulation* 123: 2292–2333.

Mozzafarian, D. 2016. Dietary and policy priorities for cardiovascular disease, diabetes,
and obesity: A comprehensive review. *Circulation* 133(2): 187–225.

Tang, G., et al. 2015. Meta-analysis of the association between whole grain intake and
coronary heart disease risk. *American Journal of Cardiology* 115(5): 625–629.

Tran, T. M., and N. M. Giang. 2014. Changes in blood pressure classification, blood pressure
goals, and pharmacological treatment of essential hypertension in medical guidelines
from 2003 to 2013. *International Journal of Cardiology Metabolic & Endocrine* 2: 1–10.

U.S. Department of Agriculture. 2015. *Scientific Report of the 2015 Dietary Guidelines
Advisory Committee* (https://www.ncbi.nlm.nih.gov/pmc/articles/PMC4717899/).

U.S. Department of Health and Human Services. 2016. *E-Cigarette Use Among Youth
and Young Adults: A Report of the Surgeon General—Executive Summary.* Atlanta,
GA: U.S. Department of Health and Human Services.

Zwald, M. L., et al. 2017. Prevalence of low high-density lipoprotein cholesterol among
adults, by physical activity: United States, 2011–2014. *NCHS Data Brief* No. 276.
Hyattsville, MD: National Center for Health Statistics.

Name _____ Section _____ Date _____

LAB 11.1 Cardiovascular Health

Part I CVD Risk Assessment

Your chances of suffering a heart attack or stroke before age 55 depend on a variety of factors, many of which are under your control. To help identify your risk factors, circle the response for each risk category that best describes you.

1. Sex and Age

    0 Female age 55 or younger; male age 45 or younger

    2 Female over age 55; male over age 45

2. Heredity/Family History

    0 Neither parent suffered a heart attack or stroke before age 60.

    3 One parent suffered a heart attack or stroke before age 60.

    7 Both parents suffered a heart attack or stroke before age 60.

3. Smoking

    0 Never smoked

    3 Quit more than 2 years ago and lifetime smoking is less than five pack-years*

    6 Quit less than 2 years ago and/or lifetime smoking is greater than five pack-years*

    8 Smoke less than 1/2 pack per day

    13 Smoke more than 1/2 pack per day

    15 Smoke more than 1 pack per day

4. Environmental Tobacco Smoke

    0 Do not live or work with smokers

    2 Exposed to ETS at work

    3 Live with smoker

    4 Both live and work with smokers

5. Blood Pressure

    (If available, use the average of the last three readings.)

    0 Below 120/80

    1 120/80–129/80

    3 Don't know blood pressure

    5 130/80–139/80

    9 140/90–169/99

    13 Above 170/100

6. Total Cholesterol

    0 Lower than 190

    1 190–210

    2 Don't know total cholesterol

    3 211–240

    4 241–270

    5 271–300

    6 Over 300

7. HDL Cholesterol

    0 Greater than or equal to 60 mg/dl

    1 50–59

    2 35–49

    3 Don't know HDL cholesterol

    5 Lower than 35

8. Exercise

    0 Exercise three times a week

    1 Exercise once or twice a week

    2 Occasional exercise less than once a week

    7 Rarely exercise

9. Diabetes

    0 No personal or family history

    2 One parent with diabetes

    6 Two parents with diabetes

    9 Type 2 diabetes

    13 Type 1 diabetes

10. Body Mass Index (kg/m^2)

    0 <21.0

    1 21.0–24.9

    2 25.0–29.9

    3 30.0–34.9

    5 35.0–39.9

    7 ≥ 40

11. Stress

    0 Relaxed most of the time

    1 Occasionally stressed and angry

    2 Frequently stressed and angry

    3 Usually stressed and angry

Scoring

Total your risk factor points. Refer to the following list to get an approximate rating of your risk of suffering an early heart attack or stroke.

Score	Estimated Risk
Less than 20	Low risk
20–29	Moderate risk
30–45	High risk
Over 45	Extremely high risk

*Pack-years can be calculated by multiplying the number of packs you smoked per day by the number of years you smoked. For example, if you smoked a pack and a half a day for 5 years, you would have smoked the equivalent of 1.5 × 5 = 7.5 pack-years.

LABORATORY ACTIVITIES

Part II Hostility Assessment

Are you too hostile? To help answer that question, Duke University researcher Redford Williams, M.D., has devised a short self-test. It's not a scientific evaluation, but it does offer a rough measure of hostility. Are the following statements true or false for you?

1. I often get annoyed at checkout cashiers or the people in front of me when I'm waiting in line.

2. I usually keep an eye on the people I work or live with to make sure they do what they should.

3. I often wonder how homeless people can have so little respect for themselves.

4. I believe that most people will take advantage of you if you let them.

5. The habits of friends or family members often annoy me.

6. When I'm stuck in traffic, I often start breathing faster and my heart pounds.

7. When I'm annoyed with people, I really want to let them know it.

8. If someone does me wrong, I want to get even.

9. I like to have the last word in any argument.

10. At least once a week, I have the urge to yell at or even hit someone.

According to Williams, five or more "true" statements suggest that you're excessively hostile and should consider taking steps to mellow out.

Using Your Results

How did you score?

(1) What is your CVD risk assessment score? Are you surprised by your score?

Are you satisfied with your CVD risk rating? If not, set a specific goal:

(2) What is your hostility assessment score? Are you surprised by the result?

Are you satisfied with your hostility rating? If not, set a specific goal:

What should you do next? Enter the results of this lab in the Preprogram Assessment column in Appendix B.
(1) If you've set a goal for the overall CVD risk assessment score, identify a risk area that you can change, such as smoking, exercise, or stress. Then list three steps or strategies for changing the risk area you've chosen.

Risk area:

Strategies for change:

(2) If you've set a goal for the hostility assessment score, begin by keeping a log of your hostile responses. Review the anger-management strategies in Chapter 10 and select several that you will try to use to manage your angry responses. Strategies for anger management:

Next, begin to put your strategies into action. After several weeks of a program to reduce CVD risk or hostility, do this lab again and enter the results in the Postprogram Assessment column of Appendix B. How do the results compare?

SOURCE: Adapted from *Life Skills* by Virginia Williams and Redford Williams.

Design elements: Evidence for Exercise box (shoes and stethoscope): Vstock LLC/Tetra Images/Getty Images; Take Charge box (lady walking): VisualCommunications/E+/Getty Images; Critical Consumer box (man): Sam74100/iStock/Getty Images; Diversity Matters box (holding devices): Robert Churchill/iStockphoto/Rawpixel Ltd/Getty Images; Wellness in the Digital Age box (Smart Watch): Hong Li/DigitalVision/Getty Images

CHAPTER 12

Cancer

LOOKING AHEAD...

After reading this chapter, you should be able to

- Explain what cancer is and how it spreads.
- Discuss causes of cancer and how they can be avoided or minimized.
- Describe common cancers.
- Describe how cancer can be detected, diagnosed, and treated.
- List actions you can take to lower your risk of cancer.

TEST YOUR KNOWLEDGE

1. Eating which of these foods may help prevent cancer?
   a. chili peppers
   b. broccoli
   c. oranges

2. Testicular cancer is the most common cancer in men between ages 15 and 35. True or false?

3. The use of condoms during sexual intercourse may prevent cancer in women. True or false?

See answers on the next page.

Pollyanna Ventura/E+/Getty Images

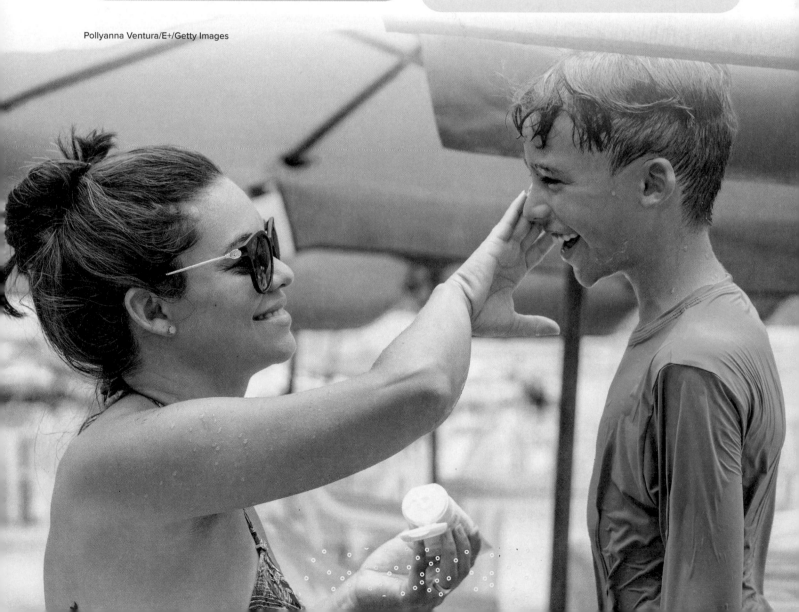

A fter heart disease, cancer is the second leading cause of death. In the United States, cancer is responsible for almost one in four deaths, claiming more than 1,600 lives every day. Evidence indicates that many cancers in the United States could be prevented by simple changes in lifestyle. Tobacco use is responsible for about 32% of all cancer deaths (Figure 12.1). Poor diet and lack of exercise, including their relationship with obesity, account for another 20% of cancer deaths. In this chapter you'll learn more about how cancer develops, common types of cancers, and steps you can take now to help reduce your risk of cancer.

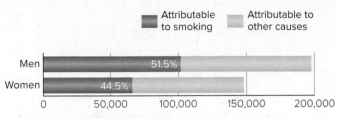

(a) Total deaths from 12 smoking-linked cancers

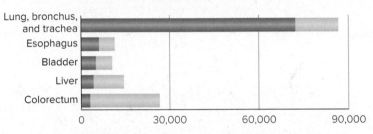

(b) Deaths from the top five smoking-linked cancers among men

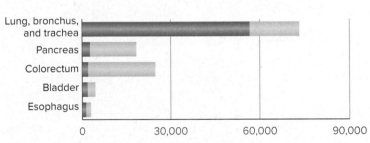

(c) Deaths from the top five smoking-linked cancers among women

VITAL STATISTICS

Figure 12.1   Cancer deaths attributable to cigarette smoking in adults age 35 and over.

SOURCE: Siegel, R. L., et al. 2015. "Deaths due to cigarette smoking for 12 smoking-related cancers in the United States," *JAMA Internal Medicine* 175, no. 9: 1574–576. (https://doi:10.1001/jamainternmed.2015.2398).

Answers (Test Your Knowledge)

1. **All three.** These and many other fruits and vegetables are rich in phytochemicals, naturally occurring substances that may have anticancer effects.
2. **True.** Although rare, testicular cancer is the most common cancer in men between ages 15 and 35. Regular self-exams may aid in its detection.
3. **True.** The primary cause of cervical cancer is infection with the human papillomavirus (HPV), a sexually transmitted pathogen. The use of condoms helps prevent HPV infection.

WHAT IS CANCER?

Cancer is the abnormal, uncontrolled multiplication of cells, which can ultimately cause death if left untreated.

Tumors

Most cancers take the form of tumors, although not all tumors are cancerous. A **tumor** (or *neoplasm*) is a mass of tissue that serves no physiological purpose. It can be benign, like a wart, or malignant, like most lung cancers.

Benign (noncancerous) **tumors** are made up of cells similar to the surrounding normal cells and are enclosed in a membrane that prevents them from penetrating neighboring tissues. They are dangerous only if their physical presence interferes with body functions. A benign brain tumor, for example, can cause death if it blocks the blood supply to the brain.

The term **malignant tumor** is synonymous with cancer. A malignant tumor can invade surrounding structures, including blood vessels, the **lymphatic system**, and nerves. It can also spread to distant sites via the blood and lymphatic circulation, producing invasive tumors in almost any part of the body. A few cancers, like leukemia (cancer of the blood) do not produce a mass but still have the fundamental property of rapid, uncontrolled cell proliferation.

Every case of cancer begins as a change in a cell that allows it to grow and divide when it should not (Figure 12.2). A malignant cell divides into new cells without regard for normal control mechanisms and gradually produces a mass of abnormal cells, or a tumor. It takes about a billion cells to make a mass the size of a pea, so a single tumor cell must go through many divisions, often taking years, before the tumor grows to a noticeable size. Eventually, a tumor produces a sign or symptom that can be detected. In an accessible location (such as a testicle), a tumor may be felt as a lump. In less accessible locations (such as the lungs), a tumor may be noticed only after considerable growth has taken place and may then be detected only by an indirect symptom, such as a persistent cough or unexplained bleeding or pain.

TERMS

cancer   Abnormal, uncontrolled multiplication of cells.

tumor   A mass of tissue that serves no physiological purpose; also called a *neoplasm*.

benign tumor   A tumor that is not cancerous.

malignant tumor   A tumor that is cancerous and capable of spreading.

lymphatic system   A system of vessels that returns proteins, lipids, and other substances from fluid in the tissues to the circulatory system.

metastasis   The spread of cancer cells from one part of the body to another.

1. Tumor development begins when a cell (light orange) is altered so that it grows and divides when it normally would not. The altered cell and its descendants look normal but continue to reproduce too much, a condition called *hyperplasia*. Over time, new mutations may arise and cause even more cell proliferation (dark orange). Hyperplasia may or may not lead to cancer.

2. After additional mutations, the descendants of the altered cells may be abnormal in shape (purple), called *dysplasia*. Dysplasia may or may not develop into cancer.

3. Over time, the affected cells may become more abnormal in shape and behavior. *In situ cancer* is diagnosed if the abnormal cells are found only in the location they first formed. The tumor may remain in this location or may acquire additional mutations (blue).

4. Abnormal cells may gain the ability to invade nearby tissues, causing *localized invasive cancer*. The function of the affected organ or tissue may be affected, but the tumor has not yet spread beyond the boundaries of the organ of origin.

5. If the tumor spreads so that it can shed malignant cells into a blood or lymphatic vessel, these cells can travel to distant sites and establish new tumors *(metastases)* throughout the body.

Altered cell   **Hyperplasia**

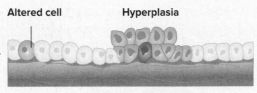

Dysplasia

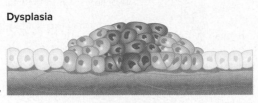

In situ cancer

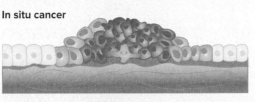

Localized invasive tumor

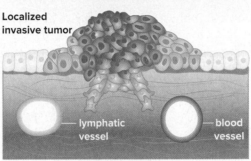

lymphatic vessel   blood vessel

Metastasis

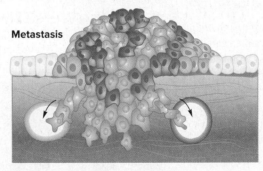

Figure 12.2   Tumor development occurs in stages.
SOURCES: Mader, S. S., and M. Windelspecht. 2018. *Human Biology,* 15e. New York: McGraw-Hill; U.S. National Institutes of Health, National Cancer Institute, *SEER Training Modules: Summary Staging Defined Main Categories.* (https://training.seer.cancer.gov/ss2k/descriptions).

Metastasis

Metastasis, the spread of cancer cells, occurs because cancer cells do not stick to each other as strongly as normal cells do and therefore may not remain at the site of the *primary tumor,* the cancer's original location. They break away and can pass through the lining of lymph or blood vessels to invade nearby tissue. They can also drift to distant parts of the body and multiply, establishing new colonies of cancer cells. This traveling and seeding

process is called *metastasizing,* and the new tumors are *secondary tumors,* or *metastases.*

The ability of cancer cells to metastasize makes early cancer detection critical. To control the cancer, every cancerous cell must be removed. Once cancer cells enter either the lymphatic system or the bloodstream, it is extremely difficult to stop their spread to other organs.

THE CAUSES OF CANCER

Although scientists do not know everything about what causes cancer, they have identified factors related to lifestyle, genetics, race/ethnicity, socioeconomics, and the environment. For example, genetic factors may explain the high rate of prostate cancer among black men. Socioeconomic factors connect low incomes and a lack of health insurance to lifestyle problems like smoking, both of which are associated with higher cancer death rates. Women from cultures in which early marriage and motherhood are common are likely to have a lower risk of breast cancer. Environmental factors include carcinogens in the water we drink and air we breathe.

Tobacco Use

Smoking is responsible for about 32% of all cancer deaths, including 83% of lung cancer deaths for men and 76% for women. In addition to lung and bronchial cancer, tobacco use is linked to cancer of the larynx, mouth, pharynx, esophagus, stomach, pancreas, kidneys, bladder, and cervix. Avoiding tobacco use and exposure to environmental tobacco smoke are key lifestyle strategies for reducing cancer risk (Figure 12.3).

Dietary Factors

One of the most complex and controversial factors in cancer prevention is diet. Your food choices can increase your cancer risk by exposing you to potentially dangerous compounds or depriving you of potentially protective ones; your choices can also act against cancer. The following dietary factors may affect cancer risk:

- *Dietary fat and meat:* Diets high in fat and meat that is red, processed, or charbroiled may increase the risk of certain cancers, including colon, stomach, and prostate cancer. Certain types of fat may be riskier than others. Too many omega-6 polyunsaturated fats are associated with a higher risk of certain cancers; omega-3 fats are not. (See Chapter 8 for more information about types of fatty acids.)

- *Alcohol:* Alcohol is associated with an increased incidence of several cancers. For example, women who have two to

AIM FOR

- A varied, plant-based diet that is high in fiber-rich foods such as legumes and whole grains

- 7–13 servings of fruits and vegetables every day, favoring foods from the following categories:
  Cruciferous vegetables
  Citrus fruits
  Berries
  Dark green leafy vegetables
  Dark yellow, orange, or red fruits and vegetables

- Regular physical activity

- A healthy weight

- Safer sex and HPV vaccination if appropriate (to avoid HPV infection)

- Skin protection from the sun with appropriate clothing and sunscreen

- Regular self-exams (skin self-exam for all, testicular self-exam for men, breast self-awareness for women)

- Recommended screening tests and discussions with your physician about any family history of cancer

AVOID

- Any tobacco or nicotine product:
  Cigarettes, electronic or traditional
  Spit tobacco
  Cigars and pipes
  Bidis and clove cigarettes

- Exposure to environmental tobacco smoke

- Occupational exposure to carcinogens

- Excessive alcohol consumption

- Charred foods (grilled in a direct flame)

- Tanning lamps and beds

LIMIT

- Fatty meats and other sources of saturated fat

- Cured and processed meats

- Salt intake

- Exposure to UV radiation from sunlight

Figure 12.3 Strategies for reducing your risk of cancer.

(beans): Corina Daniela Obertas/shopartgallerycom/123RF; (orange): Stockdisc/Getty Images; (broccoli): Stockbyte/Stockdisc/Getty Images; (sliced filet mignon): Tim Hawley/Photolibrary/Getty Images

five drinks daily have about 1.5 times the risk of women who drink no alcohol. Alcohol and tobacco interact as risk factors for oral cancer. Heavy users of both alcohol and tobacco have a risk for oral cancer many times greater than that of people who don't drink or use tobacco.

- *Foods cooked at high temperatures:* Scientists have found high levels of the chemical acrylamide (a probable human carcinogen) in starch-based foods that have been fried or baked at high temperatures, especially french fries and certain types of snack chips and crackers. Acrylamide is also found in high concentrations in tobacco. When muscle meats (beef, pork, fish, poultry) are cooked at high temperatures, such as when grilled over an open flame or pan fried, different types of cancer-causing chemicals can form.

- *Nutrients in fruits and vegetables:* Researchers have identified many mechanisms by which components in fruits and vegetables may act against cancer. Some may prevent **carcinogens** from forming in the first place or may block them from reaching or acting on target cells. Others boost enzymes that detoxify carcinogens and render them harmless. Some essential nutrients act as anticarcinogens. For example, vitamin C, vitamin E, selenium, and the **carotenoids** (vitamin A precursors) may help block cancer by acting as antioxidants. Fiber, a significant component of fruits and vegetables, may reduce cancer risk.

Many other anticancer agents in the diet fall under the broader heading of **phytochemicals**, substances in plants that help protect against chronic diseases (Table 12.1). One of the

first to be identified was sulforaphane, a potent anticarcinogen found in broccoli.

Obesity and Inactivity

The American Cancer Society (ACS) recommends maintaining a healthy weight throughout life by balancing caloric

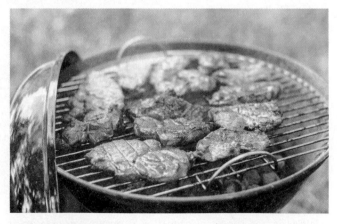

Wellness Tip Grilling meats at high temperatures can produce cancer-causing compounds. If you regularly eat grilled foods, cut away and avoid eating any charred parts. Reduce the formation of these cancer-causing chemicals by marinating before grilling, turning meat frequently, and reducing grilling time by precooking meat in the microwave before finishing on the grill.

Anastasia traveller/Alamy Stock Photo

Table 12.1

Table 12.1 Foods with Phytochemicals

FOOD	PHYTOCHEMICAL	POTENTIAL ANTICANCER EFFECTS
Chili peppers (*Note:* Hotter peppers contain more capsaicin.)	Capsaicin	Neutralizes effect of nitrosamines
Oranges, lemons, limes, onions, apples, berries, eggplant	Flavonoids	Act as antioxidants; block access of carcinogens to cells; suppress malignant changes in cells; prevent cancer cells from multiplying
Citrus fruits, cherries	Monoterpenes	Help detoxify carcinogens; inhibit spread of cancer cells
Cruciferous vegetables (broccoli, cabbage, bok choy, cauliflower, kale, brussels sprouts, collards)	Isothiocyanates	Boost production of cancer-fighting enzymes; suppress growth; block effects of estrogen on cell growth
Garlic, onions, leeks, shallots, chives	Allyl sulfides	Increase levels of enzymes that break down potential carcinogens; boost activity of cancer-fighting immune cells
Grapes, red wine, peanuts	Resveratrol	Acts as antioxidant; suppresses tumor growth
Green, oolong, and black teas (*Note:* Drinking burning hot tea may *increase* cancer risk.)	Polyphenols	Increase antioxidant activity; prevent cancer cells from multiplying; help speed excretion of carcinogens from the body
Orange, deep yellow, red, pink, and dark green vegetables; some fruits	Carotenoids	Act as antioxidants; reduce levels of cancer-promoting enzymes; inhibit spread of cancer cells
Soy foods, whole grains, flax seeds, nuts	Phytoestrogens	Block effects of estrogen on cell growth; lower blood levels of estrogen
Whole grains, legumes	Phytic acid	Binds iron, which may prevent it from creating cell-damaging free radicals

intake with physical activity; for those who are overweight or obese, losing even a small amount of weight has benefits and is recommended by the ACS. Being overweight or obese is linked with increased risk of several kinds of cancer, including endometrial, prostate, breast, and colon cancer; excess abdominal fat (apple body shape) and gaining weight over time are also associated with elevated rates of cancer (Figure 12.4). Physical activity reduces the risk of cancer of the breast, colon, and uterus, as well as advanced prostate cancer. The ACS guidelines encourage everyone to adopt a physically active lifestyle (see the box "How Does Exercise Affect Cancer Risk?").

The Role of DNA

Heredity and genetics are important factors in a person's risk of cancer. Certain genes may predispose some people to cancer, and specific gene mutations have been associated with cancer.

DNA Basics The nucleus of each cell in your body contains 23 pairs of **chromosomes**, which are made up of tightly packed coils of **DNA** (deoxyribonucleic acid). Each chromosome contains hundreds or thousands of **genes**. You have about 20,000 genes in all, each of which controls the production of a

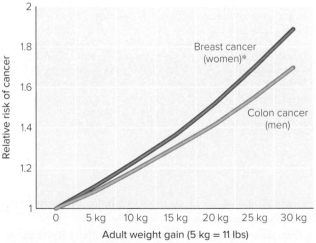

*Postmenopausal women not taking hormone replacement therapy.

VITAL STATISTICS

Figure 12.4 Adult weight gain and risk of cancer. Gaining excessive weight throughout adulthood is a risk factor for several types of cancer, including cancers of the breast and colon. Preventing weight gain during adulthood is a key lifestyle cancer prevention strategy.
SOURCE: Keum, N., et al. 2015. "Adult weight gain and adiposity-related cancers: A dose-response meta-analysis of prospective observational studies," *Journal of the National Cancer Institute* 107, no. 2: 1–14. (https://doi.org/10.1093/jnci/djv088).

TERMS

carcinogen Any substance that causes cancer.

carotenoid Any of a group of yellow-to-red plant pigments that can be converted to vitamin A by the liver; many act as antioxidants or have other anticancer effects. The carotenoids include beta-carotene, lutein, lycopene, and zeaxanthin.

phytochemical A naturally occurring substance found in plant foods that may help prevent and treat chronic diseases such as heart disease and cancer; *phyto* means "plant."

chromosomes The threadlike bodies in a cell nucleus that contain molecules of DNA; most human cells contain 23 pairs of chromosomes.

DNA Deoxyribonucleic acid, a chemical substance that carries genetic information.

gene A section of a chromosome that contains the instructions for making a particular protein; the basic unit of heredity.

THE EVIDENCE FOR EXERCISE
How Does Exercise Affect Cancer Risk?

According to statistics from the International Agency for Research on Cancer (IARC), as many as 20% of cancers are related to overweight, obesity, and physical inactivity. Increasing levels of physical activity can potentially ward off several types of cancer.

The links between exercise and cancer prevention are not entirely clear. However, studies show that people who do moderate aerobic exercise for three to four hours per week reduce their risk of colon cancer by 30%. Women who do the same amount of exercise can reduce their risk of breast cancer by as much as 40%. (Some studies suggest that women who meet certain criteria can reduce their breast cancer risk up to 80%.) Evidence also shows that, when compared with sedentary people, active people can reduce their risk of lung cancer (20%), endometrial cancer (30%), and ovarian cancer (20%). Researchers continue to study similar connections between exercise and other types of cancer.

As is the case with cardiovascular disease, physical activity appears to have an inverse relationship with the types of cancer just listed. That is, the more you exercise, the lower your risk of developing these kinds of cancer. Energy balance also seems to be a factor, at least in relation to a few types of cancer, meaning that people who burn at least as many calories as they take in may further reduce their risk of some cancers. This positive effect may be due to the fact that reducing body fat (through exercise and a healthy diet) lowers the chemical and hormonal activities of adipose (fat) tissue. (Some of the hormones and other compounds produced by adipose tissue affect cell division in ways that can potentially promote cancer.)

In addition to reducing the biological influences of adipose tissue, physical activity is known to reduce the inflammatory response and to boost immune function. Chronic inflammation, which can have many causes, leaves body tissues more vulnerable to infection. Supporting the immune system through exercise may help prevent some cancers.

Emerging data also indicate that physical activity can help improve health outcomes in people who have cancer or are cancer survivors. For example, physical activity appears to restore cardiorespiratory fitness in patients whose heart muscles have been weakened by cancer treatments. This positive outcome was found in 50 separate studies, many of which found significant improvements in heart function among cancer survivors who performed moderate-intensity exercise for 20–40 minutes three times per week. The benefits were similar across several forms of aerobic exercise, including walking, power yoga, and tai chi. Additionally, a handful of studies have found that exercise improves muscular strength and endurance and flexibility in patients whose muscles and joints have been weakened by cancer treatments.

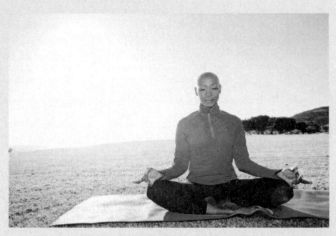

Peathegee Inc/Blend Images/Getty Images

SOURCES: Keum, N., et al. 2015. "Adult weight gain and adiposity-related cancers: A dose-response meta-analysis of prospective observational studies," *Journal of the National Cancer Institute* 10: 107(2); Mishra, S. I., et al. 2012. "Exercise interventions on health-related quality of life for people with cancer during active treatment," *Clinical Otolaryngology* 37(5): 390–392; Irwin, M. L., and S. T. Mayne. 2008. "Impact of nutrition and exercise on cancer survival," *Cancer Journal* 14(6): 435–441; Ulrich, C. M., et al., eds. 2013. *Exercise, Energy Balance, and Cancer,* Vol. 6. New York: Springer; Friedenreich C. M., et al. 2015. "Effects of a high vs moderate volume of aerobic exercise on adiposity outcomes in postmenopausal women: A randomized clinical trial," *JAMA Oncology* 1(6): 766–776.

particular protein. By making different proteins at different times, genes can act as switches to alter the ways a cell works. Some genes are responsible for controlling the rate of cell division, and these genes often play a critical role in the development of cancer.

DNA Mutations and Cancer A *mutation* is any change in the makeup of a gene. Some mutations are inherited; others are caused by environmental agents known as *mutagens.* Mutagens include radiation, certain viruses, and chemical substances in the air we breathe. When a mutagen causes cancer, it is called a *carcinogen.* Some mutations are the result of copying errors that occur when DNA replicates itself as part of cell division. A mutated gene no longer contains the proper code for producing its protein.

Genetic changes contributing to cancer often involve the following gene types:

- Proto-oncogenes, which become oncogenes
- Tumor suppressor genes
- Repair genes

Proto-oncogenes are genes that promote normal cell growth and division. If these genes are mutated, they can become **oncogenes**, which cause cells to grow and divide when they should not. Tumor suppressor genes normally limit cell growth and division. If these genes are altered, however, their control function is lost, leading to rapid and uncontrolled cell division—a precondition for the development of cancer. It usually takes several mutational changes before a normal cell takes on the properties of a cancer cell, and multiple kinds of genetic defects can be involved in the development of cancer. For example, many colon tumors involve both the activation of specific oncogenes and the inactivation of tumor suppressor genes.

Examples of tumor suppressor genes are *BRCA1* and *BRCA2* (*breast cancer gene 1* and *2*). Women who inherit a damaged copy of these genes face a significantly increased risk of breast and ovarian cancers. But having a mutation in the *BRCA1* or *BRCA2* gene is rare. Only 5–10% of breast cancers and 10–15% of ovarian cancers result from this mutation among white women in the United States (data on other ethnicities are not yet complete). Most women with the mutation are therefore advised not to opt for extreme preventive surgery. Even for women who have a mutation suggesting they will ultimately get breast or ovarian cancer, other preventive measures are available, including several medications.

Repair genes are normally involved in fixing damaged DNA; however, if these genes are altered, cells tend to develop additional mutations in other genes because there is no repair mechanism. Mutations begin to accumulate in a cell, increasing the likelihood and frequency of cancerous changes.

Cancer Promoters *Cancer promoters* make up another important piece of the cancer puzzle. These substances don't directly produce DNA mutations, but they accelerate the growth of cells, which means less time for a cell to repair DNA damage caused by other factors. Estrogen, which stimulates cellular growth in the female reproductive organs, is an example of a cancer promoter.

Race/Ethnicity and Poverty

Rates of cancer have declined among all sectors of the U.S. population in recent years, but significant disparities still exist among different racial/ethnic groups. African Americans, for example, have the highest incidence of and death rates from cancer. Hispanic women have the highest incidence of cervical cancer. Asian Americans and Pacific Islander Americans have among the highest rates of liver and stomach cancers. Koreans, especially, suffer from stomach cancer; incidence and death rates are roughly twice as high as those among Japanese, who have the next-highest rates.

No single genetic or racial/ethnic factor in cancer incidence or death is easy to isolate. An example is the higher breast cancer mortality rate among African American women. A genetic explanation grounded in tumor biology helps explain why African American women as a group have not responded as well as women with European ancestry to hormonal therapies. African American women have a higher frequency of estrogen receptor–negative breast cancer, a type of tumor more difficult to treat and

common in populations of west Africans, with whom African Americans are more likely to share ancestry than east Africans.

Confounding the genetic explanations are economic and social factors: According to the U.S. Census Bureau, blacks are more than twice as likely as whites to be poor. People of low socioeconomic status are more likely to smoke, abuse alcohol, eat unhealthful foods, and be sedentary and overweight—all factors associated with cancer. In addition, high levels of stress associated with poverty may impair the immune system, which is the body's first line of defense against cancer. People with low incomes also face health care access barriers such as diagnostic and treatment delays. A multidisciplinary approach to research, involving oncologists, population geneticists, and anthropologists, is therefore useful in uncovering the contributing causes of cancer.

Carcinogens in the Environment

Some carcinogens occur naturally in the environment, like viruses and the sun's UV rays. Others are manufactured or synthetic substances that show up occasionally in the general environment but more often in the work environments of specific industries. For a detailed discussion of environmental health, see Chapter 15.

Ingested Chemicals The food industry uses preservatives and other additives to prevent food from becoming spoiled or stale. Some of these compounds, such as citric acid, are antioxidants and may decrease any cancer-causing properties in the food. Other compounds, such as the nitrates and nitrites found in processed meats, are potentially more dangerous. Although nitrates and nitrites are not themselves carcinogenic, they can combine with dietary substances in the stomach and be converted to nitrosamines, which are highly potent carcinogens. Foods cured with nitrites, as well as those cured by salt or smoke, have been linked to esophageal and stomach cancer, and they should be eaten only in modest amounts. Vitamin C appears to prevent these carcinogens from developing.

Environmental and Industrial Pollution The best available data indicate that less than 2% of cancer deaths are caused by general environmental pollution, such as substances in our air and water. Exposure to carcinogenic materials in the workplace is another serious problem. Occupational exposure to specific carcinogens may account for about 4% of cancer deaths. With decreasing industry and government regulations since 2017, industrial sources of cancer risk may increase.

Radiation All sources of radiation are potentially carcinogenic, including medical X-rays, radioactive substances (radioisotopes), and UV rays from the sun. Most physicians and dentists are quite aware of the risk of radiation, and successful efforts have been made to reduce the amount of radiation needed for mammography, dental X-rays, and other necessary medical imaging. Sunlight is also a potential carcinogen, and care should be taken to avoid excessive exposure.

oncogene A gene involved in the transformation of a normal cell into a cancer cell. **TERMS**

Microbes About 15–20% of the world's cancers are caused by microbes, including viruses, bacteria, and parasites, although the percentage is much lower in developed countries such as the United States. Certain types of human papillomavirus (HPV) are known to cause oropharyngeal cancer, cervical cancer, and other cancers, and the *Helicobacter pylori* bacterium has been linked to stomach cancer.

The Epstein-Barr virus, best known for causing mononucleosis, is also suspected of contributing to Hodgkin disease, cancer of the nasopharynx, and some stomach cancers. Human herpesvirus 8 has been linked to Kaposi's sarcoma and certain types of lymphoma. Hepatitis viruses B and C together cause as many as 80% of the world's liver cancers.

> **? Ask Yourself**
>
> **QUESTIONS FOR CRITICAL THINKING AND REFLECTION**
>
> What do you think your risks for cancer are? Do you have a family history of cancer, or have you been exposed to carcinogens? How about your diet and exercise patterns? What can you do to reduce your risks?

COMMON CANCERS

Each year, more than 1.7 million Americans are diagnosed with cancer, and more than 600,000 die (Figure 12.5). These statistics exclude the more than 1 million cases of the curable types of skin cancer. At current rates, more than one-third of Americans will develop cancer at some point in their lives. Nearly 15.5 million living Americans have a history of cancer.

In this section we look at some of the most common cancers and their causes, prevention, and treatment.

Lung Cancer

Lung cancer is the most common cause of cancer death in the United States; it is responsible for about 143,000 deaths each year. Since 1987, lung cancer has surpassed breast cancer as the leading cause of cancer death in women.

The chief risk factor for lung cancer is tobacco smoke. When smoking is combined with exposure to other carcinogens, such as asbestos particles, the risk of cancer can be multiplied by a factor of 10 or more. Quitting substantially reduces risk, but ex-smokers remain at higher risk than those who never smoked. And the smoker is not the only one at risk. Long-term exposure to environmental tobacco smoke (ETS), or secondhand smoke, also increases risk for lung cancer. ETS causes about 7,000 lung cancer deaths in nonsmoking adults each year.

Symptoms of lung cancer usually do not appear until the disease has advanced to the invasive stage. Signals such as a persistent cough, chest pain, or recurring bronchitis may be the first indication of a tumor. Lung cancer is most often treated by a combination of surgery, radiation, and **chemotherapy**; if all the tumor cells can be removed or killed, a cure is possible. Lung cancer is usually detected only after it has begun to spread, however, and only about 15% of lung cancer patients are alive five years after diagnosis.

Colon and Rectal Cancer

Another common cancer in the United States is colon and rectal cancer (also called *colorectal cancer*). Colorectal cancer is the third most common type of cancer in both men and women. Age is a key risk factor, with the vast majority of cases diagnosed in people age 50 and older. However, younger adults can develop colorectal cancer, and rates among younger age groups have increased in recent decades. Many cancers arise from preexisting polyps, small growths on the wall of the colon that may gradually develop into malignancies. Some colon cancers may be due to inherited gene mutations.

Lifestyle also affects colon cancer risk. Regular physical activity reduces risk; obesity increases risk. Processed meats (for example, hot dogs, sausages, ham, jerky, corned beef, and smoked and canned meats) are carcinogenic and increase the risk of colorectal cancer. Consumption of red meat may also increase an individual's risk. Although the mechanisms are unclear, high intake of refined carbohydrates and simple sugars also appears to increase risk, as do excessive alcohol consumption and smoking.

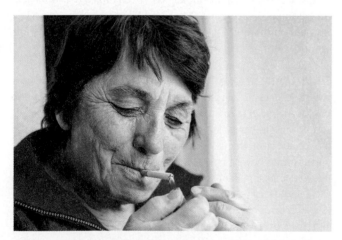

Wellness Tip Tobacco use is linked to nearly 32% of all cancer deaths. If you smoke, quit now. You can start by reviewing the resources available at http://smokefree.gov. If you don't smoke, don't start, and avoid exposure to environmental tobacco smoke whenever possible. Smoking one cigarette per day carries substantial risk of disease and early death.

sanjagrujic/iStock/Getty Images

> **chemotherapy**   The treatment of cancer with chemicals that selectively destroy cancerous cells.   **TERMS**

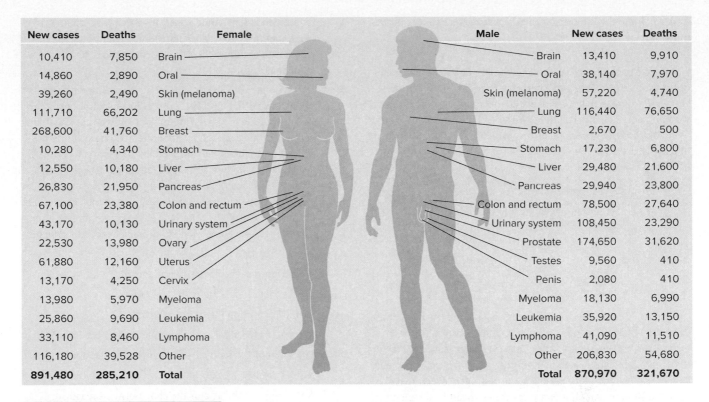

New cases	Deaths	Female	Male	New cases	Deaths
10,410	7,850	Brain	Brain	13,410	9,910
14,860	2,890	Oral	Oral	38,140	7,970
39,260	2,490	Skin (melanoma)	Skin (melanoma)	57,220	4,740
111,710	66,202	Lung	Lung	116,440	76,650
268,600	41,760	Breast	Breast	2,670	500
10,280	4,340	Stomach	Stomach	17,230	6,800
12,550	10,180	Liver	Liver	29,480	21,600
26,830	21,950	Pancreas	Pancreas	29,940	23,800
67,100	23,380	Colon and rectum	Colon and rectum	78,500	27,640
43,170	10,130	Urinary system	Urinary system	108,450	23,290
22,530	13,980	Ovary	Prostate	174,650	31,620
61,880	12,160	Uterus	Testes	9,560	410
13,170	4,250	Cervix	Penis	2,080	410
13,980	5,970	Myeloma	Myeloma	18,130	6,990
25,860	9,690	Leukemia	Leukemia	35,920	13,150
33,110	8,460	Lymphoma	Lymphoma	41,090	11,510
116,180	39,528	Other	Other	206,830	54,680
891,480	**285,210**	**Total**	**Total**	**870,970**	**321,670**

VITAL STATISTICS

Figure 12.5   Cancer cases and deaths by site and sex.

SOURCE: American Cancer Society. 2019. *Cancer Facts and Figures*. American Cancer Society: Atlanta, GA.

Protective lifestyle factors may include a diet rich in fruits, vegetables, fish, and whole grains; adequate intake of folic acid, calcium, magnesium, and vitamin D; and, in women, use of oral contraceptives. Regular use of nonsteroidal anti-inflammatory drugs such as aspirin and ibuprofen may decrease the risk of colon cancer and other cancers of the digestive tract. These agents are not currently recommended for colorectal cancer prevention, although several studies are underway to determine if the protective benefit of these drugs exceeds the risk of other negative health effects.

Polyps and early-stage cancers can be removed before they spread. Because polyps may bleed, the standard warning signs of colon cancer are bleeding from the rectum and a change in bowel habits. The ACS recommends that regular screening start at age 45. A yearly stool blood test can detect traces of blood in the stool long before obvious bleeding can be noticed. Another test is the *colonoscopy,* in which a flexible fiber-optic device is inserted through the rectum, allowing the colon to be examined and polyps to be removed (Figure 12.6). Studies show that screening could reduce the occurrence of colorectal cancer by up to 90%, but only about half of adults age 50 and over undergo these tests. Everyone, including younger adults, should immediately report any potential cancer signs to a health care provider for evaluation.

Surgery is the primary method of treatment for colon and rectal cancer. The five-year survival rate is 90% for colon and rectal cancers detected early and 65% overall.

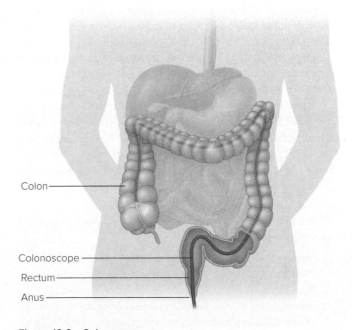

Colon

Colonoscope

Rectum

Anus

Figure 12.6   Colonoscopy.

Breast Cancer

Breast cancer is the most common cancer in women but causes about half as many deaths in women as lung cancer. In the United States, about 1 in 8 women will get breast cancer, and

1 in 38 women will die from the disease. Breast cancer occurs only rarely in men.

Risk Factors There is a strong genetic factor in breast cancer. A woman who has a mother, sister, or daughter with breast cancer is almost twice as likely to develop the disease as a woman who has no relatives with it. However, only about 5–10% of breast cancers occur in women with a family history of the disease.

Other risk factors include these:

- Early-onset menstruation or late-onset menopause
- Having no children or having a first child after age 30
- Current use of hormone replacement therapy
- Obesity
- Alcohol use
- Smoking cigarettes

The female hormone estrogen may be a common element for some of these risk factors. Estrogen promotes cell growth in responsive tissues, such as the breast and uterus, so any factor that increases estrogen exposure may raise the risk of breast cancer. Fat cells produce estrogen, and estrogen levels are higher in obese women. Alcohol can increase estrogen in the blood as well. Some studies have shown that current users of oral contraceptives have a higher risk of breast cancer, especially if they started as teenagers. Breast cancer risk declines to normal levels after 10 years without oral contraceptives.

Prevention Although some risk factors cannot be changed, important lifestyle risk factors can be controlled. Eating a healthy diet, exercising regularly, limiting alcohol intake, and maintaining a healthy body weight can minimize the chance of developing breast cancer, even for women at risk from family history or other factors.

A dietary pattern rich in fruits, vegetables, and whole grains and lower in refined carbohydrates and animal products is associated with reduced risk of breast cancer. Some studies have found that people with higher vitamin D intakes or higher blood levels of vitamin D have a lower risk of breast and certain other cancers.

Detection For women at average risk of breast cancer, the ACS recommends the following:

- *Mammography:* A **mammogram** is a low-dose breast X-ray that can spot breast abnormalities before physical symptoms arise. A newer type of mammography, called *digital mammography,* may provide more accurate results in some women, as may magnetic resonance imaging (MRI). The ACS recommends that women begin annual mammograms at age 45; at age 55, women should have mammograms every other year. However, some controversy surrounds the best age to start having mammograms. The U.S. Preventive Services Task Force (USPSTF) recommends against routine mammography before age 50, citing the anxiety and distress caused by false-positive results. The ACS

recommends that women ages 40–44 choose whether to begin mammograms, and that women over 55 choose whether to continue them. The debate about screening guidelines continues.

- *Breast awareness:* The ACS no longer recommends breast-self exams (BSE) or clinical breast exams, although some doctors still do. Studies have not yet shown that systematically examining oneself is more effective in detecting possible abnormalities than an incidental discovery. Regardless, a woman should be familiar with her breasts and alert her health care provider to any changes right away. The following are warning signs of breast cancer but can also be caused by other conditions; most breast lumps and changes are benign but should be checked by a health care provider:

  A new lump in the breast or underarm

  Thickening or swelling of part of the breast

  Irritation or dimpling of breast skin

  Redness or flaky skin in the nipple area or the breast

  Pulling in of the nipple or pain in the nipple area

  Nipple discharge other than breast milk, including blood

  Any change in the size or the shape of the breast

  Pain in any area of the breast

Women who do choose to perform BSE should review the recommended technique with their health care provider. Additional screenings may be recommended for women at increased risk for breast cancer. If a lump in the breast is detected, it can be **biopsied** or scanned by **ultrasonography** to determine whether it is cancerous.

Treatment If a lump is cancerous, one of several surgical treatments may be used, ranging from a lumpectomy (removal of the lump and surrounding tissue) to a mastectomy (removal of the breast). Chemotherapy or radiation treatment may also be used to eradicate as many cancerous cells as possible.

Several drugs have been developed for preventing and treating breast cancer. These include selective estrogen-receptor modulators (SERMs), which act like estrogen in some tissues but block estrogen's effects in others. The two best-known SERMs are tamoxifen and raloxifene. Another category of drug, called trastuzumab, is a special type of antibody that binds to a specific cancer-related target in the body. Regardless of the treatments used, social support can also affect a patient's psychological and physical wellness.

TERMS

mammogram   A low-dose X-ray of the breasts used for the early detection of breast cancer.

biopsy   The removal and examination of a small piece of body tissue for the purpose of diagnosis.

ultrasonography   An imaging method in which inaudible high-pitched sound (ultrasound) is bounced off body structures to create an image on a monitor.

If a breast cancer tumor is discovered early, before it has spread to the adjacent lymph nodes, the patient has about a 98% chance of surviving more than five years. The survival rate for all stages is 90% at five years.

Prostate Cancer

The prostate gland is situated at the base of the bladder in men; if enlarged, it can block the flow of urine. Prostate cancer is the most common cancer in men and the second leading cause of cancer death in men.

The risk factors for prostate cancer are increasing age, African ancestry, family history, and certain inherited genetic conditions. Age is the strongest predictor of risk, with about 60% of cases diagnosed in men over age 65. Inherited genetic predisposition may be responsible for 5–10% of cases; men with a family history of the disease should be vigilant about screening. Diets that are high in calories, dairy products, refined grains, and animal fats, and low in plant foods have been implicated as possible culprits, as have obesity, inactivity, and a history of sexually transmitted infections. Type 2 diabetes and insulin resistance are also associated with prostate cancer. Diet may be an important means of preventing prostate cancer. Soy foods, tomatoes, and cruciferous vegetables are being investigated for their possible protective effects.

Some cases are first detected by rectal examination during a routine physical exam. During this exam, a physician feels the prostate through the rectum to determine if the gland is enlarged or if lumps are present. Ultrasound and biopsy may also be used to detect and diagnose prostate cancer. A specialized test, called the **prostate-specific antigen (PSA) blood test**, is commonly used to detect prostate cancer and can be useful, but the test is controversial because it can yield false-positive results. The ACS recommends that men be given information about the benefits and limitations of the tests. Both the rectal exam and the PSA test should be offered annually, beginning at age 50 for men at average risk and at age 40 or 45 for men at high risk, including African Americans and those with a family history of the disease. PSA tests are not recommended after age 70.

If a malignant tumor is found, the prostate is usually removed surgically. However, a small, slow-growing tumor in an older man may be treated with watchful waiting, because he is more likely to die from another cause than from the cancer. A less-invasive treatment involves radiation of the tumor by surgically implanting radioactive seeds in the prostate gland. Radiation from the seeds destroys the tumor and much of the normal prostate tissue but leaves surrounding tissue relatively untouched. Alternative or additional treatments include external radiation, hormones that shrink tumors, cryotherapy, and chemotherapy.

Cancers of the Female Reproductive Tract

Several types of cancer can affect the female reproductive tract, and a few of these cancers are relatively common. Note that in women who use oral contraceptives, evidence shows that the risks of breast and cervical cancers are increased, whereas the risks of endometrial, ovarian, and colorectal cancers are reduced.

Cervical Cancer Cancer of the cervix occurs frequently in women in their 30s and even 20s. In the United States, almost 13,000 women are diagnosed with cervical cancer each year; the disease kills more than 4,000 women annually.

Cervical cancer is largely a sexually transmitted infection (STI). Most cases of cervical cancer stem from infection by the human papillomavirus (HPV), which causes genital warts and is transmitted during unprotected sex. Smoking, prior infection with the STIs herpes and chlamydia, and using oral contraceptives for five or more years may also be risk factors for cervical cancer. Recent studies show that birth control pills with less estrogen result in less or no risk for both cervical and breast cancers.

Screening for the changes in cervical cells that precede cancer is done chiefly by means of the **Pap test**. During a pelvic exam, loose cells are scraped from the cervix and examined. If cells are abnormal but not yet cancerous—a condition referred to as *cervical dysplasia*—the Pap test is repeated at intervals. In about one-third of cases, the cellular changes progress toward malignancy. If this happens, the abnormal cells must be removed, either surgically or by destroying them with an ultracold (cryoscopic) probe or localized laser treatment. In more advanced cases, treatment may involve chemotherapy, radiation, or hysterectomy (surgical removal of the uterus).

Because the Pap test is highly effective, all women ages 21–65 should be tested. The recommended schedule for testing depends on risk factors, the type of Pap test performed, and whether the Pap test is combined with HPV testing.

Cervical cancer can be prevented by avoiding infection with HPV. Sexual abstinence, mutually monogamous sex with an uninfected partner, and regular use of condoms can reduce the risk of HPV infection. HPV vaccines have been approved by the Food and Drug Administration (FDA) for the prevention of cervical cancer; women who are vaccinated should continue to receive routine Pap tests because the vaccine does not protect against all types of the virus. See Chapter 14 for more on HPV and other STIs.

Uterine or Endometrial Cancer Cancer of the lining of the uterus (the *endometrium*) most often occurs after age 55. Uterine cancer, also called endometrial cancer, strikes more than 60,000 American women annually and kills about 12,000 women each year. The risk factors are similar to those for

prostate-specific antigen (PSA) blood test TERMS
A diagnostic test for prostate cancer that measures blood levels of prostate-specific antigen (PSA).

Pap test A scraping of cells from the cervix for examination under a microscope to detect cancer.

breast cancer. Uterine cancer is usually detectable by pelvic examination. It is treated surgically, as well as by radiation, hormones, and chemotherapy.

Ovarian Cancer Although ovarian cancer is rare compared with uterine cancer, it causes more deaths. There are no screening tests to detect it, so it is often diagnosed late in its development. The risk factors are similar to those for breast and uterine cancers, including age, obesity, and family history. Also, because pregnancy, breastfeeding, and use of oral contraceptives lower a woman's lifetime number of ovulation cycles, they reduce the risk of ovarian cancer.

Early symptoms of ovarian cancer may include bloating, pelvic or abdominal pain, difficulty eating or feeling full quickly, and urinary problems (urgency or frequency). Women who experience these symptoms almost daily for a few weeks should see their physician. Some ovarian cancers are also detected through regular pelvic exams. Ovarian cancer is treated by surgical removal of one or both ovaries, the fallopian tubes, and the uterus.

Skin Cancer

Skin cancer is the most common cancer of all when cases of the highly curable forms are included. Of the more than 5 million cases diagnosed each year, **melanoma**, the most serious type, has about 96,000 cases occurring each year. Almost all cases of skin cancer can be traced to excessive exposure to **ultraviolet (UV) radiation** from the sun, including longer-wavelength ultraviolet A (UVA) and shorter-wavelength ultraviolet B (UVB) radiation. UVB radiation causes sunburns and can damage the eyes and immune system. UVA is less likely to cause an immediate sunburn, but it damages connective tissue and leads to premature aging of the skin. Tanning lamps and tanning salon beds emit mostly UVA radiation. Both solar and artificial sources of UVA and UVB radiation are human carcinogens that cause skin cancer.

Both severe, acute sun reactions (sunburns) and chronic low-level sun reactions (suntans) can lead to skin cancer. According to the American Academy of Dermatology, the risk of skin cancer doubles in people who have had five or more sunburns in their lifetime. Severe sunburns in childhood have been linked to a greatly increased risk of skin cancer in later life, so children in particular should be protected (see the box "Sunscreens and Sun-Protective Clothing"). People with fair skin have less natural protection against skin damage from the sun and a higher risk of skin cancer than people with naturally dark skin. Other risk factors include having many moles (particularly large ones), spending time at high altitudes, and having a family history of the disease.

There are three main types of skin cancer, named for the types of skin cell from which they develop. **Basal cell carcinomas** and **squamous cell carcinomas** together account for about 95% of the skin cancers diagnosed each year. They are usually found in chronically sun-exposed areas, such as the face, neck, hands, and arms. The carcinomas usually appear as pale, waxlike, pearly nodules, or red, scaly, sharply outlined patches. These cancers are often painless, although they may bleed, crust, and form an open sore.

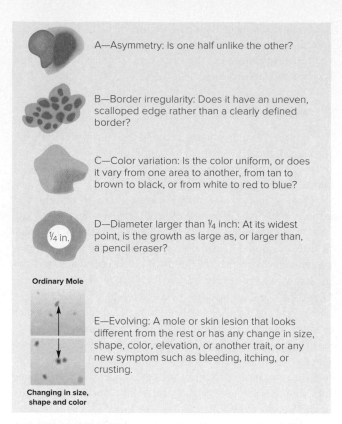

A—Asymmetry: Is one half unlike the other?

B—Border irregularity: Does it have an uneven, scalloped edge rather than a clearly defined border?

C—Color variation: Is the color uniform, or does it vary from one area to another, from tan to brown to black, or from white to red to blue?

D—Diameter larger than ¼ inch: At its widest point, is the growth as large as, or larger than, a pencil eraser?

Ordinary Mole

E—Evolving: A mole or skin lesion that looks different from the rest or has any change in size, shape, color, elevation, or another trait, or any new symptom such as bleeding, itching, or crusting.

Changing in size, shape and color

Figure 12.7   The ABCDE test for melanoma. To see a variety of photos of melanoma and benign moles, visit the National Cancer Institute's Visuals Online site (http://visualsonline.cancer.gov).

Melanoma is by far the most dangerous skin cancer because it spreads so rapidly. It can occur anywhere on the body, but the most common sites are the back, chest, abdomen, and lower legs. A melanoma (a tumor of melanin-forming cells) usually appears at the site of a preexisting mole. The mole may begin to enlarge, become mottled or varied in color (colors can include blue, pink, and white), or develop an irregular surface or irregular borders. Tissue invaded by melanoma may also itch, burn, or bleed easily. You can help with early detection by examining your skin regularly. Most of the spots, freckles, moles, and blemishes on your body are normal, but if you notice an unusual growth, discoloration, or sore that does not heal, see your physician or a dermatologist immediately. The characteristics that may signal that a skin lesion is a melanoma are illustrated in Figure 12.7.

TERMS

melanoma   A malignant tumor of the skin that arises from pigmented cells, usually a mole.

ultraviolet (UV) radiation   Light rays of a specific wavelength, emitted by the sun; most UV rays are blocked by the ozone layer in the upper atmosphere.

basal cell carcinoma   Cancer of the deepest layers of the skin.

squamous cell carcinoma   Cancer of the surface layers of the skin.

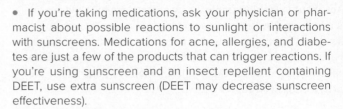

With consistent use of proper clothing, sunscreens, and common sense, you can lead an active outdoor life *and* protect your skin against most sun-induced damage.

Clothing

• Wear long-sleeved shirts and long pants. Dark-colored, tightly woven fabrics provide reasonable protection from the sun. Another good choice is clothing made from special sun-protective fabrics; these garments have an ultraviolet protection factor (UPF) rating, similar to the sun protection factor (SPF) rating for sunscreens.

• Wear a hat. A good choice is a broad-brimmed hat or a legionnaire-style cap that covers the ears and neck. Wear sunscreen on your face even if you are wearing a hat.

• Wear sunglasses. Exposure to UV rays can damage the eyes and cause cataracts.

Sunscreen

• Use a sunscreen and lip balm with an SPF of 15 or higher. An SPF rating refers to the amount of time you can stay out in the sun before you burn, compared with not using sunscreen. For example, a product with an SPF of 30 would allow you to remain in the sun without burning 30 times longer, on average, than if you didn't apply sunscreen. If you're fair-skinned, have a family history of skin cancer, are at high altitude, or will be outdoors for many hours, use a sunscreen with an even higher SPF.

• Choose a broad-spectrum sunscreen that protects against both UVA and UVB radiation. The SPF rating of a sunscreen currently applies only to UVB, but a number of ingredients, especially titanium dioxide and zinc oxide, are effective at blocking most UVA radiation. Sunscreens with the "broad-spectrum" label help protect against both UVA and UVB radiation.

• Use a water-resistant sunscreen if you swim or sweat a great deal. Under FDA regulations, sunscreens cannot be labeled as "waterproof" or "sweatproof" because these claims overstate the products' actual effectiveness. Labels for "water resistant" must specify whether they provide the labeled SPF protection for 40 or 80 minutes of swimming or sweating.

• If you have acne, look for a sunscreen that is labeled "non-comedogenic," which means that it will not cause pimples.

• Shake sunscreen before applying. Apply it 30 minutes before exposure to allow it time to bond to the skin. Reapply sunscreen frequently and generously to all sun-exposed areas (many people overlook their temples, ears, and sides and backs of their necks). Most people use less than half as much as they need to attain the full SPF rating. One ounce of sunscreen is enough to cover an average-size adult in a swimsuit. Reapply sunscreen every two hours. A higher SPF does not mean you can use less. Also be sure to reapply sunscreen after activities, such as swimming, that could remove sunscreen.

• If you're taking medications, ask your physician or pharmacist about possible reactions to sunlight or interactions with sunscreens. Medications for acne, allergies, and diabetes are just a few of the products that can trigger reactions. If you're using sunscreen and an insect repellent containing DEET, use extra sunscreen (DEET may decrease sunscreen effectiveness).

Time of Day and Location

• Avoid sun exposure between 10:00 A.M. and 2:00 P.M., when the sun's rays are most intense. Clouds allow as much as 80% of UV rays to reach your skin. Stay in the shade when you can.

• Consult the day's UV Index, which predicts UV levels on a 0–11+ scale, to get a sense of the amount of sun protection you'll need. Take special care on days with a rating of 5 or above. You can download a free UV index app from the U.S. Environmental Protection Agency or find index ratings from the National Weather Service.

• UV rays can penetrate at least three feet below the surface of water, so swimmers should wear water-resistant sunscreens. Snow, sand, water, concrete, and white-painted surfaces are also highly reflective of UV rays.

Tanning Salons

• Stay away from tanning salons! Despite advertising claims to the contrary, the lights used in tanning parlors are damaging to your skin. Tanning beds and lamps emit mostly UVA radiation, increasing your risk of premature skin aging (such as wrinkles) and skin cancer.

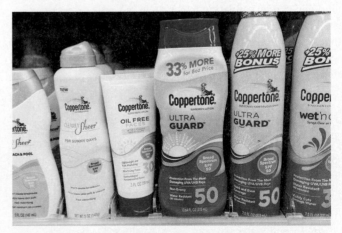

Johnny Louis/JL/Sipa USA/Newscom

To protect yourself against skin cancer, avoid overexposure to UV radiation. People of every age, including babies and children, need to be protected from the sun. If you have an unusual skin lesion, your physician will examine it and possibly perform a biopsy. If the lesion is cancerous, it is usually removed surgically, a procedure that can almost always be performed in the physician's office using a local anesthetic. Treatment is usually simple and successful when the cancer is caught early. Even for melanoma, the outlook after removal in the early stages is good, with a five-year survival rate of 98% if the tumor is localized but only 64% if the cancer has spread to adjacent lymph nodes. Most melanomas are detected in the early, localized stage.

Head and Neck Cancers

Head and neck cancers—cancers of the oral cavity, pharynx, larynx, and nasal cavity—can be traced principally to cigarette, cigar, or pipe smoking; the use of spit tobacco; and the excessive consumption of alcohol. Additionally, a subset of cancers of the tonsils and tongue base are strongly related to HPV infection. Head and neck cancer occurs more than twice as often in men as in women and most frequently in men over age 40.

Chemotherapy, radiation, and surgery are the primary methods of treatment for head and neck cancers. Patients often endure intense mouth and throat inflammation and some require disfiguring surgeries, but many can be cured. The five-year survival rate is about 65%.

Testicular Cancer

Testicular cancer is relatively rare, accounting for only 1% of cancers in men (9,560 cases per year), but it is the most common cancer in men ages 20–35. Testicular cancer is much more common among white Americans than among Latinos, Asian Americans, or African Americans. Men with undescended testicles are at increased risk for testicular cancer, and for this reason the condition should be corrected in early childhood. Self-examination may help in the early detection of testicular cancer (see the box "Testicle Self-Examination"). Tumors are treated by surgical removal of the testicle and, if the tumor has spread, by chemotherapy. The five-year survival rate is 95%.

Other Cancers

Several other cancers affect thousands of people each year. Some have identifiable risk factors (particularly smoking and obesity, which are controllable), but the causes of others are still under investigation.

- *Pancreatic cancer* causes about 46,000 deaths annually in the United States. The disease is usually well advanced before symptoms become noticeable, and no effective cure is available. About 3 out of 10 cases are linked to smoking. Other risk factors include being male, African American, or over age 60; having a family history of pancreatic

cancer; having diabetes; being inactive and obese; and eating a diet high in fat and meat and low in vegetables.

- *Bladder cancer* is three times as common in men as in women, and almost two times higher in white men than in black men. Smoking is the key risk factor. The first symptoms are likely to be blood in the urine and/or increased frequency of urination. These symptoms can also signal a urinary tract infection, but a physician evaluation is necessary. With early detection, 96% of bladder cancers are curable. There are about 80,000 new cases and 17,000 deaths each year.

- *Kidney cancer* usually occurs in people over 50. Smoking and obesity are mild risk factors, as is a family history of the disease. Symptoms may include fatigue, pain in the side, and blood in the urine. There are about 73,000 new cases each year and about 14,000 deaths.

- *Brain cancer* commonly develops for no apparent reason and can arise from most of the cell types that are found in the brain. One of the few established risk factors for brain cancer is ionizing radiation, such as X-rays of the head. Symptoms are often nonspecific and include headaches, fatigue, behavioral changes, and sometimes seizures. Some brain tumors are curable by surgery or by radiation and chemotherapy, but most are not. There are about 24,000 new cases and 17,000 deaths each year.

- *Leukemia,* cancer of the white blood cells, starts in the bone marrow but can spread to the lymph nodes, spleen, liver, other organs, and central nervous system. Some possible risk factors include smoking, radiation, certain chemicals, and infections. Most symptoms occur because leukemia cells crowd out the production of normal blood cells. The result can be fatigue, anemia, weight loss, and increased risk of infection. There are about 62,000 new cases and 23,000 deaths each year.

- *Lymphoma* is a form of cancer that begins in the lymph nodes and then may spread to almost any part of the body. There are two types—Hodgkin disease and non-Hodgkin lymphoma (NHL). NHL is the more common and more deadly form of the disease. Risk factors for NHL are not well understood but may include genetic factors, radiation, and certain chemicals and infections.

? Ask Yourself

QUESTIONS FOR CRITICAL THINKING AND REFLECTION?

Do you know anyone who has had cancer? If so, what type of cancer was it? What were its symptoms? Based on the information presented so far in this chapter, did the person have any of the known risk factors for the disease?

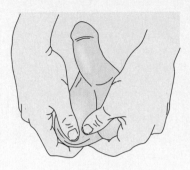

The best time to perform a testicular self-exam is after a warm shower or bath, when the scrotum is relaxed.

First, stand in front of a mirror and look for any swelling of the scrotum. Then, examine each testicle with both hands. Place the index and middle fingers under the testicle and the thumbs on top. Roll each testicle gently between the fingers and thumbs. Don't worry if one testicle seems slightly larger than the other; that's common. Also, expect to feel the *epididymis*—the soft, sperm-carrying tube at the rear of each testicle.

Perform a self-exam each month. If you find a lump, swelling, or nodule, see your doctor right away. The abnormality may not be cancer, but only a physician can make a diagnosis.

Other possible signs of testicular cancer include a change in the way a testicle feels, a sudden collection of fluid in the scrotum, a dull ache in the lower abdomen or groin, a feeling of heaviness in the scrotum, or pain in a testicle or the scrotum.

SOURCES: Testicular Cancer Resource Center. 2012. *How to Do a Testicular Self Examination* (http://tcrc.acor.org/tcexam.html); National Cancer Institute. 2010. *Testicular Cancer* (http://www.cancer.gov /cancertopics/pdq/treatment/testicular/Patient).

DETECTING AND TREATING CANCER

Early cancer detection often depends on our willingness to be aware of changes in our own body and to make sure we keep up with recommended screening tests. Although treatment success varies with individual cancers, cure rates have increased—sometimes dramatically—in this century, especially for cancers diagnosed at their early stages.

Detecting Cancer

Unlike those of some other diseases, early signs of cancer are usually not apparent to anyone but the person who has them. Even pain is not a reliable guide to early detection, because the initial stages of cancer may be painless. Self-monitoring is the first line of defense. By being aware of the risk factors in your own life, your immediate family's cancer history, and your own history, you may bring a problem to the attention of a doctor long before it would be detected at a routine physical. In addition to self-monitoring, specific screening tests for certain cancers are available. Consult the list and links in Table 12.2 for general screening guidelines from ACS; the Centers for Disease Control and Prevention (CDC), which reflect the recommendations of the USPSTF; and the National Cancer Institute (NCI). Discuss your personal risk factors, such as family history or cigarette use, with your health care provider to help determine the screening tests and schedule most appropriate for you. Digital reminders can be effective in increasing the likelihood that people follow through with cancer screening; see the box "Electronic Health Records" for more information.

Stages of Cancer

Physicians need to know the exact size and location of a tumor to treat it effectively. To confirm the type of tumor, a biopsy may be performed. Physicians can then classify the disease according to the extent of the cancer in a patient's body, whether the cancer has invaded nearby lymph nodes, and whether metastases are present. This is usually determined through imaging techniques such as MRI, computed tomography (CT) scanning, ultrasonography, or exploratory surgery. The classifying process is called *staging*, and the cancer is categorized in five stages, as shown in Table 12.3. By judging the extent of each criterion—size or extent, spread, metastases—physicians can determine the cancer's stage, establish how severe it is, and choose the most appropriate treatment based on the extent of the disease.

Treating Cancer

The ideal cancer therapy would kill or remove all cancerous cells while leaving normal tissue untouched. Sometimes this is possible, as when a surgeon removes a small superficial tumor of the skin. Typically, however, the tumor is less accessible, so some combination of treatments is used. The most common types of treatments are surgery, chemotherapy, and radiation therapy, but other treatments such as stem cell transplants and immunotherapy are used for specific cancers.

Surgery In many people, cancer is treated with surgery. If the organ containing the tumor is not essential for life, it may be partially or completely removed. For a solid tumor limited to one area, surgery can be a very effective treatment. Surgery is less effective when the tumor involves cells of the immune system, which are widely distributed throughout the body, or when the cancer has already metastasized. Surgery may also be used to remove part of a tumor to help other treatments work better or to reduce cancer symptoms caused by pain or pressure from tumors.

Chemotherapy Chemotherapy is the use of targeted drugs that destroy rapidly growing cancer cells. Many chemotherapy drugs work by interfering with DNA synthesis and replication in rapidly dividing cells. Normal cells, which usually grow slowly, are not destroyed by these drugs. However, some normal tissues such as

Table 12.2   Early Detection of Cancer in Average-Risk, Asymptomatic People

SITE/TESTS AND PROCEDURES	DESCRIPTION	LINKS FOR MORE INFORMATION
BREAST		
Mammography	Mammograms are the best way to find breast cancer early, when it is easier to treat. These imaging tests, which involve low-dose X-rays, are recommended annually for women starting at age 45 and every 1–2 years for women ages 55 and older, or as long as they are in good health.	CDC: www.cdc.gov/cancer/breast/basic_info/screening.htm NCI: www.cancer.gov/types/breast/mammograms-fact-sheet www.cancer.gov/types/breast/patient/breast-screening-pdq ACS: www.cancer.org/cancer/breast-cancer/screening-tests-and-early -detection.html
Breast awareness	Routine examination of the breasts by health care providers or by women themselves starting in their 20s has not been shown to reduce deaths from breast cancer. However, any lump or other unusual change in the breast needs to be promptly reported to a doctor.	
CERVIX		
Pap and HPV cytology tests	Pap tests can find abnormal cells in the cervix that may turn into cancer, and they can find cervical cancer early, when the chance of a cure is high. Testing every 3–5 years should begin at age 21 and end at age 65, if results have been normal. Co-testing with both Pap and HPV tests are recommended for women ages 30–65. Women who have been vaccinated against HPV still need HPV tests.	CDC: www.cdc.gov/cancer/cervical/basic_info/screening.htm NCI: www.cancer.gov/types/cervical/pap-hpv-testing-fact-sheet www.cancer.gov/types/cervical/patient/cervical-screening-pdq
COLON		
Colonoscopy and sigmoidoscopy	The ACS recommends screening for those ages 45–75; the USPSTF recommends screening begin at age 50. A sigmoidoscopy every 5 years or a colonoscopy every 10 years can reduce the likelihood of death from colorectal cancer and can detect abnormal polyps that can be removed before they turn into cancer. The virtual colonoscopy has not been shown to reduce deaths from colorectal cancer.	CDC: www.cdc.gov/cancer/colorectal/basic_info/screening/index.htm NCI: www.cancer.gov/types/colorectal/screening-fact-sheet www.cancer.gov/types/colorectal/patient/colorectal-screening-pdq ACS: www.cancer.org/cancer/colon-rectal-cancer/detection-diagnosis -staging/screening-tests-used.html
High-sensitivity fecal occult blood test (FOBT)	This yearly multiple-stool, take-home test reduces deaths from colorectal cancer. If a positive result is found, it is followed by a colonoscopy or sigmoidoscopy.	
LUNG		
Low-dose computed tomography (LDCT)	This imaging test has been shown to reduce lung cancer deaths among heavy smokers (30 pack-years*) between ages 55 and 80 who still smoke or have quit within the last 15 years.	CDC: www.cdc.gov/cancer/lung/basic_info/screening.htm NCI: www.cancer.gov/types/lung/patient/lung-screening-pdq
OVARY AND UTERUS		
CA-125 blood test, transvaginal ultrasound	There is no evidence that any screening test reduces deaths from ovarian cancer. However, these tests can help in diagnosing ovarian cancer. Women should report any unexpected bleeding or spotting to a doctor.	CDC: www.cdc.gov/cancer/ovarian/basic_info/screening.htm NCI: www.cancer.gov/types/ovarian/patient/ovarian-screening-pdq www.cancer.gov/types/uterine/patient/endometrial-screening-pdq
PROSTATE		
Prostate-specific antigen (PSA)	Although this blood test, which is often done with a digital rectal exam, can detect prostate cancer at an early stage, it can also lead to overdiagnosis and overtreatment. Starting at age 50, men should talk to a doctor about the pros and cons of this test. African American men and men whose father or brother had prostate cancer before age 65 should talk to a doctor about earlier testing.	CDC: www.cdc.gov/cancer/prostate/basic_info/screening.htm NCI: www.cancer.gov/types/prostate/psa-fact-sheet

*A pack-year is calculated by multiplying the number of packs of cigarettes smoked per day by the number of years the person has smoked. For example, smoking 2 packs per day for 10 years is equal to 20 pack-years; smoking one-half pack per day for 10 years is equal to 5 pack-years.

SOURCES: American Cancer Society (ACS). 2019. *American Cancer Society Guidelines for the Early Detection of Cancer.* (https://www.cancer.org/healthy/find-cancer-early/cancer-screening-guidelines/american-cancer-society-guidelines-for-the-early-detection-of-cancer.html) accessed May 30, 2018; Centers for Disease Control and Prevention. *Cancer Prevention and Control: Cancer Screening Tests.* (http://www.cdc.gov/cancer/dcpc/prevention/screening.htm) accessed May 2, 2018; National Cancer Institute. Screening Tests. (http://www.cancer.gov/about-cancer/screening/screening-tests) accessed January 16, 2019.

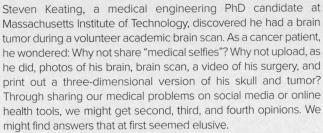

Steven Keating, a medical engineering PhD candidate at Massachusetts Institute of Technology, discovered he had a brain tumor during a volunteer academic brain scan. As a cancer patient, he wondered: Why not share "medical selfies"? Why not upload, as he did, photos of his brain, brain scan, a video of his surgery, and print out a three-dimensional version of his skull and tumor? Through sharing our medical problems on social media or online health tools, we might get second, third, and fourth opinions. We might find answers that at first seemed elusive.

Patients often have the least access to their own medical data files. Why not have a hospital "share" button? Some apps in fact have been developed toward that purpose and are being used. OpenNotes is a study enabling full patient access. Apple's ResearchKit has attracted over 50,000 people to track their symptoms using various apps to see if they are eligible for specific studies.

The Blue Button is another system that allows patients to access and share medical records. A decade ago, this initiative was launched by a partnership of private individuals, not-for-profit foundations, and the federal government. Since then, more than a million people have clicked the Blue Button to download their data through the Department of Veterans Affairs.

Unfortunately, the digital revolution in medical records has not succeeded yet. There has been patient harm from errors: Software glitches, user errors, and other system flaws are rife, and no central database yet exists to compile and study these incidents to improve safety. Patients cannot easily share computerized medical histories because competing firms have developed software that don't talk/interface with each other. Digital medical record apps require doctors to spend so much time with pulldown menus and typing that there is little time to interact with patients. And fraud is possible with the software, which can be misused to overcharge.

Electronic health records have the enormous potential to make health care better, safer, and cheaper. Once we have access to our data, we can check for accuracy of the following:

- Personal identification information

- Diagnoses—Are past health conditions correctly characterized? Has anything changed since our last patient history?

- List of medications—Does it reflect recent updates? Does it include all OTC medications we take?

- Upcoming and past screenings list of doctors and other providers

- Recorded preferences for end-of-life care

Another hopeful feature of electronic health records is a system for sending automatic cancer screening reminders. Veterans can sign up for e-mail reminders. Studies have showed that reminders—whether phone calls, e-mails, or text messages—are effective ways to get patients into clinics for regular cancer screenings. Hospitals and health maintenance organizations continue to work at switching to electronic records, but it will take time.

SOURCES: Health IT. 2019. *Blue Button* (https://www.healthit.gov/topic/health-it-initiatives/blue-button); My HealtheVet. 2019. *About My HealtheVet* (https://www.myhealth.va.gov/mhv-portal-web/web/myhealthevet/faqs#mrp1); Schulte, F. 2019. "Why the promise of electronic health records has gone unfulfilled," *National Public Radio* (https://www.npr.org/sections/health-shots/2019/03/18/704475396/why-the-promise-of-electronic-health-records-has-gone-unfulfilled).

Table 12.3	Cancer Stages

STAGE	DESCRIPTION
0	Carcinoma in situ: abnormal cells are present only in the layer of cells in which they developed; not cancer but may become cancer
I, II, and III	Higher numbers indicate more extensive disease: larger tumor size and/or spread of the cancer beyond the organ in which it first developed to nearby lymph nodes or to tissues or organs adjacent to the primary tumor
IV	Cancer that has spread to distant tissues or organs

SOURCE: National Cancer Institute. 2015. *Cancer Staging.* (http://www.cancer.gov/about-cancer/diagnosis-staging/staging/staging-fact-sheet) accessed March 9, 2015.

intestinal, hair, and blood-forming cells are always growing, and damage to these tissues produces the unpleasant side effects of chemotherapy, including nausea, vomiting, diarrhea, and hair loss. Like surgery, chemotherapy can also be used to help other treatments work better and to ease cancer symptoms by shrinking tumors.

Radiation Therapy In radiation therapy, a beam of X-rays or gamma rays is directed at the tumor, killing the tumor cells. Radiation destroys both normal and cancerous cells, but because it can often be directed precisely at the tumor, it is usually less toxic for the patient than either surgery or chemotherapy, and it can often be performed on an outpatient basis. Less commonly, radiation is delivered internally, from implanted radioactive seeds, ribbons, or capsules. This method is used in treating prostate cancer. Radiation may also be administered in liquid form as a drink, injection, or IV. Cancers of the thyroid, bones, or bone marrow respond to these forms. Radiation may be used as an exclusive treatment or in combination with surgery and/or chemotherapy.

Other Types of Cancer Treatments *Immunotherapies* boost the immune system's response to cancer and help mark cancer cells so that it is easier for the immune system to find, identify, and destroy them. One example of an immunotherapy is monoclonal antibodies, which are used to fight cancer similar to the way the immune system fights infection. All cells in the body have markers on their surfaces, and the immune system develops antibodies, or special proteins, that can recognize these markers, bind to them, and trigger destruction. Scientists carefully select cell-surface markers that are displayed on cancer cells and then administer antibodies to the patient. These monoclonal antibodies (the term *monoclonal* means they bind to only one particular cell-surface marker) target the cancer cells and enlist the help of the body's own immune system to selectively kill these cells. Another immunotherapy for some cancers are vaccines that have been developed to stimulate the immune system to attack cancer cells.

Hormone therapies are used to treat some cancers for which hormones promote the growth and spread of cancer cells, such as prostate and breast cancers. Hormone therapies usually work by blocking the body's ability to produce hormones or by interfering with how hormones act in the body. Tumor cells can be tested for the presence of hormone receptors or monitored in other ways to help determine if a hormone therapy is potentially beneficial for a particular patient.

Stem cell transplants restore blood-forming cells in people who have had their own cells destroyed by high-dosage radiation therapy or chemotherapy. They are most often used for cancers that affect the immune system or the blood, such as leukemia or lymphoma. Stem cells are taken from the patient (prior to radiation or chemotherapy) or from a compatible donor and then transplanted (after treatment) into the patient via an IV, similar to a blood transfusion. Stem cells travel to the bone marrow, where they take the place of the cells that were destroyed by prior cancer treatment; they start producing the blood cells the patient needs. Finding a compatible donor, one whose stem cells have matching sets of surface proteins, can be difficult. In some cases, a patient's own stem cells can be used. In this process, the stem cells are removed, treated to remove cancer cells, and then transplanted back into the patient.

Personalized or precision therapies are those selected based on the genetic profile of a cancer. Specific genetic changes allow cancer cells to grow and spread—and these changes may be different even for people who have the same type and stage of cancer. The hope is that treatment can be tailored to specific genetic changes, making it more effective and sparing patients from therapies that won't benefit their case. For example, some breast cancers over-express a protein called HER2, which causes cells to receive too many signals to multiply; there is a targeted therapy to block growth signals to the cell, but this therapy is only helpful for treating cancers with the HER2 gene change. Researchers hope to develop many more such precision therapies.

New Insights in Cancer Treatment. In the 1990s, a prevalent idea for treating malignant tumors was to starve them of oxygen, which every living thing needs to survive. Researchers knew that if they become hypoxic (low on oxygen), cancer cells—like healthy cells—grow new blood vessels. This replenishing of the blood and oxygen supply is called angiogenesis. If this process could be blocked (using anti-angiogenesis drugs), it seemed logical that the tumor would stop growing and eventually die.

But what most researchers and doctors did not understand was how resilient tumors are. Although lack of oxygen kills some tumor cells, other hypoxic tumor cells kick into panic mode, turning on a "subcommittee" of proteins to ensure their survival. In addition to forming new blood vessels, the stressed cells lay down highways of collagen—a stringy web that provides links over which cancer cells can move away from the "toxic neighborhood," or metastasize.

The tumor cells also develop stem-cell-like properties to repopulate the tumor. And they become more resistant to chemotherapy. Thus, what had seemed like the obvious answer—anti-angiogenesis drugs—failed. The tumors soon grew back, and even more aggressively.

One cancer researcher tried a radical approach: Rather than deprive cancer cells of oxygen, Rakesh Jain suggested infusing them with it. Trained as an engineer, Jain, a Harvard professor of tumor biology, noticed that the capillaries of tumors resembled leaky pipes, inefficient at delivering blood. His idea was to boost oxygen levels to keep tumors from entering panic mode and becoming supertumors. Instead, they would remain inefficient at best. Jain's experiments showed that well-oxygenated tumor cells could be more efficiently killed by chemotherapy.

Another researcher, David Cheresh, a pathologist from the University of California at San Diego, established that nutrient deprivation, like oxygen deprivation, makes tumors more aggressive and resistant to drugs. Cheresh and his team explained that tumor cells respond to stress by converting themselves into a kind of chemotherapy-resistant stem cell. These cells are not naturally powerful; their strength is their ability to reprogram themselves. This discovery has prompted the development of drugs, still under trial, that would block the tumor's stem-cell-like adaptation.

Another avenue of research in cancer control involves blocking tumor cell migration and metastasis. To do so, oncology professor Daniele Gilkes at Johns Hopkins University is targeting the protein that first responds to a hypoxic tumor's emergency calls and gets activated to form collagen. Stopping this process, Gilkes's lab hopes, will stop metastasis.

These ideas are still in experimental stages and need time and money to continue down their innovative paths. A more complete understanding of tumor cell responses will, eventually, allow researchers to outsmart and stop cancer.

TIPS FOR TODAY AND THE FUTURE

A growing body of research suggests that we can take an active role in preventing many cancers by adopting a wellness lifestyle.

RIGHT NOW YOU CAN

- Buy multiple bottles of sunscreen and put them in places where you will most likely need them, such as your backpack, gym bag, or car.
- Check the cancer screening guidelines in this chapter, and make sure you are up-to-date on your screenings.
- If you are a woman, develop breast self-awareness; if you are a man, do a testicular self-exam.

IN THE FUTURE YOU CAN

- Learn where to find information about daily UV radiation levels in your area, and learn how to interpret the information. Many local newspapers and television stations (and their websites) report current UV levels every day.
- Gradually add foods with abundant phytochemicals to your diet, choosing from the list shown in Table 12.1.

COMMON QUESTIONS ANSWERED

Q What is a biopsy?

A A *biopsy* is the removal and examination of a small piece of body tissue. Biopsies enable cancer specialists to carefully examine cells that are suspected of having turned cancerous. Some biopsies are fairly simple to perform, such as those on tissue from moles or skin sores. Other biopsies may require the use of a needle or probe to remove tissue from inside the body, such as in the breast or stomach.

Q What types of cancer are most common in young adults?

A Cancer is relatively rare in young adults—only about 5% of all cancer diagnoses are in young people ages 15–39—but it is one of the five leading causes of death in the age group. Certain cancers are more common in young adults than in either children or older adults, including Hodgkin lymphoma, thyroid cancer, testicular cancer, and melanoma. Rates of colorectal cancer among young adults have also increased in recent years, and researchers are trying to identify the factors that underlie this worrying trend.

The causes of most cancers in young adults aren't known. Moreover, some cancers may have unique genetic and biological features, and so younger adults may not respond as well to treatments that have been tested in older populations. The potential effects of treatments such as chemotherapy on future fertility are a special concern for young cancer patients.

Another issue is that young adults often face delays in cancer diagnosis. They may not visit health care professionals regularly, and any symptoms they do report may be attributed to causes other than cancer, given that cancer isn't common in this age group. Many symptoms of early cancer *are* much more likely to be caused by something other than cancer. But if you have unexplained symptoms—especially if they don't go away or if they get worse—seek a medical evaluation. Early signs of cancer can include an unusual lump or swelling; abnormal bleeding or easy bruising; unplanned weight loss; or ongoing pain, fever, or excessive tiredness.

SUMMARY

- Cancer is an abnormal and uncontrolled multiplication of cells; cancer cells can metastasize (spread to other parts of the body).

- The genetic basis of some cancers appears to be mutational damage to suppressor genes, which normally limit cell division.

- Cancer-promoting dietary factors include charred meat, certain types of fat, and alcohol. Dietary elements that may protect against cancer include antioxidants and phytochemicals. An inactive lifestyle is associated with some cancers.

- Some carcinogens occur naturally in the environment; others are manufactured substances. Occupational exposure is a risk for some workers.

- All sources of radiation are potentially carcinogenic, including X-rays and UV rays from the sun.

- Lung cancer kills more people than any other type of cancer; tobacco smoke is the primary cause.

- Colon and rectal cancers are linked to age, heredity, obesity, and a diet rich in red meat and low in fruits and vegetables.

- Breast cancer has a genetic component, but lifestyle and hormones are also factors. Prostate cancer is chiefly a disease of aging; diet, heredity, and ethnicity are other risk factors.

- Cancers of the female reproductive tract include cervical, uterine, and ovarian cancers. Cervical cancer is linked to HPV infection; the Pap test is an effective screening test. Vaccination is recommended for girls and young women.

- Melanoma is the most serious form of skin cancer; excessive exposure to UV radiation in sunlight is the primary cause.

- Oral cancer is caused primarily by smoking, excess alcohol consumption, and use of spit tobacco.

- Testicular cancer can be detected early through self-examination.

- Self-monitoring and regular screening tests are essential to early cancer detection.

- Methods of cancer diagnosis include MRI, CT scanning, and ultrasound.

- Cancer treatment usually consists of some combination of surgery, chemotherapy, and radiation. New methods related to boosting oxygen and nutrient supplies to tumors are under study.

FOR FURTHER EXPLORATION

American Academy of Dermatology. Provides information on skin cancer prevention.

http://www.aad.org

American Cancer Society. Provides a wide range of free materials on the prevention and treatment of cancer.

http://www.cancer.org

American Institute for Cancer Research. Provides information on lifestyle and cancer prevention, especially nutrition.

http://www.aicr.org

CureSearch National Childhood Cancer Foundation. Offers information on childhood cancers and initiatives to raise awareness and funds for research.

http://www.curesearch.org

EPA/Sunwise. Provides information about the UV Index and the effects of sun exposure, with links to sites with daily UV Index ratings for U.S. and international cities.

http://www.epa.gov/sunwise/uvindex.html

LiveStrong Foundation. Provides resources on cancer and cancer support.

http://www.livestrong.org

MedlinePlus: Breast Cancer and Genetic Testing. Provides links to reliable information about genetic testing and related topics.

https://medlineplus.gov/breastcancer.html

MedlinePlus: Cancers. Provides links to reliable cancer information.

http://www.nlm.nih.gov/medlineplus/cancers.html

National Cancer Institute. Provides information on treatment options, screening, clinical trials, and newly approved drugs.

http://www.cancer.gov

Skin Cancer Foundation. Provides information on all types of skin cancers, their prevention, and treatment.

http://www.skincancer.org

Siteman Cancer Center: Your Disease Risk. Includes interactive risk assessments as well as tips for preventing common cancers.

http://www.yourdiseaserisk.wustl.edu

World Health Organization: Cancer. Home page of WHO's worldwide anti-cancer initiative.

http://www.who.int/cancer/en

SELECTED BIBLIOGRAPHY

American Cancer Society. 2015. *Health Risks of Secondhand Smoke* (http://www.cancer.org/cancer/cancercauses/tobaccocancer/secondhand-smoke).

American Cancer Society. 2016. *Diet and Physical Activity: What's the Cancer Connection?* (http://www.cancer.org/cancer/cancercauses/dietandphysicalactivity/diet-and-physical-activity/).

American Cancer Society. 2017. *Breast Cancer Facts & Figures 2017-2018.* Atlanta, GA: American Cancer Society, Inc.

American Cancer Society. 2019. *Cancer Facts & Figures, 2019.* Atlanta, GA: American Cancer Society.

Beaber, E. F., et al. 2014. Recent oral contraceptive use by formulation and breast cancer risk among women 20 to 49 years of age. *Cancer Research* 74(15): 4078-4089.

Beavis, A. L., P. E. Gravitt, and A. F. Rositch. 2017. Hysterectomy-corrected cervical cancer mortality rates reveal a larger racial disparity in the United States. *Cancer* 123(6): 1044-1050.

Beil, L. 2017. Deflating cancer: New approaches to low oxygen may thwart tumors. *Science News* 191(4): 24-27.

Castellsagué, X., et al. 2016. HPV involvement in head and neck cancers. Comprehensive assessment of biomarkers in 3680 patients. *Journal of the National Cancer Institute* 108(6).

Connell, L. C., et al. 2017. The rising incidence of younger patients with colorectal cancer: Questions about screening, biology, and treatment. *Current Treatment Options in Oncology* 18(4): 23.

Demeyer, D., et al. 2015. Mechanisms linking colorectal cancer to the consumption of (processed) red meat: A review. *Critical Reviews in Food Science and Nutrition,* May 15.

Farvid, M. S., et al. 2016. Fruit and vegetable consumption in adolescence and early adulthood and risk of breast cancer: Population based cohort study. *British Medical Journal* 353: i2343.

Gilkes, D. M. 2016. Implications of hypoxia in breast cancer metastasis to bone. *International Journal of Molecular Sciences* 17(10): 1669.

Gram, I. T., et al. 2016. The fraction of breast cancer attributable to smoking: The Norwegian women and cancer study 1991-2012. *British Journal of Cancer* 115(5): 616-623.

Guo, F., et al. 2017. Use of *BRCA* mutation test in the U.S., 2004-2014. *American Journal of Preventive Medicine.* doi: 10.1016/j.amepre. 2017.01.027

Han, X., et al. 2015. Body mass index at early adulthood, subsequent weight change and cancer incidence and mortality. *International Journal of Cancer* 135(12): 2900-2909.

Iqbal, J., et al. 2015. Differences in breast cancer stage at diagnosis and cancer-specific survival by race and ethnicity in the United States. *Journal of the American Medical Association* 313(2): 165-173.

Joshi, A. D., et al. 2015. Meat intake, cooking methods, dietary carcinogens, and colorectal cancer: Findings from the Colorectal Cancer Family Registry. *Cancer Medicine* 4(6): 936-952.

Li, X., et al. 2016. Effectiveness of prophylactic surgeries in BRCA1 or BRCA2 mutation carriers: A meta-analysis and systematic review. *Clinical Cancer Research* 22(15): 3971-3981.

Mpekris, F., et al. 2017. Role of vascular normalization in benefit from metronomic chemotherapy. *Proceedings of the National Academy of Sciences of the United States of America* 114(8): 1994-1999.

Moore, S. C., et al. 2016. Leisure-time physical activity and risk of 26 types of cancer in 1.44 million adults. *JAMA Internal Medicine* 176(6): 816-825.

Musselwhite, L. W., et al. 2016. Racial/ethnic disparities in cervical cancer screening and outcomes. *Acta Cytologica* 60: 518-526.

National Cancer Institute. 2018. *Adolescents and Young Adults with Cancer* (https://www.cancer.gov/types/aya).

National Human Genome Research Institute. 2015. *A Brief Guide to Genomics Fact Sheet* (http://www.genome.gov/18016863).

Newman, L. A., and L. M. Kaljee. 2017. Health disparities and triple-negative breast cancer in African American women: A review. *JAMA Surgery* 152(5): 485-493.

Nunez, C., et al. 2017. Obesity, physical activity and cancer risks: Results from the Cancer, Lifestyle and Evaluation of Risk Study (CLEAR). *Cancer Epidemiology* 47: 56-63.

Oeffinger, K. C., et al. 2015. Breast cancer screening for women at average risk. *Journal of the American Medical Association* 314(15): 1599-1614.

Orlich, M. J., et al. 2015. Vegetarian dietary patterns and the risk of colorectal cancers. *JAMA Internal Medicine* 1759(5): 767-776.

Pelucchi, C., et al. 2015. Dietary acrylamide and cancer risk: An updated meta-analysis. *International Journal of Cancer* 136(12): 2912-2922.

Siegel, R. L., et al. 2017. Colorectal cancer incidence patterns in the United States, 1874-2013. *Journal of the National Cancer Institute* 109(8). doi:10.1093/jnci/djw322

Siegel, R. L., et al. 2017. Colorectal cancer statistics, 2017. *CA: A Cancer Journal for Clinicians,* Mar 1. doi:10.3322/caac.21395

Wilson, R., et al. 2016. MicroRNA regulation of endothelial TREX1 reprograms the tumour microenvironment. *Nature Communications* 7(13597). doi:10.1038/ncomms13597

Name _____ **Section** _____ **Date** _____

LAB 12.1 Cancer Prevention

This lab looks at two areas of cancer prevention over which you have a great deal of individual control—diet and sun exposure. For a detailed personal risk profile for many specific types of cancer, complete the assessments at the Washington University Siteman Cancer Center's "Your Disease Risk" site (https://siteman.wustl.edu/prevention/ydr/).

Part I Diet and Cancer

Track your diet for three days, recording the number of servings from each of the following groups that you consume.

DAY 1	DAY 2	DAY 3	POTENTIAL CANCER FIGHTERS
_____	_____	_____	Orange, deep yellow, pink, and red vegetables and some fruits (for example, apricots, cantaloupe, carrots, corn, grapefruit, mangoes, nectarines, papayas, red and yellow bell peppers, sweet potatoes, pumpkin, tomatoes and tomato sauce, watermelon, winter squash such as acorn or butternut)
_____	_____	_____	Dark green leafy vegetables (for example, broccoli rabe, chard, kale, romaine and other dark lettuces, spinach; beet, collard, dandelion, mustard, and turnip greens)
_____	_____	_____	Cruciferous vegetables (bok choy, broccoli, brussels sprouts, cabbage, cauliflower, kohlrabi, turnips)
_____	_____	_____	Citrus fruits (for example, grapefruit, lemons, limes, oranges, tangerines)
_____	_____	_____	Whole grains (for example, whole-grain bread, cereal, and pasta; brown rice; oatmeal; whole-grain corn; barley; popcorn; bulgur)
_____	_____	_____	Legumes (peas, lentils, and beans, including fava, navy, kidney, pinto, black, and lima beans)
_____	_____	_____	Berries (for example, strawberries, raspberries, blackberries, blueberries)
_____	_____	_____	Garlic and other allium vegetables (onions, leeks, chives, scallions, shallots)
_____	_____	_____	Soy products (for example, tofu, tempeh, soy milk, miso, soybeans)
_____	_____	_____	Other cancer-fighting fruits (apples, cherries, cranberries or juice, grapes, kiwifruit, pears, plums, prunes, raisins)
_____	_____	_____	Other cancer-fighting vegetables (asparagus, beets, chili peppers, eggplant, green peppers, radishes)
_____	_____	_____	**Daily totals (average for three days:_____)**

The goal is to eat at least 7 (women) or 9 (men) servings of cancer-fighting fruits and vegetables each day; the more servings, the better. (Research is ongoing, and this list of cancer fighters is not comprehensive. Remember, nearly all fruits, vegetables, and grains are healthy choices.)

Part II Skin Cancer Risk Assessment

Your risk of skin cancer from the ultraviolet radiation in sunlight depends on several factors. Take the following quiz to see how sensitive you are. The higher your UV-risk score, the greater your risk of skin cancer—and the greater your need to take precautions against too much sun. Score 1 point for each true statement:

_____ 1. I have had skin cancer before.

_____ 2. I have a family history of skin cancer.

_____ 3. I have several large or many small moles.

_____ 4. I have fair skin and/or skin that rarely tans but burns or freckles easily.

_____ 5. I have blue, green, or gray eyes.

_____ 6. I have blond, red, or light brown hair.

_____ 7. I live or vacation at high altitudes and/or in tropical or subtropical climates.

_____ 8. I have a history of one or more severe, blistering sunburns.

_____ 9. I work indoors all week but spend a lot of time in the sun on weekends.

_____ 10. I spend a lot of time outdoors.

_____ 11. I am currently taking medication that makes my skin more sensitive to sunlight.

_____ 12. I have a history of use of tanning beds or sunlamps.

_____ **Total score**

LABORATORY ACTIVITIES

SCORE	RISK OF SKIN CANCER FROM UV RADIATION
0	Low
1–3	Moderate
4–7	High
8–12	Very high

For a detailed assessment of your skin type and how your skin behaves in response to sun exposure, complete the Skin Cancer Foundation's skin type assessment (http://www.skincancer.org/prevention/are-you-at-risk/fitzpatrick-skin-quiz).

Using Your Results

How did you score?

(1) How close did you come to the goal of eating 7–9 or more servings of cancer fighters each day?

Are you satisfied with your diet in terms of cancer prevention? If not, set a specific goal for a target number of servings of cancer-fighting fruits and vegetables:

(2) What is your skin cancer risk assessment score? Does it indicate that you are at high or very high risk? Do you feel you need to take action because of your risk level?

What should you do next? Enter the results of this lab in the Preprogram Assessment column in Appendix B.

(1) If you've set a goal for the diet and cancer portion of the lab, select a target number of additional cancer fighters from the list to try over the next few days; list the foods here, along with your plan for incorporating them into your diet (as a side dish, as a snack, on a salad, as a substitute for another food, etc.).

CANCER FIGHTER TO TRY: PLAN FOR TRYING:

_____   _____

_____   _____

_____   _____

(2) You cannot control all of your risk factors for skin cancer, but you can control your behavior with regard to sun exposure. Keep a journal to track your behavior on days when you are outdoors in the sun for a significant period of time. Compare your behavior with the recommendations for skin cancer prevention described in the chapter. Record information such as time of day, total duration of exposure, UV Index for the day, clothing worn, type and amount of sunscreen used, frequency of sunscreen applications, and so on. From this record, identify ways to improve your behavior to lower your risk of skin cancer. Put together a behavior change plan.

Next, begin to put your strategies into action. After several weeks of a program to improve your diet or reduce your UV exposure, do this lab again and enter the results in the Postprogram Assessment column of Appendix B. How do the results compare?

SOURCES: Centers for Disease Control and Prevention. *What Are the Risk Factors for Skin Cancer?* (https://www.cdc.gov/cancer/ skin/basic_info/risk _factors.htm) accessed April 24, 2018; Mayo Clinic. *Skin Cancer Risk Factors.* (http://www.mayoclinic.org/diseases-conditions/skin-cancer/basics/risk -factors/con-20031606) accessed February 20, 2019; National Cancer Institute. *Skin Cancer Prevention-Patient Version.* (https://www.cancer.gov/types/skin /patient/skin-prevention-pdq) accessed April 10, 2019.

Design elements: Evidence for Exercise box (shoes and stethoscope): Vstock LLC/Tetra Images/Getty Images; Take Charge box (lady walking): VisualCommunications/E+/Getty Images; Critical Consumer box (man): Sam74100/iStock/Getty Images; Diversity Matters box (holding devices): Robert Churchill/iStockphoto/Rawpixel Ltd/Getty Images; Wellness in the Digital Age box (Smart Watch): Hong Li/DigitalVision/Getty Images

Substance Use and Misuse

LOOKING AHEAD...

After reading this chapter, you should be able to

- Define and discuss addiction.

- List the major categories of psychoactive drugs and discuss how drug abuse can be prevented and treated.

- Describe the short-term and long-term effects of alcohol use.

- Identify strategies for drinking alcohol responsibly.

- List the health hazards associated with tobacco use and exposure to environmental tobacco smoke.

- Describe strategies that can help someone stop smoking.

TEST YOUR KNOWLEDGE

1. Which of the following is the most widely used drug among college-age students?
   a. crystal meth
   b. hallucinogens
   c. marijuana
   d. heroin

2. If a man and a woman of the same weight drink the same amount of alcohol, the woman will become intoxicated more quickly than the man. True or false?

3. Electronic cigarettes are a safe alternative to tobacco cigarettes. True or false?

See answers on the next page.

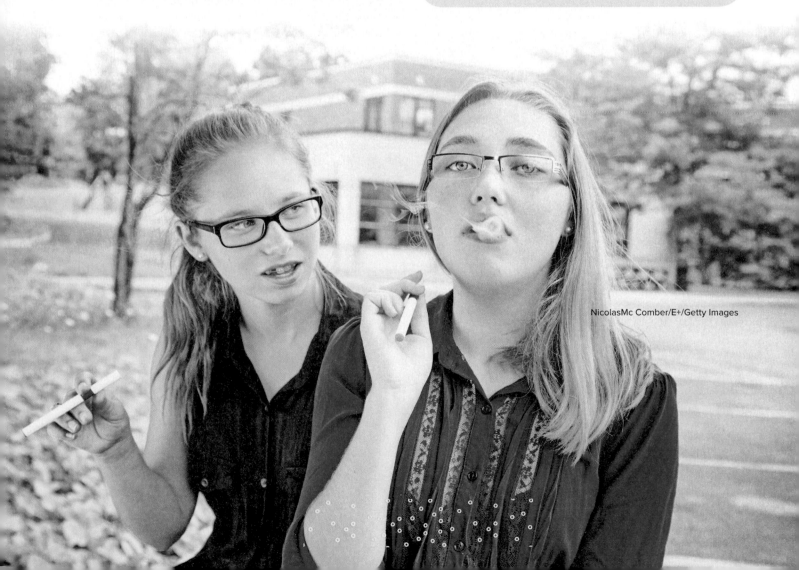

NicolasMc Comber/E+/Getty Images

The use of **drugs** for both medical and social purposes is widespread in the United States (Table 13.1). Many people believe that every problem has or should have a chemical solution. Advertisements, social pressures, and the human desire for quick solutions to life's difficult problems all contribute to the prevailing attitude that drugs can ease all pain. Unfortunately, using drugs can—and often does—have negative consequences.

Aside from death, the most serious drug-related consequences are addiction and impairment of daily activities. The drugs most often associated with addiction and impairment are **psychoactive drugs**—those that alter a person's consciousness, perception, mood, or behavior. In the short term, psychoactive drugs can cause **intoxication**, a state in which physical or mental control is markedly diminished. In the long term, recurrent drug use can have profound physical, emotional, and social effects.

This chapter examines the use of psychoactive drugs, including alcohol and tobacco, and explains their short- and long-term effects and their potential for misuse and addiction. The information provided is designed to help you make healthy, informed decisions about the role of drugs in your life.

ADDICTION

Today scientists view **addiction** as a chronic disease that involves disruption of the brain's systems related to reward, motivation, and memory. Dysfunction in these systems leads to biological, psychological, and social effects associated with pathologically pursuing pleasure or relief by substance use and other behaviors. The American Psychiatric Association (APA) defines addiction as a "complex condition, a chronic brain disease that causes compulsive substance use despite harmful consequences."

Addiction involves craving and the inability to recognize significant risk or other problems with behaviors, interpersonal relationships, and emotional response. Like other chronic diseases, addiction often involves cycles of relapse and remission. Without treatment, addiction is progressive and can result in disabling or deadly health consequences.

Although addiction is most often associated with drug use, many experts now extend the concept of addiction to other behaviors. Looking at the nature of addiction and a range of addictive behaviors can help us understand similar behaviors when they involve drugs. **Addictive behaviors** are habits that have gotten out of control, with resulting negative effects on a person's health. The loss of control is expressed as an unrelenting pursuit of a physical or psychological reward through substance use or behaviors, such as gambling, despite unwanted consequences.

The APA introduces the category of behavioral addictions, which includes gambling disorder, in the *Diagnostic and Statistical Manual of Mental Disorders* (*DSM-5*), the standard classification system used by mental health professionals. Another addictive behavior, internet addiction, is not part of the *DSM-5*, but the *DSM-5* recommends that it be studied further.

VITAL STATISTICS		
Table 13.1	**Nonmedical Drug Use Among Americans, 2017**	
	PERCENTAGE REPORTING PAST MONTH USE	
	YOUNG ADULTS (AGE 18–25)	ALL AMERICANS (AGE 12 AND OLDER)
ILLICIT DRUGS	24.2	11.2
Marijuana* and hashish	22.1	9.6
Nonmedical use of psychotherapeutics	4.5	2.2
Cocaine	1.9	0.8
Heroin	0.3	0.2
Hallucinogens	1.7	0.5
Inhalants	0.5	0.2
Methamphetamine	0.4	0.3
TOBACCO (all forms)	29.1	22.4
Cigarettes	22.3	17.9
Smokeless tobacco	4.8	3.2
Cigars	9.1	4.6
ALCOHOL	56.3	51.7
Binge alcohol use	36.9	24.5
Heavy alcohol use	9.6	6.1

*Federally illegal, but some states permit the use of marijuana.

SOURCES: SAMHSA Center for Behavioral Health Statistics and Quality. 2018. *Results from the 2017 National Survey on Drug Use and Health.* (https://www.samhsa.gov/data/sites/default/files/cbhsq-reports/NSDUHDetailedTabs2017/NSDUHDetailedTabs2017.pdf).

Answers (Test Your Knowledge)

1. **c.** Marijuana ranks first, followed (in order) by hallucinogens, cocaine, and heroin. Alcohol, however, remains by far the most popular drug among college students.

2. **True.** Women usually have a higher percentage of body fat than men and a less active form of a stomach enzyme that breaks down alcohol. Both factors cause them to become intoxicated more quickly and to a greater degree.

3. **False.** E-cigarettes produce carcinogens and other toxic chemicals.

TERMS

drug A chemical substance that affects the processes of the mind or body.

psychoactive drug A drug that can alter a person's consciousness, perception, mood, or behavior.

intoxication A state in which a person's normal functioning is impaired, usually by alcohol or drugs.

addiction A chronic disease that disrupts the brain's system of motivation and reward, characterized by a compulsive desire and increasing need for a substance or behavior, and by harm to the individual and/or society.

addictive behavior Compulsive behavior that is both rewarding and reinforcing and is often pursued to the marginalization or exclusion of other activities and responsibilities.

Internet gaming disorder involves excessive use of internet games that interferes with daily functioning.

Although experts now agree that addiction is more fully defined by behavioral characteristics, they also agree that changes in the brain underlie addiction. One such change is **tolerance**, in which the body adapts to a drug so that the initial dose no longer produces the original emotional or psychological effects. This process means the user has to take larger and larger doses of a drug to achieve the same high. The concept of addiction as a disease, based on identifiable changes to the brain, has led to many advances in the understanding and treatment of drug addiction.

The view that addiction is based in our brain chemistry does not imply that people are not responsible for their addictive behavior. Many experts believe it is inaccurate and counterproductive to think of all bad habits and excessive behaviors as diseases. All addictions involve an initial voluntary step, and other factors such as lifestyle, personality traits, and environmental factors play key roles in the development of addiction.

Diagnosing Substance Misuse and Addiction

Before we discuss addiction and substance use disorders, it's important to note that you do not have to be addicted to a drug to suffer serious consequences—you only have to misuse it once. **Substance misuse** is the use of a substance inconsistent with medical or legal guidelines. Misuse is a broad concept and can include the use of illegal drugs, prescription drugs in greater-than-prescribed amounts, another person's prescription drugs, or a legal substance such as alcohol in an unsafe manner. The situation in which a person takes prescribed painkillers to get high would be considered drug misuse. Any drug misuse carries the risk of serious and life-threatening effects.

In the *DSM-5*, the APA provides criteria for diagnosing problems associated with regular drug use. Classifying a person as having a substance use disorder is not as simple as applying a label; instead, an individual is classified based on symptoms ranging from mild to severe. Addiction is a psychological or physical dependence on a substance or behavior that has undesirable, negative consequences. According to the APA, people with addiction are focused on a particular drug or behavior to the point that it takes over their lives; they use the substance or engage in the behavior compulsively despite knowing it will cause problems.

The 11 *DSM-5* criteria for a substance use disorder are listed here; they are grouped in four categories. The severity of the disorder is determined by the number of criteria a person meets:

- 2–3 criteria indicate a mild disorder.
- 4–5 criteria point to a moderate disorder.
- 6 or more criteria are evidence of a severe disorder.

Impaired Control

1. Taking the substance in larger amounts or over a longer period than was originally intended.
2. Expressing a persistent desire to cut down on or regulate substance use but being unable to do so.

3. Spending a great deal of time getting the substance, using the substance, or recovering from its effects.
4. Craving or experiencing an intense desire or urge to use the substance.

Social Problems

5. Failing to fulfill major obligations at work, school, or home.
6. Continuing to use the substance despite having persistent or recurrent social or interpersonal problems caused or worsened by the effects of its use.
7. Giving up or reducing important social, school, work, or recreational activities because of substance use.

Risky Use

8. Using the substance in situations in which it is physically hazardous to do so.
9. Continuing to use the substance despite the knowledge of having persistent or recurrent physical or psychological problems caused or worsened by substance use.

Drug Effects

10. Developing tolerance to the substance. (When a person requires increased amounts of a substance to achieve the desired effect or notices a markedly diminished effect with continued use of the same amount, he or she has developed tolerance to the substance.)
11. Experiencing withdrawal. (In someone who has maintained prolonged, heavy use of a substance, a drop in its concentration within the body can result in unpleasant physical and cognitive **withdrawal** symptoms. Withdrawal symptoms are different for different drugs. For example, nausea, vomiting, and tremors are common withdrawal symptoms in people dependent on alcohol, opioids, or sedatives.)

The concept of withdrawal goes hand-in-hand with **dependence**—that is, misusing a drug or repeating a behavior enough that you cannot easily stop it. Note that physical dependence, in a narrow sense, can be a normal bodily response to the use of a substance.

TERMS

tolerance Lowered sensitivity to a drug so that a given dose no longer exerts the usual effect and larger doses are needed.

substance misuse The use of any substance in a manner inconsistent with legal or medical guidelines; may be associated with adverse social, psychological, or medical consequences; the use may be intermittent and with or without physical dependence.

withdrawal Physical and psychological symptoms that follow the interrupted use of a drug on which a user is physically dependent; symptoms may be mild or life threatening.

dependence Frequent or consistent use of a drug or behavior that makes it difficult for the person to get along without it; the result of physiological and/or psychological adaptation that occurs in response to the substance or behavior; typically associated with tolerance and withdrawal but can also be based solely on behavioral factors such as compulsive use.

For example, regular coffee drinkers may experience caffeine withdrawal symptoms if they reduce their intake; however, that does not mean they have a substance use disorder.

How Does an Addiction Develop?

An addiction often starts when people do something to bring pleasure or avoid pain. The activity may be drinking a beer, using the internet, or going shopping. If it makes them feel the way they want, they are likely to repeat it. They increasingly depend on the behavior, and may develop a tolerance; that is, over time, they need more of the substance or behavior to achieve the same effect. Eventually, the behavior becomes a central focus of a person's life, and other areas deteriorate, such as school performance or relationships. The behavior no longer brings pleasure, but the person needs to keep doing it to avoid the pain of going without it.

It is sometimes difficult to distinguish between a healthy habit and one that has become an addiction. Some general characteristics typically associated with addictive behaviors are the following:

- *Reinforcement:* The behavior produces pleasurable physical or emotional states or relieves negative ones.

- *Compulsion or craving:* The addict feels a compelling need to engage in the behavior.

- *Loss of control:* The addict loses control over the behavior and cannot block the impulse to do it.

- *Escalation:* More and more of the substance or activity is required to produce its desired effects.

- *Negative consequences:* The behavior continues despite serious negative consequences, such as problems with academic or job performance, difficulties with personal relationships, or health problems.

Although many common behaviors are potentially addictive, most people who engage in them don't develop problems. Risk for addiction depends on a combination of factors, including personality, lifestyle, heredity, the social and physical environment, and the nature of the substance or behavior in question. For example, nicotine (the psychoactive drug in tobacco) has a very high potential for physical addiction, but a person must be willing to try smoking—whether influenced by peer pressure, family factors, advertising, stress, or personality traits—to become addicted. Some studies have found that genetic factors play a role in risk for addiction, and some people may have a genetic predisposition for addiction to a particular drug.

Examples of Addictive Behaviors

For some people, behaviors unrelated to drugs can become addictive. Such behaviors can include eating, gambling, and playing video games. Any substance or activity that becomes the focus of a person's life at the expense of other needs and interests can be damaging to health. Behavioral or nondrug addiction symptoms such as craving, loss of control over the behavior, tolerance, withdrawal, and a repeating pattern of recovery and relapse promote changes in the brain similar to those changes associated with misuse of and addiction to alcohol, nicotine, or other drugs.

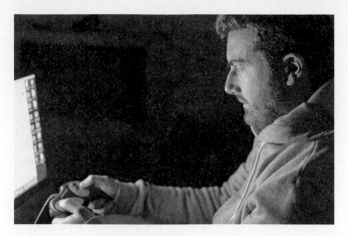

Wellness Tip Many common behaviors are potentially addictive, but most people who engage in them don't develop problems. If an activity starts becoming the focus of your life, harming relationships and academic or job performance, seek help. A counselor can help you develop healthier strategies for dealing with stress and difficult emotions.

Tommaso altamura/Alamy Stock Photo

Gambling Disorder Even in the face of personal ruin, compulsive gamblers find it difficult to resist the urge to gamble. About 1% of adult Americans are compulsive (pathological) gamblers. Some 75% of students report having gambled in the past year, and about 6% have a serious gambling problem that can result in psychological difficulties, unmanageable debt, and failing grades. The suicide rate among compulsive gamblers is 20 times higher than that of the general population.

Internet Gaming Characteristic behaviors include preoccupation with internet games, loss of interest in other activities, using gaming to relieve anxiety or guilt, and risking opportunities or relationships due to time spent gaming. The disorder is separate from gambling disorder and different from general use of social media or the internet.

Work Addiction People who are excessively preoccupied with work are often called workaholics. Work addiction, however, is based on a set of specific symptoms, including an intense work schedule; the inability to limit one's own work schedule; the inability to relax, even when away from work; and in some cases, failed attempts at curtailing the intensity of work. A person with a work addiction is likely to neglect other aspects of life. For example, she or he may exercise less, spend less time with family and friends, and avoid social activities. Work addiction typically coincides with a well-known risk factor for cardiovascular disease—personality traits of competitiveness, ambition, drive, time urgency, restlessness, hyper-alertness, and hostility.

Compulsive Buying A compulsive buyer repeatedly gives in to the impulse to buy more than he or she needs or can afford. Compulsive spenders usually buy luxury items rather than daily necessities. They are usually distressed by their behavior and its social, personal, and financial consequences. Some experts link compulsive shopping with neglect or abuse during childhood; it also seems to be associated with eating disorders, depression, and bipolar disorder.

Internet Addiction In the years since the internet became widely available, millions of Americans have become compulsive internet users—as many as 1 of 8 people. Among college students, approximately 1 of 7 fits this description. To spend more time online, internet addicts skip important school, social, or recreational activities. Compulsive internet users often spend their work time online, a fact that has led many employers to adopt strict internet usage policies. Despite negative financial, social, or academic consequences, people with this addiction don't feel able to stop.

Any substance or activity that becomes the focus of one's life at the expense of other needs can be damaging. For example, smartphones can be a source of addictive behavior. Researchers are studying cell-phone behavior in the population as a whole, as well as among its heaviest users—those under 20 years of age.

Compulsive Exercising When taken to a compulsive level, even healthy activity can turn into harmful addictions. For example, compulsive exercising is now recognized as a serious departure from normal behavior. Compulsive exercising is often accompanied by more severe psychiatric disorders such as anorexia nervosa and bulimia (see Chapter 9). Traits often associated with compulsive exercising include an excessive preoccupation and dissatisfaction with body image, use of laxatives or vomiting to lose weight, and development of other obsessive-compulsive symptoms. Other behaviors that can become addictive include eating, having sex, and watching TV.

> **? Ask Yourself**
>
> **QUESTIONS FOR CRITICAL THINKING AND REFLECTION?**
>
> Have you ever compulsively engaged in a behavior that had negative consequences? What was the behavior, and why did you continue? Were you able to bring the behavior under control? If so, how? If you feel addicted to your cell phone, what can you do about it?

PSYCHOACTIVE DRUGS

Psychoactive drugs include legal compounds such as caffeine, tobacco, alcohol, and prescription drugs, as well as illegal substances such as heroin, cocaine, and LSD. Figure 13.1 shows basic information about commonly misused drugs, which are classified according to their major effects; other drugs, especially synthetic street drugs, may not fit neatly into a single category.

Who Uses Drugs?

Drug use and abuse occur at all income and education levels, among all ethnic groups, and across all age groups. Casual or recreational use of illegal drugs is a concern because it is not possible to know when drug use will lead to abuse or addiction.

Some casual users develop substance-related problems; others do not. Some psychoactive drugs, however, are more likely than others to lead to a substance use disorder (Table 13.2).

Characteristics that place people at higher-than-average risk for trying illegal drugs or misusing prescription drugs include being male, young, a troubled adolescent, a thrill-seeker, in a dysfunctional family, in a peer group that accepts drug use, and poor; those who begin dating at a young age are also at higher risk. Drug use is less common among young people who attend school regularly, get good grades, have strong personal identities, are religious, have a good relationship with their parents, and are independent thinkers whose actions are not controlled by peer pressure. Coming from a family that has a clear policy on drug use and deals with conflicts constructively is also associated with not using drugs.

Why can some people use psychoactive drugs without becoming addicted, whereas others do? The use of drugs does not mean you have developed an addiction, nor does becoming physically dependent necessarily represent a disorder. But the boundary between normal behavior and a substance use disorder can be difficult to assess. Why some people develop addiction seems to be a combination of physical, psychological, and social factors. Some people may be born with a brain chemistry or metabolism that makes them more vulnerable to addiction. Psychological risk factors include having difficulty controlling impulses and having a strong need for excitement and immediate gratification. People may turn to drugs to numb emotional pain or to deal with difficult experiences or feelings such as rejection, hostility, or depression. Social factors that may increase the risk for substance use disorder include exposure to drug-using family members or peers, poverty, and easy access to drugs.

Opioids and Drug Overdose Deaths

The United States is in the midst of a drug overdose epidemic. Since 2000, the number of drug overdose deaths has nearly tripled, an increase driven in large part by rising rates of

Table 13.2	Psychoactive Drugs and Their Potential for Substance Use Disorder and Addiction
Very high	Heroin
High	Nicotine, morphine, opium
Moderate/high	Cocaine, methamphetamine, barbiturates
Moderate	Alcohol, Rohypnol and other benzodiazepines
Moderate/low	Caffeine, marijuana, MDMA, nitrous oxide
Low/very low	Ketamine, LSD, mescaline, psilocybin

SOURCES: Morgan, C. J. A., et al. 2013. "Harms and benefits associated with psychoactive drugs: Findings of an international survey of active drug users," *Journal of Psychopharmacology* 27(6), 497–506; Gable, R. S. 2006. *Acute Toxicity of Drugs versus Regulatory Status,* in J. M. Fish (ed.). Drugs and Society: U.S. Public Policy. Lanham, MD: Rowman & Littlefield, 149–162.

Category	Representative drugs	Street names	Appearance	Methods of use	Short-term effects
Opioids	Heroin	Dope, H, junk, brown sugar, smack	White/dark brown powder; dark tar or coal-like substance	Injected, smoked, snorted	Relief of anxiety and pain; euphoria; lethargy, apathy, drowsiness, confusion, inability to concentrate; nausea, constipation, respiratory depression
	Opium	Big O, black stuff, hop	Dark brown or black chunks	Swallowed, smoked	
	Morphine	M, Miss Emma, monkey, white stuff	White crystals, liquid solution	Injected, swallowed, smoked	
	Oxycodone, codeine, hydrocodone	Oxy, O.C., killer, Captain Cody, schoolboy, vike	Tablets, powder made from crushing tablets	Swallowed, injected, snorted	
Central nervous system depressants	Barbiturates	Barbs, reds, red birds, yellows, yellow jackets	Colored capsules	Swallowed, injected	Reduced anxiety, mood changes, lowered inhibitions, impaired muscle coordination, reduced pulse rate, drowsiness, loss of consciousness, respiratory depression
	Benzodiazepines (e.g., Valium, Xanax, Rohypnol)	Candy, downers, tranks, roofies, forget-me pill	Tablets	Swallowed, injected	
	Methaqualone	Ludes, quad, quay	Tablets	Injected, swallowed	
	Gamma hydroxy butyrate (GHB)	G, Georgia home boy, grievous bodily harm	Clear liquid, white powder	Swallowed	
Central nervous system stimulants	Amphetamine, methamphet-amine	Bennies, speed, black beauties, uppers, chalk, crank, crystal, ice, meth	Tablets, capsules, white powder, clear crystals	Injected, swallowed, smoked, snorted	Increased and irregular heart rate, blood pressure, metabolism; increased mental alertness and energy; nervousness, insomnia, impulsive behavior; reduced appetite
	Cocaine, crack cocaine	Blow, C, candy, coke, flake, rock, toot, snow	White powder, beige pellets or rocks	Injected, smoked, snorted	
	Ritalin	JIF, MPH, R-ball, Skippy	Tablets	Injected, swallowed, snorted	
	Synthetic cathinones ("bath salts")	Bliss, Blue Silk, Flakka, Ivory Wave, Meow Meow, Vanilla Sky, White Lightning	Fine white, off-white, or slightly yellow-colored powder or crystals; can be tablets or capsules	Swallowed, smoked, vaporized, sniffed, snorted, injected	Increased blood pressure, rapid heart rate, panic attacks in some people
Marijuana and other cannabis products	Marijuana	Dope, grass, joints, Mary Jane, reefer, skunk, weed, pot	Dried leaves and stems	Smoked, swallowed	Euphoria, slowed thinking and reaction time, confusion, anxiety, impaired balance and coordination, increased heart rate
	Hashish	Hash, hemp, boom, gangster	Dark, resin-like compound formed into rocks or blocks	Smoked, swallowed	
	K-2, Spice	Black Mamba, Bliss, Bombay Blue, Fake Weed, Genie, Spice, Zohai	Dried leaves	Smoked, teas	Increased blood pressure and heart rate, paranoia, panic attacks
Hallucinogens	LSD	Acid, boomers, blotter, yellow sunshines	Blotter paper, liquid, gelatin tabs, pills	Swallowed, absorbed through mouth tissues	Altered states of perception and feeling; nausea; increased heart rate, blood pressure; delirium; impaired motor function; numbness, weakness
	Mescaline (peyote)	Buttons, cactus, mesc	Brown buttons, liquid	Swallowed, smoked	
	Psilocybin	Shrooms, magic mushrooms	Dried mushrooms	Swallowed	
	Ketamine	K, special K, cat valium, vitamin K	Clear liquid, white or beige powder	Injected, snorted, smoked	
	PCP	Angel dust, hog, love boat, peace pill	White to brown powder, tablets	Injected, swallowed, smoked, snorted	
	MDMA (ecstasy)	X, peace, clarity, Adam, Molly	Tablets	Swallowed	
Inhalants	Solvents, aerosols, nitrites, anesthetics	Laughing gas, poppers, snappers, whippets	Household products, sprays, glues, paint thinner, petroleum products	Inhaled through nose or mouth	Stimulation, loss of inhibition, slurred speech, loss of motor coordination, loss of consciousness

Figure 13.1 **Commonly misused drugs and their effects.**

SOURCES: The Partnership for a Drug-Free America. 2016. *Drug Guide.* (http://www.drugfree.org/drug-guide); National Institute on Drug Abuse. *Commonly Abused Drugs Chart.* (https://www.drugabuse.gov/drugs-abuse/commonly-abused-drugs-charts) accessed July 2018.

misuse of prescription and illicit opioids. Prescription opioids such as morphine, codeine, and oxycodone treat moderate to severe pain. But they are often misused because in addition to controlling pain, they produce euphoria. If taken in large doses or combined with other drugs, opioids can cause respiratory depression (slow and shallow breathing), coma, and death.

What's driving the epidemic? The amount of opioids prescribed is six times the amount in 1999. By 2013, enough opioids were prescribed for every American adult to have a bottle of pills. Greater exposure led to an increase in the number of people addicted to opioids and to more drug overdose deaths. Changes made in response to the epidemic, including greater controls on prescription practices, appear to have prompted people with opioid addiction to switch to heroin and synthetic opioids such as fentanyl. (Fentanyl is a prescription opioid similar to morphine but up to 100 times more powerful; illegally made fentanyl may be mixed with heroin.) Sold on the street, heroin and fentanyl are often less expensive and more easily obtained than prescription opioids, but they are even more dangerous. Heroin and fentanyl are responsible for much of the recent spike in overdose deaths (Figure 13.2).

Opioid use has also affected the college-age population. In one survey of eight colleges conducted by Ohio State University, 1 in 10 undergraduates had used prescription painkillers for nonmedical reasons. Additionally, 68% of those who responded said they had intentionally misused these drugs on more than one occasion, and 13% reported doing so at least 40 times.

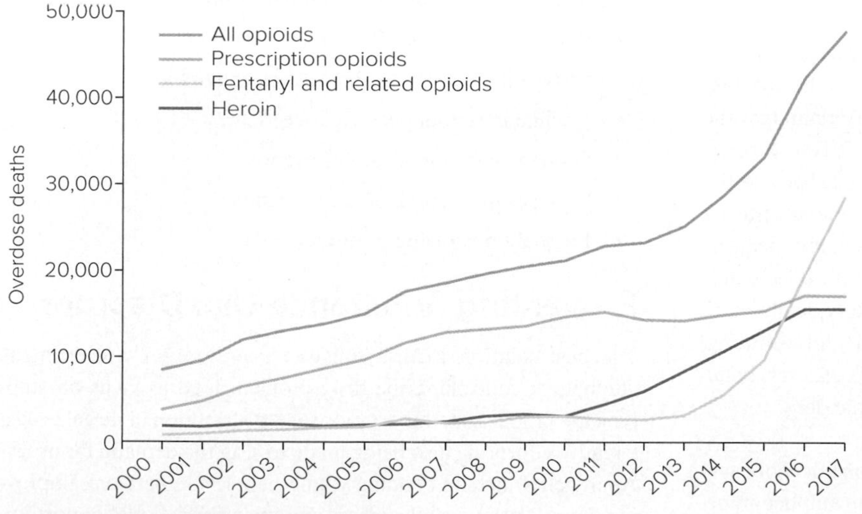

Strategies for preventing opioid overdose deaths include the following:

- Improve opioid-prescribing practices to reduce exposure to the drugs.
- Expand access to naloxone, a drug used to safely reverse opioid overdose.
- Provide access to treatment for people with opioid addiction.
- Expand substance misuse prevention programs.
- Increase research into non-opioid treatment strategies for chronic pain.

Kratom, a plant in the coffee family, has both stimulant properties (e.g., khat) and opioid-like properties. It has been used to aid in opioid withdrawal and to act as a substitute in opioid addiction. In February 2018, the Food and Drug Administration (FDA) echoed the declaration of the Drug Enforcement Administration (DEA) five years earlier that there are no known medical uses of kratom, and little is known about its safety.

Other Current Illicit Drugs of Concern

With almost 24 million users in 2016, marijuana is the most widely used federally illegal drug in the United States. As of 2019, marijuana use is illegal under federal law, but 33 states and the District of Columbia have legalized medical marijuana, and 10 plus DC have regulated recreational use. Despite the new laws, marijuana use among high schoolers is the lowest in two decades. At the same time, however, marijuana use among college students in 2016 was found to be at its highest rate since the mid-1980s.

THC (tetrahydrocannabinol) is the main active ingredient in marijuana; the concentration of THC in marijuana can vary from 1% up to 8%. The short-term effects of marijuana are described in Figure 13.1. Of particular note is the potential impact of THC on the parts of the brain controlling balance, coordination, and reaction time. Marijuana use impairs driving performance and is even more dangerous when combined with alcohol.

Other illicit drugs tend to vary in popularity over time based on social, economic, and legal factors. The makeup of drugs also changes as their chemical structures are altered to avoid regulation and reduce the cost of manufacturing. Substitute drugs are often sold in place of street drugs, putting users at risk for taking dangerous combinations of unknown substances. Some current drugs of concern are described briefly in this section.

VITAL STATISTICS

Figure 13.2 U.S. opioid overdose deaths, 2000–2017. Overdose deaths from opioids increased significantly since 2000. As deaths from prescription opioids began to level off in the early 2010s, overdoses from first heroin and then fentanyl increased dramatically, with fentanyl-related deaths increasing more than 10-fold between 2012 and 2017. In 2017, opioids were responsible for two-thirds of all drug overdose deaths.

SOURCE: Centers for Disease Control and Prevention, National Center for Health Statistics. 2018. *Multiple cause of death 1999–2017*. CDC WONDER Online Database (https://wonder.cdc.gov/mcd.html).

Prescription Stimulant Misuse According to the most recent National College Health Assessment survey, under 5% of college students reported using a prescription stimulant in the past year that was not prescribed to them. This category of drugs includes stimulants for treating attention-deficit/hyperactivity disorder (ADHD), such as Adderall, Concerta, and Ritalin. Most college students who misuse Adderall or other stimulants get the drug from a friend or classmate who received a prescription for the drug for treatment of ADHD. Misuse of stimulant drugs occurs more frequently among full-time college students than part-time students or nonstudents.

MDMA (Ecstasy) Taken in pill form, MDMA (methylene-dioxymethamphetamine), or Ecstasy, is a stimulant with mildly hallucinogenic and amphetamine-like effects. Tolerance to MDMA develops quickly, leading users to take the drug more frequently, use higher doses, or combine MDMA with other drugs to enhance the drug's effects. High doses can cause anxiety, delusions, and paranoia. It can produce dangerously high body temperature and potentially fatal dehydration; several cases have been reported of low total body salt concentrations (hyponatremia). Some users experience confusion, depression, anxiety, paranoia, muscle tension, involuntary teeth clenching, blurred vision, and seizures. Even low doses can affect a person's concentration and driving ability. Use during pregnancy is linked to increased risk of birth defects. Chronic use of MDMA may produce long-lasting, perhaps permanent, damage to the neurons that release serotonin. This may explain why heavy use is associated with persistent problems with learning and verbal and visual memory. MDMA users perform worse than nonusers on complex cognitive tasks of memory, attention, and general intelligence.

LSD A potent hallucinogen, LSD (lysergic acid diethylamide) is sold in tablets or capsules, in liquid form, or on small squares of paper called blotters. LSD increases heart rate and body temperature and may cause hallucinations, mood changes, nausea, tremors, sweating, numbness, and weakness.

Synthetic Marijuana "Spice," "K2," and "Genie" are just a few names given to synthetic cannabinoids, which typically consist of dried, shredded plant materials with chemical additives that produce psychoactive effects. Packaging labels may claim that the product is safe and natural, but current research fails to support the claim. The effects of these drugs are unpredictable because the chemicals being used change, and there are no manufacturing standards or regulations. Depending on the type and concentration of chemical additive(s) in a product, short-term effects may be similar to those from using marijuana, but are typically more potent. They include anxiety, agitation, nausea and vomiting, rapid heart rate, elevated blood pressure, tremors, seizures, hallucinations, cognitive impairment, psychosis, and suicide.

Bath Salts Drugs called "bath salts" contain one or more synthetic cathinones, which are chemicals related to an amphetamine-like stimulant found in the khat plant. Bath salts are inhaled, injected, or taken orally; they may have both stimulant and hallucinatory effects. Use of the drugs has been linked to an increase in emergency room visits, with people experiencing dangerous cardiovascular symptoms (high heart rate and blood pressure, chest pains) as well as psychiatric symptoms such as panic attacks and extreme paranoia and agitation. Frequent use may lead to tolerance, dependence, and strong withdrawal symptoms.

Club Drugs (GHB, Rohypnol, Ketamine) Club drugs are a diverse group of drugs that tend to be misused by young adults in club and party settings. GHB, Rohypnol, and ketamine have sedative effects and can be dangerous when taken alone and fatal if combined with alcohol. GHB and Rohypnol can cause anterograde amnesia, meaning users cannot remember events they experienced while under the influence of the drug. Because of their effects, these drugs have been used to commit drug-assisted sexual assaults and are sometimes referred to as "date rape drugs." Congress in 1996 passed the Drug-Induced Rape Prevention and Punishment Act, which increased penalties for use of any controlled substance to aid in sexual assault. (Alcohol, described in the next section of the chapter, is the drug most commonly used to facilitate sexual assault.)

Treatment for Substance Use Disorder and Addiction

Various types of programs are available to help people break their drug habits, but there is no single best method of treatment. The relapse rate is high for all types of treatment, but receiving treatment is better than not. Professional treatment programs usually take the form of drug substitution programs or treatment centers. Nonprofessional self-help groups and peer counseling are also available. To be successful, a treatment program must deal with the reasons behind users' drug abuse and help them develop behaviors, attitudes, and a social support system that will help them remain drug free. For resources related to treatment, see "For Further Exploration" at the end of the chapter.

Young people with drug problems are often unable to seek help on their own. In such cases, friends and family members may need to act on their behalf. One or more of the following signals may suggest serious drug misuse:

- Sudden withdrawal or emotional distance
- Rebellious or unusually irritable behavior
- Loss of interest in usual activities or hobbies
- Decline in school performance
- Sudden change in group of friends
- Changes in sleeping or eating habits
- Frequent borrowing of money

Preventing Substance Use Disorder

The best solution to drug misuse is prevention. Government attempts at controlling the drug problem tend to focus on stopping the production, importation, and distribution of illegal drugs. Creative efforts are also being made to stop the demand for drugs. Approaches include building young people's self-esteem, improving their academic skills, increasing their recreational opportunities, providing them with honest information about the effects of drugs, and teaching them strategies for resisting peer pressure.

The Role of Drugs in Your Life

Whatever your experience has been up to now, it is likely that you will encounter drugs at some point in your life. Contemplate the following questions; your answers may help you establish the inner resources needed to resist peer pressure and make your own decisions.

- *What are the risks involved?* Many drugs carry an immediate risk of injury or death or legal consequences. Most carry long-term risks of abuse and dependence.

- *Is using the drug compatible with your goals?* Consider how drug use will affect your education and career objectives, your relationships, your future happiness, and the happiness of those who love you.

- *What are your ethical beliefs about drug use?* Consider whether using a drug conflicts with your personal ethics, religious beliefs, social values, or family responsibilities.

- *What are the financial costs?* Many drugs are expensive, especially if you become dependent on them.

- *Are you trying to solve a deeper problem?* Drugs will not make emotional pain go away. In the long run, they make it worse. If you are feeling depressed or anxious, seek help from a mental health professional instead of self-medicating with drugs.

ALCOHOL

You have probably noticed that alcohol affects people in different ways. One person seems to get drunk after one or two drinks, while another is able to tolerate a great deal of alcohol without apparent effect. These differences help explain the many misconceptions about alcohol use. In the following sections we describe how alcohol works in the body, as well as the short- and long-term effects of alcohol use and misuse.

Chemistry and Metabolism

Ethyl alcohol is the psychoactive ingredient in all alcoholic beverages. The concentration of alcohol varies with the type of beverage; it is indicated by the **proof value**, which is two times the percentage concentration. For example, if a beverage is 80 proof,

it contains 40% alcohol. When we discuss alcohol consumption, **one drink** (a *standard drink*) refers to a 12-ounce bottle of beer, a 5-ounce glass of wine, or a cocktail with 1.5 ounces of 80-proof liquor. Each of these drinks contains approximately 0.6 ounce of alcohol (Figure 13.3).

When consumed, alcohol is absorbed into the bloodstream from the stomach and small intestine. Once in the bloodstream, alcohol is distributed throughout the body's tissues, affecting nearly every body system (Figure 13.4). The main site of alcohol metabolism is the liver, which transforms alcohol into energy and other products.

Immediate Effects of Alcohol

Blood alcohol concentration (BAC)—the amount of alcohol in a person's blood—is a primary factor determining the effects of alcohol. BAC is determined by the amount of alcohol consumed and by individual factors such as heredity, body weight, and amount of body fat. A woman drinking the same amount of alcohol as a man will typically have a higher BAC because of her smaller size, greater percentage of body fat, and less-active alcohol-metabolizing stomach enzymes.

Typically, the body can metabolize about half a drink in an hour. If a person drinks slightly less than that each hour, BAC remains low. People can drink large amounts of alcohol this way

TERMS

ethyl alcohol The intoxicating ingredient in fermented liquors; a colorless, pungent liquid.

proof value Two times the percentage of alcohol in a beverage, measured by volume; a 100-proof beverage contains 50% alcohol.

one drink The amount of a beverage that typically contains about 0.6 ounce of alcohol; also called a standard drink.

blood alcohol concentration (BAC) The amount of alcohol in the blood in terms of weight per unit volume; used as a measure of intoxication.

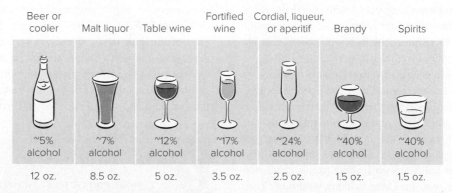

Beer or cooler	Malt liquor	Table wine	Fortified wine	Cordial, liqueur, or aperitif	Brandy	Spirits
~5% alcohol	~7% alcohol	~12% alcohol	~17% alcohol	~24% alcohol	~40% alcohol	~40% alcohol
12 oz.	8.5 oz.	5 oz.	3.5 oz.	2.5 oz.	1.5 oz.	1.5 oz.

Figure 13.3 One standard drink contains about 0.6 ounce of alcohol. To determine the drink size of other beverages, use the National Institutes of Health drink size calculator (http://rethinkingdrinking.niaaa.nih.gov/Tools/Calculators/drink-size-calculator.aspx) or do your own calculation by dividing 0.6 by the percentage alcohol volume of the beverage, expressed as a decimal. For example, to calculate the size of a standard drink of beer labeled as having 5% alcohol content: 0.6 oz of alcohol = amount of alcohol in a standard drink If beer = 5% alcohol, the amount of beer that contains 0.6 oz alcohol is 0.6 / 0.05 = 12 oz beer = 1 standard drink of alcohol

SOURCE: National Institute on Alcohol Abuse and Alcoholism. 2016. *Rethinking Drinking: Alcohol and Your Health*, NIH Publication No. 15-3770. Rockville, MD: National Institute on Alcohol Abuse and Alcoholism.

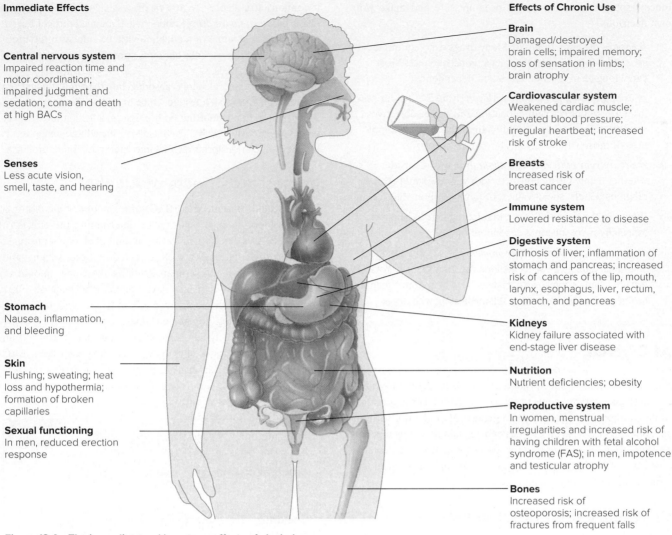

Immediate Effects

Central nervous system
Impaired reaction time and
motor coordination;
impaired judgment and
sedation; coma and death
at high BACs

Senses
Less acute vision,
smell, taste, and hearing

Stomach
Nausea, inflammation,
and bleeding

Skin
Flushing; sweating; heat
loss and hypothermia;
formation of broken
capillaries

Sexual functioning
In men, reduced erection
response

Effects of Chronic Use

Brain
Damaged/destroyed
brain cells; impaired memory;
loss of sensation in limbs;
brain atrophy

Cardiovascular system
Weakened cardiac muscle;
elevated blood pressure;
irregular heartbeat; increased
risk of stroke

Breasts
Increased risk of
breast cancer

Immune system
Lowered resistance to disease

Digestive system
Cirrhosis of liver; inflammation of
stomach and pancreas; increased
risk of cancers of the lip, mouth,
larynx, esophagus, liver, rectum,
stomach, and pancreas

Kidneys
Kidney failure associated with
end-stage liver disease

Nutrition
Nutrient deficiencies; obesity

Reproductive system
In women, menstrual
irregularities and increased risk of
having children with fetal alcohol
syndrome (FAS); in men, impotence
and testicular atrophy

Bones
Increased risk of
osteoporosis; increased risk of
fractures from frequent falls

Figure 13.4   The immediate and long-term effects of alcohol use.

over a long period of time (for example, two drinks over a four-hour period) without becoming noticeably intoxicated; however, they still run the risk of significant long-term health problems. But if people consume more alcohol than they can metabolize (for example, two drinks within 30 minutes), the BAC will increase steadily, and they will likely be noticeably drunk (Figure 13.5).

Drinking makes some people so uncomfortable that they are unlikely to develop an alcohol use disorder. Some people, primarily those of Asian descent, inherit ineffective or inactive variations of alcohol dehydrogenase, the enzyme that breaks down alcohol. Other people, including some of African and Jewish descent, have forms of this enzyme that metabolize alcohol very quickly. Either way, toxic acetaldehyde builds up when these people drink alcohol. They experience a reaction called flushing syndrome. Their skin feels hot; their heart and respiration rates increase; and they may get a headache, vomit, or break out in hives.

The combination of impaired judgment, weakened sensory perception, reduced inhibitions, impaired motor coordination, and often increased aggressiveness and hostility that comes with alcohol intoxication can be dangerous or even deadly. Alcohol

use contributes to over 40% of all murders, assaults, and rapes. Alcohol is frequently found in the bloodstreams of victims as well as perpetrators. Eighty percent of arrests happen for alcohol- and drug-related offenses (domestic violence, driving under the influence of alcohol, public drunkenness, and property offenses). Alcohol use is also a significant risk factor for suicide and for alcohol poisoning: Drinking large amounts of alcohol over a short time can rapidly raise the BAC into the lethal range (see the box "Dealing with an Alcohol Emergency").

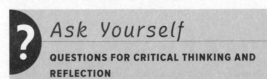

? Ask Yourself

QUESTIONS FOR CRITICAL THINKING AND REFLECTION

Have you ever decided to drive after having too much to drink? Who was with you, and what were the circumstances? What was your experience like? What would you tell someone else who was planning to drive despite having too much to drink?

Being very drunk is potentially life-threatening. Helping a drunken friend could save a life.

- Be firm but calm. Don't engage the person in an argument or discuss her drinking behavior while she is intoxicated.

- Get the person out of harm's way. Don't let him drive or wander outside. Don't let him drink any more alcohol.

- If the person is unconscious, don't assume she is just "sleeping it off." Place her on her side with her knees up. This position helps prevent choking if she vomits.

- Stay with the person; you need to be ready to help if he vomits or stops breathing.

- Don't try to give the person anything to eat or drink, including coffee or other drugs. Don't give cold showers or try to make her walk around. None of these things help to sober up someone, and they can be dangerous.

Call 9-1-1 immediately in any of the following instances:

- You can't wake up the person even by shouting or shaking.

- The person is taking fewer than eight breaths per minute, or his breathing seems shallow or irregular.

- You think the person took other drugs in addition to alcohol.

- The person has had an injury, especially a blow to the head.

- The person drank a large amount of alcohol within a short time and then became unconscious. Death from alcohol poisoning most often occurs when the blood alcohol level rises very quickly due to rapid ingestion of alcohol.

If you aren't sure what to do, call 9-1-1. You may save a life.

Alcohol Use Disorder: From Mild to Severe

Alcohol misuse is recurrent alcohol use that has potentially negative consequences, such as drinking in dangerous situations (for example, before driving), or drinking patterns that result in academic, professional, interpersonal, or legal difficulties. **Alcohol use disorder** involves more extensive problems such as physical tolerance and withdrawal. The important point is that one does not have to have a severe alcohol use disorder to have problems with alcohol. The person who drinks only once a month, perhaps after an exam, but then drives while intoxicated is a dangerous alcohol user. (Lab 13.1 includes an assessment to help you determine if alcohol is a problem in your life.)

Warning signs of problem alcohol use include drinking alone or secretively, using alcohol to deal with negative feelings or

> **TERMS**
>
> **alcohol misuse**   The use of alcohol to a degree that causes physical damage, impairs functioning, or results in harm to others.
>
> **alcohol use disorder**   A chronic psychological disorder characterized by excessive and compulsive drinking, and measured as mild, moderate, or severe.

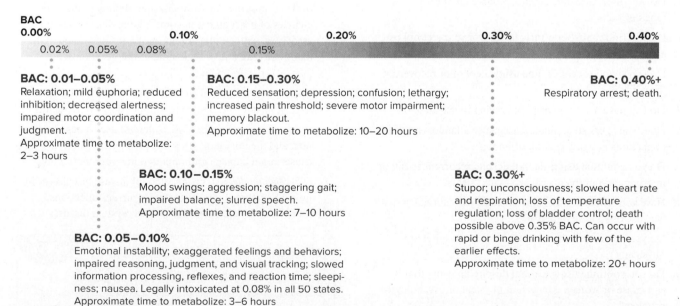

Figure 13.5   Effects of alcohol at different blood alcohol concentrations (BAC). The approximate number of hours required to metabolize the amount of alcohol consumed is also given for each stage of intoxication.

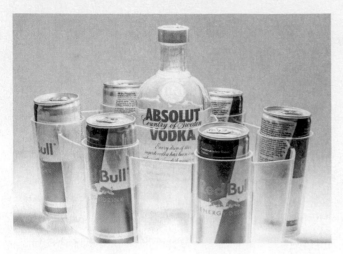

Wellness Tip Don't mix alcohol and energy drinks. College students who combine them are more likely to engage in risky behaviors than those who consume alcohol alone. Research has found that those who combine alcohol with energy drinks are more likely to drive drunk (despite knowing they have had too much alcohol to drive safely) and are more likely to knowingly ride with an intoxicated driver.

Dejan Krsmanovic/Alamy Stock Photo

difficult situations, feeling uncomfortable if alcohol is not available, and escalating alcohol consumption. How can you tell if you or someone you know has an alcohol use disorder? As described earlier in the chapter, the *DSM-5* provides specific criteria for identifying and classifying the severity of an alcohol use disorder. If a person meets two of the following criteria, she or he has an alcohol use disorder; two to three symptoms indicate a mild disorder; four to five, a moderate disorder; and six or more, a severe disorder. To determine a person's place on the disorder spectrum, ask these questions:

1. Do you often consume alcohol in large amounts over a long period?

2. Do you find that your efforts to control your alcohol use are unsuccessful?

3. Do you spend excessive time using alcohol or recovering from its effects?

4. Do you have a strong desire or craving to use alcohol?

5. Does your persistent alcohol use cause a failure to fulfill obligations at work, school, or home?

6. Do you continue using alcohol despite recurrent social or interpersonal problems caused by its effects?

7. Have you reduced important social or recreational activities because of your alcohol use?

8. Do you persist in using alcohol in situations that are physically risky?

9. Do you continue using alcohol despite knowing that it can cause or worsen a recurrent physical or psychological problem?

10. Do you have a need for increased amounts of alcohol to achieve a desired effect (increased tolerance)?

11. Do you experience symptoms of withdrawal, such as an unusual amount of any of the following: sweating, increased pulse rate, hand tremors, insomnia, nausea, and anxiety?

Severe alcohol use disorder, also sometimes referred to as *alcoholism,* is usually characterized by tolerance and withdrawal. Everyone who drinks—even nonalcoholics—develops tolerance to alcohol after repeated use. When alcoholics stop drinking or cut their intake significantly, they have withdrawal symptoms, which can range from unpleasant to serious and even life-threatening distress. Symptoms of alcohol withdrawal include trembling hands (shakes, or jitters), a rapid pulse and breathing rate, insomnia, nightmares, anxiety, and gastrointestinal upset. Less common are seizures and the severe reaction known as the **DTs (delirium tremens)**, characterized by confusion and vivid, usually unpleasant, hallucinations.

Some alcoholics recover without professional help, but the majority do not. Treatment is difficult. However, many kinds of programs exist, including those that emphasize group and friend support, those that stress lifestyle management, and those that use drugs and chemical substitutes as therapy. Although treatment is not successful for all alcoholics, many achieve permanent abstinence.

Effects of Alcohol Use Disorder

On average, people with an alcohol use disorder have a life span that is 15 years shorter than people without one. Potential health effects of chronic alcohol use include the following:

- *Cirrhosis:* In **cirrhosis**, liver cells are destroyed and replaced with fibrous scar tissue; cirrhosis is a major cause of death in the United States.

- *Digestive problems:* Alcohol can inflame the pancreas, causing nausea, vomiting, abnormal digestion, and severe abdominal pain.

- *Cardiovascular problems:* Although moderate doses of alcohol (one drink or less per day for women, and one to two drinks per day for men) may slightly reduce the chances of heart attack in some people, high doses are associated with cardiovascular problems, including high blood pressure and a weakening of the heart muscle.

- *Cancer:* Alcohol is a known human carcinogen and is causally related to oral cancer; cancers of the esophagus, liver, stomach, and pancreas; and possibly breast cancer.

- *Psychiatric problems:* Excessive alcohol use can cause paranoia and memory gaps. In some people, chronic drinking causes brain damage and impaired mental functioning.

- *Other health effects:* Chronic alcohol misuse has also been linked to asthma, gout, diabetes, recurrent infections, nutritional deficiencies, and nervous system diseases.

TERMS

DTs (delirium tremens)   A state of confusion brought on by the reduction of alcohol intake in an alcohol-addicted person; other symptoms are sweating, trembling, anxiety, hallucinations, and seizures.

cirrhosis   A disease in which the liver is severely damaged by alcohol, other toxins, or infection.

Maternal drinking during pregnancy can result in miscarriage, stillbirth, or **fetal alcohol syndrome (FAS)**. Children with this syndrome are small at birth, are likely to have heart defects, and often have abnormal features such as small, wide-set eyes. Many are mentally impaired; others exhibit more subtle problems with learning and fine motor coordination. FAS is the most common preventable cause of developmental disabilities in the Western world, occurring in 2 to 9 infants for every 10,000 live births in the United States. Many more babies are born with alcohol-related neurodevelopmental disorder (ARND). These children appear physically normal but often have learning and behavioral problems and are more likely as adults to develop substance abuse and legal problems. Excessive drinking just one time during the final three months of pregnancy, when the fetus's brain cells are developing rapidly, can cause fetal brain damage. The safest course of action is to abstain from alcohol during pregnancy.

Drinking and Driving

People who drink are unable to drive safely because their judgment is impaired, their reaction time is slower, and their coordination is reduced. While deaths from drunk driving have fallen in recent decades, the National Highway Transportation Safety Administration (NHTSA) reports that someone is killed in an alcohol-related crash every 48 minutes. Based on current rates, the chance of being involved in an alcohol-impaired crash at some point in your life is 1 in 3—as a driver, a passenger, a pedestrian, or an occupant of another vehicle. Drivers between the ages of 16 and 24 make up 40% of drivers involved in alcohol-related crashes; adults ages 25–34 make up another 33%, with much higher rates among men.

In addition to increasing the risk of injury and death, driving while intoxicated can have serious legal consequences. Offenders face stiff penalties for drunk driving, including fines, loss of license, confiscation of vehicle, and jail time. The legal limit for BAC in Utah is 0.05%. In all other states, the District of Columbia, and Puerto Rico the limit is 0.08%; however, alcohol impairs the user even at much lower BACs (Figure 13.6). Many states now have zero-tolerance laws regarding alcohol use by drivers under age 21. Under these laws, young drivers who have consumed any alcohol can have their licenses suspended.

Binge Drinking

The National Institute on Alcohol Abuse and Alcoholism (NIAAA) defines **binge drinking** as a pattern of rapid, periodic alcohol use that brings a person's BAC up to 0.08% or above (typically five drinks for men or four drinks for women), consumed within about two hours. Binge drinking is most common among people aged 18–24 years, and most people under age 21 report binge drinking when they drink at all. One in six adults reports binge drinking about four times a month.

In 2017, 36.9% of Americans aged 18–25 reported that they engaged in binge drinking in the past month; 9.6% reported that they engaged in heavy drinking in the past month. Binge drinking has a profound effect on students' lives. Every year, more than 1,800 college students ages 18–24 die from alcohol-related injuries. Another 600,000 sustain unintentional alcohol-related injuries, 700,000 are assaulted by other students who have been drinking, and close to 100,000 are victims of alcohol-related date rape or sexual assault. Binge drinkers have also been found more likely to miss classes, fall behind in schoolwork, and argue with friends. The more frequent the binges, the more problems the students encountered. Despite their experiences, fewer than 1% of the binge drinkers identify themselves as problem drinkers.

Drinking and Responsibility

The responsible use of alcohol means drinking in a way that keeps your BAC low and your behavior under control. See the box "Drinking Behavior and Responsibility" for specific suggestions.

> **fetal alcohol syndrome (FAS)** A characteristic **TERMS** group of birth defects caused by alcohol consumption by the mother, including facial deformities, heart defects, and physical and mental impairments.
>
> **binge drinking** Periodically drinking alcohol to the point of severe intoxication.

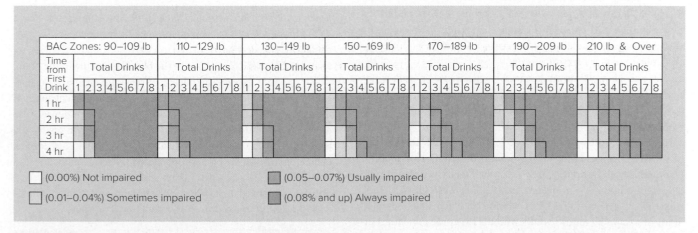

BAC Zones: 90–109 lb								110–129 lb								130–149 lb								150–169 lb								170–189 lb								190–209 lb								210 lb & Over							
Time from First Drink	Total Drinks								Total Drinks								Total Drinks								Total Drinks								Total Drinks								Total Drinks								Total Drinks							
	1	2	3	4	5	6	7	8	1	2	3	4	5	6	7	8	1	2	3	4	5	6	7	8	1	2	3	4	5	6	7	8	1	2	3	4	5	6	7	8	1	2	3	4	5	6	7	8	1	2	3	4	5	6	7	8
1 hr																																																								
2 hr																																																								
3 hr																																																								
4 hr																																																								

☐ (0.00%) Not impaired   ▨ (0.05–0.07%) Usually impaired
☐ (0.01–0.04%) Sometimes impaired   ▨ (0.08% and up) Always impaired

Figure 13.6 Approximate blood alcohol concentration and body weight. This chart shows the BAC an average person of a given weight would reach after drinking the specified number of drinks in the time shown. The legal limit for BAC is 0.08%. For drivers under 21 years of age, many states have zero-tolerance laws that set BAC limits of 0.01% or 0.02%.

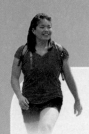
TOBACCO

According to the U.S. Surgeon General, smoking is the leading preventable cause of illness and death in the United States. Each year, nearly 500,000 Americans die prematurely from smoking-related causes; tobacco use is related to nearly 1 of every 5 adult deaths. Millions of Americans suffer chronic illnesses (such as cancer and heart disease) as a result of smoking. Tobacco use in any form—cigarettes, e-cigarettes, cigars, pipes, chewing tobacco, clove cigarettes, or snuff—is unsafe.

Despite its well-known hazards, tobacco use is still widespread in our society. More than 1 in 4 adults uses at least one form of tobacco, and about 40% of people who use tobacco use more than one product; the most common combination is standard cigarettes plus e-cigarettes. Overall, cigarettes remain the most commonly used tobacco product. According to the CDC National Health Interview Survey, 14% of Americans ages 18 and older (34 million) were cigarette smokers in 2017 (Table 13.3). About 16% of men and 12% of women reported that they currently smoked cigarettes. Adults with a 12th-grade education or less were much more likely to smoke cigarettes than were those with a college degree. Other groups with higher-than-average smoking rates include those living below the poverty level, those without health insurance, and those who have a physical disability or serious psychological disorder. The number of people in the United States who smoke (every day or some days) has decreased overall, however, by about 16% recently and 67% since 1965. The largest decrease has been in adults ages 18–24.

Nicotine Addiction

Regular tobacco use—especially cigarette smoking—is not just a habit but an addiction, involving physical dependence on the psychoactive drug **nicotine**. Addicted tobacco users must keep a steady amount of nicotine circulating in the blood and going to the brain, where the drug triggers the release of powerful chemical messengers and causes a wide range of physical and emotional changes. If nicotine intake falls below a certain level, they experience withdrawal symptoms that can include cravings, insomnia, confusion, tremors, difficulty concentrating, fatigue, muscle pains, headache, nausea, irritability, anger, and depression. Nicotine addiction can start within a few days of smoking and after just a few cigarettes. You can get hooked on nicotine much faster than you might think—a good reason to avoid trying tobacco in the first place.

> **nicotine** A poisonous, addictive substance found in tobacco and responsible for many of the effects of tobacco. **TERMS**

VITAL STATISTICS

Table 13.3 — Who is Using Tobacco?

	PERCENTAGE OF SMOKERS		
	ANY TOBACCO PRODUCT	CIGARETTES	E-CIGARETTES
Race/Ethnicity			
Non-Hispanic white	21.4	15.2	3.3
Non-Hispanic black	20.4	14.9	2.2
Non-Hispanic Asian	8.9	7.1	0.9
Non-Hispanic American Indian/ Alaskan Native	29.8	24.0	–
Hispanic	12.7	9.9	1.8
Non-Hispanic multirace	27.4	20.6	5.6
Education			
0–12 years (no diploma)	26.1	23.1	2.1
GED	42.6	36.8	7.2
High school diploma	24.3	18.7	3.1
Associate degree	20.4	15.5	2.7
Undergraduate degree	12.5	7.1	1.7
Graduate degree	8.3	4.1	0.9

SOURCE: Wang, T. W., et al. 2018. "Tobacco product use among adults—United States, 2017," *Morbidity and Mortality Weekly Report 67*, no. 44: 1225–1232.

Health Hazards of Cigarette Smoking

Cigarette smoking has negative effects on nearly every part of the body and increases the risk of many life-threatening diseases. At least 69 chemicals in tobacco smoke are linked to cancer. Some, such as benzo(a)pyrene and urethane, are carcinogens—that is, they directly cause cancer. Other chemicals, such as formaldehyde, are cocarcinogens; they do not themselves cause cancer but combine with other chemicals to stimulate the growth of certain cancers, at least in laboratory animals. Other substances in tobacco cause health problems because they damage the lining of the respiratory tract or decrease the lungs' ability to fight off infection.

Carbon monoxide, the deadly gas in automobile exhaust, is present in cigarette smoke in concentrations 400 times greater than the safety threshold set in workplaces. Low-tar and low-nicotine cigarettes deliver just as dangerous a dose of these chemicals as regular cigarettes because smokers inhale more deeply and frequently.

The effects of nicotine on smokers vary, depending on the size of the dose and the smoker's past smoking behavior. Nicotine can either excite or tranquilize the nervous system, generally resulting in stimulation that gives way to tranquility and then depression. Figure 13.7 summarizes the immediate effects and long-term health risks of smoking.

In the short term, smoking interferes with the functions of the respiratory system and often leads rapidly to shortness of breath and the conditions known as smoker's throat, smoker's

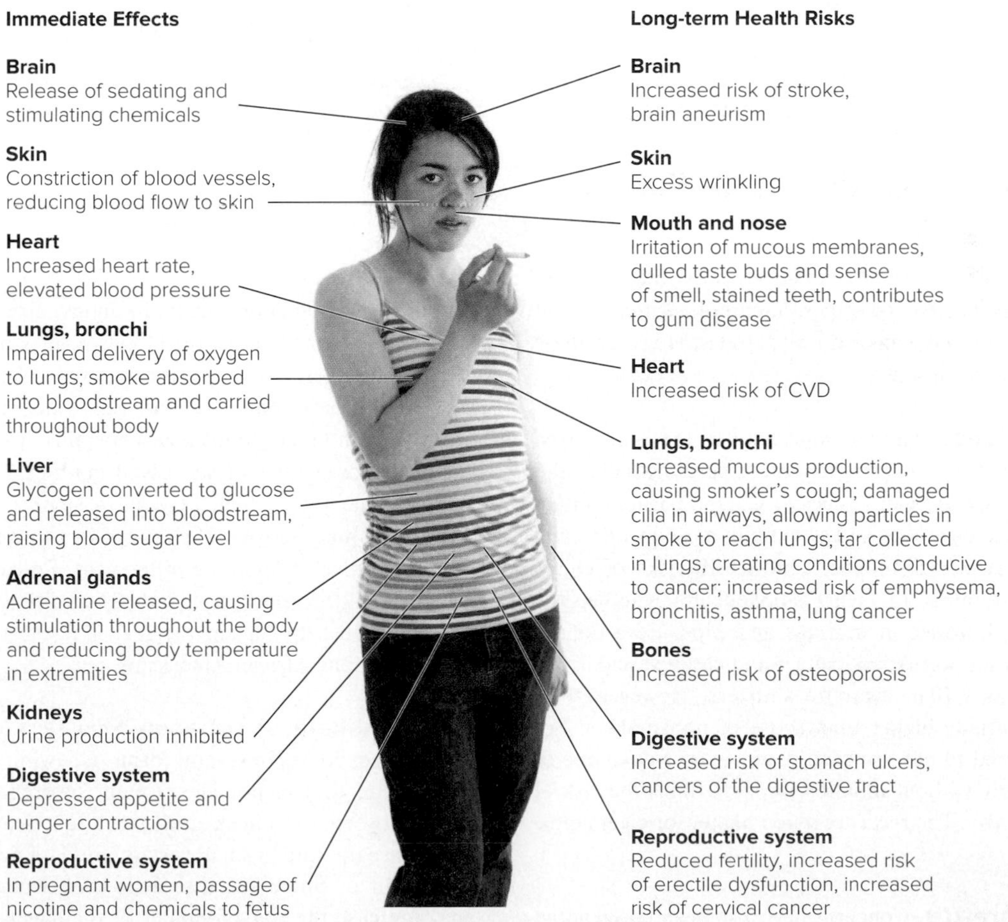

Immediate Effects

Brain
Release of sedating and stimulating chemicals

Skin
Constriction of blood vessels, reducing blood flow to skin

Heart
Increased heart rate, elevated blood pressure

Lungs, bronchi
Impaired delivery of oxygen to lungs; smoke absorbed into bloodstream and carried throughout body

Liver
Glycogen converted to glucose and released into bloodstream, raising blood sugar level

Adrenal glands
Adrenaline released, causing stimulation throughout the body and reducing body temperature in extremities

Kidneys
Urine production inhibited

Digestive system
Depressed appetite and hunger contractions

Reproductive system
In pregnant women, passage of nicotine and chemicals to fetus

Long-term Health Risks

Brain
Increased risk of stroke, brain aneurism

Skin
Excess wrinkling

Mouth and nose
Irritation of mucous membranes, dulled taste buds and sense of smell, stained teeth, contributes to gum disease

Heart
Increased risk of CVD

Lungs, bronchi
Increased mucous production, causing smoker's cough; damaged cilia in airways, allowing particles in smoke to reach lungs; tar collected in lungs, creating conditions conducive to cancer; increased risk of emphysema, bronchitis, asthma, lung cancer

Bones
Increased risk of osteoporosis

Digestive system
Increased risk of stomach ulcers, cancers of the digestive tract

Reproductive system
Reduced fertility, increased risk of erectile dysfunction, increased risk of cervical cancer

Figure 13.7   Tobacco use: Immediate effects and long-term health risks.
Tim Large–Youth Social Issues/Alamy Stock Photo

cough, and smoker's bronchitis. It raises blood pressure, accelerates heart rate, and requires the heart to pump more blood. Other common short-term effects are loss of appetite, diarrhea, fatigue, hoarseness, weight loss, stomach pains, insomnia, and impaired visual acuity, especially at night.

Long-term effects fall into two general categories. The first is premature death: Life expectancy for smokers is at least 10 years shorter than for nonsmokers. The second category involves quality of life. Smokers have higher rates of acute and chronic diseases than those who have never smoked. The more people smoke, and the deeper and more often they inhale, the greater the risk of disease and other complications. Cigarette smoking increases the risk of all the following:

- Cardiovascular disease (coronary heart disease, heart attack, stroke, hypertension, high cholesterol levels), lung disease (emphysema, chronic bronchitis), osteoporosis, diabetes, and many types of cancer (lung, trachea, mouth, pharynx, esophagus, larynx, pancreas, bladder, kidney, breast, cervix, stomach, liver, colon)

- Tooth decay, gum disease, bad breath, colds, ulcers, hair loss, facial wrinkling, and discolored teeth and fingers

- Menstrual disorders, early menopause, impotence, infertility, stillbirth, and low birth weight (see the box "Gender and Tobacco Use")

- Motor vehicle crashes (smoking causes a serious distraction) and fire-related injuries

When smokers quit, health improvements begin almost immediately. The younger people are when they stop smoking, the more pronounced are these improvements (Table 13.4).

Risks Associated with Other Forms of Tobacco Use

Many smokers have switched from cigarettes to other forms of tobacco, such as cigars and pipes, menthol cigarettes, spit (smokeless) tobacco, hookahs, and e-cigarettes. However, these alternatives are far from safe.

Cigars and Pipes Cigar and pipe smokers are at increased risk for many health problems, including cardiovascular and respiratory diseases and many types of cancer. Cigars contain more tobacco than cigarettes and so contain more nicotine and produce more tar when smoked. The health risks of cigars depend on the number of cigars smoked and whether the smoker inhales. Because most cigar and pipe users do not inhale, they have a lower risk of cancer and cardiovascular and respiratory diseases than cigarette smokers. However, their risks are substantially higher than those of nonsmokers. For example, compared to nonsmokers, people who smoke one or two cigars per day without inhaling have six times the risk of cancer of the larynx. The risks are much higher for cigar smokers who inhale.

Menthol Cigarettes Concerns have also been raised about menthol cigarettes. Menthol is a bronchodilator; as mentioned

Table 13.4	Benefits of Quitting Smoking
TIME SINCE QUITTING SMOKING	CHANGES AND BENEFITS
20 minutes	• Heart rate and blood pressure drop to normal. • The temperature of your hands and feet increases to normal.
8–12 hours	• Carbon monoxide in blood drops to normal; blood oxygen levels increase to normal.
24–48 hours	• Risk of sudden heart attack goes down. • Nerve endings begin to regrow. • Senses of smell and taste begin to return to normal.
2 weeks to 3 months	• Heart attack risk begins to drop. • Circulation and lung function improve. • Wounds heal more quickly.
1–9 months	• Coughing and shortness of breath decrease. • Energy levels increase. • Fewer illnesses, colds, and asthma attacks.
1 year	• Added risk of coronary heart disease drops to half that of smokers.
5 years	• Stroke risk is reduced to nearly that of nonsmokers. • Risk of cancer of the mouth, throat, esophagus, and bladder are cut in half.
10 years	• Lung cancer death rate drops to about half that of smokers. • Risk of larynx and pancreatic cancer decreases.
15 years	• Risk of coronary heart disease is close to that of nonsmokers.

SOURCES: U.S. Department of Health and Human Services n.d. *Get on a Path to a Healthier You.* (http://betobaccofree.hhs.gov/gallery/quit.html) accessed 2016; National Library of Medicine. 2015. *Benefits of Quitting Tobacco.* (http://www.nlm.nih.gov/medlineplus/ency/article/007532) accessed 2015.htm.

earlier, bronchodilators open the lungs' airways and make it easier for nicotine to enter the bloodstream. About 70% of black smokers use these cigarettes, as compared to 30% of white smokers. Studies have found that African Americans absorb more nicotine than other groups and metabolize it more slowly; they also have lower rates of successful quitting. The anesthetizing effect of menthol, which may allow smokers to inhale more deeply and hold smoke in their lungs for a longer period, may be partly responsible for these differences. Research is needed to determine if the effects of menthol and differences in smoking behavior can help explain the higher rates of smoking-related diseases among African Americans.

Spit (Smokeless) Tobacco Smokeless tobacco, which is not burned, comes in several forms. Chewing tobacco is cured (aged) and sold in pouches. Often flavored, it is chewed or held between the cheek and gums to release the nicotine. Snuff, usually sold in small tins, is cured tobacco that has been finely cut or processed into a powder. Long-term snuff use may increase the risk of cancer of the cheek and gums by as much as 50 times.

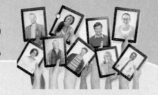

American men are currently more likely than women to smoke, but the rate of smoking among women is not far behind that of men, as are rates of tobacco-related illness and death. Lung cancer, emphysema, and cardiovascular diseases sicken and kill both men and women who smoke, and more American women now die each year from lung cancer than from breast cancer.

Although overall risks for tobacco-related illness are similar for women and men, sex appears to make a difference in some diseases. Women, for example, are more at risk for smoking-related blood clots and strokes than are men, and the risk is even greater for women who use oral contraceptives. Among men and women with the same smoking history, the odds of developing three major types of cancer, including lung cancer, are 1.2–1.7 times higher for women than men. Women may also have a greater biological vulnerability to lung cancer. Women who smoke have

higher rates of osteoporosis (a bone-thinning disease that can lead to fractures), thyroid-related diseases, and depression.

Tobacco use is associated with sex-specific health problems. Men who smoke increase their risk of erectile dysfunction and infertility. Women who smoke have greater menstrual bleeding, greater duration of painful menstrual cramps, and more variability in menstrual cycle length. Smokers have a more difficult time becoming pregnant, and they reach menopause on average a year or two earlier than nonsmokers. They face increased chances of miscarriage, placental disorders, premature delivery, ectopic pregnancy, preeclampsia, and stillbirth. Smoking is a risk factor for cervical cancer, too.

Women are less successful than men in quitting. Women report more severe withdrawal symptoms when they stop smoking and are more likely than men to report cravings in response to social and behavioral cues associated with

smoking. For men, relapse to smoking is often associated with work or social pressure; women are more likely to relapse when sad or depressed or concerned about weight gain. Women and men also respond differently to medications: Nicotine replacement therapy appears to work better for men, whereas the non-nicotine medication bupropion appears to work better for women.

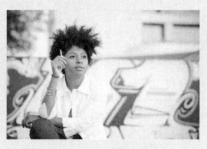

Eugenio Marongiu/Cultura/Getty Images

Spit tobacco causes bad breath, tooth decay, and gum disease. One of the most serious effects of chewing tobacco is the increased risk of oral cancer—cancers of the lip, tongue, cheek, throat, gums, roof and floor of the mouth, and larynx.

Hookahs The practice of puffing flavored tobacco through a waterpipe (*hookah*) has grown in the United States in recent years, particularly among college students. In the 2018 ACHA college survey, 12.4% of college students have used a hookah at least once. The smoker inhales through a hose, drawing air over a piece of burning charcoal, heating the tobacco, and producing smoke that travels through the body of the pipe, an urn filled with water, and the hose.

Many people assume that hookahs provide a safer way of using tobacco, but research has found that the smoke from these pipes contains many harmful chemicals, including 10 times more carbon monoxide than the smoke from a single cigarette. The amount of smoke inhaled during a typical hookah session, which lasts 30–60 minutes, can be more than 150 times the smoke inhaled from a cigarette. Smoke from both tobacco and nontobacco hookah products contains toxic compounds that increase the risk for smoking-related cancers, heart disease, and lung disease. Depending on which toxic compound is measured, a single hookah session is the equivalent of smoking between 1 and 50 cigarettes.

E-Cigarettes The electronic cigarette, also known as an e-cigarette or e-cig, is a battery-powered device that resembles a real cigarette. Instead of containing tobacco, the device uses a changeable filter that contains one or more chemicals, such as nicotine, flavorings, and other compounds. The user "smokes" or "vapes" an e-cig by sucking the filtered end; the device's battery heats the chemicals to create an inhalable vapor. During use, the device's tip even glows like the burning end of a real cigarette.

Because they deliver nicotine in a vapor instead of smoke, electronic cigarettes have been advertised as a safe alternative to traditional cigarettes. They have also been touted as a smoking-cessation product, like nicotine gums and patches. But e-cigs get hot enough to produce carcinogens and other toxic chemicals such as formaldehyde, found in traditional cigarettes, and diethylene glycol, a toxic chemical in antifreeze. They also produce nanoparticles, which have been linked to inflammation leading to asthma, stroke, and heart disease. No evidence submitted to the FDA supports the claim that e-cigarettes are being used as a smoking-cessation product.

E-cigarettes are of special concern because of their appeal to and growing use among youth. The U.S. Department of Health and Human Services marked a 900% increase in e-cigarette use among high school students from 2011–2015. Between 2017 and 2018, vaping among high schoolers surged again by 78%, and among middle schoolers by 48%. In real numbers, this means that in 2018, 3.6 million kids used e-cigarettes. Amid a deadly 2019 outbreak of a severe lung disease linked to vaping, state and federal legislators are fighting to ban flavored e-cigarettes.

Studies have linked nicotine use during this period to long-term cognition and attention problems, and an increased risk for mood disorders. Furthermore, early nicotine exposure increases the chance of nicotine dependence later in life and the likelihood of using other dependence-producing substances.

Environmental Tobacco Smoke

Environmental tobacco smoke (ETS), commonly called *secondhand smoke,* consists of **mainstream smoke**, the smoke exhaled by smokers, and **sidestream smoke**, the smoke from the burning end of the cigarette, cigar, or pipe. Of the 7,000 chemicals in tobacco smoke, hundreds are toxic, and 70 can cause cancer. Sidestream smoke is unfiltered by a cigarette filter or a smoker's lungs, so it contains significantly higher concentrations of toxic and carcinogenic compounds than mainstream smoke.

Nearly 85% of the smoke in a room where someone is smoking is sidestream smoke. Even though such smoke is diffuse, the concentrations can be considerable. Where several people are smoking, levels of carbon monoxide, for instance, can exceed those permitted by federal Air Quality Standards for outside air. The Centers for Disease Control and Prevention estimates that 58 million nonsmokers in the United States, including 15 million children, are exposed to ETS.

Thirdhand Smoke

A further complicating factor is thirdhand smoke, the toxic residues and chemicals that linger on indoor surfaces, curtains, and furniture, and in dust. Although it may seem like only a stale smell, thirdhand smoke contains the chemicals of secondhand smoke from tobacco: gases and particulate matter, including carcinogens and heavy metals such as arsenic, lead, and cyanide. Highly toxic particulates like nicotine can cling to walls and ceilings; gases can be absorbed into dust, fabrics, and upholstery. These toxic mixes can then recombine to form harmful compounds that remain at high levels long after smoking has stopped.

The transition from secondhand to thirdhand smoke is gradual, so the distinct chronic effects of each are not yet clear. The predicted health damage caused by thirdhand smoke ranges from 5% to 60% of total harm, much of which may currently be attributed to secondhand smoke. We do know that nicotine in thirdhand smoke forms carcinogens that are then inhaled, absorbed, or ingested, increasing the risk of respiratory illnesses. Young children who crawl and put objects in their mouths are more likely to come in contact with contaminated surfaces and are therefore the most vulnerable to thirdhand smoke's harmful effects. Homes of former smokers remained polluted with thirdhand smoke for months after residents quit smoking. Nicotine could be measured in the bodies of nonsmokers who moved into homes that had been smoked in, cleaned, and left empty several months.

Effects of ETS

ETS is a known human carcinogen. Each year in people who do not smoke, ETS causes about 7,300 lung cancer deaths and 34,000 deaths from heart disease. ETS also aggravates respiratory conditions such as allergies and asthma.

Measuring changes in the bloodstreams of healthy young nonsmokers who spent three hours in a smoke-filled room, researchers found that after just 30 minutes of exposure to ETS, the function in the coronary arteries was reduced to the same level as that of smokers. Carcinogens in the blood had reached levels capable of producing lung-tissue damage and promoting tumors. The harmful effects of ETS can remain with people hours after they have left a smoky environment. Carbon monoxide, for example, lingers in the bloodstream for up to 12 hours.

Children and ETS

Infants and children are particularly vulnerable to the harmful effects of ETS. Because they breathe faster than adults, they inhale more air and more of the pollutants it contains. Because they weigh less than adults, children inhale proportionately more pollutants per unit of body weight.

ETS triggers bronchitis, pneumonia, and other respiratory infections in infants and toddlers up to 18 months old, resulting in as many as 15,000 hospitalizations each year. Older children suffer, too. ETS can induce asthma in children and exacerbate symptoms in children who already have asthma.

Avoiding ETS

If you are a nonsmoker, you have the right to breathe clean air, free from tobacco smoke. Try these strategies to keep the air around you safe:

- *Speak up tactfully:* Try something like, "Would you mind putting your cigarette out or moving to another spot? The smoke is bothering me."

- *Don't allow smoking in your home or room:* Get rid of ashtrays, and ask smokers to light up outside.

- *Open a window:* If you cannot avoid being in a room with smokers, try to provide some ventilation.

- *Fight for a smoke-free environment:* For your sake and that of others, join with others either to eliminate all smoking indoors or to confine it to certain outdoor areas.

- *Make sure schools and daycares are tobacco-free:* Teach children to stay away from secondhand smoke.

- *Research quitting strategies:* Social pressure is a major factor in many former smokers' decision to quit.

Smoking and Pregnancy

Smoking almost doubles a pregnant woman's chance of having a miscarriage, and women who smoke also face an increased risk

> **environmental tobacco smoke (ETS)** Smoke **TERMS** that enters the atmosphere from the burning end of a cigarette, cigar, or pipe, as well as smoke that is exhaled by smokers; also called *secondhand smoke.*
>
> **mainstream smoke** Smoke that is inhaled by a smoker and then exhaled into the atmosphere.
>
> **sidestream smoke** Smoke that enters the atmosphere from the burning end of a cigarette, cigar, or pipe.

Each year, millions of Americans visit their doctors in the hope of finding a drug that will help them stop smoking. Although pharmacological options are limited, the few available drugs have proved successful.

Chantix (Varenicline)

The newest smoking cessation drug, marketed under the name Chantix, works on neurotransmitters in the brain by reducing nicotine cravings, easing the withdrawal process, and blocking the pleasant effects of nicotine.

Zyban (Bupropion)

Bupropion is an antidepressant (prescribed as Wellbutrin) as well as a smoking cessation aid (prescribed as Zyban). As a smoking cessation aid, bupropion acts on neurotransmitter receptors in the brain, easing the symptoms of nicotine withdrawal and reducing the urge to smoke.

Nicotine Replacement Products

The most widely used smoking cessation products replace the nicotine that the user would normally get from tobacco. The user continues to get nicotine, so withdrawal symptoms and cravings are reduced. Although still harmful, nicotine replacement products provide a cleaner form of nicotine, without the poisons and tars produced by burning tobacco. Nicotine doses are gradually lowered until users are able to cease nicotine use altogether.

Nicotine replacement products come in several forms, including patches, gum, lozenges, nasal sprays, and inhalers. They are available in a variety of strengths and can be worked into many different smoking cessation strategies. Most are available without a prescription.

---

of ectopic pregnancy, in which the fertilized egg implants itself in an oviduct rather than in the uterus. Maternal smoking causes hundreds of infant deaths in the United States each year, primarily due to premature delivery and smoking-related problems with the placenta, the organ that delivers blood, oxygen, and nutrients to the fetus. Maternal smoking is a major factor in low birth weight, which puts newborns at high risk for infections and other serious problems. If a nonsmoking mother is regularly exposed to ETS, her infant is also at greater risk for low birth weight.

Babies born to mothers who smoke more than two packs a day perform poorly on developmental tests in the first hours after birth, compared to babies of nonsmoking mothers. Later in life, obesity, hyperactivity, short attention span, and lower scores on spelling and reading tests all occur more frequently in children whose mothers smoked during pregnancy than in those born to nonsmoking mothers. Prenatal tobacco exposure has also been associated with behavioral problems in children.

Giving Up Tobacco

Giving up tobacco is a long-term, difficult process, usually accompanied by psychological craving and physical withdrawal. Research shows that most tobacco users move through predictable stages—from being uninterested in stopping, to thinking about change, to making a concerted effort to stop, to finally maintaining abstinence. Most users attempt to quit several times before they finally succeed. Relapse is a normal part of the process, as with most behavior change plans. Quitting is an ongoing process, not a single event.

Quitting requires a strategy for success. Some people quit cold turkey, whereas others taper off slowly. Over-the-counter and prescription products exist that help many people (see the box "Smoking Cessation Products"). Behavioral factors that have been shown to increase the chances of a smoker's

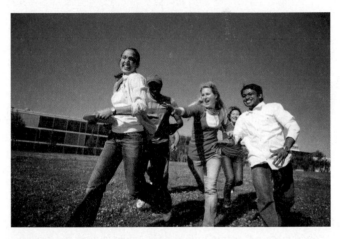

Wellness Tip Regular physical activity and social support can make it easier to stop smoking.
Holger Hill/fStop/Getty Images

permanent smoking cessation are support from others and regular exercise (see the box "How Does Exercise Help a Smoker Quit?"). Support can come from friends and family, websites, and/or formal group programs sponsored by organizations such as the American Cancer Society and the American Lung Association or by a college health center or community hospital.

If you are trying to quit, keeping track of cravings and urges in a health journal can help you deal with them. (Lab 13.2 can help identify your smoking triggers.) When you have an urge to use tobacco, use a relaxation technique, take a brisk walk, chew gum, or substitute some other activity. Practice stress management and time management so that you don't get overwhelmed at school or work. Eat sensibly and get enough sleep. Quitting can be hard, but the benefits are lifelong.

THE EVIDENCE FOR EXERCISE
How Does Exercise Help a Smoker Quit?

Most research on smoking cessation has not found any difference in quit rates between smokers who exercise and those who don't. However, many experts believe that health care providers should prescribe an appropriate level of physical activity to their patients who want to quit smoking. The reason for this is a growing body of evidence that exercise reduces withdrawal symptoms and cravings during smoking cessation—making it easier for people to stick to their quit plan.

In one study of young adults, combining exercise with use of a nicotine lozenge significantly and immediately reduced the craving for cigarettes. Another study showed that smokers' withdrawal symptoms and nicotine cravings decreased significantly during a single bout of aerobic exercise and remained measurably lower for nearly an hour after exercising. The positive effects were seen whether participants exercised vigorously or at a low level of exertion. The reason for these effects may lie in brain chemistry: Researchers in one study used MRI scans to look at activity in the parts of the brain focused on reward, motivation, and attention. After only 10 minutes of moderate-intensity exercise, smokers reported lower cravings in response to smoking images, and the scans showed less activation in associated parts of the brain. This confirmed other findings and provided evidence of a shift in brain activation in response to smoking cues following exercise. Although 10 minutes of activity was enough to have a measurable effect, other studies found that the more smokers exercised, the less likely they were to resume smoking. All these studies support the idea that physical activity can aid smokers in efforts to quit.

As described in the chapter, the physical benefits of quitting smoking are tremendous. Regular physical activity enhances some of these benefits, such as improved lung function, blood pressure, and overall fitness. Even in smokers who can't or won't quit, regular exercise reduces the risk of death from all causes, cardiovascular disease, and cancer by 30%.

Many smokers worry about weight gain associated with quitting. Although most ex-smokers gain a few pounds, at least temporarily, incorporating exercise and a healthy diet into a new, tobacco-free lifestyle lays the foundation for healthy weight management. Research findings vary on the effect of exercise on weight gain after quitting smoking, but at least one recent study shows that although exercise might not reduce short-term weight gain among new ex-smokers, physical activity, when accompanied by a healthy dietary pattern, does produce weight loss over the long term. Regardless, the health risks of adding a few pounds are far outweighed by the risks of continued smoking. According to one estimate, an ex-smoker would have to gain 75–100 pounds to equal the health risks of smoking a pack of cigarettes a day.

SOURCES: O'Donovan, G., et al. 2017. "Relationships between exercise, smoking habit and mortality in more than 100,000 adults," *International Journal of Cancer* 140(8): 1819–1827; Tritter, A., et al. 2015. "The effect of acute exercise on cigarette cravings while using a nicotine lozenge," *Psychopharmacology* 232(14): 2531–2539; Parsons, A. C., et al. 2009. "Interventions for preventing weight gain after smoking cessation," *Cochrane Database of Systematic Reviews* (Online) (1): CD006219; Taylor, A. H., et al. 2007. "The acute effects of exercise on cigarette cravings, withdrawal symptoms, affect and smoking behavior: A systematic review," *Addiction* 102(4): 534–543; Van Rensburg, J. K., et al. 2009. "Acute exercise modulates cigarette cravings and brain activation in response to smoking-related images: An fMRI study," *Psychopharmacology* 203(3): 589–598.

Action Against Tobacco

Individuals and communities have taken action against this major health threat. An assessment made in 2019 found that over 81% of Americans live in municipalities that restrict or ban smoking in public buildings, workplaces, restaurants, and bars. Over 2,000 colleges and universities now have totally smoke-free campuses; most prohibit both smoking and use of smokeless tobacco, both indoor and outdoor, as well as e-cigarettes. In 2016, the Obama administration banned smoking inside all public housing. As local nonsmoking laws proliferate, evidence mounts that environmental restrictions are effective in encouraging smokers to quit.

At the state level, many tough anti-tobacco laws have been passed. As of March 2017, 28 states and the District of Columbia had met the American Lung Association's Smokefree Air Challenge, which means they have passed laws prohibiting smoking in all public places and workplaces. California has one of the most aggressive—and successful—tobacco control programs, combining taxes on cigarettes, graphic advertisements, and bans on smoking in the workplace, bars, and restaurants. As of 2019, seven states and 441 cities and the District of Columbia have raised the minimum age to purchase tobacco products from 18 to 21. Fifteen states, including California, prohibit e-cigarettes in many public places and the workplace.

Until 2009, the FDA did not have the power to regulate tobacco products. That changed when Congress passed the Family Smoking Prevention and Tobacco Control Act, giving the FDA broad regulatory powers over the production, marketing, and sale of tobacco products. The law gives the FDA the power to eliminate or control levels of the thousands of chemical additives used to make tobacco more appealing and addictive. Under the legislation, manufacturers are required to use larger warning labels on cigarette packages, list cigarette ingredients on packages, and disclose changes in products as well as research findings. In March 2018, the FDA began the first steps toward a new regulatory effort to decrease the level of nicotine in tobacco products to make them less addictive.

Many states, as well as the federal government, have filed lawsuits against the tobacco industry to reclaim money spent on tobacco-related health care. A 1998 agreement requires tobacco companies to pay states $206 billion over 25 years. For these and other reasons, tobacco consumption in the United States is declining among some groups. In response, the U.S. tobacco industry has increased its efforts to sell in foreign markets, especially in developing nations with few restrictions on tobacco advertising.

COMMON QUESTIONS ANSWERED

Q What can I do for someone who I know has a drug problem?

A If you believe a friend or family member has a drug problem, obtain information about resources for drug treatment available on your campus or in your community. Communicate your concern, provide information about treatment options, and offer your support during treatment.

If the person denies having a problem, you may want to talk with an experienced counselor about an intervention—a formal, structured confrontation designed to end denial by having family, friends, and other caring individuals present their concerns to the drug user. Participants in an intervention point out the ways in which the person is hurting others as well as him- or herself. If your friend or family member agrees to treatment, support him or her to maintain the regimen.

In addition, examine your relationship with the person for signs of codependency. A *codependent* is someone whose actions help or enable a person to remain dependent on a drug by removing or softening the effects of the drug use on the user. Common actions by codependents include making excuses or lying for someone, loaning money to someone to continue drug use, and not confronting someone who is obviously intoxicated or high on a drug.

Enabling behavior can prevent a person from experiencing the consequences of her or his behavior and so delay recovery. If you see yourself developing a codependent relationship, get help for yourself. Al-Anon and Alateen are organizations dedicated to helping people who are affected by someone else's drinking.

Q Does drinking coffee help an intoxicated person sober up more quickly?

A No. Once alcohol is absorbed into the body, there is no way to accelerate its breakdown. The rate of alcohol metabolism varies among individuals, largely as a result of heredity, but it is not affected by caffeine, exercise, fresh air, or other stimulants. To sober up, you simply have to wait until your body has had sufficient time to metabolize all the alcohol consumed.

Q Can marijuana be used medically?

A Yes, although its use is restricted. Even though marijuana is considered an illegal drug at the federal level in the United States, at the time of writing, 33 states and Washington, D.C., have legalized marijuana to treat certain illnesses and medical conditions. Research shows benefits for treating muscle spasms in multiple sclerosis and cancer-related pain that is not otherwise relieved by opioid medications. Many cancer patients and people with AIDS use marijuana because they find it effective in relieving nausea and restoring appetite. Additional research is under way to find ways to target symptoms, standardize doses, and administer the drug so that the user is not subjected to the hazards of smoking marijuana, such as potential lung damage associated with long-term heavy use.

TIPS FOR TODAY AND THE FUTURE

The best treatment for dependence is prevention—not starting in the first place—but it's never too late to regain control of your life.

RIGHT NOW YOU CAN
- Carefully consider your use of drugs, alcohol, or tobacco—if any—and decide whether this is the time for you to stop. If it is, throw away the offending products. Keep in mind that substance cessation is difficult, and waiting for the "perfect time" to quit may only prolong an addiction.
- List five rewarding things you can do instead of giving in to the temptation to use a drug, alcohol, or tobacco.

IN THE FUTURE YOU CAN
- Look for local resources that can help you stop using drugs, alcohol, or tobacco. On campus, the student health center or counseling center may offer counseling or support services, such as a smoking cessation program. It can also be informative and inspiring to attend an Alcoholics Anonymous (AA) meeting.
- Track your progress toward quitting for good. Use a journal to record your cravings or urges and to describe the tactics you use to overcome them.

SUMMARY

- Addictive behaviors involve the loss of ability to recognize significant risk or other ways they negatively impact a person's health. Characteristics of addictive behaviors include reinforcement, craving, loss of control, escalation, and negative consequences.

- Substance misuse is use of a substance that is not consistent with medical or legal guidelines. Misuse can include use of illegal drugs; prescription drugs in greater-than-prescribed amounts; another person's prescription drug; or a legal substance, such as alcohol, in an unsafe manner.

- Addiction is a chronic disease that involves brain system disruptions relating to reward, motivation, and memory. Further disruptions occur in a person's body, emotional behavior, and social relationships.

- Factors to consider when deciding whether to try a psychoactive drug include short- and long-term risks of drug use, your future goals, ethical beliefs, the financial cost of the drug, and your reasons for drug use.

- At low doses, alcohol causes relaxation; at higher doses, it interferes with motor and mental functioning and is associated with injuries; at very high doses, alcohol poisoning, coma, and death can occur.

- Continued alcohol use has negative effects on the digestive and cardiovascular systems and increases cancer risk and overall mortality.

- Women who drink while pregnant risk giving birth to children with fetal alcohol syndrome.

- Alcohol use disorder involves drinking to clinically significant impairment. Severe alcohol use disorder, or alcoholism, is characterized by more severe problems with alcohol, usually involving tolerance and withdrawal.

- Binge drinking is a common form of alcohol misuse on college campuses that has negative effects on both drinking and nondrinking students.

- Nicotine is the addictive psychoactive drug in tobacco products.

- In the short term, smoking can either excite or tranquilize the nervous system; it also interferes with the functions of the respiratory system. Long-term effects of smoking include higher rates of acute and chronic diseases and reduced life expectancy.

- Other forms of tobacco use—cigars, pipes, clove cigarettes, e-cigarettes, and spit tobaccos—also have serious associated health risks.

- Environmental tobacco smoke contains toxic and carcinogenic compounds in high concentrations. It causes health problems, including cancer and heart disease, in nonsmokers exposed to it; infants and children are especially at risk.

- Many approaches and products are available to aid people in quitting smoking, and local, state, and federal efforts are aimed at combating smoking.

FOR FURTHER EXPLORATION

Action on Smoking and Health (ASH). Provides statistics, news briefs, and other information about smoking.

  http://www.ash.org

Al-Anon Family Group Headquarters. Provides information and referrals to local Al-Anon and Alateen groups.

  http://www.al-anon.org

Alcoholics Anonymous (AA). Provides information on AA, literature on alcoholism, and information about AA meetings.

  http://www.aa.org

American Cancer Society (ACS). Sponsor of the annual Great American Smokeout; provides information on the dangers of tobacco, as well as tools for preventing and stopping the use of tobacco products.

  http://www.cancer.org

American Lung Association. Provides information on lung diseases, tobacco control, and environmental health.

  http://www.lung.org

American Psychiatric Association: Help with Addiction and Substance Use Disorders. Blog posts and APA resources that cover a variety of mental health issues for patients and families.

  https://www.psychiatry.org/patients-families/addiction

Centers for Disease Control and Prevention: Smoking and Tobacco Use. Provides educational materials and tips on how to quit smoking.

  http://www.cdc.gov/tobacco

Education Development Center. Links to projects, experts, and resources for prevention and intervention programs.

  http://www.edc.org/body-work/opioid-and-other-substance-abuse
  -prevention

National Institute on Alcohol Abuse and Alcoholism (NIAAA). Provides booklets and other publications on a variety of alcohol-related topics, including fetal alcohol syndrome, alcoholism treatment, and alcohol use and minorities.

  http://www.niaaa.nih.gov

National Institute on Drug Abuse. Develops and supports research on drug abuse prevention programs; fact sheets on drugs of abuse are available on the website.

  http://www.drugabuse.gov

Quitnet. Provides interactive tools and questionnaires, support groups, a library, and the latest news on tobacco issues.

  https://quitnet.meyouhealth.com

Smokefree.gov. Provides step-by-step strategies for quitting as well as expert support via telephone or instant messaging.

  http://www.smokefree.gov

The following hotlines provide support and referrals:

  800-ALCOHOL

  800-622-HELP

SELECTED BIBLIOGRAPHY

American College Health Association. 2018. *American College Health Association-National College Health Assessment: Reference Group Data Report Fall 2018.* Hanover, MD: American College Health Association.

American Lung Association. 2017. *Smokefree Air Laws* (https://www.lung.org/our-initiatives/tobacco/smokefree-environments/smokefree-air-laws.html).

American Psychiatric Association. 2013. *Diagnostic and Statistical Manual of Mental Disorders,* 5th ed. Washington, DC: American Psychiatric Association.

Araújo, A. M., et al. 2015. Raising awareness of new psychoactive substances: Chemical analysis and in vitro toxicity screening of "legal high" packages containing synthetic cathinones. *Archives of Toxicology* 89(5): 757–771.

Ashrafioun, L., et al. 2016. Patterns of use, acute subjective experiences, and motivations for using synthetic cathinones ("bath salts") in recreational users. *Journal of Psychoactive Drugs* 48(5): 336–343.

Bhatnagar, A., et al. 2019. AHA Scientific Statement: Water pipe (hookah) smoking and cardiovascular disease risk. *Circulation* 139(19): e917–e936.

Bhatnagar, A., et al. 2019. New and emerging tobacco products and the nicotine endgame: The role of robust regulation and comprehensive tobacco control and prevention. *Circulation* 139(19): e937–e958.

Brandon, T. H., et al. 2015. Electronic nicotine delivery systems: A policy statement from the American Association for Cancer Research and the American Society of Clinical Oncology. *Journal of Clinical Oncology* 33(8): 952–963.

Carbonneau, R., et al. 2015. Trajectories of gambling problems from mid-adolescence to age 30 in a general population cohort. *Psychology of Addictive Behaviors,* July 13.

Castaneto, M. S., et al. 2014. Synthetic cannabinoids: Epidemiology, pharmacodynamics, and clinical implications. *Drug and Alcohol Dependence* 144: 12–41.

Center for Behavioral Health Statistics and Quality. 2016. *Impact of the DSM-IV to DSM-5 Changes on the National Survey on Drug Use and Health.* Rockville, MD: Substance Abuse and Mental Health Services Administration.

Centers for Disease Control and Prevention. 2015. *CDC Vital Signs: Secondhand Smoke: An Unequal Danger* (http://www.cdc.gov/vitalsigns/tobacco/index.html).

Centers for Disease Control and Prevention. 2016. Increases in drug and opioid-involved overdose deaths—United States, 2010–2015. *MMWR* 65(50-51): 1445–1452.

Centers for Disease Control and Prevention. 2016. *Smoking and tobacco Use: Hookahs* (https://www.cdc.gov/tobacco/data_statistics/fact_sheets/tobacco_industry/hookahs).

Centers for Disease Control and Prevention. 2017. *Motor Vehicle Safety: Impaired Driving* (https://www.cdc.gov/motorvehiclesafety/impaired_driving/impaired-drv_factsheet.html).

Centers for Disease Control and Prevention. 2018. *Opioid Overdose* (https://www.cdc.gov/drugoverdose).

Centers for Disease Control and Prevention. 2018. Tobacco use among middle and high school students—United States, 2011–2017. *MMWR* 67(22): 629–633.

CollegeGambling.org. 2014. *Fact Sheet: Gambling Disorders.* National Center for Responsible Gambling (http://www.collegegambling.org/facts-and-stats/just-facts)

De-Sola Gutierrez, J., F. Rodriguez de Fonseca, and G. Rubio. 2016. Cell phone addiction: A review. *Frontiers in Psychiatry* 7: 175.

Dubois, S., et al. 2015. The combined effects of alcohol and cannabis on driving: Impact on crash risk. *Forensic Science International* 248: 94–100.

Fiore, M. C., et al. 2008. *Treating Tobacco Use and Dependence: 2008 Update.* Content last reviewed October 2014. Rockville, MD: Agency for Healthcare Research and Quality (http://www.ahrq.gov/professionals/clinicians-providers/guidelines-recommendations/tobacco/clinicians/update/correctadd.html).

Ford, B. M., et al. 2017. Synthetic pot: Not your grandfather's marijuana. *Trends in Pharmacological Sciences* 38(3): 257–276.

Hart, C., and C. Ksir. 2015. *Drugs, Society, and Human Behavior,* 16th ed. New York: McGraw-Hill.

Kalkhoran, S., and S. A. Glantz. 2016. E-cigarettes and smoking cessation in real-world and clinical settings: A systematic review and meta-analysis. *Lancet Respiratory Medicine* 4(2): 116–128.

Kasza, K. A., et al. 2017. Tobacco-product use by adults and youths in the United States in 2013 and 2014. *New England Journal of Medicine* 376(4): 342–353.

Miech, R., et al. 2017. E-cigarette use as a predictor of cigarette smoking: Results from a 1-year follow-up of a national sample of 12th grade students. *Tobacco Control.* doi:10.1136/tobaccocontrol-2016-053291

National Center for Health Statistics. 2017. Electronic cigarette use among adults: United States, 2014. *NCHS Data Brief* No. 217. Hyattsville, MD: National Center for Health Statistics.

National Center for Health Statistics. 2018. Drug overdose deaths in the United States, 1999–2017. *NCHS Data Brief,* no 329. Hyattsville, MD: National Center for Health Statistics.

National Highway Traffic Safety Administration. 2018. *Alcohol-Impaired Driving* (https://crashstats.nhtsa.dot.gov/Api/Public/ViewPublication/812630).

National Institute on Alcohol Abuse and Alcoholism. 2015. *College Drinking Fact Sheet* (http://pubs.niaaa.nih.gov/publications/CollegeFactSheet/CollegeFactSheet.pdf).

National Institute on Alcohol Abuse and Alcoholism. 2018. *Alcohol Overdose: The Dangers of Drinking Too Much* (https://pubs.niaaa.nih.gov/publications/alcoholoverdosefactsheet/overdosefact.htm).

National Institute on Drug Abuse. 2014. *Club Drugs (GHB, Ketamine, and Rohypnol)* (https://www.drugabuse.gov/sites/default/files/drugfacts_clubdrugs_12_2014.pdf).

National Institute on Drug Abuse. 2019. *DrugFacts: What Is Kratom?* (https://www.drugabuse.gov/publications/drugfacts/kratom).

National Institute on Drug Abuse. 2019. *Overdose Death Rates* (https://www.drugabuse.gov/related-topics/trends-statistics/overdose-death-rates).

National Institutes of Health, Fogarty International Center. 2014. NIH shows hookahs pose risks. *Global Health Matters,* Mar/Apr 2014.

Parrott, A. C., et al. 2014. MDMA, cortisol, and heightened stress in recreational ecstasy users. *Behavioural Pharmacology* 25(5–6): 458–472.

ProCon.org. 2018. *33 Legal Medical Marijuana States and DC* (http://medicalmarijuana.procon.org/view.resource.php?resourceID=000881).

Reilly, M. T., et al. 2014. Perspectives on the neuroscience of alcohol from the National Institute on Alcohol Abuse and Alcoholism. *Handbook of Clinical Neurology* 125: 15–29.

Ribeiro, L. I. G., and P. W. Ind. 2016. Effect of cannabis smoking on lung function and respiratory symptoms: A structured literature review. *Primary Care Respiratory Medicine* 26(16071). doi:10.1038/npjpcrm.2016.71

Rostron, B. L., B. Wang, and S. T. Liu. 2019. Waterpipe or hookah-related poisoning events among U.S. adolescents and young adults. *Journal of Adolescent Health* 64(6): 800–803.

Sayette, M. A. 2016. The role of craving in substance use disorders: Theoretical and methodological issues. *Annual Review of Clinical Psychology* 12: 407–433.

Smith, P. H., et al. 2015. Gender differences in medication use and cigarette smoking cessation: Results from the International Tobacco Control Four Country Survey. *Nicotine and Tobacco Research* 17(4): 463–472.

Soneji, S., et al. 2015. Associations between initial water pipe tobacco smoking and snuff use and subsequent cigarette smoking: Results from a longitudinal study of US adolescents and young adults. *JAMA Pediatrics* 169(2): 129–136.

U.S. Department of Health and Human Services. 2014. *The Health Consequences of Smoking: 50 Years of Progress. A Report of the Surgeon General.* Atlanta, GA: U.S. Department of Health and Human Services.

U.S. Department of Health and Human Services. 2016. *E-Cigarette Use Among Youth and Young Adults. A Report of the Surgeon General.* Atlanta, GA: U.S. Department of Health and Human Services.

Valente, M. J., et al. 2014. Khat and synthetic cathinones: A review. *Archives of Toxicology* 88(1): 15–45.

Van Amsterdam, J., T. Brunt, and W. van den Brink. 2015. The adverse health effects of synthetic cannabinoids with emphasis on psychosis-like effects. *Journal of Psychopharmacology* 29(3): 254–263.

Volkow, N. D., and A. T. McLellan. 2016. Opioid abuse in chronic pain—misconceptions and mitigation strategies. *New England Journal of Medicine* 371: 1253–1263.

Weinstein, A., et al. 2015. Internet addiction is associated with social anxiety in young adults. *Annals of Clinical Psychiatry* 27(1): 4–9.

Woolsey, C. L., et al. 2015. Combined use of alcohol and energy drinks increases participation in high-risk drinking and driving behaviors among college students. *Journal of Studies on Alcohol and Drugs* 76(4): 615–619.

Young, K. S., and C. de Abreu, eds. 2011. *Internet Addiction: A Handbook and Guide to Evaluation and Treatment.* Hoboken, NJ: Wiley.

Zhang, J., et al. 2017. Facial flushing after alcohol consumption and the risk of cancer: A meta-analysis. *Medicine* 96(13): e6506.

Name _____ Section _____ Date _____

LAB 13.1   Is Alcohol a Problem in Your Life?

Part I Is Your Drinking Pattern Low Risk?

1. On any day in the past year, have you ever had (circle one):

Yes   No   For men: More than 4 drinks?*

Yes   No   For women: More than 3 drinks?*

2. During a typical week:

On average, how many days a week do you drink alcohol?   _____ days

How many drinks do you typically have?   X _____ drinks

_____

Multiply to determine your typical weekly consumption: _____ weekly average

According to the National Institutes of Health, low-risk drinking limits for men and women are as follows. To stay low risk, you must be within both the single-day and weekly limits. How does your drinking pattern compare?

*   For men: No more than 4 drinks on any day AND no more than 14 drinks per week.

*   For women: No more than 3 drinks on any day AND no more than 7 drinks per week.

*If you need to review what counts as a drink, visit http://rethinkingdrinking.niaaa.nih.gov/Tools/Calculators/drink-size-calculator.aspx.

Part II Do You Have Signs of an Alcohol Use Disorder?

Check any statement that is true for you. Over the past year, have you:

_____ 1. Had times when you ended up drinking more, or longer, than you intended?

_____ 2. More than once wanted to cut down or stop drinking, or tried to, but couldn't?

_____ 3. Spent a lot of time drinking or recovering from its effects?

_____ 4. Experienced a strong need, or urge, to drink—you wanted a drink so badly you couldn't think of anything else?

_____ 5. Found that drinking or its effects interfered with taking care of your home or family? Or caused troubles at school or your job?

_____ 6. Continued to drink even though it was causing trouble with your family or friends?

_____ 7. Given up or cut back on social or recreational activities that were important or interesting to you, or gave you pleasure, in order to drink?

_____ 8. More than once gotten into physically risky situations while or after drinking (such as driving, swimming, using machinery, or having unsafe sex)?

_____ 9. Continued to drink even though it was making you feel depressed or anxious or adding to another health problem? Or after having had a memory blackout?

_____ 10. Developed tolerance to alcohol and had to drink much more than you once did to get the effect you want or found that your usual number of drinks had much less effect than before?

_____ 11. Found that when the effects of alcohol were wearing off, you had withdrawal symptoms, such as sweating, increased pulse, shakiness, insomnia, nausea, irritability, anxiety, or depression?

If you have any symptoms, then alcohol may already be a cause for concern. According to the American Psychiatric Association, if a person meets two of the criteria, she or he has an alcohol use disorder; two to three symptoms indicate a mild disorder; four to five, a moderate disorder; and six or more, a severe disorder. A health professional can look at the number, pattern, and severity of symptoms and help decide the best course of action.

LABORATORY ACTIVITIES

Part III Are You Troubled by Someone's Drinking?

Millions of people are affected by the excessive drinking of someone close to them. The following questions are designed to help you decide whether you need Al-Anon. If you answer yes to any question, put a check next to it.

_____ 1. Do you worry about how much someone else drinks?

_____ 2. Do you have money problems because of someone else's drinking?

_____ 3. Do you tell lies to cover up for someone else's drinking?

_____ 4. Do you feel that if the drinker cared about you, he or she would stop drinking to please you?

_____ 5. Do you blame the drinker's behavior on his or her companions?

_____ 6. Are plans frequently upset or canceled or meals delayed because of the drinker?

_____ 7. Do you make threats, such as, "If you don't stop drinking, I'll leave you?"

_____ 8. Do you secretly try to smell the drinker's breath?

_____ 9. Are you afraid to upset someone for fear it will set off a drinking bout?

_____ 10. Have you been hurt or embarrassed by a drinker's behavior?

_____ 11. Are holidays and gatherings spoiled because of drinking?

_____ 12. Have you considered calling the police for help because of fear of abuse?

_____ 13. Do you search for hidden alcohol?

_____ 14. Do you often ride in a car with a driver who has been drinking?

_____ 15. Have you refused social invitations out of fear or anxiety?

_____ 16. Do you feel like a failure because you can't control the drinker?

_____ 17. Do you think that if the drinker stopped drinking, your other problems would be solved?

_____ 18. Do you ever threaten to hurt yourself to scare the drinker?

_____ 19. Do you feel angry, confused, or depressed most of the time?

_____ 20. Do you feel there is no one who understands your problems?

If you answered yes to three or more of these questions, Al-Anon or Alateen may be able to help. See the "For Further Exploration" section of this chapter.

Using Your Results

How did you score? (1) Is your drinking pattern low-risk? Do you have any signs of an alcohol use disorder? Are you surprised by the results of the evaluations of your alcohol use?

(2) Did the Al-Anon quiz indicate that you are affected by someone else's excessive drinking? Are you surprised by the result?

What should you do next? If your alcohol use pattern isn't low-risk, if the alcohol use disorder assessment indicates a problem, or if you are encountering drinking-related problems with your academic performance, job, relationships, or health, or with the law, you should consider seeking help. Check for campus or community resources, including counseling, self-help groups, AA, and formal treatment programs.

If you are troubled by someone else's drinking, you can contact Al-Anon or Alateen by looking in your local telephone directory or contacting Al-Anon's main office (1600 Corporate Landing Parkway, Virginia Beach, VA 23454; 800-344-2666; http://www.al-anon.org).

SOURCES: Part I: National Institutes of Health, National Institute on Alcohol Abuse and Alcoholism. 2016. _Rethinking Drinking: What's Your Pattern?_ (https://www.rethinkingdrinking.niaaa.nih.gov/How-much-is-too-much/Is-your-drinking-pattern-risky/Whats-Your-Pattern.aspx); Part II: National Institutes of Health, National Institute on Alcohol Abuse and Alcoholism. 2017. _Alcohol Use Disorder_ (https://www.niaaa.nih.gov/alcohol-health/overview-alcohol-consumption/alcohol-use-disorders); American Psychiatric Association. 2013. _Diagnostic and Statistical Manual of Mental Disorders,_ 5th ed. Washington, DC: American Psychiatric Association; Part III: Al-Anon Family Group Headquarters, Inc. 1980. _Are You Troubled by Someone's Drinking?_ Reprinted by permission of Al-Anon Family Group Headquarters, Inc. (https://al-anon.org/pdf/S17.pdf).

Name _____ Section _____ Date _____

LAB 13.2   For Smokers Only: Why Do You Smoke?

Although smoking cigarettes is physiologically addictive, people smoke for reasons other than nicotine craving. What kind of smoker are you? Knowing what your motivations and satisfactions are can ultimately help you quit. This test is designed to provide you with a score on each of six factors that describe many people's smoking. Read the statements and then circle the number that represents how often you feel this way when you smoke cigarettes. Be sure to answer each question.

		Always	Frequently	Occasionally	Seldom	Never
A.	I smoke cigarettes to keep myself from slowing down.	5	4	3	2	1
B.	Handling a cigarette is part of the enjoyment of smoking it.	5	4	3	2	1
C.	Smoking cigarettes is pleasant and relaxing.	5	4	3	2	1
D.	I light up a cigarette when I feel angry about something.	5	4	3	2	1
E.	When I have run out of cigarettes, I find it almost unbearable until I can get them.	5	4	3	2	1
F.	I smoke cigarettes automatically without even being aware of it.	5	4	3	2	1
G.	I smoke cigarettes for stimulation, to perk myself up.	5	4	3	2	1
H.	Part of the enjoyment of smoking a cigarette comes from the steps I take to light up.	5	4	3	2	1
I.	I find cigarettes pleasurable.	5	4	3	2	1
J.	When I feel uncomfortable or upset about something, I light up a cigarette.	5	4	3	2	1
K.	I am very much aware of the fact when I am not smoking a cigarette.	5	4	3	2	1
L.	I light up a cigarette without realizing I still have one burning in the ashtray.	5	4	3	2	1
M.	I smoke cigarettes to get a "lift."	5	4	3	2	1
N.	When I smoke a cigarette, part of the enjoyment is watching the smoke as I exhale it.	5	4	3	2	1
O.	I want a cigarette most when I am comfortable and relaxed.	5	4	3	2	1
P.	When I feel "blue" or want to take my mind off cares and worries, I smoke cigarettes.	5	4	3	2	1
Q.	I get a real gnawing hunger for a cigarette when I haven't smoked for a while.	5	4	3	2	1
R.	I've found a cigarette in my mouth and didn't remember putting it there.	5	4	3	2	1

LABORATORY ACTIVITIES

How to Score

Enter the numbers you have circled in the spaces provided. Total the scores on each line. Total scores can range from 3 to 15. Any score of 11 or above is high; any score of 7 or below is low.

					Totals
_____ A	+	_____ G	+	_____ M	= _____ Stimulation
_____ B	+	_____ H	+	_____ N	= _____ Handling
_____ C	+	_____ I	+	_____ O	= _____ Pleasurable relaxation
_____ D	+	_____ J	+	_____ P	= _____ Crutch: tension reduction
_____ E	+	_____ K	+	_____ Q	= _____ Craving: strong physiological or psychological addiction
_____ F	+	_____ L	+	_____ R	= _____ Habit

Using Your Results

How did you score? For which factors did you score the highest? Are you surprised by the results of the assessment?

What should you do next? Use the information from this assessment to help plan a successful approach for quitting. The six factors measured by this test describe ways of experiencing or managing certain kinds of feelings. The higher your score on a particular factor, the more important that factor is in your smoking, and the more useful the following tips will be in your attempt to quit. Highlight or make a list of the strategies that seem most helpful to you and post the list in a prominent place.

Stimulation: If you score high on this factor, it means you are stimulated by a cigarette—you feel that it helps wake you up, organize your energies, and keep you going. If you try to give up smoking, you may want a safe substitute—a brisk walk or moderate exercise, for example—whenever you feel the urge to smoke.

Handling: Handling things can be satisfying, but there are many ways to keep your hands busy without lighting up or playing with a cigarette. Try doodling or toying with a pen, a pencil, or another small object.

Pleasurable relaxation: Those who do get real pleasure from smoking often find that an honest consideration of the harmful effects of their habit is enough to help them quit. They substitute social or physical activities and find they do not seriously miss their cigarettes.

Crutch: Many smokers use cigarettes as a kind of crutch in moments of stress or discomfort, and occasionally it may work; but heavy smokers are apt to discover that cigarettes do not help them deal with their problems effectively. When it comes to quitting, this kind of smoker may find it easy to stop when everything is going well but may be tempted to start again in a time of crisis. Physical exertion or social activity may serve as a useful substitute for cigarettes.

Craving: Quitting smoking is difficult for people who score high on this factor. It may be helpful for them to smoke more than usual for a day or two, so that the taste for cigarettes is spoiled, and then isolate themselves completely from cigarettes until the craving is gone.

Habit: These smokers light up frequently without even realizing it; they no longer get much satisfaction. They may find it easy to quit and stay off if they can break the habit patterns they have built up. The key to success is becoming aware of each cigarette when it's smoked. Ask, "Do I really want this cigarette?"

SOURCES: National Institutes of Health. 1990. *Why Do You Smoke?* NIH Pub. no. 90-1822. U.S. Department of Health and Human Services. Public Health Service.

Design elements: Evidence for Exercise box (shoes and stethoscope): Vstock LLC/Tetra Images/Getty Images; Take Charge box (lady walking): VisualCommunications/E+/Getty Images; Critical Consumer box (man): Sam74100/iStock/Getty Images; Diversity Matters box (holding devices): Robert Churchill/iStockphoto/Rawpixel Ltd/Getty Images; Wellness in the Digital Age box (Smart Watch): Hong Li/DigitalVision/Getty Images

LOOKING AHEAD...

After reading this chapter, you should be able to

- Explain how HIV is transmitted, diagnosed, and treated.

- Discuss the symptoms, risks, and treatments of other major STIs.

- List strategies for protecting yourself from STIs.

TEST YOUR KNOWLEDGE

1. Worldwide, which of the following is the primary means of spreading HIV infection?
   a. injection drug use
   b. sex between men
   c. mother-to-child transmission
   d. heterosexual sex

2. A man with an STI is more likely to transmit the infection to a female partner than vice versa. True or false?

3. After you have had an STI once, you become immune to that disease and cannot get it again. True or false?

See answers on the next page.

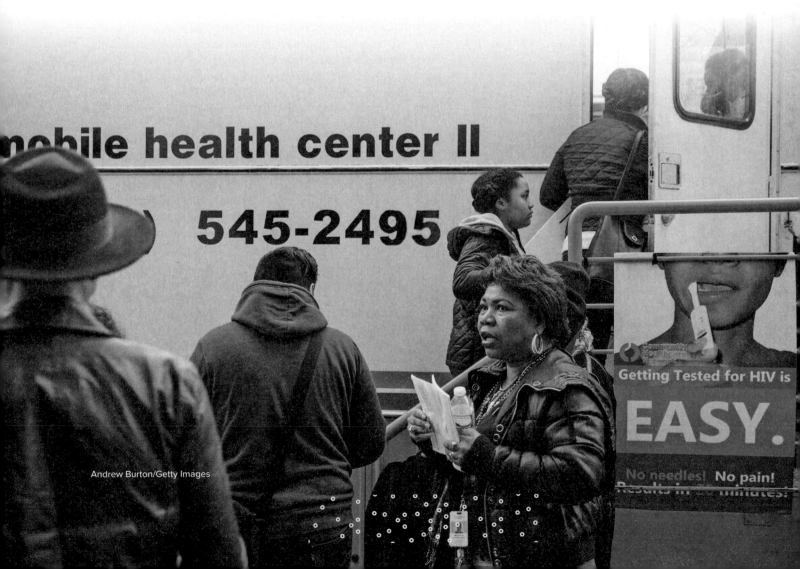

Andrew Burton/Getty Images

Considering the intimate nature of sexual activity, it is not surprising that it allows for the transmission of many infections. Of course, colds, influenza, and other infections can spread from one sexual partner to another, but sexual contact is not the primary means of transmission for these illnesses. **Sexually transmitted infections (STIs)**—also still called **sexually transmitted diseases (STDs)**—spread from person to person mainly through sexual activity. STIs are a particularly insidious group of illnesses because a person can be infected and be able to transmit a disease, yet not look or feel sick; this is why the term *sexually transmitted infection* has come into common use.

STIs can be prevented. Many STIs can also be cured if treated early and properly. This chapter introduces the major forms of STIs. It also provides information about healthy, safer sexual behavior to help you reduce the further spread of these diseases.

THE MAJOR STIs

The following seven STIs pose major health threats:

- HIV/AIDS
- Chlamydia
- Gonorrhea
- Human papillomavirus (HPV)
- Herpes
- Hepatitis
- Syphilis

These diseases are considered major threats because they cause serious complications if left untreated, and they pose risks to a fetus or newborn. STIs often result in long-term consequences, including chronic pain, infertility, stillbirths, genital cancers, and death.

All these diseases have a relatively high incidence among Americans (Table 14.1). In fact, the United States has one of the highest rates of STIs of any industrialized nation; young people ages 15–24 account for half of STI cases in the United States. Several of the most common STIs, including chlamydia, gonorrhea, and syphilis, are on the rise. The Centers for Disease Control and Prevention (CDC) estimates that 110 million Americans are infected with an STI, and over 20 million Americans become newly infected each year. Some STIs are treatable or resolve on their own, but others persist or are incurable.

Table 14.1	Estimated Annual New Cases of Selected STIs in the United States

STI	NEW CASES*
HPV	14,000,000
Chlamydia	2,860,000
Trichomoniasis	1,090,000
Gonorrhea	820,000
Herpes simplex virus (HSV 2)	776,000
Syphilis	101,600
Hepatitis B	43,000
HIV infection	38,300

*For many STIs, the estimated number of new infections significantly exceeds the number of cases formally diagnosed.

SOURCES: Centers for Disease Control and Prevention. "Sexually Transmitted Diseases (STDs)." (https://www.cdc.gov/std/default.htm) accessed 2019; Centers for Disease Control and Prevention. 2017. *HIV Surveillance Report 29* (http://www.cdc.gov/hiv/library/reports/hiv-surveillance.html); U.S. Department of Health and Human Services. n. d. "Hepatitis B." (https://www.hhs.gov/opa/reproductive-health/fact-sheets/sexually-transmitted-diseases/hepatitis-b/index.html) accessed 2019.

STIs and Sexual Anatomy

Both men and women are affected by STIs, but the symptoms and outcomes can vary between the sexes. For example, chlamydia may cause inflammation of the oviducts in women and the epididymis in men. Figures 14.1 and 14.2 provide basic information about male and female sexual anatomy as a point of reference throughout the discussion of STIs. As will be described later in the chapter, women tend to experience STIs as more problematic than men, for both biological and social reasons.

HIV Infection and AIDS

The **human immunodeficiency virus (HIV)** causes **acquired immunodeficiency syndrome (AIDS)**, a disease that without treatment is fatal. With the best treatment, someone with HIV infection will live almost as long as people not infected. Worldwide, adequate treatment for HIV is not available, and most infected persons die within 8–10 years.

An estimated 78 million people have been infected since the epidemic began in 1981—over 1% of the world's population—and tens of millions of those people have died. Currently, about 36.9 million people are infected with HIV/AIDS worldwide.

The number of people living with HIV infection has leveled off. Many experts believe that the global HIV epidemic peaked in the late 1990s, at about 3.5 million new infections per year, compared with an estimated 1.8 million new infections in 2017. Despite a slowing of the epidemic, however, AIDS remains a primary cause of death in Africa and continues to be a major cause of mortality around the world.

In the United States, about 1.1 million people are living with HIV infection; about 40,000 cases of HIV infection are

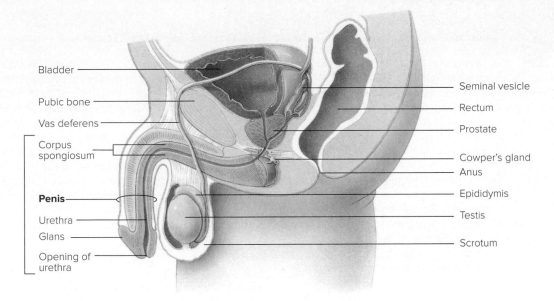

Figure 14.1   Male sexual anatomy.

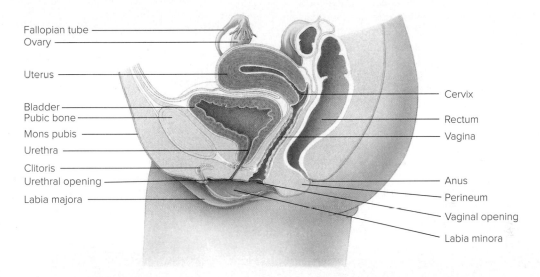

Figure 14.2   Female sexual anatomy.

diagnosed each year. Today, 1 in 7 Americans infected with HIV are unaware of their infection. More than 670,000 Americans have died from AIDS since the start of the epidemic.

What Is HIV Infection? **HIV infection** is a chronic disease that progressively damages the body's immune system, making an otherwise healthy person less able to resist a variety of infections and disorders. Normally, when a virus or other pathogen enters the body, it is targeted and destroyed by the immune system. But HIV attacks the immune system itself, taking over immune system cells and forcing them to produce new copies of HIV. It also makes them incapable of performing their immune functions (see the box "Does Exercise Help Our Immune System?").

The destruction of the immune system is signaled by the loss of **CD4 T cells**. As the number of CD4 T cells declines, an infected person may begin to experience mild to moderately

TERMS

sexually transmitted infection (STI)
or **sexually transmitted disease (STD)**   A disease that can be transmitted by sexual contact; some can also be transmitted by other means.

human immunodeficiency virus (HIV)   The virus that causes HIV infection and AIDS.

acquired immunodeficiency syndrome (AIDS)   A generally fatal, incurable, sexually transmitted viral disease.

HIV infection   A chronic, progressive viral infection that damages the immune system.

CD4 T cell   A type of white blood cell that helps coordinate the activity of the immune system; the primary target for HIV infection. A decrease in the number of these cells correlates with the risk and severity of HIV-related illness.

THE EVIDENCE FOR EXERCISE
Does Exercise Help Our Immune System?

A strong immune system can help defend your body against infections, including STIs, if only by keeping the infection at bay and minimizing damage until medical therapy (such as antibiotics) can be started. When an infection is detected, the immune system's white blood cells jump into action. They invade pathogens and infected body cells, and they prime the immune system for future infections by the same agent.

Many lifestyle factors, including nutrition, sleep, and stress management, are known to support immune function. The effects of physical activity and exercise on the immune system are more complex. It appears that effects vary depending on the intensity of the activity. Research has demonstrated that moderate-intensity exercise tends to improve immune function, whereas vigorous-intensity exercise tends to impair immunity temporarily.

Patients with HIV/AIDS can exercise at low to moderate intensity and not increase their risk for developing other infections. Study results showed that aerobic exercise and resistance training improved cardiovascular and muscle endurance and also prevented muscle wasting due to HIV. Resistance training has also been shown to improve strength in frail older adults with HIV. It is possible that strength training increases CD4 cell counts. Other studies have examined the effects of exercise on specific components of the immune system (such as natural killer cells, neutrophils, and dendritic cells) and found that the overall immune system response to physical activity is positive.

Intense interval training (see Chapter 3) provides immediate short-term benefits to the immune system. Intensive training for long periods has mixed short- and long-term effects. Studies have found that people who exercise vigorously, for prolonged periods, or without proper nutrition, experience temporary declines in immune system function; full function is then typically recovered in a matter of hours or days. But longitudinal studies (those conducted repeatedly over months or years) also show that vigorous exercise offers important anti-inflammatory benefits. For most of us, the evidence strongly indicates that regular moderate-intensity exercise promotes immune system function in many ways.

SOURCES: Durrer, C., et al. 2017. "Acute high-intensity interval exercise reduces human monocyte Toll-like receptor 2 expression in type 2 diabetes," *American Journal of Physiology Integrative Comparative Physiology* 312(4): R529–R538; Moro-García Marco, A. 2013. "Effects of maintained intense exercise throughout the life on the adaptive immune response in elderly and young athletes," *British Journal of Sports Medicine* 47: e3; de Souza, P. M. L., et al. 2011. "Effect of progressive resistance exercise on strength evolution of elderly patients living with HIV compared to healthy controls," *Clinics* (São Paulo) 66(2): 261–266; Giraldo, E., et al. 2009. "Exercise intensity-dependent changes in the inflammatory response in sedentary women: Role of neuroendocrine parameters in the neutrophil phagocytic process and the pro-/anti-inflammatory cytokine balance," *Neuroimmunomodulation* 16(4): 237–244.

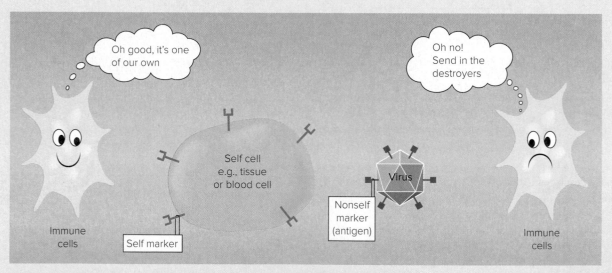

Immune cells learn to ignore cells marked "self" and to attack nonself antigens introduced into the body.

severe symptoms. A person is diagnosed with AIDS when CD4 T cells in the blood drop below a certain level (200/µ1), or when certain secondary, or opportunistic, infections are present. People with AIDS are vulnerable to a number of serious—often fatal—secondary, or opportunistic, infections.

The asymptomatic or incubation period of HIV—the time between the initial viral infection and the onset of disease symptoms—may range from months to 20 years, with an average of 11 years in untreated adults. Most infected people experience flu-like symptoms shortly after the initial infection, but most remain generally healthy for years. During this time, however, the virus is progressively infecting and destroying the cells of the immune system. People infected with HIV can pass the virus to others—even if they have no symptoms and especially if they do not know they have been infected.

Transmitting the Virus HIV lives only within cells and body fluids, not outside the body. It is transmitted by blood and **blood products**, semen, preejaculate, vaginal and cervical secretions, rectal fluid, and breast milk. It cannot live in air, water, or saliva, or on objects or surfaces such as toilet seats, eating utensils, or telephones. A person is not at risk of getting HIV infection by being in the same classroom, dining room, or even household with someone who is infected.

There are three main routes of HIV transmission:

• Specific kinds of sexual contact

• Direct exposure to infected blood

• Contact between an HIV-infected woman and her child during pregnancy, childbirth, or breastfeeding

These means of transmission are discussed in the following sections.

SEXUAL CONTACT HIV is more likely to be transmitted through unprotected vaginal or anal intercourse than by other sexual activities. During vaginal intercourse, male-to-female transmission is more likely to occur than female-to-male transmission. HIV has been found in preejaculatory fluid, so transmission can occur before ejaculation. Any trauma or irritation of tissues, such as those that can occur through rough or unwanted intercourse or through the overuse of spermicides, increases the risk of HIV transmission. The presence of lesions or blisters from other STIs also makes it easier for the virus to be passed.

Oral-genital contact carries some risk of transmission, although less than vaginal or anal intercourse. The risk of HIV transmission during oral sex increases if a participant has oral sores, even if from poor oral hygiene practice (which can include bleeding gums from vigorous flossing or brushing just before or after oral sex). Some evidence suggests that drinking alcohol before oral sex may make the cells that line the mouth more susceptible to infection with HIV.

Although the majority of HIV infection cases worldwide result from heterosexual contact, the most common means of HIV exposure among Americans is sexual activity between men (MSM); heterosexual contact and injection drug use (IDU) are the next most common means of exposure in the United States (Figure 14.3).

CONTACT WITH INFECTED BLOOD Needles used to inject drugs are usually contaminated with the user's blood. If needles are shared, small amounts of one person's blood are injected into another person's bloodstream. About 6% of all new U.S. cases of HIV are caused through the sharing of drug injection equipment contaminated with HIV. HIV can be transmitted through subcutaneous and intramuscular injection as well, from needles or blades used in acupuncture, tattooing, ritual scarring, and piercing of any body part.

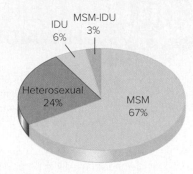

MSM = Men who have sex with men
IDU = Injection drug users

Figure 14.3 Routes of HIV transmission among Americans newly diagnosed with HIV infection in 2017.
SOURCE: Centers for Disease Control and Prevention. *HIV Surveillance Report* vol. 29. (http://www.cdc.gov/hiv/library/reports/hiv-surveillance.html) accessed November 2018.

CONTACT BETWEEN MOTHER AND CHILD The final major route of HIV transmission is mother to child, also called *vertical,* or *perinatal, transmission,* which can occur during pregnancy, childbirth, or breastfeeding. The number of new cases of HIV/AIDS among American infants has declined more than 90% since 1992 because of testing and treatment of infected women with anti-HIV drugs. Treatment is expensive, however, and vertical transmission

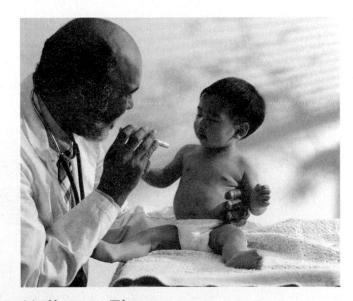

Wellness Tip The CDC recommends HIV screening for all pregnant women at the first prenatal visit to protect the health of mothers and their infants. Currently available treatments can significantly increase the chance that this baby, born to an HIV-infected mother, will be free of the virus.

Don Mason/Corbis/Getty Images

blood products Elements of whole blood such as plasma, platelets, and red blood cells that are used in replacement therapy. **TERMS**

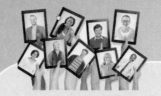

DIVERSITY MATTERS
HIV/AIDS Around the World

HIV continues to disproportionately affect nonwhite racial and ethnic populations and the poor. Adolescent girls and young women are at particularly high risk; HIV was among the top five causes of death for girls aged 10–14 in 2017. The gender imbalance is even more pronounced in sub-Saharan Africa, the hardest-hit region, where girls and young women aged 15–24 accounted for one in five new infections, despite being just 10% of the population. Factors at the root of this disparity include harmful gender norms and inequalities, violence, poverty, and lack of access to sexual and reproductive health services. Other key populations at risk worldwide include gay men and other men who have sex with men, people who inject drugs, sex workers, clients of sex workers, transgender people, prisoners, and other sex partners of at-risk populations. These groups are often marginalized and stigmatized, reducing their access to services, which in turn increases rates of infection.

Efforts to combat AIDS are complicated by political, economic, and cultural barriers. Education and prevention programs are often hampered by resistance from social and religious institutions and by the taboo on openly discussing sexual issues. Condoms are not commonly used in many countries, and women in many societies do not have the necessary control over sexual situations to insist that men use condoms. Empowering women is a crucial priority in reducing the spread of HIV. In particular, reducing sexual violence against women, promoting financial independence, and increasing women's education and employment opportunities are essential.

Despite the ongoing tragedy of the epidemic, strides have been made in treatment and prevention. By 2017, an estimated 21.7 million people were accessing treatment, compared with 8 million in 2010. Due to these scaled-up efforts, the rates of new infections and deaths have declined in some regions. Treating HIV with effective drugs not only prolongs life and decreases suffering, but it also reduces the spread of the virus because individuals who have received treatment are generally much less infectious than those who have not.

Successful prevention approaches include STI treatment and education, public education campaigns about safer sex, improved access to condoms, and syringe-exchange programs for injection drug users. In addition, male circumcision has been shown to reduce the risk of heterosexually acquired HIV infection in men by about 60%; the World Health Organization (WHO) recommends voluntary adult male circumcision as part of prevention programs in

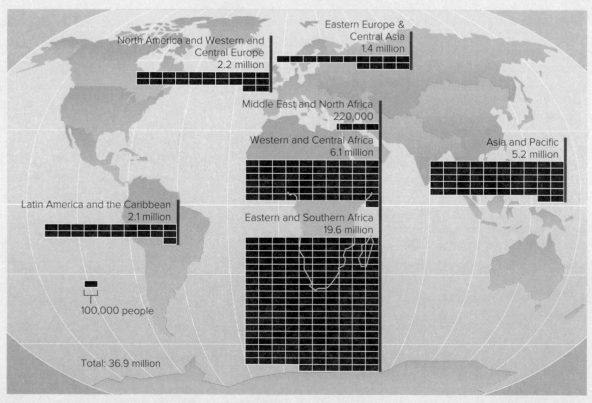

Approximate number of people living with HIV/AIDS in 2017.

continues to be a major threat worldwide (see the box "HIV/AIDS Around the World"). Cesarean delivery further reduces the risk of HIV transmission in women with high blood levels of HIV.

Symptoms Within a few days or weeks of infection with HIV, some victims develop symptoms of *primary HIV infection.* These can include fever, fatigue, rashes, headache, swollen lymph nodes, body aches, night sweats, sore throat, nausea, and ulcers in the mouth. Because the symptoms of primary HIV infection are similar to those of many common viral illnesses, the condition often goes undiagnosed.

Because the immune system is weakened, people with HIV infection are highly susceptible to other infections, both common and uncommon. The infection most often seen among people with HIV is *Pneumocystis* pneumonia, a fungal infection. Kaposi's sarcoma, a once-rare form of cancer, is common in HIV-infected men. Women with HIV infection often have frequent and difficult-to-treat vaginal yeast infections. Cases of tuberculosis are also increasingly being reported in people with HIV.

Diagnosis Three general types of HIV diagnostic tests are currently available:

- *HIV antibody tests,* performed on blood or oral fluids, check whether the body is producing antibodies against the HIV virus; these tests usually detect infection within 3–12 weeks after exposure.

- *Combination HIV antigen/antibody* tests look both for antibodies and for an HIV antigen known as p24 (part of the virus itself). Because the antigen is produced before antibodies develop, combination blood tests can detect HIV earlier in the course of infection (usually two to six weeks after exposure), compared to antibody-only tests.

- *Nucleic acid tests (NATs)* test directly for HIV RNA in the blood and can usually detect HIV within one to four weeks after infection; the test is expensive and not routinely used for initial screening.

A positive result is always confirmed with follow-up tests. Because it takes time for HIV RNA, p24 antigens, and HIV antibodies to become detectable, it is important to consider the timing of testing. The window period—the time between infection with HIV and when a test can accurately detect it—varies with the type of test and with the individual. If you get an HIV test within three months after a potential HIV exposure and the result is negative, get tested again in three months. Testing for HIV is recommended for everyone (see the box "Getting an HIV Test").

If a person is diagnosed as **HIV positive**, the next step is to determine the severity of the disease to plan appropriate treatment. The infection can be monitored by tracking the amount of virus in the body (the viral load).

Treatment Although there is no known cure for HIV infection, medications can significantly alter the course of the disease and extend life. The drop in the number of U.S. AIDS deaths that has occurred since 1996 is due in large part to the increasing use of combinations of new drugs. Treatment can reduce viral loads to undetectable levels, which helps keep patients healthy and greatly reduces the risk of transmitting the infection.

The main types of antiviral drugs used against HIV/AIDS are reverse transcriptase inhibitors, protease inhibitors, integrase inhibitors, and entry inhibitors. These drugs either block HIV from replicating itself or prevent it from infecting other cells. More than 30 drugs are now available to treat HIV, including two once-a-day tablets (containing three combined HIV medications). In addition to antiviral drugs, most patients with low CD4 T cell counts take a variety of antibiotics to help prevent opportunistic infections such as pneumonia, tuberculosis, and other bacterial and fungal infections.

In some cases, medications are used to prevent infection in people who have been exposed to HIV, such as victims of sexual assault and health care workers with potential exposure to

HIV positive A diagnosis resulting from the presence of HIV antibodies in the bloodstream; also referred to as *seropositive.*

TERMS

CRITICAL CONSUMER
Getting an HIV Test

Who and How Often?

The CDC recommends that everyone between the ages of 13 and 64 be tested for HIV at least once as part of routine health care. Routine HIV testing will increase the likelihood that people with HIV will be diagnosed earlier. People with certain risk factors should be tested more often. The CDC recommends testing at least once a year for anyone who answers yes to any of the following questions:

- Are you a man who has had sex with another man?

- Have you had sex—anal or vaginal—with an HIV-positive partner?

- Have you had more than one sex partner since your last HIV test?

- Have you injected drugs and shared needles or works (for example, water or cotton) with others?

- Have you exchanged sex for drugs or money?

- Have you been diagnosed with or sought treatment for another sexually transmitted infection?

- Have you been diagnosed with or treated for hepatitis or tuberculosis (TB)?

- Have you had sex with someone who could answer yes to any of the above questions or with someone whose sexual history you don't know?

In addition, CDC guidelines state that sexually active gay and bisexual men may benefit from more frequent testing (every three to six months). If you decide to get an HIV test, you can either visit a physician or health clinic or take a home test.

Physician or Clinic Testing

Your physician, student health clinic, Planned Parenthood, public health department, or local AIDS association can arrange your HIV test. Testing usually costs $50–$100, but public clinics often charge little or nothing. The standard test involves drawing a sample of blood that is sent to a lab, which checks using one or more of the available test types. For accuracy and early diagnosis, the CDC recommends laboratory tests done in the following sequence:

1. Combination test; if it is positive for antibodies and/or p24 antigen, this is followed by

2. Specialized antibody test, which confirms which type of HIV is present

3. If findings from the second test are indeterminate or contradictory, the NAT test is done to confirm if HIV RNA is present.

It takes three weeks or more for results of these tests to become available, and you'll be asked to phone or come in personally to obtain your results, which should also include appropriate counseling. Alternative tests are available at some clinics. The OraSure test uses oral fluid, which is collected by placing a treated cotton pad in the mouth. Rapid tests are also available at some locations. These tests involve the use of blood or oral fluid and

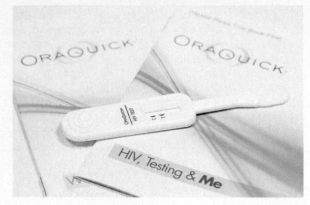

Kristoffer Tripplaar/Alamy Stock Photo

can provide results in as little as 20 minutes. If a rapid test is positive for HIV infection, a confirmatory test will be performed.

Before getting tested, be sure you understand what will be done with the results. Results from confidential tests may become part of your medical record or be reported to state and federal public health agencies. If you decide you want to be tested anonymously, ask your physician or counselor about an anonymous test, or use a home test.

Home Testing

Home HIV test kits are available and cost about $40–$70. Use OraQuick, a home test kit with FDA approval, rather than other tests sold on the internet. Similar to the OraSure clinic test, the OraQuick test uses a sample taken from the mouth and returns results in 20 minutes. Anyone testing positive should call their health care professional or the OraQuick Consumer Support Center for counseling and routes to care. The results of home test kits are completely anonymous.

Understanding the Results

A negative test result means that no evidence of infection was found—no antibodies or, if you had a combination test, p24 antigens. However, as noted earlier, it may take three weeks or even longer for the infection to be detectable. Therefore, an infected person may get a false-negative result. If you think you've been exposed to HIV, get a test immediately; if it's negative but your risk of infection is high, ask about a NAT test, which allows very early diagnosis. If you engage in any risky behaviors, get retested frequently.

A positive result means that you are infected. It is important to seek medical care and counseling immediately. Rapid progress is being made in treating HIV, and treatments are potentially much more successful when begun early. For more information on testing, visit the National HIV and STI Testing Resources website (https://gettested.cdc.gov/).

SOURCES: Centers for Disease Control and Prevention. 2018. *HIV Basics: Testing* (http://www.cdc.gov/hiv/basics/testing.html); AIDS.gov. 2018. *HIV Test Types* (https://www.aids.gov/hiv-aids-basics/prevention /hiv-testing /hiv-test-types/index.html); Centers for Disease Control and Prevention. 2019. *Home Tests* (https://www.cdc.gov/hiv/testing/hometests.html).

HIV-infected blood or body fluids. This type of treatment, called postexposure prophylaxis (PEP), should begin as soon as possible after exposure, but always within 72 hours.

The cost of treatment for HIV continues to be an area of major concern. Pharmaceutical companies, the World Bank, and the international community are working to lower drug costs and provide aid for developing regions. The high cost of drugs in the United States, especially in the case of HIV therapy, helps explain why the U.S. rate of viral load suppression is so much lower than in other high-income countries. The HIV viral suppression rate, reflecting the proportion of people with HIV considered healthy and noncontagious, is estimated to be about 54% in the United States, compared to 84% in the United Kingdom and 76% in Germany. The U.S. viral suppression rate is also lower than in African countries such as Kenya and Zimbabwe. HIV treatment is also challenging because taking the combination drugs is complicated, and the drugs have short-term side effects that may cause people to stop taking them. The drugs can also have long-term side effects, including serious health problems in some individuals.

The best hope for stopping the spread of HIV worldwide rests with the development of a safe, effective, and inexpensive vaccine. Many approaches to the development of an AIDS vaccine are currently under investigation, and human trials have begun on several vaccines. However, no vaccine is likely to be ready for widespread use within the next decade. Researchers are making more rapid progress in producing a microbicide that could be used to prevent HIV and other STIs. A microbicide in the form of a cream, gel, sponge, or suppository could function as a kind of chemical condom.

Prevention Although AIDS is currently incurable, it is preventable. Approaches to prevention include abstinence, consistent condom use with all sexual acts, and needle exchange programs for persons who use intravenous drugs. The FDA has approved a drug to be taken by people who do not have HIV but are at high risk for it. It is called a preexposure prophylaxis (PrEP), meaning that it is a prevention method intended to be used with other methods for reducing HIV risk.

You can protect yourself by avoiding behaviors that may bring you into contact with HIV. This means making careful choices about sexual activity (Figure 14.4) and not sharing needles if you inject drugs.

Anal and vaginal intercourse are the sexual activities associated with the highest risk of HIV infection. If you have intercourse, always use a condom (see the box "Using Male Condoms"). The use of a lubricated condom reduces the risk of transmitting HIV during all forms of intercourse. Condoms are not perfect, and they do not provide risk-free sex. When used properly, however, a condom provides a high level of protection against HIV and other STIs. Experts also suggest the use of latex squares and dental dams, devices that can be used as barriers during oral-genital or oral-anal sexual contact. Also, avoid using lubricants and lubricated condoms that contain the spermicide nonoxynol-9 (N-9). This spermicide has been shown to cause tissue irritation, which can make STI transmission more likely.

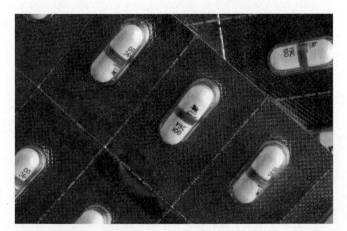

Wellness Tip If you have a possible exposure to HIV, talk to your doctor immediately (within three days) about the possibility of short-term treatment, known as postexposure prophylaxis. Starting medicine immediately and taking it for four weeks can reduce (but not eliminate) your chance of getting HIV.

Will & Deni McIntyre/Science Source

High Risk

Unprotected anal sex is the riskiest sexual behavior, especially for the receptive partner.

Unprotected vaginal intercourse is the next riskiest, especially for women, who are much more likely to be infected by an infected male partner than vice versa.

Oral sex is probably considerably less risky than anal and vaginal intercourse but can still result in HIV transmission.

Sharing of sex toys can be risky because they can carry blood, semen, or vaginal fluid.

Use of a condom reduces risk considerably but not completely for any type of intercourse. Anal sex with a condom is riskier than vaginal sex with a condom; oral sex with a condom is less risky, especially if the man does not ejaculate.

Hand-genital contact and deep kissing are less risky but could still theoretically transmit HIV; the presence of cuts or sores increases risk.

Sex with only one uninfected and totally faithful partner is without risk but effective only if both partners are uninfected and completely monogamous.

Activities that don't involve the exchange of body fluids carry no risk: hugging, massage, closed-mouth kissing, masturbation, phone sex, and fantasy.

Abstinence is without risk. For many people, it can be an effective and reasonable method of avoiding HIV infection and other STDs during certain periods of life.

No Risk

Figure 14.4 What's risky and what's not: The approximate relative risk of HIV transmission of various sexual activities.

Although they're not 100% effective as a contraceptive or as protection from STIs—only abstinence is—condoms improve your chances on both counts. Use them properly:

- **Buy latex condoms.** If you're allergic to latex, use a polyurethane condom or wear a lambskin condom under a latex one.

- **Buy and use condoms while they are fresh.** Packages have an expiration date or a manufacturing date. Don't use condoms beyond the expiration date or more than five years after the manufacturing date (two years if they contain spermicide).

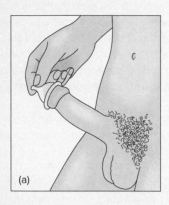

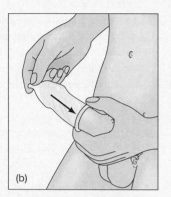

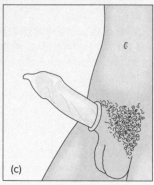

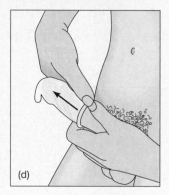

- **Try different styles and sizes.** Male condoms come in a variety of textures, colors, shapes, lubricants, and sizes. Shop around until you find a brand that's right for you. Condom widths and lengths vary by about 10–20%. A condom that is too tight may be uncomfortable and more likely to break; one that is too loose may slip off.

- **Don't remove the condom from its individual, sealed wrapper until you're ready to use it.** Open the packet carefully. Don't use a condom if it is gummy, dried out, or discolored.

- **Store condoms correctly.** Don't leave condoms in extreme heat or cold, and don't carry them in a pocket or wallet.

- **Use only water-based lubricants such as K-Y Jelly.** Never use oil-based lubricants like Vaseline or hand lotion; they may cause the condom to break. Avoid oil-based vaginal products.

- **Avoid condoms with lubricants containing the spermicide nonoxynol-9 (N-9).** N-9 causes tissue irritation that increases the risk of STI transmission.

- **Practice.** Condoms aren't hard to use, but practice helps. Take one out of the wrapper; examine it and stretch it to see how strong it is. Practice by yourself and with your partner.

Open the discussion of using condoms with your partner *before* you have sex. Despite the embarrassment most people feel at bringing up the subject, at least one study has shown that even if you have to *insist* on using condoms, your partner will feel more comfortable.

Use of the Male Condom

(a) Place the rolled-up condom over the head of the erect penis. Hold the top half-inch of the condom (with air squeezed out) to leave room for semen. (b) While holding the tip, unroll the condom onto the penis. Gently smooth out any air bubbles. (c) Unroll the condom down to the base of the penis. (d) To avoid spilling semen after ejaculation, hold the condom around the base of the penis as the penis is withdrawn. Remove the condom away from your partner, taking care not to spill any semen.

Chlamydia

Chlamydia trachomatis causes **chlamydia**, the most prevalent bacterial STI in the United States. According to the CDC, about 2.8 million new chlamydia infections occur each year, half of them undiagnosed and untreated. For women, the highest rates of infection occur among 15–24 year olds. For men, the highest rates occur among 20–24 year olds. Black men and women have chlamydia infection rates nearly six times higher than those of white men and women.

C. trachomatis can be transmitted by sexual contact with the penis, vagina, mouth, or anus of an infected partner. Ejaculation does not have to occur for chlamydia to be transmitted or acquired. If a mother has untreated chlamydia, it can be transmitted to the newborn perinatally (during the birthing process),

leading to neonatal conjunctivitis (a type of eye infection) and pneumonia. Having a chlamydia infection increases the risk of HIV transmission.

Both men and women are susceptible to chlamydia, but women bear the greater burden because of possible complications and consequences of the disease. If left untreated, chlamydia can lead to *pelvic inflammatory disease (PID),* a serious infection that can cause infertility. PID is discussed later in this chapter.

Chlamydia can also lead to infertility in men, although not as often as in women. In men under age 35, chlamydia is the most

chlamydia An STI transmitted by the bacterium *Chlamydia trachomatis.*

common cause of *epididymitis*—inflammation of the sperm-carrying ducts. In men, up to half of all cases of urethritis—inflammation of the urethra—are caused by chlamydia.

Symptoms Most people experience few or no symptoms from chlamydia infection, increasing the likelihood that they will inadvertently spread the infection to their partners. In men, symptoms can include painful urination, a watery discharge from the penis, and sometimes pain around the testicles.

Women may notice increased vaginal discharge, burning with urination, pain or bleeding with intercourse, and lower abdominal pain. Because infection rates are high and most women are asymptomatic, annual screening is recommended for sexually active young women.

Diagnosis and Treatment Chlamydia is diagnosed through a urine test or laboratory examination of fluid from the urethra or cervix. After chlamydia has been diagnosed, the infected person and his or her partner(s) are given antibiotics—usually doxycycline, erythromycin, or a newer drug, azithromycin, which can cure chlamydia in a single dose. It is important for the infected person's partner to be tested and treated. If a one-dose treatment is used, couples should wait seven days after taking their medication to resume sexual activity. The CDC now recommends that women and men who have been treated for chlamydia be retested three months after treatment is completed.

Gonorrhea

Gonorrhea is caused by the bacterium *Neisseria gonorrhoeae,* which flourishes in mucous membranes. It is transmitted in the same way as chlamydia. The CDC estimates that there are more than 820,000 new gonorrhea infections each year in the United States. The highest incidence is among 15–24-year-olds. Like chlamydia, untreated gonorrhea can cause PID in women and urethritis and epididymitis in men. It can also cause arthritis and rashes, and it occasionally affects internal organs. An infant passing through the birth canal of an infected mother may contract *gonococcal conjunctivitis,* an infection in the eyes that can cause blindness if not treated.

Symptoms In men, the incubation period for gonorrhea is brief, generally two to seven days. The first symptoms are due to urethritis, which causes urinary discomfort and a thick, yellowish-white or yellowish-green discharge from the penis. The lips of the urethral opening may become inflamed and swollen. In some cases, the lymph glands in the groin become enlarged and swollen. Many men have very minor symptoms or none at all.

Most women with gonorrhea are asymptomatic. Those who have symptoms often experience urinary pain, increased vaginal discharge, and severe menstrual cramps. Women may also develop painful abscesses in the Bartholin's glands, a pair of glands located on either side of the opening of the vagina. Up to 40% of women with untreated gonorrhea develop PID.

Gonorrhea can also infect the throat of people who engage in oral sex or the rectum of people who engage in anal sex. Gonorrhea symptoms in the throat may be a sore throat or pus on the tonsils, and those in the rectum may be pus or blood in the feces or rectal pain and itching.

Diagnosis and Treatment Gonorrhea is detectable by several tests. Depending on the test, samples of urine or vaginal, cervical, urethral, throat, or rectal fluids may be collected by the patient or provider. Antibiotics are used to treat gonorrhea, but increasing drug resistance is a major concern. People with gonorrhea often also have chlamydia, requiring additional antibiotics to treat that infection.

Pelvic Inflammatory Disease

Pelvic inflammatory disease (PID) is a major complication in 10–40% of women who have been infected with either chlamydia or gonorrhea and have not received treatment. PID occurs when the initial infection travels upward, often along with other bacteria, beyond the cervix into the uterus, oviducts, ovaries, and pelvic cavity. PID is often serious enough to require hospitalization and sometimes surgery. Even if the disease is treated successfully, about 25% of affected women will have long-term problems such as a continuing susceptibility to infection, ectopic pregnancy, infertility, and chronic pelvic pain. PID is the leading cause of infertility in young women. An estimated 2.5 million American women ages 18–44 have been diagnosed with PID.

Symptoms Symptoms of PID vary greatly. Some women, especially those with PID from chlamydia, may be asymptomatic;

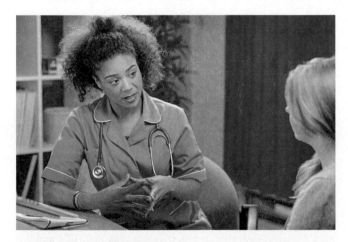

Wellness Tip Like many other STIs, chlamydia and gonorrhea are often symptomless. For this reason alone, it's a good idea to talk to your doctor about your risks and the need for STI testing. If you don't have a regular source of health care, visit https://gettested.cdc.gov to find a testing center near you.

Sturti/E+/Getty Images

> **gonorrhea** An STI transmitted by the bacterium *Neisseria gonorrhoeae.*
>
> **pelvic inflammatory disease (PID)** An infection that progresses from the vagina and cervix to the uterus, oviducts, and pelvic cavity.
>
> **TERMS**

others may feel very ill with abdominal pain, fever, chills, nausea, and vomiting. Early symptoms are essentially the same as those described for chlamydia and gonorrhea. Symptoms often begin or worsen during or soon after a woman's menstrual period. Many women have abnormal vaginal bleeding—either bleeding between periods or heavy and painful menstrual bleeding.

Diagnosis and Treatment Diagnosis of PID is made on the basis of symptoms, physical examination, ultrasound, and laboratory tests. **Laparoscopy** may be used to confirm the diagnosis and obtain material for cultures.

Treatment should begin as quickly as possible to minimize damage to the reproductive organs. Antibiotics are usually started immediately; in severe cases, the woman may be hospitalized and antibiotics given intravenously. It is especially important that an infected woman's partners be treated. As many as 60% of the male contacts of women with PID are infected but asymptomatic.

Human Papillomavirus (HPV)

Human papillomavirus (HPV) infection causes several human diseases, including common warts, **genital warts**, and genital cancers. HPV also causes virtually all cervical cancers, as well as anal, penile, vulvar, vaginal, and some forms of oropharyngeal cancers. Genital HPV is usually spread through sexual activity, including oral sex. HPV is the most common STI in the United States, and 80% of sexually active people are infected at some point in their lives. The body clears the infection within 2 years in most cases, but in others, infection persists. It is estimated that 42% of adults ages 18–59 have active genital HPV infections, and 7% have active oral HPV infections. A person with an active infection, even if she or he has no symptoms, can transmit the virus to a partner. HPV is especially common in young people, with some of the highest infection rates among college students.

The types of HPV that cause warts do not cause cancer. Infection with a high-risk HPV strain, if it persists, can cause cancer. HPV vaccination can prevent most HPV-linked cancers from occurring. Currently, only one vaccine, Gardasil 9, is available in the United States. The vaccine protects against seven cancer-causing HPVs, two of which are responsible for 70% of cervical cancers, as well as two HPVs that cause 90% of genital warts. The CDC recommends routine vaccination for all boys and girls at 11–12 years of age, although the vaccine can be given as early as age 9. The vaccine is most effective when given before exposure to genital HPV, and this virus is so common that many young people will be exposed to it shortly after becoming sexually active. Vaccination is recommended for women through 26 years of age and men through 21. HPV vaccine is also recommended up to age 26 for the following people if they did not receive it when they were younger:

- Young men who have sex with men
- Young adults who are transgender
- Young adults with conditions that compromise their immune systems

Symptoms HPV-infected tissue often appears normal; it may also look like anything from a small bump on the skin to a large warty growth. Untreated warts can grow together to form a cauliflower-like mass. In males, they appear on the penis and often involve the urethra, appearing first at the opening and then spreading inside. The growths may cause irritation and bleeding, leading to painful urination and a urethral discharge. Warts may also appear around the anus or within the rectum.

In women, warts may appear on the labia or vulva and may spread to the *perineum,* the area between the vagina and the anus. If warts occur only on the cervix, the woman will generally have no symptoms or awareness that she has HPV.

The incubation period ranges from 1 month to 2 years from the time of contact. People can be infected with the virus and be capable of transmitting it to their sex partners without having any symptoms at all. The vast majority of people with HPV infection have no visible warts or symptoms of any kind.

Diagnosis and Treatment Genital warts are usually diagnosed based on the appearance of the lesions. Frequently, HPV infection of the cervix is detected on routine Pap tests.

Treatment of genital warts focuses on reducing the number and size of warts. The currently available treatments do not eradicate HPV infection. Warts may be removed by cryosurgery (freezing), electrocautery (burning), or laser surgery. Direct applications of a cytotoxic acid may be used, and there are treatments that patients can use at home.

Even after treatment and the disappearance of visible warts, the individual may continue to carry HPV in healthy-looking tissue and can probably still infect others. Anyone who has ever had HPV should inform all partners. Condoms should be used, even though they do not provide total protection. As with HIV, circumcision may provide some protection against HPV.

Genital Herpes

Genital herpes affects about 1 in 6 adults in the United States. Two types of herpes simplex viruses, HSV 1 and HSV 2, cause genital herpes and oral-labial herpes (cold sores). Both types of virus are spread by skin-to-skin contact with infected areas, often during vaginal, anal, or oral sex, and by kissing. Sores found around the genitals, anus, or inner thighs are called genital herpes and are usually caused by HSV 2; those around the lips, mouth, and throat are called oral herpes, and are usually caused by HSV 1. Oral sex can transmit both types between the mouth and genital regions. Infection with HSV is generally lifelong;

TERMS

laparoscopy   A method of examining the internal organs by inserting a tube containing a small light through an abdominal incision.

human papillomavirus (HPV)   The virus that causes human warts, including genital warts, and is responsible for many genital cancers.

genital warts   A sexually transmitted viral infection characterized by growths on the genitals; caused by HPV.

genital herpes   A sexually transmitted infection caused by the herpes simplex virus.

after infection, the virus lies dormant in nerve cells and can reactivate at any time. Because the virus dies quickly outside the body, you can't get herpes from hugging, holding hands, coughing, sneezing, or sitting on toilet seats.

HSV 1 infection is so common that 50–80% of adults have antibodies to HSV 1 (indicating previous exposure to the virus). Most people are exposed to HSV 1 during childhood. HSV 2 infection usually occurs during adolescence and early adulthood, most commonly between ages 18 and 25. About 16% of adults have antibodies to HSV 2.

HSV 2 is almost always sexually transmitted, including during oral sex. The infection spreads readily whether people have active sores or are completely asymptomatic. If you have ever had an outbreak of genital herpes (that is, the appearance of genital sores), you should consider yourself always contagious and inform your partners. Avoid intimate contact when any sores are present, and use condoms during all sexual contact, including times when you have no symptoms. One study showed that using condoms for every act of intercourse results in a 30% decrease in the transmission of herpes compared with no condom use.

Newborns can occasionally be infected with HSV, usually during passage through the birth canal of an infected mother. Without treatment, 65% of newborns with HSV will die, and most who survive will have some degree of brain damage. Pregnant women who have ever been exposed to genital herpes should inform their physician so that appropriate precautions can be taken to protect the baby from infection.

Symptoms Most people who are infected with HSV have no symptoms. Those who develop symptoms often first notice them within 2–20 days of having sex with an infected partner. The first episode of genital herpes frequently causes flu-like symptoms in addition to genital lesions. The lesions usually heal within three weeks, but the virus remains alive in an inactive state within nerve cells. A new outbreak of herpes can occur at any time. On average, newly diagnosed people will experience five to eight outbreaks a year, with a decrease in the frequency of outbreaks over time. Outbreaks can be triggered by a number of events, including stress, illness, fatigue, sun exposure, sexual intercourse, and menstruation.

Diagnosis and Treatment Genital herpes can be diagnosed on the basis of symptoms; a sample of fluid from the lesions may also be sent to a laboratory for evaluation. Several blood tests can detect the presence of HSV antibodies in the blood and may alert many asymptomatic people to the fact that they are infected.

There is no cure for herpes. Once infected, a person carries the virus for life. Antiviral drugs such as acyclovir can be taken at the beginning of an outbreak to shorten the severity and duration of symptoms. Support groups are available to help people learn to cope with herpes. There is no vaccine to prevent herpes infection, but research is ongoing.

Hepatitis B

Hepatitis (inflammation of the liver) can cause serious and sometimes permanent damage to the liver, which can result in death in severe cases. One of the many types of hepatitis is caused by hepatitis B virus (HBV). Hepatitis B virus can be spread through nonsexual close contact.

HBV is found in all body fluids, including blood and blood products, semen, saliva, urine, and vaginal secretions. It is easily transmitted through any sexual activity that involves the exchange of body fluids, the use of contaminated needles, and any blood-to-blood contact, including the use of contaminated razor blades, toothbrushes, and eating utensils. Note that HBV is not usually spread by hugging, coughing, food or water, sharing eating utensils or drinking glasses, or casual contact.

Symptoms Many people infected with HBV never develop symptoms; they have what is known as a silent infection. The normal incubation period is 30–180 days. Mild cases of hepatitis cause flu-like symptoms. As the illness progresses, there may be nausea, vomiting, dark-colored urine, abdominal pain, and jaundice.

People with hepatitis B sometimes recover completely, but they can also become chronic carriers of the virus, capable of infecting others for the rest of their lives. Some chronic carriers remain asymptomatic, while others develop chronic liver disease. Chronic hepatitis can cause cirrhosis, liver failure, and a deadly form of liver cancer. In 2016, approximately 1,700 Americans died from hepatitis B. Worldwide, the annual death toll from hepatitis B exceeds 780,000.

Diagnosis and Treatment Blood tests can diagnose hepatitis by analyzing liver function and detecting the infecting organism. There is no cure for hepatitis B and no specific treatment for acute infections; antiviral drugs and immune system modulators may be used for chronic HBV infection to help delay or reverse liver damage. For people exposed to HBV, treatment with hepatitis B immunoglobulin can provide protection against the virus.

The vaccine for hepatitis B is safe and effective. Immunization is recommended for everyone under age 19 and for all adults at increased risk, including people who have more than one sex partner in six months, men who have sex with other men, those who inject drugs, and health care workers who are exposed to blood and body fluids.

Syphilis

Syphilis, a disease that once caused death and disability for millions, can now be treated effectively with antibiotics. Rates in the United States hit a low in 2001 but have increased steadily since then. In 2017, over 30,000 new cases of primary and secondary syphilis (the earliest and most transmissible stages) were reported in the United States.

TERMS

hepatitis Inflammation of the liver, which can be caused by infection, drugs, or toxins; some forms of infectious hepatitis can be transmitted sexually.

syphilis A sexually transmitted infection caused by the bacterium *Treponema pallidum*.

Syphilis is caused by a corkscrew-shaped bacterium called *Treponema pallidum.* It requires warmth and moisture to survive, and it dies very quickly outside the human body. The bacterium passes through any break or opening in the skin or mucous membranes and can be transmitted by kissing, vaginal or anal intercourse, or oral-genital contact.

The rate of syphilis has increased over 72% since 2013. Rates among men are far higher than for women, and the majority of new cases occur among MSM. Congenital syphilis—syphilis passed from pregnant women to their babies—has also sharply increased; the rates for infants born to black or Latina mothers was three and six times higher, respectively, compared to white mothers.

Symptoms Syphilis progresses through several stages. *Primary syphilis* is characterized by an ulcer called a **chancre** that appears within about 10–90 days after exposure. The chancre is usually found at the site where the organism entered the body. Chancres contain large numbers of bacteria and make the disease highly contagious when present; they are often painless and typically heal on their own within a few weeks.

Secondary syphilis is usually marked by mild, flu-like symptoms and a skin rash that appears three to six weeks after the chancre, often on the palms of the hands and soles of the feet.

If the disease remains untreated, the symptoms of secondary syphilis may recur over a period of several years. Affected individuals may then lapse into an asymptomatic latent stage in which they experience no further consequences of infection. However, in about 15% of cases of untreated syphilis, the individual develops *late,* or *tertiary syphilis,* with symptoms that can appear 10–20 years after infection. Late syphilis can damage many organs of the body, possibly causing severe dementia, cardiovascular damage, blindness, and death.

In infected pregnant women, syphilis can cross the placenta. If the mother is not treated, the probable result is stillbirth, prematurity, or congenital deformity. In some cases, the infant is born infected *(congenital syphilis)* and requires treatment.

Diagnosis and Treatment Syphilis is diagnosed by examination of infected tissues and with blood tests. All stages can be treated with antibiotics, but damage from late syphilis can be permanent.

Other STIs

A few other infections are transmitted sexually, but they can be avoided by practicing responsible sexual behavior.

Trichomoniasis, often called *trich,* is the most prevalent nonviral STI in the United States and is estimated to affect some 3.7 million individuals. The single-celled organism that causes trich, *Trichomonas vaginalis,* thrives in warm, moist conditions, making women particularly susceptible to these infections in the vagina. Women who become symptomatic with trich develop a yellowish-green, diffuse, or foul-smelling vaginal discharge and severe itching and vulvar irritation. Men may develop inflammation of the urethra, epididymis, or prostate. Prompt treatment with oral metronidazole (Flagyl) is important because studies suggest that trich may increase the risk of HIV transmission and,

in pregnant women, premature delivery. Although trich is treatable, reinfection is common.

Bacterial vaginosis (BV) is the most common cause of abnormal vaginal discharge in women of reproductive age. BV occurs when healthy bacteria that normally inhabit the vagina become displaced by unhealthy species. BV is clearly associated with sexual activity and often occurs after a change in partners. Symptoms of BV include vaginal discharge with a fishy odor and sometimes vaginal irritation. BV is treated with topical and oral antibiotics.

Lymphogranuloma venereum (LGV) is an infection of the lymphatic system caused by three strains of the bacteria *Chlamydia trachomatis* (not the same strain that causes the genital STI chlamydia). LGV is more common in men than in women; the main risk factor is being HIV positive. The first symptom is an ulcer at the site of sexual penetration that appears 3–30 days after exposure; there may also be swollen glands in the genital area. Among those who practice anal receptive intercourse, symptoms may include rectal ulcers, bleeding, and pain. If the infection is untreated, chronic symptoms may develop, so individuals with symptoms should see a physician. If you have this infection, your partner should be referred for testing and treatment.

Pubic lice (commonly known as *crabs*) and **scabies** are highly contagious parasitic infections. Treatment is generally easy, although lice infestation can require repeated applications of medications.

WHAT YOU CAN DO ABOUT STIs

Because STIs can have serious, long-term effects, be vigilant about exposure, treatment, and prevention.

Education

Many schools have STI counseling and education programs. These programs allow students to practice communicating with potential sex partners and negotiating for safer sex, to engage in role-playing to build self-confidence, and to learn how to use condoms.

You can find free pamphlets and other literature about STIs at public health departments, health clinics, physicians' offices,

---

TERMS

chancre The sore produced by syphilis in its earliest stage.

trichomoniasis A protozoal infection caused by *Trichomonas vaginalis;* transmitted sexually and externally.

bacterial vaginosis (BV) A condition caused by an overgrowth of certain bacteria inhabiting the vagina.

lymphogranuloma venereum (LGV) An infection of the lymphatic system caused by three strains of the bacteria *Chlamydia trachomatis,* transmitted sexually.

pubic lice Parasites that infest the hair of the pubic region; commonly called *crabs.*

scabies A contagious skin disease caused by burrowing parasitic mites.

- **Abstinence.** The only truly foolproof way to protect yourself from STIs is abstinence—abstaining from sexual relations with other people. Remember that it is okay to say no to sex.

- **Monogamy.** Next to abstinence, the most effective way to protect yourself is monogamy—having sex exclusively with one partner, who engages in sex with no one else but you, and who does not have an STI.

- **Communication.** If you choose to be sexually active, protect yourself by practicing open and honest communication and insisting on the same from your partner. Be truthful about your past, and ask your partner to do the same. Remember that you are indirectly exposing yourself to all of your partner's prior sexual contacts.

- **Safer sexual activities.** Know which sexual activities are risky (see Figure 14.4). Safer alternatives to intercourse include fantasy, hugging, massage, rubbing clothed bodies together, mutual masturbation, and closed-mouth kissing.

- **Condoms.** Always use latex condoms during every act of vaginal intercourse, anal intercourse, and oral sex. Multiple studies show that regular condom use can reduce the risk of several diseases, including HIV, chlamydia, and genital herpes.

- **Activities to avoid.** Don't drink or use drugs in sexual situations. Mood-altering drugs can affect your judgment and make you more likely to engage in risky behaviors. Limit your number of sexual partners; having multiple partners is associated with increased risk of STIs. Avoid sexual contact with partners who have an STI or have had unprotected sex in the past. Avoid sexual contact that could cause tears or cuts in the skin or tissue. Don't inject drugs; don't share needles, syringes, or anything that might have blood on it. Decontaminate needles and syringes with household bleach and water. If you are at risk for HIV infection, don't donate blood, sperm, or organs.

- **Other preventive measures.** Get tested for HIV during your next routine medical examination. Have periodic screenings for STIs if you are at risk. Make sure all your vaccinations are up-to-date; if appropriate for you, get vaccinated against HPV and/or hepatitis B.

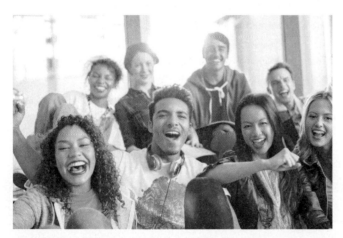

Wellness Tip All STIs are preventable. You can greatly reduce your risk of exposure to STIs by following the guidelines given throughout this chapter and by making responsible sexual choices.

Caia Images/Glow Images

student health centers, and Planned Parenthood; easy-to-understand books are available in libraries and bookstores. National hotlines provide free, confidential information and referral services to callers anywhere in the country (see "For Further Exploration" at the end of the chapter).

Diagnosis and Treatment

Early diagnosis and treatment of STIs can help you avoid complications and can also help prevent the spread of infection. If you are sexually active, be alert and seek treatment for any sign or symptom of disease, such as a rash, a discharge, sores, or unusual pain. Many STIs can be asymptomatic, however, so a professional examination and testing are recommended following any risky sexual encounter—even in the absence of symptoms.

Prevention

The only sure way to avoid exposure to STIs is to abstain from sexual activity. If you choose to be sexually active, think about prevention before you have a sexual encounter or find yourself in the "heat of the moment." Plan ahead for safer sex. For tips and strategies, see the box "Protecting Yourself from STIs." Remember that asking questions and being aware of signs and symptoms show that you care about yourself and your partner. Concern about STIs is an essential and mutually beneficial part of a sexual relationship.

If you are diagnosed as having an STI, begin treatment as quickly as possible. Inform your partner(s) and avoid any sexual activity until your treatment is complete.

? *Ask Yourself*

QUESTIONS FOR CRITICAL THINKING AND REFLECTION?

Have you ever engaged in sexual activities you regretted later? If so, what were the circumstances, and what influenced you to act the way you did? Were there any negative consequences? What preventive strategies can you use in the future to make sure it doesn't happen again?

TIPS FOR TODAY AND THE FUTURE

RIGHT NOW YOU CAN

- Make an appointment with your health care provider if you are worried about possible STI infection.
- Resolve to discuss condom use with your partner if you are sexually active and are not already using condoms.

IN THE FUTURE YOU CAN

- Learn how to communicate effectively with a partner who resists safer sex practices or is reluctant to discuss his or her sexual history. Support groups and classes can help.
- Make sure all your vaccinations are up-to-date; ask your doctor if you should be vaccinated against any STIs.
- Follow instructions for treatment carefully and take all medication as prescribed.

SUMMARY

- HIV damages the immune system and causes AIDS. People with AIDS are vulnerable to often-fatal opportunistic infections.

- HIV is carried in blood and blood products, semen, vaginal and cervical secretions, and breast milk; it is transmitted through the exchange of these fluids.

- Drugs have been developed to slow the course of HIV infection and to prevent or treat certain secondary infections, but there is no cure.

- Chlamydia is a bacterial infection that causes epididymitis and urethritis in men and can lead to PID in women.

- Untreated, gonorrhea can cause PID in women and epididymitis in men, leading to infertility. In infants, untreated gonorrhea can cause blindness.

- Pelvic inflammatory disease (PID), a complication of untreated chlamydia or gonorrhea, is an infection of the uterus and oviducts that may extend to the ovaries and pelvic cavity. It can lead to infertility, ectopic pregnancy, and chronic pelvic pain.

- Infection with human papillomavirus (HPV) can cause genital warts as well as cervical and other cancers. Treatment does not eradicate the virus, but a vaccine is available.

- Genital herpes is a common incurable viral infection characterized by outbreaks of lesions and periods of latency.

- Hepatitis B is a viral infection of the liver transmitted through sexual and nonsexual contact. Some people become chronic carriers of the virus and may develop serious, potentially fatal, complications.

- Syphilis is a highly contagious bacterial infection that can be treated with antibiotics. If left untreated, it can lead to deterioration of the central nervous system and death.

- Other common STIs include trichomoniasis, bacterial vaginosis, pubic lice, and scabies.

- Successful diagnosis and treatment of STIs involves being alert for symptoms, getting tested, informing partners, and following treatment instructions.

- All STIs are preventable; the key is practicing responsible sexual behaviors.

FOR FURTHER EXPLORATION

American College Health Association. Offers information on STIs, alcohol use, acquaintance rape, and other issues.

http://www.acha.org/

American Sexual Health Association (ASHA). Provides information and referrals on STIs; sponsors support groups for people with herpes and HPV.

http://www.ashasexualhealth.org/

The Body: The Complete HIV/AIDS Resource. Provides information about prevention, testing, and treatment, and includes an online risk assessment.

http://www.thebody.com

Centers for Disease Control and Prevention: National Prevention Information Network. Provides extensive information and links on AIDS and other STIs.

https://npin.cdc.gov/

Centers for Disease Control and Prevention: National STI and AIDS Hotlines. Callers can obtain information, counseling, and referrals for testing and treatment. The hotlines offer information on more than 20 STIs and include Spanish and TTY service.

800-342-AIDS or 800-227-8922; 800-344-SIDA (Spanish) 800-243-7889 (TTY, deaf access)

HIV InSite: Gateway to AIDS Knowledge. Provides information about prevention, education, treatment, statistics, clinical trials, and new developments.

http://hivinsite.ucsf.edu

Joint United Nations Program on HIV/AIDS (UNAIDS). Provides statistics and information on the international HIV/AIDS situation.

http://www.unaids.org

MedlinePlus: Sexually Transmitted Diseases. Maintained by the CDC; a clearinghouse of links and information on STIs and other sexual health topics.

http://www.nlm.nih.gov/medlineplus/sexualhealthissues.html

Planned Parenthood Federation of America. Provides information on STIs, family planning, and contraception.

http://www.plannedparenthood.org

Smarter Sex. Designed for college students; provides tips and information on safer sex practices, relationships, STIs, and more.

http://smartersex.org/index.asp

COMMON QUESTIONS ANSWERED

Q **Why do young people, including college students, have high rates of STIs?**

A Half of all STI cases in the United States are accounted for by young people. Contributing factors may include the following:

• *College students underestimate their risk of STIs and HIV.* Although students may know about STIs, they often believe the risks do not apply to them. One study of students with a history of STIs showed that more than half had unprotected sex while they were infected, and 25% of them continued to have sex without ever informing their partner(s).

• *Risky sexual behavior is common.* In the 2018 American College Health Association survey of undergraduates, two-thirds of students reported that they had been sexually active during the past year, and 25% reported having multiple partners. However, the percentage of students who reported consistent use of condoms and other protective barriers was low. Another study found that 19% of male students and 33% of female students had consented to sexual intercourse simply because they felt awkward refusing. Many young adults are sexually active but not yet in long-term monogamous relationships; they are more likely to have more than one partner over time and to have a partner with an STI.

• *Alcohol and drug use play an important role.* Between one-third and one-half of college students report participating in sexual activity as a direct result of being intoxicated. Students who binge drink are more likely to have multiple partners, use condoms inconsistently, and delay seeking treatment for STIs than students who drink little or no alcohol. Sexual assaults occur more frequently when either the perpetrator or the victim has been drinking.

Q **Does the success of the new AIDS drugs mean that I don't need to worry about HIV infection anymore?**

A No. The new combination drug therapy has had dramatic effects for some people infected with HIV. In the United States, the number of HIV-infected people who progress to AIDS each year is declining, as is the death rate from AIDS. But the new drugs are expensive, can have serious side effects, and are not effective for everyone. Scientists do not yet know how long the drugs will keep HIV at bay, and no treatment has yet been shown to permanently eradicate HIV from the body. AIDS is still an incurable, fatal disease.

Q **Which contraceptive methods protect best against STIs?**

A Latex male condoms are the best known protection against HIV and other STIs. Condoms are not foolproof, however, and they do not protect against the transmission of diseases from sores that they do not cover.

Other contraceptive methods may provide some protection against certain STIs. The diaphragm and cervical cap cover the cervix and may offer some protection against diseases that involve the infection of cervical cells. Combining these barrier methods with a condom can provide even greater protection.

Hormonal methods such as oral contraceptives do not protect against STIs in the lower reproductive tract but do provide some protection against PID. If vaginal irritation occurs from the use of spermicides, the risk of infection with HIV and other STIs may actually increase.

Q **Why are women hit harder by STIs than men?**

A Sexually transmitted infections cause suffering for all who are infected, but in many ways, women and girls are the hardest hit, for both biological and social reasons:

• *Male-to-female transmission of many infections is more likely to occur than female-to-male transmission.* This is particularly true of HIV.

• *Young women are even more vulnerable to STIs than older women because the less mature cervix is more susceptible to injury and infection.* As a woman ages, the cells at the opening of the cervix gradually change so that the tissue becomes more resistant to infection. Young women are also more vulnerable for social and emotional reasons: Lack of control in relationships, fear of discussing condom use, and having an older sex partner are all linked to increased STI risk.

• *Once infected, women tend to suffer more consequences of STIs than men.* For example, gonorrhea and chlamydia can cause PID and permanent damage to the oviducts in women, while these infections tend to have less serious effects in men. HPV infection causes nearly all cases of cervical cancer. HPV infection is also associated with penile cancer in men, but penile cancer is much less common than cervical cancer. Women also have the added concern of the potential effects of STIs during pregnancy.

• *Women with HIV infection often face greater challenges when they are ill.* Women may become sicker at lower viral loads compared to men. Women and men with HIV do about as well if they have similar access to treatment, but in many cases women are diagnosed later in the course of HIV infection, receive less treatment, and die sooner. In addition, they may be caring for family members who are also infected and ill. The proportion of new AIDS cases in women is increasing both in the United States and globally.

• *Worldwide, social and economic factors play a large role in the transmission and consequences of AIDS and other STIs for women.* Practices such as very early marriage for women, often to much older men who have had many sexual partners, place women at risk for infection. Cultural gender norms that promote premarital and extramarital relationships for men, combined with women's lack of power to negotiate safe sex, make infection a risk even for women who are married and monogamous. In some parts of the world, the stigma of AIDS hits women harder. In addition, lack of education and limited economic opportunities can force women into commercial sex work, placing them at high risk for all STIs. Solutions to the STI crisis in women include greater access to health care as well as empowerment in the social sphere.

SELECTED BIBLIOGRAPHY

Alcaid, M. L., et al. 2016. The incidence of Trichomonas vaginalis infection in women attending nine sexually transmitted diseases clinics in the USA. *Sexually Transmitted Infections* 92(1): 58–62.

American College Health Association. 2018. *American College Health Association–National College Health Assessment: Undergraduate Reference Group Executive Summary Fall 2017.* Hanover, MD: American College Health Association.

American Sexual Health Association. 2015. *Herpes Testing* (http://www.ashasexualhealth.org/stdsstis/herpes/herpes-testing/).

American Sexual Health Association. 2015. *HPV* (http://www.ashasexualhealth.org/stdsstis/hpv/).

Centers for Disease Control and Prevention. 2014. *Laboratory Testing for the Diagnosis of HIV Infection: Updated Recommendations.* Atlanta, GA: Centers for Disease Control and Prevention.

Centers for Disease Control and Prevention. 2015. *Hepatitis B Information for Health Professionals* (http://www.cdc.gov/hepatitis/hbv/).

Centers for Disease Control and Prevention. 2016. *Vaccine Information Statements: Human Papillomavirus VIS* (https://www.cdc.gov/vaccines/hcp/vis/vis-statements/hpv.html).

Centers for Disease Control and Prevention. 2017. *Syphilis—CDC Fact Sheet (Detailed)* (https://www.cdc.gov/std/syphilis/stdfact-syphilis-detailed.htm).

Centers for Disease Control and Prevention. 2017. *STD Facts: Chlamydia* (http://www.cdc.gov/std/chlamydia/stdfact-chlamydia.htm)

Centers for Disease Control and Prevention. 2018. *Expedited Partner Therapy* (http://www.cdc.gov/std/ept/default.htm).

Centers for Disease Control and Prevention. 2018. *HIV Basics: PEP* (https://www.cdc.gov/hiv/basics/pep.html).

Centers for Disease Control and Prevention. 2018. *Sexually Transmitted Disease Surveillance, 2017.* Atlanta, GA: U.S. Department of Health and Human Services.

Centers for Disease Control and Prevention. 2018. *Viral Hepatitis Statistics and Surveillance* (http://www.cdc.gov/hepatitis/Statistics/).

Centers for Disease Control and Prevention. 2018. *Adolescent and School Health: Sexual Risk Behaviors: HIV, STD, & Teen Pregnancy Prevention* (https://www.cdc.gov/healthyyouth/sexualbehaviors).

Choopanya, K., et al. 2013. Antiretroviral prophylaxis for HIV infection in injecting drug users in Bangkok, Thailand (the Bangkok Tenofovir Study): A randomized, double-blind, placebo-controlled phase 3 trial. *Lancet* 381: 2083–2090.

de Voux A., et al. 2017. State-specific rates of primary and secondary syphilis among men who have sex with men—United States, 2015. *MMWR* 66: 349–354.

Ginocchio, C. C., et al. 2012. Prevalence of Trichomonas vaginalis and coinfection with Chlamydia trachomatis and Neisseria gonorrhoeae in the United States as determined by the Aptima Trichomonas vaginalis nucleic acid amplification assay. *Journal of Clinical Microbiology* 50(8): 2601–2608.

Hay, P. E., et al. 2015. Which sexually active young female students are most at risk of pelvic inflammatory disease? A prospective study. *Sexually Transmitted Infections* 92(1): 63–66.

Hutton, H. E., et al. 2013. Alcohol use, anal sex, and other risky sexual behaviors among HIV-infected women and men. *AIDS and Behavior* 17(5): 1694.

International AIDS Vaccine Initiative. 2013. *State of the Field* (http://www.iavi.org/What-We-Do/Science/Progress/Pages/default.aspx).

Kaiser Family Foundation. 2019. *HIV Viral Suppression Rate in U.S. Lowest Among Comparable High-Income Countries* (https://www.kff.org/hivaids/slide/hiv-viral-suppression-rate-in-u-s-lowest-among-comparable-high-income-countries).

Kreisel, K., et al. 2017. Prevalence of pelvic inflammatory disease in sexually experienced women of reproductive age—United States, 2013–2014. *MMWR* 66: 80–83.

Markowitz, L. E., et al. 2013. Reduction in human papillomavirus (HPV) prevalence among young women following HPV vaccine introduction in the United States, National Health and Nutrition Examination Surveys, 2003–2010. *Journal of Infectious Diseases* 208(3): 385–393.

McQuillan, G., et al. 2017. Prevalence of HPV in adults aged 18–69: United States, 2011–2014. *NCHS Data Brief* No. 280. Hyattsville, MD: National Center for Health Statistics.

Petrosky E., et al. 2015. Use of 9-valent human papillomavirus (HPV) vaccine: Updated HPV vaccination recommendations of the Advisory Committee on Immunization Practices. *MMWR* 64(11): 300–304.

Planned Parenthood. 2019. *Oral & Genital Herpes* (https://www.plannedparenthood.org/learn/stds-hiv-safer-sex/herpes).

Rosenberg, T. 2018. HIV drugs cost $75 in Africa, $39,000 in the U.S. Does it matter? *The New York Times*, September 18.

Saraceni, S., et al. 2014. High prevalence of HPV multiple genotypes in women with persistent Chlamydia trachomatis infection. *Infectious Agents and Cancer* 9: 30.

Tobian, A., et al. 2009. Male circumcision for the prevention of HSV-2 and HPV infections and syphilis. *New England Journal of Medicine* 360: 1298–1309.

UNAIDS. 2018. *Fact Sheet: Latest Statistics on the Status of the AIDS Epidemic* (http://www.unaids.org/en/resources/fact-sheet).

U.S. Department of Health and Human Services. 2018. *AIDS Global Statistics* (https://www.aids.gov/hiv-aids-basics/hiv-aids-101/global-statistics/).

U.S. Food and Drug Administration. 2018. *Information Regarding the OraQuick In-Home HIV Test* (http://www.fda.gov/BiologicsBloodVaccines/BloodBloodProducts/ApprovedProducts/PremarketApprovalsPMAs/ucm311895.htm).

Wellings, K., et al., ed. 2012. *Sexual Health: A Public Health Perspective.* Berkshire, England: Open University Press.

World Health Organization. 2018. *Hepatitis* (https://www.who.int/hepatitis/en/).

World Health Organization. 2018. *HIV/AIDS* (https://www.who.int/en/news-room/fact-sheets/detail/hiv-aids).

Name _____ Section _____ Date _____

LAB 14.1 Behaviors and Attitudes Related to STIs

Part I Risk Assessment

To identify your risk factors for STIs, read the following list of statements and mark whether they're true or false for you. *Note:* The statements in this assessment are worded in a way that assumes current sexual activity. If you have never been sexually active, you are not now at risk for STIs. Respond to the statements in the quiz based on how you realistically believe you would act. If you are currently in a mutually monogamous relationship with an uninfected partner or are not currently sexually active (but have been in the past), you are at low risk for STIs at this time. Respond to the statements in the quiz according to your attitudes and past behaviors. (For more on your risk factors for STIs, take the online assessment available at www.thebody.com.)

True	False	
_____	_____	1. I have only one sex partner.
_____	_____	2. I always use a latex condom for each act of intercourse, even if I am fairly certain my partner has no infections.
_____	_____	3. I do not use oil-based lubricants with condoms.
_____	_____	4. I discuss STIs and prevention with new partners before having sex.
_____	_____	5. I do not use alcohol or another mood-altering drug in sexual situations.
_____	_____	6. I would tell my partner if I thought I had been exposed to an STI.
_____	_____	7. I am familiar with the signs and symptoms of STIs.
_____	_____	8. I regularly perform genital self-examination to check for signs and symptoms of STIs.
_____	_____	9. When I notice any sign or symptom of any STI, I consult my physician immediately.
_____	_____	10. I have been tested for HIV or plan to be tested at my next routine medical exam.
_____	_____	11. I obtain screenings for STIs regularly. In addition (if female), I obtain recommended pelvic exams and Pap tests.
_____	_____	12. I have been vaccinated for hepatitis B and, if recommended for my age, for HPV.
_____	_____	13. When diagnosed with an STI, I inform all recent partners.
_____	_____	14. When I have a sign or symptom of an STI that goes away on its own, I still consult my physician.
_____	_____	15. I do not use drugs prescribed for friends or partners or left over from other illnesses to treat STIs.
_____	_____	16. I do not share syringes or needles to inject drugs.

Using Your Results

How did you score? False responses indicate attitudes and behaviors that may put you at risk for contracting STIs or for suffering serious medical consequences from them. How many false responses did you give? Are you satisfied that you're doing everything you can to protect yourself from STIs?

What should you do next? Any false response indicates a factor that you could change to reduce your risk for STIs. Choose one as the focus of a behavior change program.

LABORATORY ACTIVITIES

Part II Communication

Good communication with sex partners or potential sex partners is a critical component of STI prevention. Regardless of your responses to the risk assessment, complete this communication exercise to help build your communication skills.

1. List three ways to bring up the subject of STIs with a new partner. How would you ask whether he or she has been exposed to any STIs or engaged in any risky behaviors? (Remember that, because many STIs can be asymptomatic, it is important to know about past behaviors even if no STI was diagnosed.)

   a. _____

   b. _____

   c. _____

2. List three ways to bring up the subject of condom use with your partner. How might you convince someone who does not want to use a condom?

   a. _____

   b. _____

   c. _____

3. If you have had an STI in the past that you might possibly still pass on (e.g., herpes, genital warts), how would you tell your partner(s)?

   _____

   _____

4. If you were diagnosed with an STI that you believe was given to you by your current partner, how would you begin a discussion of STIs with her or him?

   _____

   _____

Design elements: Evidence for Exercise box (shoes and stethoscope): Vstock LLC/Tetra Images/Getty Images; Take Charge box (lady walking): VisualCommunications/E+/Getty Images; Critical Consumer box (man): Sam74100/iStock/Getty Images; Diversity Matters box (holding devices): Robert Churchill/iStockphoto/Rawpixel Ltd/Getty Images; Wellness in the Digital Age box (Smart Watch): Hong Li/DigitalVision/Getty Images

CHAPTER 15

Environmental Health

LOOKING AHEAD...

After reading this chapter, you should be able to

- Explain how population growth affects the earth's environment.

- Discuss the causes and effects of air and water pollution.

- Discuss the impact of solid waste on the environment and human health.

- Identify key sources of chemical and radiation pollution, and discuss methods for preventing such pollution.

- Explain the impact of energy use on the environment and strategies for using energy more efficiently.

TEST YOUR KNOWLEDGE

1. The world's current population is approximately
   a. 760 million
   b. 7.6 billion
   c. 76 billion
   d. 760 billion

2. Air pollution can be naturally occurring, as well as human made. True or false?

3. Light-emitting diode (LED) bulbs can last 40 times longer than standard incandescent light bulbs. True or false?

See answers on the next page.

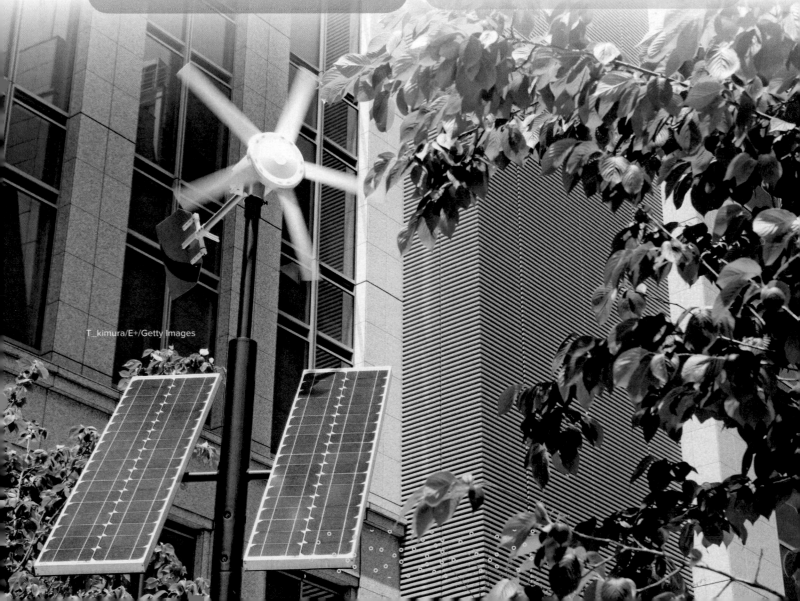

T_kimura/E+/Getty Images

We have always had to struggle against our **environment** to survive. Although the planet provides us with food, water, air, and everything else that sustains life, it also presents us with natural occurrences—earthquakes, tsunamis, hurricanes, drought, climate changes—that destroy life and disrupt society. Today, in addition to dealing with natural disasters, we also have to find ways to protect the environment and ourselves from the by-products of our way of life.

This chapter introduces the concept of environmental health and explains how the environment affects us. It also discusses the ways humans affect the planet and its resources, and the steps you can take to improve your personal environmental health while reducing your impact on the earth.

ENVIRONMENTAL HEALTH DEFINED

The field of **environmental health** grew out of efforts to control communicable diseases. When certain insects and rodents were found to carry microorganisms that cause disease in humans, campaigns were enacted to eradicate or control this pestilence. Scientists also recognized that *pathogens* (microorganisms that can produce diseases) could be transmitted in sewage, drinking water, and food. These discoveries led to systematic garbage collection, sewage treatment, filtration and chlorination of drinking water, food inspection, and the establishment of public health enforcement agencies.

These efforts to control and prevent communicable diseases changed the health profile of the industrialized world. Americans rarely contract cholera, typhoid fever, plague, diphtheria, or other diseases that once killed large numbers of people, but these diseases have yet to be eradicated worldwide. The importance of vaccine can be seen in the recent rise in measles: Because fewer Americans are getting the vaccine, the greatest number of cases has been reported in the United States since 1994 and since measles was declared eliminated in 2000. Every time we venture beyond the boundaries of our everyday world, whether traveling to a poorer country or camping in the wilderness, we are reminded of the importance of these basics: clean water, sanitary waste disposal, safe food, and insect and rodent control.

> **TERMS**
>
> **environment**   The natural and human-made surroundings in which we spend our lives.
>
> **environmental health**   The collective interactions of humans with the environment that promote human health and well-being and foster safe communities.

Answers (Test Your Knowledge)

1. **b.** The world's current population is about 7.6 billion, and it is expected to reach 9.7 billion by 2050.
2. **True.** There are many types of naturally occurring air pollution, such as smoke from forest fires and dust from dust storms.
3. **True.** Compared to regular light bulbs, LED bulbs use 10% as much energy and last up to 42 times longer.

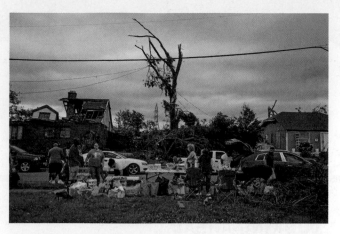

Wellness Tip Natural disasters—such as the central U.S. tornado outbreak in May 2019—expose harmful chemicals in destroyed buildings and wipe out essential services, leading to contaminated water and soil. Visit www.ready.gov and Appendix A to find out more about how to prepare for an emergency in your area, including putting together a basic disaster kit.

Megan Jelinger/SOPA Images/ZUMA Wire/Alamy Live News/Alamy Stock Photo

Rapid population growth (more than doubling in the past 50 years) has resulted in more people consuming and competing for resources and, thus, increasing human environmental impact. Although many environmental problems are complex and seem beyond the control of the individual, every person can find ways to make a difference to the future of the planet. Our responsibility is to pass on a world no worse, and preferably better, than the one we live in today.

Ask Yourself

QUESTIONS FOR CRITICAL THINKING AND REFLECTION?

How often do you think about the environment's impact on your personal health? In what ways do your immediate surroundings (your home, neighborhood, school, workplace) affect your well-being? In what ways do you influence the health of your personal environment?

POPULATION GROWTH AND CONTROL

Throughout most of human history, we have caused a minor pressure on the planet. About 300 million people were alive in the year 1 CE; by the time Europeans were settling in the Americas 1,600 years later, the world population had increased gradually to a little over half a billion. But then it began rising exponentially—zooming to one billion by about 1800, more than doubling by 1930, and then doubling again in just 40 years (Figure 15.1).

The world's population, currently about 7.6 billion, is increasing at a rate of about 80 million per year—approximately

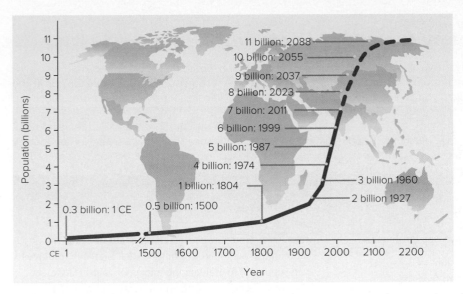

Figure 15.1 World population growth. The United Nations estimates that the world's population will continue to increase dramatically until it stabilizes above 11 billion people in 2100.
SOURCE: United Nations Population Division. 2017. *World Population Prospects: The 2017 Revision.* New York: United Nations. (https://population.un.org/wpp/DataQuery); US Census Bureau.

157 people every minute. The United Nations projects that world population will reach 9.7 billion by 2050.

The average number of children per woman fell from 5 in 1950 to half that (2.5) in 2010. This decline began in Western countries decades ago and is now happening in poor countries. In sub-Saharan Africa, Asia, and Latin America, women with more education have fewer children; these regions nevertheless contribute the most to population growth. Changes are also projected for the world's age distribution: For the first time in history, there are more older people than young children. By 2050, there will be 3.4 times more people aged 60 and over than children aged 4 and under.

Despite a slowing rate of expansion, the population is still always expanding. This rapid expansion of population, particularly in the past 50 years, is generally believed to be responsible for most of the stress humans put on the environment. A large and rapidly growing population makes it more difficult to provide the basic components of environmental health discussed earlier, including clean and disease-free food and water. It is also a driving force behind many of the relatively more recent environmental health concerns, including chemical pollution, global warming, and the thinning of the atmosphere's ozone layer.

Factors That Contribute to Population Growth

Although population growth poses significant challenges, population trends are difficult to influence and manage. A variety of interconnecting factors fuel the current population explosion:

- *High birth rates:* The combination of poverty, high child mortality rates, and a lack of social provisions of every

type is associated with high birth rates in the developing world. Families have many children to ensure that enough survive childhood to work for the household and care for parents in old age. Most countries, whether economically emerging or stable, have experienced significant reductions in birth rates as contraceptive use has increased. China offers a remarkable example of population control: Since 1979 its government limited couples to only one child. However, effective 2016, with its working-age population declining, the government increased the one-child policy to two children. Still, overall, the majority of economically emerging countries have fertility levels that ensure substantial population growth. In a small number of countries, which are among the poorest, birth rates continue to be very high.

- *Lack of family planning resources:* Half the world's couples don't use any form of family planning or contraceptives.

- *Lower death rates:* Although death rates remain relatively high in the developing world, they have decreased in recent years because of public health measures and improved medical care.

Changes in any of these factors can affect population growth, but the issues are complex. Increasing death rates through disease, famine, or war might slow population growth, but few people would argue in favor of these as methods of population control. Although the increased availability of family planning services is a crucial part of population management, cultural, political, and religious factors also need to be considered. To be successful, population management policies must change the condition of people's lives, especially poverty, to remove the pressures to have large families.

A report of the secretary general of the United Nations, prepared for the 50th session of the Commission on Population in 2017, found that internal migration can attenuate the impacts of an aging population. The report encourages countries to enable young people to move around, within their homelands and abroad. Other research indicates that the combination of improved health, better education, and increased literacy and employment opportunities for women works together with family planning to decrease birth rates.

How Many People Can the World Hold?

No one knows how many people the world can support, but most scientists agree that there is a limit. One estimate from the Global Footprint Network is that the population's demand for resources already exceeds the earth's capacity by 70%.

The primary factors that may eventually put a cap on human population are the following:

- *Food:* Enough food is currently produced to feed the world's entire population, but economic and sociopolitical factors have led to food shortages and famine. Food production can be expanded in the future, but better distribution of food will be needed as the world's population keeps growing. The makeup of the world's diet may also need to change. Some populations have eaten insects and used them to feed livestock for centuries, promoting them as a sustainable protein source. New technology for meatless burgers may also reduce our dependence on livestock. A current controversy is the use of "golden rice," a crop genetically modified to contain vitamin A and provide extra nutrition to economically emerging countries. Although many people oppose the use of genetically modified organisms (GMOs), others believe that GMOs can help solve the food crisis.

- *Available land and water:* Forests are cut for wood, soil is depleted, and water is withdrawn at ever-increasing rates. These trends contribute to local hardships and to many global environmental problems, including habitat destruction and species extinction.

- *Energy:* Currently, most of the world's energy comes from nonrenewable sources: oil, coal, natural gas, and nuclear power. As these sources are depleted, the world will have to shift to renewable (sustainable) energy sources, such as hydropower and solar, geothermal, wind, biomass, and ocean power. Supporting a growing population, maintaining economic productivity, and stemming environmental degradation will require both greater energy efficiency and an increased use of renewable energy sources.

- *Minimum acceptable standard of living:* The mass media have exposed the entire world to the American lifestyle and raised people's expectations of living at a comparable level. But such a lifestyle is supported by levels of energy consumption that the earth cannot support indefinitely. The United States has about 5% of the world's population but uses 25% of the world's energy. In contrast, India has 16% of the population but uses only 3% of the energy. China's energy consumption is increasing rapidly, and that nation accounts for 20% of the world's population. If all people are to enjoy a minimally acceptable standard of living, the population must be limited to a number that available resources can support. (To evaluate the impact of your lifestyle, see the box "Checking Your Environmental Footprint.")

AIR QUALITY AND POLLUTION

Air pollution is not a human invention or even a new problem. The air is polluted naturally with every forest fire, pollen bloom, and dust storm, as well as with countless other natural pollutants. Humans contribute to pollution with the by-products of our activities.

Air pollution is linked to a wide range of health problems, and the very young and the elderly are among the most vulnerable to its effects. For people with chronic ailments such as diabetes or heart failure, even relatively brief exposure to particulate air pollution can increase the risk of death by nearly 40%. Recent studies have linked exposure to air pollution to reduced lung capacity in teens, and atherosclerosis (thickening of the arteries) in adults. Further, the children of pregnant women exposed to air pollution in urban environments have reduced birth weight, reduced IQ, and increased instances of obesity. Combustion emissions cause about 200,000 deaths per year for those Americans with chronic illness.

Air Quality and Smog

The U.S. Environmental Protection Agency (EPA) uses a measure called the **Air Quality Index (AQI)** to indicate whether air pollution levels pose a health concern. The AQI is used for five major air pollutants:

- *Carbon monoxide (CO):* An odorless, colorless gas, CO forms when the carbon in **fossil fuels** does not burn completely. The primary sources of CO are vehicle

Air Quality Index (AQI) A measure of local air quality and explanation of its relationship to health.

fossil fuels Buried deposits of decayed animals and plants that are converted into carbon-rich fuels by exposure to heat and pressure over millions of years; oil, coal, and natural gas are fossil fuels.

TERMS

exhaust and fuel combustion in industrial processes. CO binds to blood cells in place of oxygen, depriving the body of oxygen and causing headaches, fatigue, and impaired vision and judgment. It also aggravates cardiovascular disease (CVD).

- *Sulfur dioxide (SO_2):* SO_2 is produced by the burning of sulfur-containing fuels such as coal and oil, during metal smelting, and by other industrial processes; power plants are a major source. In humans, SO_2 narrows the airways, which may cause wheezing, chest tightness, and shortness of breath, particularly in people with asthma. SO_2 may also aggravate symptoms of CVD.

- *Nitrogen dioxide (NO_2):* NO_2 is a reddish-brown, highly reactive gas formed when nitric oxide combines with oxygen in the atmosphere; major sources include motor vehicles and power plants. In people with respiratory diseases such as asthma, NO_2 affects lung function and causes symptoms such as wheezing and shortness of breath. NO_2 exposure may also increase the risk of respiratory infections.

- *Particulate matter (PM):* Particles of different sizes are released into the atmosphere from a variety of sources, including combustion of fossil fuels, crushing or grinding operations, industrial processes, and dust from roadways. PM can accumulate in the respiratory system, aggravate cardiovascular and lung diseases, and increase the risk of respiratory infections.

- *Ground-level ozone:* At ground level, ozone is a harmful pollutant. Where it occurs naturally in the upper atmosphere, it shields the earth from the sun's harmful ultraviolet rays. (The health hazards from the thinning of this protective ozone layer are discussed later in the chapter.) Ground-level ozone is formed when pollutants emitted by cars, power plants, industrial plants, and other sources react chemically in the presence of sunlight (photochemical reactions). Ozone can irritate the respiratory system, reduce lung function, aggravate asthma, increase susceptibility to respiratory infections, and damage the lining of the lungs. Short-term elevations of ozone levels have also been linked to increased death rates.

AQI values run from 0 to 500; the higher the AQI, the greater the level of pollution and associated health danger. When the AQI exceeds 100, air quality is considered unhealthy, for groups sensitive to pollution, and for everyone as AQI values rise over 150. For local areas, AQI values are calculated for each of the five pollutants listed earlier, and the highest value becomes the AQI rating for that day. Depending on the AQI value, local officials may issue precautionary health advice. Local AQI information is often available in newspapers, on television and radio, from state and local telephone hotlines, and from airnow.gov.

The term **smog** was first used in the early 1900s in London to describe the combination of smoke and fog. What we typically call smog today is a mixture of pollutants; ground-level ozone is the key ingredient. Heavy motor vehicle traffic, high temperatures, and sunny weather can increase the production of ozone.

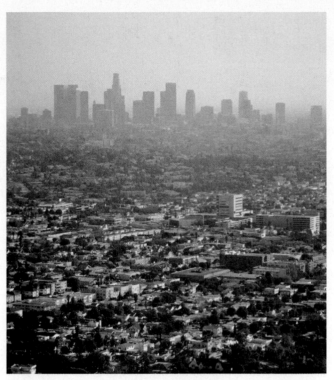

Fitness Tip Smog tends to form over cities because of great amounts of motor vehicle exhaust in the air and geographical features that restrict wind and airflow. Exercising in polluted outdoor air can reduce lung function, at least temporarily. When the air quality outside is bad, exercise indoors.

Izzy Schwartz/Photodisc/Getty Images

Pollutants are also more likely to build up in areas with little wind or where a topographic feature such as a mountain range or valley prevents the wind from pushing out stagnant air.

The Greenhouse Effect and Global Warming

Life on earth depends on a process known as the **greenhouse effect**, which contributes to a warm atmosphere. The temperature of the earth's atmosphere depends on the balance between the amount of energy the planet absorbs from the sun (mainly as high-energy ultraviolet radiation) and the amount of energy lost back into space as lower-energy infrared radiation. Key components of temperature regulation are carbon dioxide (CO_2), water vapor, methane, and other **greenhouse gases**—so named because,

---

TERMS

smog Hazy atmospheric conditions resulting from increased concentrations of ground-level ozone and other pollutants.

greenhouse effect A process that occurs when gases in earth's atmosphere trap the sun's heat.

greenhouse gas A gas (such as carbon dioxide) or vapor that traps infrared radiation instead of allowing it to escape through the atmosphere, resulting in a warming of the earth (the greenhouse effect).

Table 15.1	Sources of Greenhouse Gases
GREENHOUSE GAS	SOURCES
Carbon dioxide	Fossil fuel and wood burning, factory emissions, car exhaust, deforestation
Chlorofluorocarbons (CFCs)	Refrigeration and air conditioning, aerosols, foam products, solvents
Methane	Cattle, wetlands, rice paddies, landfills, gas leaks, coal and gas industries
Nitrous oxide	Fertilizers, soil cultivation, deforestation, animal feedlots and wastes
Ozone and other trace gases	Photochemical reactions, car exhaust, power plant emissions, solvents

like the glass panes in a greenhouse, they let through visible light from the sun but trap some of the resulting infrared radiation and reradiate it back to the earth's surface. This greenhouse effect causes a buildup of heat that raises the temperature of the lower atmosphere.

There is scientific consensus that this natural process has been disrupted by human activity, causing **global warming**, or *climate change*. The concentration of heat-trapping greenhouse gases is increasing because of human activity, especially the combustion of fossil fuels and emissions from agricultural production (Table 15.1). Carbon dioxide levels in the atmosphere have increased rapidly in recent decades and, for the first time in recorded history, exceeded 411 parts per million in 2018. The use of fossil fuels pumps more than 20 billion tons of CO_2 into the atmosphere every year. Experts believe CO_2 may account for about 60% of the greenhouse effect. Analysis of ice core samples shows that CO_2, methane, and nitrous oxide levels are now higher than at any time in at least the past 800,000 years. The United States is responsible for one-third of the world's total emissions of CO_2. Deforestation, often by burning, also releases CO_2 into the atmosphere and reduces the number of trees available to convert CO_2 into oxygen.

The year 2016 was the warmest since recordkeeping began in 1880. The global temperature has risen by about 2.0°F since the late 19th century. Most scientists agree that temperatures will continue to rise, although estimates vary as to how much they will change. If global warming persists, experts say the impact may be devastating (Figure 15.2). The effects of global warming are already having devastating consequences; current and potential future impacts include the following:

- Increased rainfall and flooding in some regions, increased drought in others. Coastal zones, where half the world's people live, would be severely affected.

- Increased mortality from heat stress, urban air pollution, and tropical diseases. Deaths from weather events such as hurricanes, tornadoes, droughts, and floods might also increase.

- A poleward shift of about 50–350 miles (150–550 km) in the location of vegetation zones, affecting crop yields, irrigation demands, and forest productivity.

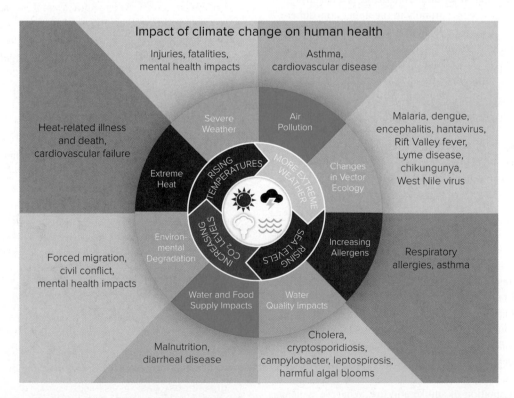

Figure 15.2 Climate effects on health. Climate change can influence health and disease in many ways; the effects may vary based on a person's location, age, socioeconomic status, and other factors.

SOURCE: Centers for Disease Control and Prevention. 2017. *Climate Effects on Health.* (http://www.cdc.gov/climateandhealth/effects); Fourth National Climate Assessment, vol. II. 2018. *Impacts, Risks, and Adaptation in the United States.* Washington, DC: U.S. Global Change Research Program.

- Alterations of ecosystems, resulting in possible species extinction.

- Increasingly rapid and drastic melting of the earth's polar ice caps. Arctic ice melts to some extent during the summer each year, but melting has increased by 20% since 1979. Extensive melting could mean increased flooding in the Northern Hemisphere, further changes in weather patterns, and the elimination of habitat for species that live in the Arctic.

According to EPA estimates, the earth's average surface temperature is likely to increase 4.0–8.0°F (7.2–14.4°C) by the end of the 21st century. Warming will not be evenly distributed around the globe. Land areas will warm more than oceans in part due to water's ability to store heat. High latitudes will warm more than low ones in part due to the effects of melting ice.

At the 2015 United Nations Climate Change Conference in Paris, France, a landmark agreement was made to limit average global warming to 2°C above pre-industrial temperatures, striving for a limit of 1.5°C, if possible. According to the Paris Agreement, each country is in charge of setting its own greenhouse emissions limits, so countries must pledge sufficient reductions in order for the agreement to be effective. President Obama considered the adoption of this agreement between the 195 participating countries a "turning point for the world." In June 2017, however, the new administration announced it would withdraw the United States from the Paris Agreement.

U.S. Greenhouse Gas Sources The primary economic sectors responsible for emissions of greenhouse gases in the United States are electricity production (28%), transportation (28%), industry (22%), commercial and residential (11%), and agriculture (9%). Across all these sectors, fossil fuel combustion is the major greenhouse gas source, accounting for 76% of all carbon dioxide emissions, which in turn account for 82% of total U.S. greenhouse gas emissions. Other sources of greenhouse gases include chemical reactions during industrial processes as well as management of waste and wastewater from homes and businesses. Agriculture contributes to greenhouse gas emissions in multiple ways, including the methane-producing digestive processes of cattle and other livestock; fertilizer use; manure and soil management; rice cultivation; and deforestation needed for cattle grazing and feed.

Should We Get Rid of Meat? If you like meat, a juicy burger can be one of your favorite meals. Scientists who specialize in creating plant-based foods have not been able to copy it—until now. The Impossible Burger and the Beyond Burger taste very close to meat. The texture and aroma are so close to beef that you don't know you are eating pea and wheat protein. Several fast-food restaurants now offer these burgers. If they catch on, the implication for the health of the environment is enormous.

Thinning of the Ozone Layer

Another air pollution problem is the thinning of the **ozone layer** of the atmosphere, a fragile, invisible layer about 10–30 miles above the earth's surface that shields the planet from the sun's hazardous ultraviolet (UV) rays. Since the mid-1980s, scientists have observed the seasonal appearance and growth of a hole in the ozone layer over Antarctica. More recently, thinning over other areas has been noted.

The ozone layer is being destroyed primarily by **chlorofluorocarbons (CFCs)**, industrial chemicals used as coolants in refrigerators and air conditioners, as foaming agents in some rigid foam products, as propellants in some kinds of aerosol sprays (most of which were banned in 1978), and as solvents. When CFCs rise into the atmosphere, winds carry them toward the polar regions. During winter, circular winds form a vortex that keeps the air over Antarctica from mixing with air from elsewhere. CFCs react with airborne ice crystals, releasing chlorine atoms, which destroy ozone. When the polar vortex weakens in the summer, winds richer in ozone from the north replenish the lost Antarctic ozone.

The largest and deepest ozone hole, recorded in 2000, measured 11.5 million square miles, larger than the surface of North America. Although the ozone hole has been consistently smaller since then, it neared that size again in 2015. The Antarctic ozone layer has begun to show signs of healing, but because of the long lifetimes of ozone-depleting substances in the atmosphere, it will likely not return to its early 1980s state until about 2050. More recent concern is for the thinning ozone layer at midlatitudes, where most people live. The chemicals that eat away at ozone come from natural and human-made sources. Because of an international agreement that regulates the production of ozone-depleting chemicals, overall atmospheric ozone is no longer decreasing. The gradual overall recovery will include annual variations caused by weather fluctuations over Antarctica.

Without the ozone layer to absorb the sun's UV radiation, life on earth would be impossible. The potential effects of increased long-term exposure to UV light for humans include skin cancer, wrinkling and aging of the skin, cataracts and blindness, and reduced immune response. Some scientists blame ozone loss for many cases of melanoma. UV radiation levels under the Antarctic hole were high enough to cause sunburn within seven minutes.

UV light may interfere with photosynthesis and cause lower crop yields; it may also kill phytoplankton and krill, the basis of the ocean food chain. And because heat generated by the absorption of UV rays in the ozone layer helps create stratospheric winds, the driving force behind weather patterns, a drop in the concentration of ozone may have already begun to alter the earth's climate systems.

TERMS

global warming An increase in the earth's atmospheric temperature when averaged across seasons and geographical regions; also called climate change.

ozone layer A layer of ozone molecules (O_3) in the upper atmosphere that screens out UV rays from the sun.

chlorofluorocarbons (CFCs) Chemicals used as spray-can propellants, refrigerants, and industrial solvents; implicated in the destruction of the ozone layer.

Energy Use and Air Pollution

Americans are now the second biggest energy consumers in the world; Chinese are first. We use energy to create electricity, transport us, power our industries, and run our homes. About 80% of the energy we use comes from fossil fuels—oil, coal, and natural gas. The remainder comes from nuclear power and renewable energy sources such as hydroelectric, wind, and solar power.

Energy consumption is at the root of many environmental problems. Automobile exhaust and the burning of oil and coal by industry and by electric power plants are primary causes of smog and acid precipitation. The mining of coal and the extraction and transportation of oil cause pollution on land and in the water; the 2010 oil spill in the Gulf of Mexico was the worst environmental disaster in American history and one of the largest oil spills ever to occur. Nuclear power generation creates hazardous wastes and carries the risk of dangerous releases of radiation.

Two key strategies for controlling energy use are conservation and the development of nonpolluting, renewable sources of energy. Although the use of renewable energy sources has increased in recent years, renewables still supply only a small proportion of our energy, in part because of their cost. Some countries have chosen to promote energy efficiency by removing subsidies or adding taxes on the use of fossil fuels. This strategy is reflected in the varying prices drivers pay for gasoline. For example, drivers in France, Germany, and England pay more than twice per gallon than drivers in the United States, where more than 70% of commuters drive alone to work, and low-fuel-economy sport utility vehicles (SUVs) remain popular. The largest SUVs increase greenhouse gas emissions by six-plus tons more per year than an average car.

Alternative Fuels The U.S. Department of Energy (DOE) is encouraging researchers and automobile manufacturers to produce vehicles that can handle alternative fuels such as

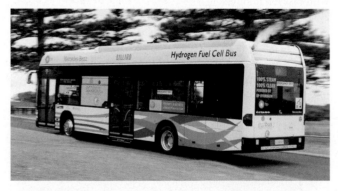

Wellness Tip Your transportation choices can help reduce air pollution. Bike, walk, or use public transportation whenever possible; public transit may provide a choice of vehicles, including hybrid and electric options. When selecting your own vehicle, research your choices at fueleconomy.gov.

Paul Kane/Getty Images

ethanol. Ethanol, a form of alcohol, is a renewable fuel produced from fermenting plant sugars in corn, sugarcane, and other starchy agricultural products. Ethanol use reduces the amount of oil required to produce gasoline, reduces overall greenhouse gas emissions from automobiles, and supports the U.S. agricultural industry. Ethanol has been mixed with gasoline for years in the United States, but several other countries (such as Brazil) use ethanol much more extensively.

Ethanol, however, has its critics, who say the alternative fuel may do more harm than good. For one thing, some reports show that corn-based ethanol requires more energy to produce than it yields when burned as fuel. Other reports dispute this point, and improvements in manufacturing processes may reduce the amount of energy required to make the fuel. Ethanol made from sugarcane and other plant matter may be far more energy efficient, say some experts.

Potential drawbacks of ethanol are the diversion of corn crops from the food supply to produce the fuel, and the billion-dollar federal subsidies to farmers for ethanol production. These practices have been blamed for skyrocketing food prices and food shortages around the world, which have led to food riots in several countries. Food-related concerns prompted the United Nations to call for a moratorium on food-based ethanol production until nonfood sources of alternative fuels could be developed.

Another alternative fuel is biodiesel, a fuel made primarily from vegetable oils, fats, or greases—most famously from recycled restaurant grease. It is the fastest-growing alternative fuel in the United States, is biodegradable, and produces lower levels of most air pollutants than petroleum-based products. Biodiesel, like ethanol, can be problematic depending on its material source. The plants used to make it, such as soybeans and palm oil trees, absorb carbon dioxide as they grow, which can offset the carbon dioxide produced while making and using biodiesel. In such cases, the biodiesel is carbon neutral. Most of the biodiesel used in the United States is made from soybean oil that is a by-product of processing soybeans for animal feed and numerous other food and nonfood products, and from waste animal fat and grease. But in some parts of the world, natural vegetation and forests have been cleared and burned to grow soybeans and palm oil trees to make biodiesel, and these negative environmental and social effects can outweigh any benefit.

Hybrid and Electric Vehicles Hybrid vehicles use two or more distinct power sources to propel the vehicle, such as an on-board energy storage system (batteries, for example) and an internal combustion engine and electric motor. The hybrid vehicle typically realizes greater fuel economy than a conventional car does and produces fewer polluting emissions. Hybrids also tend to run with less noise than conventional vehicles. Many hybrid models are currently available in the United States, but they typically cost several thousand dollars more than their conventional gas-powered counterparts. Still, hybrids are gaining popularity with consumers and are being used more commonly in both corporate and government vehicle fleets.

Another type of alternative vehicle is all-electric. In these vehicles, electricity is stored in battery packs and then converted into mechanical power that runs the vehicle. After a given number of miles, the batteries must be recharged. These vehicles do not produce tailpipe emissions, but generators that produce the electricity for the batteries do emit pollutants. All-electric vehicles are gaining credibility and popularity. Changing consumer perceptions regarding trip use and distance capacity have led to growth in "quick-charging station" infrastructure and a new generation of all-electric vehicles with better battery storage. Researchers hope that hybrid and battery technologies can be extended to all classes of vehicles.

Indoor Air Pollution

Although most people associate air pollution with the outdoors, your home may also harbor potentially dangerous pollutants. Some of these compounds trigger allergic responses, and others have been linked to cancer and developmental problems in children. Common indoor pollutants include the following:

- *Environmental tobacco smoke (ETS),* a human carcinogen that also increases the risk of asthma, bronchitis, and cardiovascular disease. The definition of ETS has broadened to include toxic residues of thirdhand smoke, chemicals that linger on indoor surfaces and in dust long after smoking stops. Most states and cities have passed legislation known as clean indoor air acts, which state that enclosed, indoor areas used by the public shall be smoke-free except for certain designated areas.

- *Carbon monoxide and other combustion by-products,* which can cause chronic bronchitis, headaches, dizziness, nausea, fatigue, and even death. Common sources in the home are woodstoves, fireplaces, kerosene heaters and lamps, and gas ranges. Gas stoves produce nitrogen dioxide, carbon monoxide, and formaldehyde, which can cause health problems. In poverty-stricken areas, especially in Asia and Africa, people commonly burn solid fuels like coal for cooking and heating their homes. The World Health Organization says the smoke and by-products from these indoor fires kill about 1.5 million people annually—mostly children. Solid fuels are the primary heating source for about 6.5 million Americans.

- *Volatile organic compounds (VOCs),* gases emitted from certain solids and liquids, including formaldehyde gas, which can cause eye, nose, and throat irritation; shortness of breath; headaches; nausea; dizziness; lethargy; and, over the long term, cancer. VOCs are found in paints, lacquers, cleaning supplies, aerosols, construction materials, dry-cleaned clothing, furnishings, and office equipment. No regulatory standards have been set for VOCs in nonindustrial environments.

- *Biological pollutants,* including bacteria, dust mites, mold, and animal dander, which can cause allergic reactions and other health problems. These allergens are typically found in bathrooms, damp or flooded basements, humidifiers, air conditioners, and even some carpets and furniture.

- *Indoor mold,* fungi that grow in damp places, such as on shower tiles and damp basement walls. More than 100 common indoor molds have been classified as potentially hazardous to people, but only a few are serious threats to human health. One of the most common of these is *Stachybotrys* mold, commonly known as "toxic black mold." It is greenish black in color and appears slimy when wet. Toxic mold spores permeate the air and can cause health problems when inhaled, especially for people with asthma and other respiratory conditions.

Preventing Air Pollution

You can do a great deal to reduce air pollution. Here are a few ideas:

- Cut back on driving. Ride your bike, walk, use public transportation, or carpool in a fuel-efficient vehicle. When carbon monoxide, nitrogen dioxide, and particulate matter pollution were reduced in Los Angeles County, the number of hospitalizations for asthma decreased.

- Keep your car tuned and well maintained. Tires inflated at recommended pressures reduce tailpipe emissions of CO_2. To save energy when driving, avoid quick starts, stay within the speed limit, limit the use of air conditioning, and don't let your car idle unless absolutely necessary. Have your car's air conditioner checked and serviced by a station that uses environmentally friendly refrigerants (automotive air conditioners made before 1994 are a major source of CFCs).

- Buy energy-efficient appliances and use them only when necessary. Run the washing machine, dryer, and dishwasher only when you have full loads, and do laundry in warm or cold water instead of hot; don't overdry your clothes. Clean refrigerator coils and clothes dryer lint screens frequently. Towel or air-dry your hair rather than using an electric dryer.

- Use energy-efficient lighting: halogen, light-emitting diode (LED), or compact fluorescent bulbs (not fluorescent tubes). For more information, see the box "Energy-Efficient Lighting."

- Make sure your home is well insulated with ozone-safe agents; use insulating shades and curtains to keep heat in during winter and out during summer.

- Plant and care for trees in your yard and neighborhood. They recycle carbon dioxide, so trees work against global warming. They also provide shade and cool the air, so less air conditioning is needed.

- Before discarding a refrigerator, air conditioner, or dehumidifier, check with the waste hauler or your local

Energy-Efficient Lighting

Lighting accounts for about 6% of all residential electricity use. Switching to energy-efficient lighting is a good way to cut your home's energy use, lower your energy bills, and reduce your environmental footprint.

The Energy Independence and Security Act (EISA) of 2007 set national performance standards for light bulbs for the first time, requiring that basic bulbs be at least about 25% more efficient; the standards were phased in between 2012 and 2014. Traditional incandescent light bulbs did not meet these new efficiency standards, so use of other lighting choices has grown:

- **Halogen incandescents:** More energy-efficient incandescent bulbs that also last up to three times longer than traditional bulbs.

- **Compact fluorescent light bulbs (CFLs):** Long-lasting fluorescents that work in many types of household fixtures. These bulbs contain a very small amount of mercury and require special handling if they are broken (visit epa.gov/cfl for specific clean-up and recycling instructions).

- **Light-emitting diodes (LEDs):** Rapidly expanding in household use, LEDs use only about 20% of the energy and last up to 25 times longer than traditional bulbs.

Although the newer styles of light bulbs are more expensive than traditional incandescents, over the long term, they save money for the user. The savings come from two differences between incandescent bulbs and high-efficiency bulbs. First, high-efficiency bulbs use much less energy by requiring less electricity to produce light. For example, a 17W LED bulb produces as much light as a 75W incandescent light bulb. Second, they last longer: CFLs last up to 10 times longer than conventional light bulbs, and some LED bulbs have useful lives of more than 22 years.

To aid consumers in selecting bulbs, the Federal Trade Commission mandated Lighting Facts labels on all bulbs. Using these labels, you can compare different types of bulbs and select the most appropriate bulb for your planned use. The brightness comparison is based on lumens rather than watts, because energy-efficient bulbs produce a brighter light with less energy— more lumens per watt than a traditional incandescent bulb.

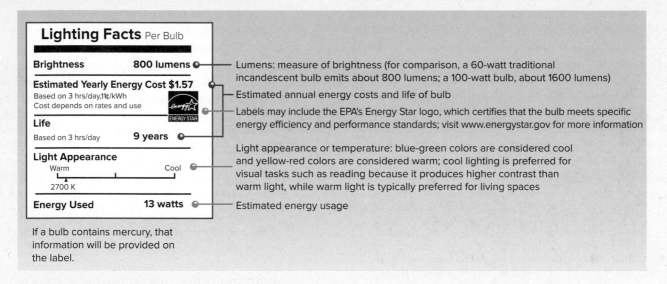

If a bulb contains mercury, that information will be provided on the label.

SOURCES: U.S. Energy Information Administration. 2019. *How Much Electricity is Used for Lighting in the United States?* (http://www.eia.gov/tools/faqs/faq.cfm?id=99&t=3); Office of Energy Efficiency & Renewable Energy. 2014. *How Energy-Efficient Light Bulbs Compare with Traditional Incandescents* (http://energy.gov/energysaver/articles/how-energy-efficient-light-bulbs-compare-traditional-incandescents); Federal Trade Commission. 2011. *Shopping for Lightbulbs* (http://www.consumer.ftc.gov/articles/0164-shopping-light-bulbs).
(Energy Star Logo) Source: Energy Star Logo. Environmental Protection Agency.

government to ensure that ozone-depleting refrigerants will be removed prior to disposal.

- Keep your house adequately ventilated and buy some houseplants; they naturally rid the air of harmful pollutants.

- Keep paints, cleaning agents, and other chemical products tightly sealed in their original containers.

- Don't smoke, and don't allow others to smoke in your room, apartment, or home. If these rules are too strict for your situation, limit smoking to a single, well-ventilated room.

- Clean and inspect chimneys, furnaces, and other appliances regularly. Install carbon monoxide detectors.

- Always use an outside-venting hood when cooking.

- Use paints with low or no VOCs, and ventilate well when using high-VOC products. Pregnant women should avoid painting.

- Keep areas mold free by fixing any leaks from the bathroom, roof, or basement.

- Use a HEPA air filter.

WATER QUALITY AND POLLUTION

Few parts of the world have enough safe, clean drinking water, and yet few things are as important to human health.

Water Contamination and Treatment

Many cities rely at least in part on wells that tap local groundwater, but often it is necessary to tap lakes and rivers to supplement wells. Because such surface water is more likely to be contaminated with both organic matter and pathogenic microorganisms, it is purified in water treatment plants before being piped into the community. At treatment facilities, the water is subjected to various physical and chemical processes, including screening, filtration, and disinfection (often with chlorine), before it is introduced into the water supply system. **Fluoridation**, a water-treatment process that reduces tooth decay by 15–40%, has been used successfully in the United States since 1945.

In most areas of the United States, water systems have adequate, dependable supplies, are able to control waterborne disease, and provide water without unacceptable color, odor, or taste. However, problems do occur. In 1993, more than 400,000 people became ill and 100 died when Milwaukee's drinking water was contaminated with the bacterium *Cryptosporidium.* The Centers for Disease Control and Prevention estimates that 1 million Americans become ill and 900–1,000 die each year from microbial illnesses from drinking water. Pollution by hazardous chemicals from manufacturing, agriculture, and household wastes is another concern. (Chemical pollution is discussed later in the chapter.) Worldwide, 1.6 million people, mostly children, die from water-related diseases each year.

Water Shortages

Water shortages are a growing concern in many regions of the world. Some parts of the United States are experiencing a combination of severe drought and rapid population growth that outstrips the ability of local systems to provide adequate water to all. Many proposals are being discussed to relieve these shortages, including long-distance transfers; conservation; the recycling of some water, such as the water in office-building air conditioners; and the sale of water by regions with large supplies to areas with less available water.

According to the World Health Organization, 844 million people do not have safe drinking water and 2.6 billion do not have access to basic sanitation, such as toilets and latrines. Less than 1% of the world's fresh water—about 0.007% of all the water on earth—is readily accessible for direct human use.

Groundwater pumping and the diversion of water from lakes and rivers for irrigation are further reducing the amount of water available to local communities. In some areas, groundwater is being removed at twice the rate at which it is replaced. Due to agricultural diversions, the Yellow River ran dry for the first time in China's 3,000-year history in 1972, failing to reach the sea for 15 days that year; now, the dry period extends for more than half of each year. In the United States, the Colorado River is now diverted to the extent that it no longer flows into the ocean.

Sewage

Prior to the mid-19th century, many people contracted diseases such as typhoid, cholera, and hepatitis A by direct contact with human feces, which were disposed of at random. After the links between sewage and disease were discovered, practices began to change. People learned how to build sanitary outhouses and how to locate them so that they would not contaminate water sources.

As plumbing moved indoors, sewage disposal became more complicated. In rural areas, the **septic system**, a self-contained sewage disposal system, worked quite well. Today, many rural homes still rely on septic systems; however, many old tanks are leaking contaminants into the environment.

Different approaches became necessary as urban areas developed. Most cities have sewage-treatment systems that separate fecal matter from water in huge tanks and ponds and stabilize it so that it cannot transmit infectious diseases. After the water is treated and is biologically safe, it is released back into the environment. The sludge that remains behind is often contaminated with **heavy metals** such as lead, cadmium, copper, tin, mercury, **polychlorinated biphenyls (PCBs)**, and other toxins. Studies have linked exposure to these chemicals with long-term health consequences, including cancer and damage to the central nervous system. Many cities have therefore expanded sewage-treatment measures to remove heavy metals and other hazardous chemicals from sludge, though the technology is still developing and the costs involved are immense. Decontaminated sludge is used as agricultural fertilizer around the world, including in the United States, although scientists and some government agencies are discouraging this practice due to safety concerns, and it is not permitted in organic agriculture.

Protecting the Water Supply

By reducing your own water use, you help preserve your community's valuable supply and lower your monthly water bill. By taking steps to keep the water supply clean, you reduce pollution overall and help protect the land, wildlife, and other people from illness. Here are some simple steps you can take to protect your water supply:

- Take showers, not baths, to minimize your water consumption. Don't let water run when you're not actively using it while brushing your teeth, shaving, or handwashing clothes or dishes. Don't run a dishwasher or washing machine until you have a full load.

> **TERMS**
>
> **fluoridation** The addition of fluoride to the water supply to reduce tooth decay.
>
> **septic system** A self-contained sewage disposal system, often used in rural areas, in which waste material is decomposed by bacteria.
>
> **heavy metal** A metal with a high specific gravity, such as lead, copper, or tin.
>
> **polychlorinated biphenyl (PCB)** An industrial chemical used as an insulator in electrical transformers and linked to certain human cancers; banned worldwide since 1977 but persistent in the environment.

- Install sink faucet aerators and water-efficient shower-heads, which use two to five times less water with no noticeable decrease in performance.

- Purchase a water-saver toilet, or put a displacement device in your toilet tank to reduce the amount of water used with each flush.

- Fix leaky faucets in your home. Leaks can waste thousands of gallons of water per year.

- Don't pour toxic materials such as cleaning solvents, bleach, or motor oil down the drain. Store them until you can take them to a hazardous waste collection center.

- Don't pour old medicines down the drain or flush them down the toilet. Some pharmacies will take back unused or expired medications for disposal, and many communities have drop-off days for these drugs.

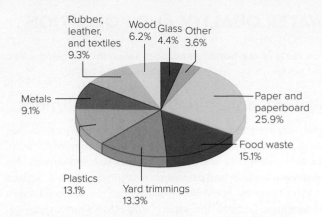

Figure 15.3 Components of municipal solid waste, by weight, before recycling.
SOURCE: Environmental Protection Agency. 2018. *Advancing Sustainable Materials Management: 2015 Tables and Figures* (https://www.epa.gov/sites/production/files/2018-07/documents/smm_2015_tables_and_figures_07252018_fnl_508_0.pdf.)

SOLID WASTE POLLUTION

Humans generate huge amounts of waste, which must be handled appropriately if the environment is to be kept safe.

Solid Waste

The bulk of the organic food garbage produced in American kitchens is now dumped in the sewage system by way of the mechanical garbage disposal. The garbage that remains is not very hazardous from the standpoint of infectious disease because it contains very little food waste, but it does represent an enormous disposal and contamination problem.

What's in Our Garbage? In 2015, Americans generated about 262 million tons of trash; of these, about 67 million tons were recycled or composted, about 25% of the total. As individuals, we generate over 4 pounds of trash a day. The biggest single component of household trash by weight is paper products, including corrugated boxes, newspapers, office papers, and mail (Figure 15.3). Yard waste, plastic, metals, and glass are other significant components. About 1% of the solid waste is toxic; a major source of toxic waste is the disposal of computer components in both household and commercial waste. Burning, as opposed to burial, reduces the bulk of solid waste, but it can release hazardous material into the air, depending on what is being burned. Solid waste is not limited to household products. Manufacturing, mining, and other industries all produce large amounts of potentially dangerous materials that cannot simply be dumped.

Disposing of Solid Waste Since the 1960s, billions of tons of solid waste have been buried in **sanitary landfill** disposal sites. Potential landfill sites are thoroughly studied to ensure they are not near sources of water that could be contaminated by leakage from the landfill. Sometimes protective liners are used around the site, and nearby monitoring wells are now

required in most states. Layers of solid waste are regularly covered with thin layers of dirt until the site is filled. Some communities then plant grass and trees and convert the site into a park. Landfill is relatively stable; almost no decomposition occurs in the solidly packed waste.

Burying solid waste in landfills has several disadvantages. Burial is expensive and requires huge amounts of space. Waste can also contain chemicals, such as pesticides, paints, and oils that, despite precautions, sometimes leak into the surrounding soil and groundwater.

Biodegradability *Biodegradation* is the process by which organic substances are decomposed naturally by living organisms. These organic materials—including plant and animal matter, substances originating from living organisms, or artificial materials similar in nature to plants and animals—are put to use by microorganisms. The term **biodegradable** means that certain products can break down naturally, safely, and quickly into the raw materials of nature, then disappear back into the environment. Table 15.2 shows the amount of time required for specific materials to biodegrade.

Recycling Because of the expense and potential chemical hazards of any form of solid waste disposal, many communities encourage individuals and businesses to recycle their trash. In **recycling**, many kinds of waste materials are collected and used

---

TERMS

sanitary landfill A disposal site where solid wastes are buried.

biodegradable The ability of some materials to break down naturally and disappear back into the environment.

recycling The use of waste materials as raw materials in the production of new products.

Table 15.2	How Long Items Take to Biodegrade	
ITEM	**TIME REQUIRED TO BIODEGRADE**	
Banana peel	2–10 days	
Paper	2–5 months	
Rope	3–14 months	
Orange peel	6 months	
Wool sock	1–5 years	
Cigarette butt	1–12 years	
Plastic-coated milk carton	5 years	
Aluminum can	80–100 years	
Plastic six-pack holder ring	450 years	
Glass bottle	1 million years	
Plastic bottle	Forever	

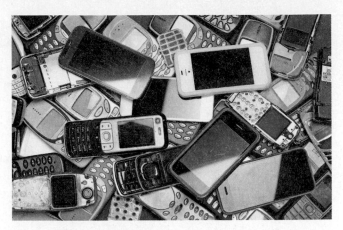

Wellness Tip Each year, millions of pounds of electron waste are discarded; about 40% is recycled, but much more could be. If you have a cell phone, computer, or other electronic device to dispose of, look for an e-waste recycling program in your area. Look for a "green" program or one that is certified by e-stewards, an organization that advocates for responsible e-waste recycling (www.e-stewards.org).

Peter Dazeley/Photographer's Choice/Getty Images

as raw materials in the production of new products. For example, waste paper can be recycled into new paper products, or an old bicycle frame can be melted down and used in the production of appliances. The number of recycling opportunities is almost limitless. Recycling is a good idea for two reasons. First, it puts unwanted objects back to good use. Second, it reduces the amount of solid waste sitting in landfills, some of which takes decades or centuries to decay naturally. Some cities offer curbside pickup of recyclables; others have recycling centers where people can bring their waste. These materials are not limited to paper, glass, and cans but also include things such as discarded tires and used oils.

Recycling surged in popularity starting in the late 1980s. From 1980–2015, the recycling rate increased from about 10% to 34%; however, recent changes in the handling of recyclables have affected rates. In the past, around 40% of recyclables in the United States were sold to China, but in 2018, China banned these imports because of contamination with too much trash. As a result, recycling costs have soared, and recycling programs in many U.S. cities have imposed greater restrictions on what they collect or have ceased altogether; vast amounts of recyclable waste is now being incinerated (creating energy in energy recovery plants, but also air pollution) or buried in landfills.

Discarded Technology: e-Waste A newer solid waste disposal problem involves the discarding of old computers, televisions, cell phones, MP3 players, and other electronic devices. Americans scrap about 400 million consumer electronic devices each year. In 2015, only about 40% of e-waste was recycled. This e-waste is the fastest-growing portion of our waste stream. Junked electronic devices are toxic because they contain varying amounts of lead, mercury, and other heavy metals. Many components of electronic devices are valuable, however, and can be recycled and reused.

Reducing Solid Waste

By reducing your consumption, recycling more, and throwing away less, you can conserve landfill space and put more reusable items back into service. Here are some ideas to help you reduce solid waste:

- Limit your purchase and use of plastic products, including micro plastics, which can be found in soaps (microbeads).

- Buy products with the least amount of packaging, or buy products in bulk (see the box "How to Be a Green Consumer"). For example, buy large jars of juice, not individually packaged juice drinks; buy a water filter, not individual bottles of drinking water. Buy products packaged in recyclable containers.

- Buy recycled or recyclable products. Avoid disposables; instead, use long-lasting or reusable products such as refillable pens and rechargeable batteries.

- Bring your own ceramic coffee mug and metal spoon to work or wherever you drink coffee or tea. Pack your lunch in reusable containers, and use a cloth or plastic lunch sack or a lunch box.

- To store food, use reusable plastic or glass containers rather than foil and plastic wrap.

- Recycle your newspapers, glass, cans, paper, and other recyclables. If you receive something packaged with foam pellets, take them to a commercial mailing center that accepts them for recycling.

- Do not throw electronic items, batteries, or fluorescent lights into the trash. Take these items to state-approved recycling centers; check with your local disposal service for more information.

- Start a compost pile for your organic garbage (non-animal food and yard waste) if you have a yard. If you live in an apartment, you can create a small composting system using earthworms, or take your organic wastes to a community composting center. Some cities now collect kitchen scraps for recycling into compost, which is sold to farms and wineries.

It may seem like a hassle to consider the environmental impact of the things you buy, but a few simple choices can make a big difference without compromising your lifestyle.

- Remember the four Rs of green consumerism:

  - **Reduce** the amount of trash and pollution you generate by consuming and throwing away less.

  - **Reuse** as many products as possible—either yourself or by selling them or donating them to charity.

  - **Recycle** all appropriate materials and buy recycled products whenever possible.

  - **Respond** by educating others about reducing waste and recycling, by finding creative ways to reduce waste and toxicity, and by making your preferences known.

- Choose products packaged in refillable, recycled, reusable containers or in readily recyclable materials, such as paper, cardboard, aluminum, or glass. Don't buy products that are excessively packaged or wrapped.

- Look for products made with the highest possible content of recycled paper, metal, glass, plastic, and other materials.

- Choose simple products containing the lowest amounts of bleaches, dyes, and fragrances. Look for organically grown foods and clothes made from organically grown cotton, from Fox Fibre, or another naturally colored type of cotton.

- Buy high-quality appliances that have an Energy Star seal from the EPA or some other type of certification indicating that they are energy and water efficient.

- Reuse your shopping bags, whether cloth or plastic. One study reports that the best reusable ones are made from polyester or plastics such as polypropylene. Don't bag items that don't need to be bagged.

- Don't buy what you don't need—borrow, rent, or share. Take good care of the things you own, repair items when they break, and replace them with used rather than new items whenever possible.

- Look beyond the products to the companies that make them. Support those with good environmental records. If some of your favorite products are overpackaged or contain harmful ingredients, contact the manufacturer.

- Keep in mind that doing something is better than doing nothing. Even if you can't be a perfectly green consumer, doing your best on any purchase will make a difference.

SOURCES: Rosalsky, G. 2019. *Are Plastic Bag Bans Garbage?* Planet Money, National Public Radio (https://www.npr.org/sections/money/2019/04/09/711181385/are-plastic-bag-bans-garbage); U.S. Natural Resources Defense Council. 2012. *NRDC's Smarter Living* (http://www.nrdc.org/living/default.asp).

CHEMICAL POLLUTION AND HAZARDOUS WASTE

Chemical pollution is by no means a new problem. The ancient Romans were plagued by lead poisoning, and industrial chemicals have claimed countless lives over the past few centuries.

Today, new chemical substances are constantly being introduced into the environment—as pesticides, herbicides, solvents, and hundreds of other products. More people and wildlife are exposed to them than ever before. See the box "Endocrine Disruption" for more information on one new type of chemical hazard.

The pivotal publication of Rachel Carson's *Silent Spring* in 1962 drew attention to the problems of chemical pollution and prompted the formation of the Environmental Protection Agency (EPA). In the 1970s the EPA established the Superfund program to clean up the nation's uncontrolled hazardous waste sites. A national list prioritizes 1,803 sites for cleanup. To date, the EPA has completed cleanups at 375 sites. As the Superfund program matures, so does the size, complexity, and cost of cleanup work. The EPA also pushes industrial polluters to pay the costs of cleanups.

Asbestos

A mineral-based compound, asbestos was widely used for fire protection and insulation in buildings until the late 1960s. Microscopic asbestos fibers can be released into the air when this material is applied or when it later deteriorates or is damaged. These fibers can lodge in the lungs, causing **asbestosis**, lung cancer, and other serious lung diseases. Similar conditions expose workers to risk in the coal mining industry, from coal and silica dust (black lung disease), and in the textile industry, from cotton fibers (brown lung disease).

Asbestos can pose a danger in homes and apartment buildings, about 25% of which are thought to contain some. Areas where it is most likely to be found are in insulation around water and steam pipes, ducts, and furnaces; boiler wraps; vinyl flooring; floor, wall, and ceiling insulation; roofing and siding; and fireproof board.

> **asbestosis** A lung condition caused by inhalation of microscopic asbestos fibers, which inflame the lung and can lead to lung cancer. **TERMS**

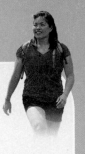

Endocrine Disruption: A "New" Toxic Threat

In the 1970s and 1980s, scientists began to document strange occurrences in wildlife: disrupted reproduction, birth defects, tumors, and behavioral changes in birds, fish, and reptiles. It was also becoming apparent that a drug given to pregnant women in the 1950s (a potent synthetic estrogen, DES) was causing infertility and rare reproductive cancers in their adult daughters.

Researchers noted that low amounts of these toxic chemicals over a long period of time can cause disease. Even more distressing was the evidence that exposure during gestation of a fetus can cause lasting changes and possible future disease in adults.

These chemicals, known as **endocrine disrupting chemicals (EDCs)**, were disturbing the hormone systems of organisms. Most systems in the body rely on hormones, which are chemical signals that initiate a variety of effects in the immune, metabolic, nervous, and other body systems. Low levels of EDCs can disrupt these systems by mimicking or blocking natural hormones. EDC exposure before and after birth may cause lifelong effects, including fertility problems, cancers, cardiovascular disease, obesity, and mental disorders. These effects have been proven in laboratory animals and supported by observational (epidemiological) studies in humans.

Various synthetic chemicals, some in everyday products such as plastic, cosmetics, food packaging, flame retardants, pesticides, and others, are proven EDCs. Bisphenol A (BPA) is a chemical present in #7 plastic—in water bottles, the lining of canned foods, dental fillings, and cash register receipts. In the United States, manufacturers have removed BPA from many infant products, but some scientists believe it should be regulated more stringently.

What can you do?

- Educate yourself about the personal-care and household products you use.

- Eat organic foods. Eat lower on the food chain (more plant-based, less red meat).

- Avoid plastic, especially in contact with food and drinks. Do not microwave plastic containers.

- Dust, vacuum, and wipe down surfaces often.

- Avoid nonstick cookware and products.

- Avoid flame-retardant clothes and furniture.

- Avoid handling cash-register receipts. If you must, use gloves.

- Be especially cautious about exposing pregnant women, infants, and children to EDCs.

- Support legislation that will provide adequate testing and regulation of potential EDCs.

For more information and a list of EDCs, visit the websites of the Endocrine Disruption Exchange (www.endocrinedisruption.org) and the National Institute of Environmental Health Sciences (www.niehs.nih.gov).

Lead

Although lead poisoning is less of a problem now than in the past, the Centers for Disease Control and Prevention (CDC) estimates that approximately half a million U.S. children ages 1–5 years have blood lead levels above the cutoff at which CDC recommends public health action. Many of these children live in poor, inner-city areas (see the box "Poverty and Environmental Health"). No safe blood lead level has been identified for children. When lead is ingested or inhaled, it can permanently damage the central nervous system, cause mental impairment, hinder oxygen transport in the blood, and create kidney and digestive problems. Severe lead poisoning may cause coma or death. Lead exposure has been linked to attention-deficit/hyperactivity disorder (ADHD) in children. Lead can also build up in bones, where it may be released into the bloodstream during pregnancy or when bone mass is lost from osteoporosis.

Most environmental lead comes from lead-based paints. They were banned from residential use in 1978, but as many as 57 million American homes still contain them. Guidelines require contractors to take special lead containment measures when doing renovations, repairs, or painting in certain buildings. The use of lead in plumbing is now also banned, but some old pipes and faucets contain it; if these pipes and fixtures corrode, lead can leach into the water. The presence of lead pipes contributed to the drinking water crisis in Flint, Michigan. In 2014, the city changed water supplies to one that had higher levels of corrosive compounds but failed to add a required anticorrosive agent. Lead from aging pipes leached into the drinking water, and researchers found that the incidence of elevated blood levels doubled in children in Flint after the water source change.

Pesticides

Pesticides are chemicals that kill unwanted pests. Herbicides (plant killers) and insecticides (insect killers) are used

---

endocrine disrupting chemicals (EDCs) **TERMS**
Chemicals that disrupt the hormone systems of organisms.

pesticides Chemicals used to prevent the spread of diseases transmitted by insects and to maximize food production by killing insects that eat crops.

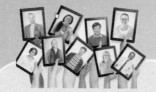

DIVERSITY MATTERS
Poverty and Environmental Health

Residents of poor and minority communities are often exposed to more environmental toxins than residents of wealthier communities, and they are more likely to suffer from health problems caused or aggravated by pollutants.

Poor neighborhoods are often located near highways and industrial areas that have high levels of air and noise pollution; they are also common sites for hazardous waste production and disposal. Residents of substandard housing are more likely to come into contact with lead, asbestos, carbon monoxide, pesticides, and other hazardous pollutants associated with peeling paint, old plumbing, and poorly maintained insulation and heating equipment.

Poor people are more likely to have jobs that expose them to asbestos, silica dust, and pesticides, and they are more likely to catch and consume fish contaminated with PCBs, mercury, and other toxins.

The most thoroughly researched and documented link among poverty, the environment, and health is lead poisoning in children. During the Flint, Michigan, water crisis, the highest blood lead levels in children were found in the most socioeconomically disadvantaged neighborhoods with aging infrastructure.

A 2013 study showed that whether they lived in a rural or urban environment, blacks and Latinos were more likely to be exposed to lead from contaminated soils than were non-minorities. This was true for children age 6 and under, which is important because children are especially vulnerable to lead exposure. The CDC and the American Academy of Pediatrics recommend annual testing of blood lead levels for all children under age 6.

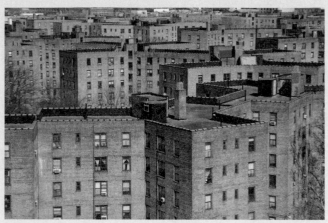

dbimages/Alamy Stock Photo

SOURCES: Hatta-Attisha, M., et al. 2016. "Elevated blood lead levels in children associated with the Flint drinking water crisis: A spatial analysis of risk and public health response," *American Journal of Public Health* 106(2): 283–290; Akinbami, L. J., A. E. Simon, and L. M. Rosen. 2016. "Changing trends in asthma prevalence among children," *Pediatrics* 137(1); Aelion, C. M., et al. 2013. "Associations between soil lead concentrations and populations by race/ethnicity and income-to-poverty ratio in urban and rural areas," *Environmental Geochemistry and Health* 35(1): 1–12.

extensively in agriculture, and they often have toxic effects in unwanted targets, such as beneficial insects and birds. Insecticides are used primarily for two purposes: to prevent the spread of insect-borne diseases and to maximize food production by killing crop pests. Pesticide use has risks and benefits. For example, DDT was extremely effective in controlling mosquito-borne diseases in tropical countries and in increasing crop yields throughout the world, but it was found to harm birds, fish, and reptiles. DDT also builds up in the food chain, increasing in concentration as larger animals eat smaller ones, a process known as **biomagnification**. DDT bioaccumulation was linked to eggshell thinning in predatory birds, contributing to the decline of species such as the peregrine falcon. DDT was banned in the United States in 1972.

Mercury

A naturally occurring metal, mercury is a toxin that affects the brain and nervous system and may damage the kidneys and gastrointestinal tract, and increase blood pressure, heart rate, and heart attack risk. Mercury slows fetal and child development and causes irreversible deficits in brain function. Coal-fired power plants are the largest producers of

mercury; other sources include mining and smelting operations and the disposal of consumer products containing mercury.

Mercury persists in the environment, and like pesticides, it is bioaccumulative. In particular, large, long-lived fish may carry high levels of mercury.

Other Chemical Pollutants

There are tens of thousands of chemical pollutants, and the extent of their toxic effects are just beginning to be understood. As mentioned earlier, potentially hazardous materials are commonly found in the home and should be handled and disposed of properly. They include automotive supplies (motor oil, antifreeze, transmission fluid), paint supplies (turpentine, paint thinner, mineral spirits), art and hobby supplies (oil-based paint, solvents, acids and alkalis, aerosol sprays), insecticides, batteries, computer and electronic

> **biomagnification** The accumulation of a substance in a food chain.

TERMS

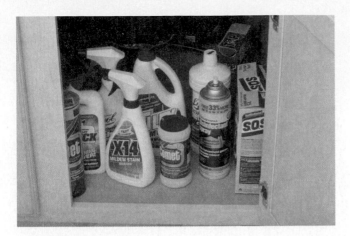

Wellness Tip Hazardous chemicals accumulate in many homes, as well as in business and industrial sites. Dispose of your household hazardous wastes properly. If you don't know how to dispose of an item, contact your local environmental health office or health department for information.

Tony Freeman/PhotoEdit

components, and household cleaners containing sodium hydroxide (lye) or ammonia. These chemicals are dangerous when inhaled or ingested, when they contact the skin or the eyes, or when they are burned or dumped. Many cities provide guidelines about approved disposal methods and have hazardous waste collection days.

Preventing Chemical Pollution

You can take steps to reduce the chemical pollution in your community. Just as important, by reducing and eliminating the number of chemicals in your home, you may save the life of a child or animal who might encounter one of those chemicals.

- When buying cleansers, disinfectants, polishes, and other personal and household products, read the labels, and choose the least toxic, non-petrochemical ones available. Download the "GoodGuide" app to aid in purchasing nontoxic personal care, household, and food items (www .goodguide.com/about/mobile).

- Dispose of your household hazardous wastes properly. If you are not sure whether something is hazardous or don't know how to dispose of it, contact your local environmental health office or health department.

- Eat and live organically. Avoid using chemical pesticides (weed, insect, and rodent killers) in the home and garden.

- Buy organic produce or produce that has been grown locally.

- If you must use pesticides or toxic household products, store them in a locked place where children and pets can't get to them. Don't measure chemicals with food-preparation utensils, and wear gloves whenever handling them.

- If you have your house fumigated for pest control, be sure to hire a licensed exterminator. Keep everyone, including pets, out of the house while the crew works and, if possible, for a few days after.

RADIATION POLLUTION

Radiation comes in several forms, such as ultraviolet rays, microwaves, or X-rays, and from several sources, such as the sun, uranium, and nuclear weapons (Figure 15.4). These forms of

> **radiation** Energy transmitted in the form of rays, waves, or particles. **TERMS**

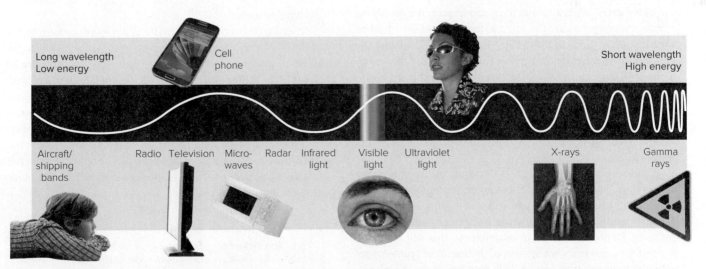

Figure 15.4 Electromagnetic radiation. Electromagnetic radiation takes the form of waves that travel through space. The length of the wave determines the type of radiation: The shortest waves are high-energy gamma rays; the longest are radio waves and extremely low-frequency waves used for communication between aircraft, ships, and submarines. Different types of electromagnetic radiation have different effects on health.

(cell phone): Mark Dierker/McGraw-Hill Education; (person with sunglass): Stockbyte/Getty Images; (child watching TV): Imagery Majestic/Cutcaster; (microwave): Stockbyte/Getty Images; (eye): Barbara Penoyar/Photodisc/Getty Images; (x-ray): itsmejust/Shutterstock; (gamma rays): Martin Diebel/fStop/Getty Images

electromagnetic radiation differ in wavelength and energy, with shorter waves having the highest energy levels.

Of most concern to health are gamma rays, which are produced by radioactive sources such as nuclear weapons, nuclear energy plants, and radon gas. These high-energy waves are powerful enough to penetrate objects and break molecular bonds. Gamma radiation cannot be seen or felt, but its effects at high doses can include **radiation sickness** and death. At lower doses, chromosome damage, sterility, tissue damage, cataracts, and cancer can occur. Other types of radiation can also affect health. For example, exposure to UV radiation from the sun or from tanning salons can increase the risk of skin cancer. The effects of some sources of radiation, such as cell phones, remain controversial.

Nuclear Weapons and Nuclear Energy

Nuclear weapons pose a health risk of the most serious kind to all species. Public health associations have cautioned that in the event of a discharge of these weapons, there could be millions of casualties. Reducing the stockpiles of nuclear weapons is a challenge and a goal for the 21st century.

Power-generating plants that use nuclear fuel also pose health problems. When **nuclear power** was first developed as an alternative to oil and coal, it was promoted as clean, efficient, inexpensive, and safe. In general, this has proven to be the case. Power systems in several parts of the world rely on nuclear power plants. However, despite all the built-in safeguards and regulating agencies, accidents in nuclear power plants do happen, many due to human error (as at Three Mile Island in the United States and Tokaimura in Japan), and the consequences of such accidents are far more serious than those of similar accidents in other types of power-generating plants. The 1986 fire and explosion at the Chernobyl nuclear power station in Ukraine caused hundreds of deaths and increased rates of genetic mutation and cancer; the long-term effects are not yet clear. The zone around Chernobyl could be unsafe for the next 24,000 years. In 2011, a 9.0 magnitude earthquake 15 miles below Japan's Honshu Island, followed by a powerful tsunami, severely damaged the Fukushima Daiichi nuclear power plant complex, resulting in the largest release of radiation into the Pacific Ocean in history. All nuclear plants in Japan were shut down until August 2015. Fisheries in the nearby area were also closed due to concern of exposure to radiation.

Another, enormous problem is disposing of the radioactive wastes these plants generate. They cannot be dumped in a sanitary landfill because the amount and type of soil used to cap a sanitary landfill are not sufficient to prevent radiation from escaping. Deposit sites have to be developed that will be secure not just for a few years but for tens of thousands of years—longer than the total recorded history of human beings on this planet. To date, no storage method has been devised that can provide infallible, infinitely durable shielding for nuclear waste. Despite these problems, nuclear power is gaining favor again as an alternative to fossil fuels.

Medical Uses of Radiation

Another area of concern is the use of radiation in medicine, primarily the X-ray. The development of machines that could produce images of internal bone structures was a major advance in medicine. Chest X-rays were routinely used to screen for tuberculosis, and children's feet were even X-rayed in shoe stores to make sure their new shoes fit properly. As time passed, studies revealed that X-ray exposure is cumulative and that no level of exposure is absolutely safe.

Early X-ray machines are no longer used because of the high amounts of radiation. Each new generation of X-ray machines has used less radiation more effectively. From a personal health point of view, no one should ever have a "routine" X-ray examination; each such exam should have a definite purpose, and its benefits and risks should be carefully weighed.

Radiation in the Home and Workplace

Recently, there has been concern about electromagnetic radiation associated with common modern devices such as microwave ovens, computer monitors, and even high-voltage power lines. These forms of radiation do have effects on health, but research results are inconclusive.

Another controversial issue today is the effect of radiation from cell phones on health. The California Department of Public Health recently issued a fact sheet on the possible risks of cell phone use and how to reduce radiation exposure. Cell phones use electromagnetic waves (radio frequency radiation) to send and receive signals. This radiation is not directional, meaning that it travels in all directions equally, including toward the user. Factors such as the type of digital signal coding in the network, the antenna and handset design, and the position of the phone relative to the head all determine how much radiation is absorbed by a user.

Specific absorption rate (SAR) is a way of measuring the quantity of radio frequency energy that is absorbed by the body. If you're concerned about limiting your exposure to possible radiation from your cell phone, look for a phone with a low SAR (some municipalities require phone manufacturers to provide this information on packaging). You can also text instead of call, use a wired headset or speakerphone whenever possible, and carry your phone at least one inch from your body. Studies to date have not provided conclusive evidence that cell phone use actually exposes users to harmful levels of radiation.

> **TERMS**
>
> **radiation sickness** An illness caused by excessive radiation exposure, marked by low white blood cell counts and nausea; possibly fatal.
>
> **nuclear power** The use of controlled nuclear reactions to produce steam, which in turn drives turbines to produce electricity.

Avoiding Radiation

The following steps can help you avoid unneeded exposure to radiation:

- If your physician orders an X-ray, ask why it is necessary. Only get X-rays that you need, and keep a record of the date and location of every X-ray exam. Don't have a full-body CT scan for routine screening; the radiation dose of one full-body CT scan is nearly 100 times that of a typical mammogram.

- Follow government recommendations for radon testing.

- Find out if there are radioactive sites in your area. If you live or work near such a site, form or join a community action group to get the site cleaned up.

- Use sunscreen to protect yourself from the sun's UV radiation.

NOISE POLLUTION

We are increasingly aware of the health effects of loud or persistent noise in the environment. Concerns focus on two areas: hearing loss and stress. Prolonged exposure to sounds above 80–85 **decibels** (a measure of the intensity of a sound wave) can cause permanent hearing loss (Figure 15.5). Hearing damage can occur after eight hours of exposure to sounds louder than 80 decibels. Regular exposure for longer than one minute to more than 100 decibels can cause permanent hearing loss. Children may suffer damage to their hearing at lower noise levels than those at which adults suffer damage.

Two common sources of excessive noise are the workplace and large gatherings of people at sporting events, rock music and other concerts, and movie theaters. The Occupational Safety and Health Administration (OSHA) sets legal standards for noise in the workplace, but no laws exist regulating noise levels at concerts, which can be much louder than most workplaces.

Here are some ways to avoid exposing yourself to excessive noise:

- Wear ear protectors when working around noisy machinery.

- When listening to music on a headset with a volume range of 1–10, keep the volume no louder than 6. Your headset is too loud if you are unable to hear people around you speaking in a normal tone of voice. Earmuff-style headphones may be easier on the ears than earbuds, which are inserted into the ear canal. Experts warn that earbuds should not be used more than 30 minutes a day unless the volume is set below 60% of maximum; headphones can be used up to one hour. It is good to put covers over your earbuds because this can reduce the decibel level a little. Do not push your earbuds in too far. Keep the volume quite a bit lower than you think you need because the sound is far louder than you realize.

- Avoid toys for children that make loud noise.

> **decibel**   A unit for expressing the relative intensity of sounds on a scale from 0 for the average least perceptible sound to about 120 for the average pain threshold.   **TERMS**

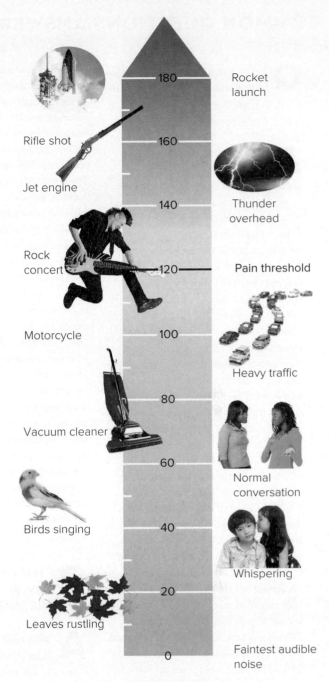

Figure 15.5   The intensity of selected sounds.

(rocket): Source: Space Shuttle Highlights Gallery/NASA; (gun): Stockbyte/Getty Images; (lightning): JupiterImages/Comstock Images/Getty Images; (guitar player): Daxiao Productions/Shutterstock; (cars): Stockbyte/Getty Images; (vacuum): Brand X Pictures/Getty Images; (conversation): Ken Karp/McGraw-Hill Education; (bird): xpixel/Shutterstock; (whispering): Phasin Sudjai/123RF; (leaves): Siede Preis/Photodisc/Getty Images

- Avoid loud music. Don't sit or stand near speakers or amplifiers at a concert, and don't play a car radio or stereo so loud that you can't hear the traffic.

- Avoid exposure to painfully loud sounds, and avoid repeated exposure to any sounds above 80 decibels.

COMMON QUESTIONS ANSWERED

Q Are newer sources of fossil fuel, such as oil extraction from tar sands, safe for the environment?

A That is a difficult question to answer because there are many unknowns, but all fossil fuel extraction processes have potential environmental costs. As supplies of easily accessible oil dwindle, some energy companies have turned to what are often called unconventional or "extreme" energy sources. This term describes fossil fuels that are relatively difficult to access and extract from the environment. Examples include deepwater oil rigs, tar sands oil extraction, and drilling and hydrofracking of natural gas. Accessing these energy sources requires new technologies and practices. Critics worry that these technologies have been insufficiently studied and regulated and may pose significant new environmental risks.

The Deepwater Horizon oil rig that exploded in April 2010 in the Gulf of Mexico was a deepwater rig. It took three months to plug the leak, after nearly 5 million barrels of oil were released into the Gulf. The combination of the oil and the chemicals used to clean it up killed thousands of birds and marine mammals, and the long-term health effects to the remaining wildlife are not known. The Gulf's ecosystems may need generations to recover fully, and some parts of it may never recover. Researchers have discovered trace amounts of oil in some fish and shellfish, leading to concerns that oil could reach the human food chain.

Tar sands (or oil sands) are sand deposits that are saturated with a dense form of petroleum called bitumen. The largest deposits are found in Canada, Kazakhstan, and Russia. Making liquid fuel from the oil in tar sands is a very energy-intensive process. When used as fuel, the resulting molasses-like product produces two to four times the amount of greenhouse gases per barrel compared to other conventional oils. In addition, Canada's tar sands oil will need to travel by pipeline and ship, which poses a risk to wildlife habitats on land and at sea.

Hydraulic fracturing, or "fracking," uses pressurized mixes of fluids to create cracks in rock formations deep underground, releasing natural gas. The term *fracking* is commonly used to describe both the drilling and fracturing processes in natural gas extraction. New technology and techniques have recently prompted the mining of deposits in certain areas of the United States. However, critics have raised concerns about the safety of the technique, especially because many of these wells are in residential areas, near homes and schools. The specific chemicals used have not been publicly disclosed by energy companies using this technique, and reports of groundwater contamination have been verified by independent third parties. In addition, the disposal of wastewater from the fracking process (which is done by injecting the fluid deep in the ground) can induce earthquakes and has been linked to a dramatic increase in earthquakes in the central United States. Further, there has been little environmental assessment of the possible air pollution from natural gas extraction, which can come from trucks, chemicals used for cleaning and running equipment, and emissions from the process itself.

Q What is renewable energy, and what are its advantages?

A With fossil fuels becoming increasingly problematic politically, economically, and environmentally, interest and investment in renewable energy sources have grown in recent years. Renewable energy sources are those sources that are naturally replenished and essentially inexhaustible, such as wind and water. Together with technologies that improve energy efficiency, renewable energy sources contribute to sustainability—the capacity of natural or human systems to endure and maintain well-being over time. A common definition of sustainable development is development that meets society's present needs without compromising the ability of future generations to meet their needs.

Renewable energy sources include wind power, solar power, water and wave power, geothermal power, and biomass and biofuels from renewable sources, among others.

- Wind power uses the energy of the wind to turn blades that run a turbine, which spins a generator, which produces electricity.

- Solar power uses the heat and light of the sun to produce energy via a variety of technologies. One solar technology is the concentrating solar power (CSP) system, which use mirrors, dishes, or towers to reflect and collect solar heat to generate steam, which runs a turbine to produce electricity. Another solar technology is the photovoltaic (solar cell) system, which converts sunlight directly into electricity by means of semiconducting materials.

- Geothermal power taps the heat in the earth's core. It may be in the form of hot water or steam, which can be used to run a turbine to produce electricity. In some geologically unstable parts of the planet, including Yellowstone Park and parts of northern California, geothermal energy is close to the surface.

- Biomass is plant material, including trees. When biomass is burned, it produces energy. If the plants are produced and harvested sustainably, they are a renewable source of energy.

- Biofuels are fuels based on natural materials. Bioethanol is made primarily from sugar and starch crops like corn, although trees and grasses may be used in the future. Ethanol can be used as a fuel for vehicles or added to gasoline. Biodiesel is made from vegetable oils or animal fats and can be used either in a pure form to power vehicles or added to diesel to reduce carbon emissions.

Capacity for solar-powered electricity has grown immensely, producing 1% of the electricity used worldwide at the end of 2015. In the same year, wind power generation capacity reached 7%, and bioenergy (traditional and modern biomass as well as biofuels) reached 11% of the global energy supply. Renewable energy accounted for 12% of total energy consumption in the United States in 2018, the highest since the 1930s, with the greatest growth coming from wind and solar.

TIPS FOR TODAY AND THE FUTURE

Environmental health involves protecting ourselves from environmental dangers and protecting the environment from the dangers created by humans.

RIGHT NOW YOU CAN

- Turn off the lights and electronics in any unoccupied rooms.
- Turn off power strips when not in use. Don't leave seldom-used devices on and in standby mode.
- Turn down the heat a few degrees and put on a sweater, or turn off the air conditioner and change into cooler clothes.
- Check your trash for recyclable items and take them out for recycling. If your town does not provide curbside pickup for recyclable items, find out the location of the nearest community recycling center.

IN THE FUTURE YOU CAN

- Replace light bulbs with high-efficiency light bulbs as your existing bulbs burn out.
- Have your car checked to make sure it runs as well as it can and puts out the lowest amount of polluting emissions possible.
- Go online and find one of the many calculators available that can help you estimate your environmental footprint. After calculating your footprint, figure out ways to reduce it.

SUMMARY

- Environmental health encompasses all the interactions of humans with their environment and the health consequences of those interactions.

- The world's population is increasing rapidly, especially in the developing world. Factors that may eventually limit human population are food, availability of land and water, energy, and minimum acceptable standard of living.

- Increased amounts of air pollutants are especially dangerous for children, older adults, and people with chronic health problems.

- Factors contributing to the development of smog include heavy motor vehicle traffic, hot weather, and stagnant air.

- Carbon dioxide and other natural gases act as a greenhouse around the earth, increasing the temperature of the atmosphere. Levels of these gases are rising through human activity; as a result, the world's climate is changing.

- The ozone layer that shields the earth's surface from the sun's UV rays has thinned and developed holes in certain regions.

- Environmental damage from energy use can be limited through energy conservation and the development of nonpolluting, renewable sources of energy.

- Indoor pollutants can trigger allergies and illness in the short term and cancer in the long term.

- Concerns with water quality focus on pathogenic organisms and hazardous chemicals from industry and households, as well as on water shortages.

- Sewage treatment prevents pathogens, heavy metals, and hazardous chemicals from contaminating drinking water.

- The amount of garbage is growing all the time; paper is the biggest component. Recycling can help reduce solid waste disposal problems.

- Potentially hazardous chemical pollutants include asbestos, lead, pesticides, mercury, and many household products. Proper handling and disposal are critical.

- Radiation can cause radiation sickness, chromosome damage, and cancer, among other health problems.

- Loud or persistent noise can lead to hearing loss and/or stress; two common sources of excessive noise are the workplace and music concerts.

FOR FURTHER EXPLORATION

CDC National Center for Environmental Health. Provides brochures and fact sheets on a variety of environmental issues.

https://www.cdc.gov/nceh/default.htm

Colin Beavan: A Fulfilling Life and a Better World. A blog by Beavan, an activist for environmental and quality-of-life issues. Features his 2009 book and movie *No Impact Man.*

http://www.colinbeavan.com/

Earth Times. An international online newspaper devoted to global environmental issues.

http://www.earthtimes.org

Ecological Footprint. Calculates your personal ecological footprint based on your diet, transportation patterns, and living arrangements.

http://www.myfootprint.org

Fuel Economy. Provides information on the fuel economy of cars made since 1985 and tips on improving gas mileage.

http://www.fueleconomy.gov

Indoor Air Quality Information Hotline. Answers questions, provides publications, and makes referrals.

(800) 438-4318

National Lead Information Center. Provides information packets and specialist advice.

https://www.epa.gov/lead

National Oceanic and Atmospheric Administration (NOAA): Climate. Provides information on a variety of issues related to climate, including global warming, drought, and El Niño and La Niña.

http://www.noaa.gov/climate.html

National Safety Council. Provides information on lead, radon, indoor air quality, hazardous chemicals, and other environmental issues.

http://www.nsc.org/pages/home.aspx

Power Shift Network. A coalition of student and youth environmental groups working to mitigate climate change.

    http://www.powershift.org

United Nations. Several U.N. programs are devoted to environmental problems on a global scale; the websites provide information on current and projected trends and on international treaties developed to deal with environmental issues.

    http://www.un.org/popin (Population Information Network)

    http://www.unep.org (Environment Programme)

U.S. Department of Energy: Energy Efficiency and Renewable Energy (EERE). Provides information about alternative fuels and tips for saving energy at home and in your car.

    https://energy.gov/eere/office-energy-efficiency-renewable-energy

U.S. Environmental Protection Agency (EPA). Provides information about EPA activities and many consumer-oriented materials. The website includes special sites devoted to global warming, ozone loss, pesticides, and other areas of concern.

    http://www.epa.gov

Worldwatch Institute. A public policy research organization focusing on emerging global environmental problems and the links between the world economy and the environment.

    http://www.worldwatch.org

There are many national and international organizations working on environmental health problems. A few of the largest and best known are listed below:

Greenpeace: 800-326-0959; http://www.greenpeace.org

National Audubon Society: 212-979-3000; http://www.audubon.org

National Wildlife Federation: 800-822-9919; http://www.nwf.org

Nature Conservancy: 800-628-6860; http://www.nature.org

Sierra Club: 415-977-5500; http://www.sierraclub.org

World Wildlife Fund—U.S.: 800-960-0993; http://www.worldwildlife.org

SELECTED BIBLIOGRAPHY

Aelion, C. M. 2013. Associations between soil lead concentrations and populations by race/ethnicity and income-to-poverty ratio in urban and rural areas. *Environmental Geochemistry and Health* 35(1): 1–12.

Bourne, J. 2015. *The End of Plenty: The Race to Feed a Crowded World.* Melbourne, Australia: Scribe Publications.

CDC National Center for Environmental Health. 2018. *Lead* (http://www.cdc.gov /nceh/lead/).

Centers for Disease Control and Prevention. 2017. Surveillance for waterborne disease outbreaks associated with drinking water—United States, 2013–2014. *MMWR Surveillance Summaries* 66(44): 1216–1221.

Centers for Disease Control and Prevention. 2017. Childhood blood levels in children aged <5 years—United States, 2009–2014. *MMWR* 66(3): 1–10.

Centers for Disease Control and Prevention. 2017. *Over 70 years of community water fluoridation.* (https://www.cdc.gov/fluoridation/basics/70-years.htm).

Centers for Disease Control and Prevention. 2019. *Measles Cases and Outbreaks* (https://www.cdc.gov/measles/cases-outbreaks.html).

Cunningham, W. P., et al. 2013. *Environmental Science: A Global Concern,* 12th ed. New York: McGraw-Hill.

Delamater, P. L., et al. 2012. An analysis of asthma hospitalizations, air pollution, and weather conditions in Los Angeles County, California. *Science of the Total Environment* 425: 110–118.

Environmental Protection Agency. 2014. *Municipal Solid Waste* (http://www.epa.gov /waste/nonhaz/municipal/index.htm).

Environmental Protection Agency. 2016. *Volatile Organic Compounds' Impact on Indoor Air Quality* (https://www.epa.gov/indoor-air-quality-iaq/volatile-organic-compounds -impact-indoor-air-quality#main-content).

Environmental Protection Agency. 2019. *Sources of Greenhouse Gas Emissions* (https:// www.epa.gov/ghgemissions/sources-greenhouse-gas-emissions).

Global Footprint Network. 2018. Earth Overshoot Day 2018 is August 1 (https://www .footprintnetwork.org/2018/07/23/earth-overshoot-day-2018-is-august-1-the-earliest -date-since-ecological-overshoot-started-in-the-early-1970s-2/).

Hwang, B. F., et al. 2015. Relationship between exposure to fine particulates and ozone and reduced lung function in children. *Environmental Research* 137: 382–390.

Intergovernmental Panel on Climate Change. 2015. *Climate Change 2014: Synthesis Report* (https://www.ipcc.ch/report/ar5/syr/).

NASA. 2012. *2012 Antarctic Ozone Hole Second Smallest in 20 Years* (http://www.nasa .gov/topics/earth/features/ozone-hole-2012.html).

NASA Earth Observatory. 2015. *World of Change: Antarctic Ozone Hole* (http:// earthobservatory.nasa.gov/Features/WorldOfChange/ozone.php).

National Center for Environmental Information. 2014. *State of the Climate: Summary Information* (http://www.ncdc.noaa.gov/sotc/summary-info/global/201412).

National Oceanic and Atmospheric Administration. 2014. *Billion Dollar U.S. Weather Disasters, 1980–2012* (http://www.ncdc.noaa.gov/billions/events).

Patz, J. A., et al. 2014. Climate change: Challenges and opportunities for global health. *Journal of the American Medical Association* 312(15): 1565–1580.

Public Affairs. 2015. Does that cellphone in your pocket pose a health risk? *Berkeley News,* May 21 (http://news.berkeley.edu/2015/05/21/opinion-does-that-cellphone -in-your-pocket-pose-a-health-risk/)

Reese, A. 2018. Disturbing losses of protective ozone near Earth's equator may be tied to short-lived chemicals. *Science.* doi:10.1126/science.aat2233 (https://www .sciencemag.org/news/2018/02/ozone-hole-s-repair-belies-thinning-planet-s-ultraviolet -shield-closer-equator).

Rogalsky, D. K., et al. 2014. Estimating the number of low-income Americans exposed to household air pollution from burning solid fuels. *Environmental Health Perspectives* 122(8): 806–810.

Sadler, R. C., J. LaChance, and M. Hanna-Atti. 2017. Social and built environmental correlates of predicted blood lead levels in the Flint water crisis. *American Journal of Public Health.* doi:10.2105/AJPH.2017.303692

Shah, A. S., et al. 2013. Global association of air pollution and heart failure: A systematic review and meta-analysis. *Lancet* 382(9897): 1039–1048.

UNICEF and World Health Organization. 2015. *Progress on Sanitation and Drinking Water—2015 Update and MDG Assessment.* Geneva: WHO.

United Nations Population Division. 2017. Ten key findings and recommendations. *Report of the Secretary-General on the 50th Session on Population and Development.* New York: United Nations (https://www.un.org/development/desa/publications /world-population-prospects-the-2017-revision.html).

United Nations Population Division. 2015. *World Population Prospects: The 2015 Revision.* New York: United Nations.

U.S. Energy Information Agency. 2019. *In 2018, the United States Consumed More Energy Than Ever Before* (https://www.eia.gov/todayinenergy/detail .php?id=39092).

U.S. Energy Information Administration. 2015. *International Energy Statistics* (http:// www.eia.gov/cfapps/ipdbproject/IEDIndex3.cfm?tid=44&pid=44&aid=2).

U.S. Environmental Protection Agency. 2014. *Motor Vehicle Air Conditioning Refrigerant Transition & Environmental Impacts* (http://www.epa.gov/ozone/title6/609/transition .html).

World Energy Council. 2016. *World Energy Resources Summary Report 2016.* London: World Energy Council.

World Health Organization. 2018. Cholera annual report 2017. *Weekly Epidemiological Record* 93(38): 489–500.

World Health Organization (WHO) and the United Nations Children's Fund (UNICEF). 2017. *Progress on Drinking Water, Sanitation and Hygiene: 2017 Update and SDG Baselines.* Geneva (https://apps.who.int/iris/bitstream/handle/10665/258617 /9789241512893-eng.pdf;jsessionid=D434C6891270E70D40C498E8D6A8C3C4 ?sequence=1).

World Nuclear Association. 2018. *Fukushima Accident 2011* (http://world-nuclear.org /info/Safety-and-Security/Safety-of-Plants/Fukushima-Accident/).

Name _____ Section _____ Date _____

LAB 15.1 Environmental Health Checklist

The following list of statements relates to your effect on the environment. Check the statements that are true for you.

Conserving Energy and Reducing Air Pollution

_____ I ride my bike, walk, use public transportation, or carpool whenever possible.

_____ I keep my car tuned up and well maintained.

_____ My vehicle is fuel efficient (city: _____ MPG; highway: _____ MPG).

_____ My car tires are inflated at the proper pressure.

_____ I avoid quick starts and I drive within the speed limit.

_____ I don't use my car's air conditioner when opening the window would suffice.

_____ My residence is well insulated and energy efficient.

_____ I use the most energy-efficient bulb available for each use in my residence (LEDs, halogens, or compact fluorescent bulbs).

_____ I turn off lights and unplug appliances and electronics when they are not in use.

_____ I avoid turning on heat or air conditioning whenever possible.

_____ I run the washing machine, clothes dryer, and dishwasher only when they have full loads.

_____ I wash clothes in warm or cold water rather than hot.

_____ I run the clothes dryer only as long as it takes my clothes to dry.

_____ I dry my hair with a towel rather than a hair dryer.

_____ I clean refrigerator coils and clothes drying lint screens frequently.

_____ I keep my car's air conditioner in good working order and have it serviced by a service station that recycles chlorofluorocarbons (CFCs).

_____ I have energy-efficient appliances (refrigerator, washer, dryer, dishwasher), which I keep in good working order.

Improving Indoor Air

_____ I don't smoke, and I don't allow smoking in my residence.

_____ I have houseplants.

_____ I keep cleaning and other chemical products tightly closed when not in use, stored in their original containers.

_____ When painting or using cleaning or other products that give off VOCs, I have adequate ventilation.

_____ I vacuum often using a vacuum cleaner with a HEPA filter.

_____ My residence has carbon monoxide detectors.

Reducing Garbage

_____ When shopping, I choose products with the least amount of packaging.

_____ I choose recycled and recyclable products.

_____ I avoid products packaged in plastic and unrecycled aluminum.

_____ I store food in reusable/glass containers.

_____ I take my own bag along when I go shopping.

_____ Whenever possible, I use long-lasting or reusable products (such as refillable soap dispensers, rechargeable batteries).

_____ I use a ceramic mug and metal spoon for coffee and tea rather than disposable cups and stirrers.

_____ I recycle newspapers, glass, cans, paper, and other recyclables.

_____ I have a compost pile or bin for my organic garbage, or I take my organic garbage to a community composting center.

Reducing Chemical Pollution and Avoiding Radiation

_____ When shopping, I read labels and try to buy the least toxic products available.

_____ I dispose of household hazardous wastes, including e-waste, properly.

_____ I take unused medications to an appropriate disposal site.

_____ If I am unsure of the proper way to dispose of something, I contact my local health department or environmental health office.

_____ Whenever possible, I buy organic produce or produce that is in season and has been grown locally.

_____ I get only medically necessary X-rays and CT scans.

_____ I follow government recommendations for radon testing.

_____ I use sunscreen to protect my skin from ultraviolet radiation.

Saving Water

_____ I take showers instead of baths.

_____ I take short showers and switch off the water when I'm not actively using it.

_____ I do not run the water while brushing my teeth, shaving, or handwashing dishes or clothes.

_____ My faucets have aerators installed in them.

_____ My shower has a low-flow showerhead.

_____ I have a water-saving toilet, or I have a water-displacement device in my toilet.

_____ I fix any faucets that leak.

Avoiding Noise Pollution

_____ I avoid exposure to painfully loud sounds and wear ear protectors when working around loud noises.

_____ I keep the volume on headphones and earbuds at a safely low level.

_____ I keep the volume of my car's audio system at a safely low level.

Preserving Wildlife and the Natural Environment

_____ I snip or rip plastic six-pack rings before I throw them out.

_____ I don't buy products made from endangered species.

_____ When hiking or camping, I never leave anything behind.

Using Your Results

Statements you have not checked can help you identify behaviors you can change to improve environmental health. Select one behavior from the list and describe strategies for changing it to a more environmentally friendly habit.

Design elements: Evidence for Exercise box (shoes and stethoscope): Vstock LLC/Tetra Images/Getty Images; Take Charge box (lady walking): VisualCommunications/E+/Getty Images; Critical Consumer box (man): Sam74100/iStock/Getty Images; Diversity Matters box (holding devices): Robert Churchill/iStockphoto/Rawpixel Ltd/Getty Images; Wellness in the Digital Age box (Smart Watch): Hong Li/DigitalVision/Getty Images

APPENDIXES

RESOURCES FOR FINDING NUTRITIONAL CONTENT OF COMMON FOODS

If you are developing a behavior change plan to improve your diet, or if you simply want to choose healthier foods, you may want to know more about the nutritional content of common food items.

- USDA FoodData Central (**https://fdc.nal.usda.gov/index.html**) provides detailed nutritional data on a wide variety of foods.
- ChooseMyPlate (**https://www.choosemyplate.gov**) provides information on making healthy choices within food groups, including how to count servings from each group, how to identify whole grains, and how to place vegetables in the five vegetable subgroups.
- Dietary Guidelines for Americans (**https://health.gov/dietaryguidelines/2015/guidelines**) includes appendixes with good food sources of nutrients of concern for many Americans— potassium, calcium, vitamin D, and dietary fiber.
- Users of McGraw-Hill Connect can track and analyze their diet using NutritionCalcPlus, available from the home page of a Connect section.

Resources for Finding Nutritional Content of Popular Items from Fast-Food Restaurants

Although most foods served at fast-food restaurants are high in calories, fat, saturated fat, cholesterol, sodium, and sugar, some items are healthier than others. If you eat at fast-food restaurants, knowing the nutritional content of various items can help you make better choices. Fast-food restaurants provide nutritional information both online and in print brochures available at most restaurant locations. To learn more about the items you order, visit the restaurants' websites:

Arby's:	**arbys.com**	Papa John's Pizza:	**www.papajohns.com**
Burger King:	**bk.com**	Pizza Hut:	**www.pizzahut.com**
Chipotle:	**chipotle.com**	Starbucks:	**www.starbucks.com**
Domino's Pizza:	**www.dominos.com**	Subway:	**www.subway.com**
Hardees:	**www.hardees.com**	Taco Bell:	**www.tacobell.com**
KFC:	**www.kfc.com**	Wendy's:	**www.wendys.com**
McDonald's:	**www.mcdonalds.com**	White Castle:	**www.whitecastle.com**

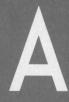

Unintentional injuries are the leading cause of death in the United States for people under age 45. Injuries are generally classified into four categories, based on where they occur: motor vehicle injuries, home injuries, leisure injuries, and work injuries. The greatest number of disabling injuries occur in the home; falls are the leading cause of nonfatal, unintentional injuries that are treated in hospital emergency departments. Violent crimes, including assault, rape, and terrorism, are other sources of injury, as are natural disasters. In all these areas, your preparation for emergency situations can make a significant difference.

MOTOR VEHICLE INJURIES

According to the Centers for Disease Control and Prevention, there are more than 35,000 deaths and 2 million injuries in motor vehicle crashes in the United States each year. These numbers have increased significantly in recent years. Those most affected by motor vehicle crashes are people 15–24 years of age. Motor vehicle injuries also result in the majority of cases of paralysis due to spinal injuries, and they are the leading cause of severe brain injury in the United States.

Factors in Motor Vehicle Injuries

Driving Habits   Nearly two-thirds of motor vehicle injuries are caused by bad driving, especially speeding. As speed increases, momentum and force of impact increase and the time available for the driver to react decreases. Speed limits are posted to establish the safest *maximum* speed limit for a given area under *ideal* conditions. Aggressive driving—characterized by speeding, frequent and abrupt lane changes, tailgating, and passing on the shoulder—also increases the risk of crashes.

Distracted driving contributes to 25–50% of all crashes. Anything that distracts a driver—sleepiness, bad mood, children or pets in the car, use of a cell phone—can increase the risk of a crash. Sleepiness reduces reaction time, coordination, and speed of information processing and can be as dangerous as drug and alcohol use. Even mild sleep deprivation causes a deterioration in driving ability comparable to that caused by a 0.05% blood alcohol concentration.

Cell phone users respond to hazards about 20% slower than undistracted drivers and are about twice as likely to rear-end a braking car in front of them. According to the National Safety Council (NSC), drivers who use cell phones are nearly four times as likely to be involved in a crash as drivers who don't. Hands-free devices do not help significantly; the mental distraction of talking, rather than the act of holding a phone, is the factor in crashes. Text-messaging (texting) on a cell phone while driving is even more dangerous than talking; a texting driver is 8–23 times more likely than a non-texting driver to be involved in a crash. Estimates provided by the NSC attribute 1.3 million traffic crashes (about 24% of all crashes) to the use of cell phones and

text messaging. Many cities and states have outlawed the use of cell phones while driving.

Safety Belts and Air Bags   A person who doesn't wear a safety belt is twice as likely to be injured in a crash as a person who does wear one. Safety belts not only prevent occupants from being thrown from the car at the time of the crash but also provide protection from the "second collision," which occurs when the occupant of the car hits something inside the car, such as the steering column or windshield. The safety belt also spreads the stopping force of a collision over the body.

Since 1998, all new cars have been equipped with dual air bags—one for the driver and one for the front passenger seat. Air bags provide supplemental protection in a collision but are most useful in head-on collisions. (Many newer vehicles feature side air bags to offer protection in a side-impact crash.) They also deflate immediately after inflating and so do not provide protection in collisions involving multiple impacts. To ensure that air bags work as intended, follow these guidelines:

- Place infants in rear-facing infant seats in the back seat.
- Transport children age 12 and under in the back seat.
- Always use safety belts or appropriate safety seats.
- Keep at least 10 inches between the air bag cover and the breastbone of the driver or passenger.

If you cannot comply with these guidelines, you can apply to the National Highway Traffic Safety Administration for permission to install an on-off switch that temporarily disables the air bag.

Alcohol and Other Drugs   Alcohol is involved in about 3 out of 10 fatal crashes. Alcohol-impaired driving, defined by blood alcohol concentration (BAC), is illegal. As of 2018, the legal BAC limit is 0.08% in all states except Utah, where it is 0.05%, but driving ability is impaired at much lower BACs. All psychoactive drugs have the potential to impair driving ability.

Preventing Motor Vehicle Injuries

About 75% of all motor vehicle collisions occur within 25 miles of home and at speeds lower than 40 mph. These crashes often occur because the driver believes safety measures are not necessary for short trips. Clearly, the statistics prove otherwise.

To prevent motor vehicle injuries:

- Obey the speed limit. If you have to speed to get to your destination on time, then you're not allowing enough time.
- Always wear a safety belt and ask passengers to do the same. Strap infants and toddlers into government-approved car seats in the back seat. Children who have outgrown child safety seats but who are

still too small for adult safety belts alone (usually ages 4–8) should be secured using booster seats. All children under age 12 should ride in the back seat.

- Never drive under the influence of alcohol or other drugs or with a driver who is.
- Do not drive when you are sleepy or have been awake for 18 or more hours.
- Avoid using your cell phone while driving—your primary obligation is to pay attention to the road. If you do make calls, follow laws set by your city or state. Place calls when you are at a stop, and keep them short. Pull over if the conversation is stressful or emotional.
- Never text while driving.
- Keep your car in good working order. Regularly inspect tires, oil and fluid levels, windshield wipers, spare tire, and so on.
- Always allow enough following distance. Follow the "3-second rule": When the vehicle ahead passes a reference point, count out 3 seconds. If you pass the reference point before you finish counting, drop back and allow more following distance.
- Always increase following distance and slow down if weather or road conditions are poor.
- Choose major highways rather than rural roads. Highways are much safer because of better visibility, wider lanes, fewer surprises, and other factors.
- Always signal before turning or changing lanes.
- Stop completely at stop signs. Follow all traffic laws.
- Take special care at intersections. Always look left, right, and then left again. Make sure you have plenty of time to complete your maneuver in the intersection.
- Don't pass on two-lane roads unless you are in a designated passing area and have a clear view ahead.

Motorcycles and Scooters

About 1 of every 7 traffic fatalities among people ages 15–34 involves someone riding a motorcycle. Injuries from motorcycle collisions are generally more severe than those involving automobiles because motorcycles provide little, if any, protection. Scooter riders face additional challenges. Motorized scooters usually have a maximum speed of 30–35 mph and have less power for maneuverability.

To prevent motorcycle and scooter injuries:

- Make yourself easier to see by wearing light-colored clothing, driving with your headlights on, and correctly positioning yourself in traffic.
- Develop the necessary skills. Lack of skill, especially when evasive action is needed to avoid a collision, is a major factor in motorcycle and moped injuries. Skidding from improper braking is the most common cause of loss of control.
- Wear a close-fitting helmet, one marked with the symbol DOT (for Department of Transportation).
- Protect your eyes with goggles, a face shield, or a windshield.
- Drive defensively and never assume that other drivers see you.

Pedestrians and Bicycles

Injuries to pedestrians and bicyclists are considered motor vehicle related because they usually involve motor vehicles. About 1 in 7 motor vehicle deaths involves pedestrians, and more than 160,000 pedestrians are injured each year.

To prevent injuries when walking or jogging:

- Walk or jog in daylight.
- Make yourself easier to see by wearing light-colored, reflective clothing.
- Face traffic when walking or jogging along a roadway, and follow traffic laws.
- Avoid busy roads or roads with poor visibility.
- Cross only at marked crosswalks and intersections.
- Don't use headphones while walking or jogging.
- Don't hitchhike. Hitchhiking places you in a potentially dangerous situation.

Bicycle injuries result primarily from not knowing or understanding the rules of the road, failing to follow traffic laws, and not having sufficient skill or experience to handle traffic conditions. Bicycles are considered vehicles; bicycle riders must obey all traffic laws that apply to automobile drivers, including stopping at traffic lights and stop signs.

To prevent injuries when riding a bike:

- Wear safety equipment, including a helmet, eye protection, gloves, and proper footwear. Secure the bottom of your pant legs with clips and secure your shoelaces so that they don't get tangled in the chain.
- Make yourself easier to see by wearing light-colored, reflective clothing. Equip your bike with reflectors and use lights, especially at night or when riding in wooded or other dark areas.
- Ride with the flow of traffic, not against it, and follow traffic laws. Use bike paths when they are available.
- Ride defensively; never assume that drivers can see you. Be especially careful when turning or crossing at corners and intersections. Watch for cars turning right.
- Stop at all traffic lights and stop signs. Know and use hand signals.
- Continue pedaling at all times when moving (don't coast) to help keep the bike stable and to maintain your balance.
- Properly maintain your bike.

Aggressive Driving

Aggressive driving, known as *road rage,* has increased more than 50% since 1990. Aggressive drivers increase the risk of crashes for themselves and others. They further increase the risk of injuries if they stop their vehicles and confront each other. Even if you are successful at controlling your own aggressive driving impulses, you may still encounter an aggressive driver.

To avoid being the victim of an aggressive driver:

- Always keep distance between your car and others. If you are behind a very slow driver and can't pass, slow down to increase distance in case that driver does something unexpected. If you are being tailgated, do not increase your speed; instead, let the other driver pass you. If you are in the left lane when being tailgated, signal and pull over to let the other driver go by, even if you are traveling at the speed limit. When you are merging, make sure you have plenty of room. If you are cut off by a merging driver, slow down to make room.
- Be courteous, even if the other driver is not. Use your horn rarely, if ever. Avoid making gestures of irritation, even shaking your head.

When parking, let the other driver have the space that both of you found.

- Refuse to join in a fight. Avoid eye contact with an angry driver. If someone makes a rude gesture, ignore it. If you think another car is following you and you have a cell phone, call the police. Otherwise, drive to a public place and honk your horn to get someone's attention.
- If you make a mistake while driving, apologize. Raise or wave your hand or touch or knock your head with the palm of your hand to indicate "What was I thinking?" You can also mouth the words "I'm sorry."

HOME INJURIES

Contrary to popular belief, home is one of the most dangerous places to be. The most common fatal home injuries are caused by falls, poisoning, fires, suffocation and choking, and incidents involving firearms.

Falls

About 90% of fatal falls involve people age 45 and older, but falls are a significant cause of unintentional death for people under age 25. Most deaths occurring from falls involve falling on stairs or steps or from one level to another. Falls also occur on the same level, from tripping, slipping, or stumbling. Alcohol is a contributing factor in many falls.

To prevent injuries from falls:

- Install handrails and nonslip surfaces in the shower and bathtub. Place skidproof backing on rugs and carpets.
- Keep floors, stairs, and outside areas clear of objects or conditions that could cause slipping or tripping, such as heavy wax coating, electrical cords, and toys.
- Put a light switch by the door of every room so that no one has to walk across a room to turn on a light. Use night lights in bedrooms, halls, stairways, and bathrooms.
- Outside the house, clear dangerous surfaces created by ice, snow, fallen leaves, or rough ground.
- Install handrails on stairs. Keep stairs well lit and clear of objects.
- When climbing a ladder, use both hands. Never stand higher than the third step from the top. When using a stepladder, make sure the spreader brace is in the locked position. With straight ladders, set the base out 1 foot for every 4 feet of height. Don't stand on chairs to reach things.
- If there are small children in the home, place gates at the top and bottom of stairs. Never leave a baby unattended.

Poisoning

More than 2 million nonfatal poisonings and 60,000 fatal poison-related incidents occur each year in the United States; this category includes drug overdoses.

To prevent poisoning:

- Store all medicines out of the reach of children. Use medicines only as directed on the label or by a physician. Don't mix alcohol and other drugs; get treatment for any substance use disorder.
- Use cleaners, pesticides, and other dangerous substances only in areas with proper ventilation. Store them out of the reach of children.

- Never operate a vehicle in an enclosed space. Have your furnace inspected yearly. Use caution with any substance that produces potentially toxic fumes, such as kerosene. If appropriate, install carbon monoxide detectors.
- Keep poisonous plants out of the reach of children. These include azalea, oleander, rhododendron, wild mushrooms, daffodil and hyacinth bulbs, mistletoe berries, apple seeds, morning glory seeds, wisteria seeds, and the leaves and stems of potato, rhubarb, and tomato plants.

To be prepared in case of poisoning:

- Keep the number of the nearest Poison Control Center (or emergency room) in an accessible location. A call to the national poison control hotline (800-222-1222) will be routed to a local center.

Emergency first aid for poisonings:

1. Remove the poison from contact with eyes, skin, or mouth, or remove the victim from contact with poisonous fumes or gases.
2. Call the Poison Control Center immediately for instructions. Have the container with you.
3. Do not follow emergency instructions on labels. Some may be out-of-date and carry incorrect treatment information.
4. If you are instructed to go to an emergency room, take the poisonous substance or its container with you.

Guidelines for specific types of poisons:

- *Swallowed poisons.* Call the Poison Control Center or a physician for advice. Do not induce vomiting.
- *Poisons on the skin.* Remove any affected clothing. Flood affected parts of the skin with warm water, wash with soap and water, and rinse. Then call for advice.
- *Poisons in the eye.* For children, flood the eye with lukewarm water poured from a pitcher held 3–4 inches above the eye for 15 minutes; alternatively, irrigate the eye under a faucet. For adults, get in the shower and flood the eye with a gentle stream of lukewarm water for 15 minutes. Then call for advice.
- *Inhaled poisons.* Immediately carry or drag the person to fresh air and, if necessary, give rescue breaths (Figure A.1). If the victim is not breathing easily, call 9-1-1 for help. Ventilate the area. Then call the Poison Control Center for advice.

Fires

Each year, about 85% of fire deaths and 65% of fire injuries occur in the home. Careless smoking is the leading cause of home fire deaths. Cooking is the leading cause of home fire injuries.

To prevent fires:

- Dispose of all cigarettes in ashtrays. Never smoke in bed.
- Do not overload electrical outlets. Do not place extension cords under rugs or where people walk. Replace worn or frayed extension cords.
- Place a wire screen in front of fireplaces and woodstoves. Remove ashes carefully and store them in airtight metal containers, not paper bags.
- Properly maintain electrical appliances, kerosene heaters, and furnaces. Clean flues and chimneys annually.

EMERGENCY CARE FOR CHOKING

- If the victim is coughing, encourage the coughing to clear the object from the airway.
- If the victim is not coughing, follow the steps in "Choking Care for Responsive Adult or Child."

Choking Care for Responsive Adult or Child

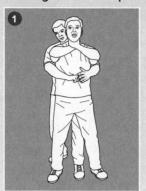

1 Stand behind an adult victim with one leg forward between the victim's legs. (With a child, kneel behind the victim.) Keep your head slightly to one side. Reach around the abdomen with both arms. Make a fist with one hand and place the thumb side of the fist against the abdomen just above the navel.

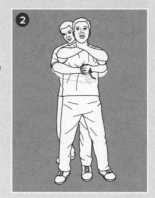

2 Grasp your fist with your other hand and thrust inward and upward into the victim's abdomen with quick jerks. Continue abdominal thrusts until the victim expels the object or becomes unresponsive. If the victim becomes unresponsive lower the victim to the floor onto his or her back, and follow the steps in "Choking Care for Unresponsive Adult or Child." If you are not comfortable performing abdominal thrusts, perform back blows: Standing behind the victim with one arm around his or her chest, lean the person forward until the trunk is parallel to the floor. Use the heel of your other hand to deliver firm blows between the shoulder blades.

Choking Care for Unresponsive Adult or Child: CPR

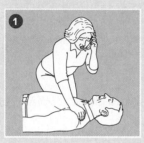

1 Call 9-1-1 and begin first aid and CPR. Check for any object in the victim's mouth that might be causing the choking. Open the person's mouth by placing your thumb over the tongue and your index finger under the chin. If you see a loose object, remove it

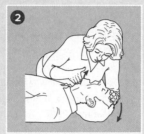

2 Open the airway to see if the victim is breathing. Use the "head tilt–chin lift" maneuver to open the airway: Push down on the forehead and lift the chin. Check for breathing by putting your ear close to the person's mouth and watching for chest movement. Listen and look for breathing for 5 seconds.

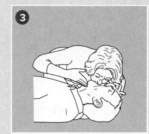

3 If the victim is not breathing, give two rescue breaths, each lasting 1 second. Pinch the victim's nose shut and blow a normal breath into the victim's mouth. If the first breath does not go in (the chest does not rise), reposition the head to open the airway and try again. Each time you give a rescue breath, look for an object in the victim's mouth and remove it if present.

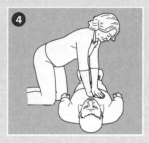

4 If the obstruction remains, begin chest compressions. Place the heel of one hand in the center of the chest between the nipples and the other hand on top of the first. Position your shoulders over your hands and lock your elbows. Give 30 chest compressions at a rate of 100–120 per minute. The chest should go down by at least 2, but not more than 2.4, inches. Then give two breaths, looking in the mouth for an expelled object. Continue chest compressions until help arrives. **Remember: Push hard and push fast at a rate of 100–120 compressions per minute.**

EMERGENCY CARE FOR CARDIAC ARREST

1 Call 9-1-1.

2 Start CPR (100–120 compressions per minute, stopping every 30 compressions to give 2 rescue breaths).

3 If an automated external defibrillator (AED) is available, or as soon as one arrives, give one shock to restart the victim's heart.

4 Go back to CPR immediately after the shock. Continue until prompted by the AED to check heart rhythm and possibly shock again.

Hands-Only CPR

If you are untrained in CPR, the American Heart Association Heart Association recommends providing compression-only CPR.

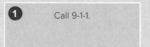

1 Call 9-1-1.

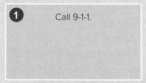

2 Push hard and fast in the center of the chest at a rate of 100–120 compressions per minute.

Don't wait for an emergency to learn how to use an AED or perform CPR. To find a course in your area, contact the American Heart Association (1-877-AHA-4CPR) or the American Red Cross (1-800-REDCROSS or http://www.redcross.org/ux/take-a-class).

Figure A.1   Emergency care for choking and for cardiac arrest.

SOURCES: Neumar, R. W., et al. 2015. "2015 American Heart Association guidelines update for cardiopulmonary resuscitation and emergency cardiovascular care," *Circulation* 132: S315–S367; MedlinePlus. 2015. *Choking - Adult or Child Over 1 Year.* (https://medlineplus.gov/ency/article/000049.htm); American Heart Association. 2015. *Highlights of the 2015 American Heart Association Guidelines Update for CPR and ECC* (http://eccguidelines.heart.org/wp-content/uploads/2015/10/2015-AHA-Guidelines-Highlights-English.pdf).

- Keep portable heaters at least three feet away from curtains, bedding, towels, or anything that might catch fire. Never leave operating heaters unattended.

To be prepared for a fire:

- Plan at least two escape routes out of each room. Designate a location outside the home as a meeting place. Stage a home fire drill.
- Install a smoke detection device on every level of your home. Clean the detectors and test batteries once a month, and replace the batteries at least once a year.
- Keep a fire extinguisher in your home and know how to use it.

To prevent injuries from fire:

- Get out as quickly as possible and go to the designated meeting place. Don't stop for a keepsake or a pet. Never hide in a closet or under a bed. Once outside, count heads to see if everyone is out. If you think someone is still inside the burning building, tell the firefighters. Never go back inside a burning building.
- If you're trapped in a room, feel the door. If it is hot or if smoke is coming in through the cracks, don't open it; use the alternative escape route. If you can't get out of a room, go to the window and shout or wave for help.
- Avoid inhaling smoke. Smoke inhalation is the largest cause of death and injury in fires. To avoid inhaling smoke, crawl along the floor away from the heat and smoke. Cover your mouth and nose, ideally with a wet cloth, and take short, shallow breaths.
- If your clothes catch fire, don't run. Drop to the ground, cover your face, and roll back and forth to smother the flames. Remember: Stop-drop-roll.

Suffocation and Choking

Suffocation and choking account for nearly 7,000 deaths annually in the United States. Children can suffocate if they put small items in their mouths, get tangled in their crib bedding, or get trapped in airtight appliances like old refrigerators. Keep small objects out of reach of children under age 3, and don't give them raw carrots, hot dogs, popcorn, peanuts, or hard candy. Examine toys carefully for small parts that could come loose; don't give plastic bags or balloons to small children.

Adults can also become choking victims, especially if they fail to chew food properly, eat hurriedly, or try to talk and eat at the same time. Many choking victims can be saved with abdominal thrusts, also called the Heimlich maneuver (see Figure A.1). Infants who are choking can be saved with blows to the upper back, followed by chest thrusts if necessary.

Incidents Involving Firearms

Firearms pose a significant threat of unintentional injury, especially to people between ages 5 and 29.

To prevent firearm injuries:

- Always treat a gun as though it were loaded, even if you know it isn't.
- Never point a gun—loaded or unloaded—at something you do not intend to shoot.
- Always unload a firearm before storing it. Store unloaded firearms under lock and key, away from ammunition.
- Inspect firearms carefully before handling them.

- If you own a gun, buy and use a gun lock designed specifically for that weapon.
- If you ever plan to handle a gun, take a firearms safety course first.

LEISURE INJURIES

Leisure injuries take place in public places but do not involve motor vehicles. Many injuries in this category involve such recreational activities as boating and swimming, playground activities, in-line skating, and sports.

Drowning and Boating Injuries

Although most drownings are reported in lakes, ponds, rivers, and oceans, more than half the drownings of young children take place in residential pools. Among adolescents and adults, alcohol plays a significant role in many boating injuries and drownings.

To prevent drowning and boating injuries:

- Develop adequate swimming skill and make sure children learn to swim.
- Make sure residential pools are fenced and that children are never allowed to swim without supervision.
- Don't swim alone or in unsupervised places.
- Use caution when swimming in unfamiliar surroundings or for an unusual length of time. To avoid being chilled, don't swim in water colder than 70°F.
- Don't swim or boat under the influence of alcohol or other drugs. Don't chew gum or eat while in the water.
- Check the depth of water before diving.
- When on a boat, use a life jacket (personal flotation device).

In-Line Skating and Scooter Injuries

Most in-line skating injuries occur because users are not familiar with the equipment and do not wear appropriate safety gear. Injuries to the wrist and head are the most common. To prevent injuries while skating, wear a helmet, elbow and knee pads, wrist guards, a long-sleeved shirt, and long pants.

Wearing a helmet and knee and elbow pads is also important for preventing scooter injuries. The rise in popularity of lightweight scooters has seen a corresponding increase in associated injuries. Scooters should not be viewed as toys, and young children should be closely supervised. Be sure that handlebars, the steering column, and all nuts and bolts are securely fastened. Ride on smooth, paved surfaces away from motor vehicle traffic. Avoid streets and surfaces with water, sand, gravel, or dirt.

Sports Injuries

Since more people have begun exercising to improve their health, there has been an increase in sports-related injuries.

To prevent sports injuries:

- Develop the skills required for the activity. Recognize and guard against the hazards associated with it.
- Always warm up and cool down.
- Make sure facilities are safe.
- Follow the rules and practice good sportsmanship.

- Use proper safety equipment, including, where appropriate, helmets, eye protection, knee and elbow pads, and wrist guards. Wear correct footwear.
- When it is excessively hot and humid, avoid heat stress by following the guidelines given in Chapter 3.

WORK INJURIES

Many aspects of workplace safety are monitored by the Occupational Safety and Health Administration (OSHA), a federal agency. The Bureau of Labor Statistics estimates that 2.8 million Americans suffered injuries on the job in 2017. The highest rate of work-related injuries occurs among laborers, whose jobs usually involve extensive manual labor and lifting—two areas not addressed by OSHA safety standards. Back injuries are the most common work injury.

To protect your back when lifting:

- Don't try to lift beyond your strength. If you need it, get help.
- Get a firm footing, with your feet shoulder-width apart. Get a firm grip on the object.
- Keep your torso in a relatively upright position, bending slightly at the knees and hips. Avoid bending at the waist. To lift, stand up or push up with your leg muscles. Lift gradually, keeping your arms straight. Keep the object close to your body.
- Don't twist. If you have to turn with an object, change the position of your feet.
- Put the object down gently, reversing the rules for lifting.

Another type of work-related injury is damage to the musculoskeletal system from repeated strain on the hand, arm, wrist, or other part of the body. Such repetitive-strain injuries are proliferating due to increased use of computers. One type, carpal tunnel syndrome, is characterized by pain and swelling in the tendons of the wrists and sometimes numbness and weakness.

To prevent carpal tunnel syndrome:

- Maintain good posture at the computer. Use a chair that provides back support and place your feet flat on the floor or on a footrest.
- Position the screen at eye level and the keyboard so that your hands and wrists are straight.
- Take breaks periodically to stretch and flex your wrists and hands to lessen the cumulative effects of stress.

VIOLENCE AND INTENTIONAL INJURIES

According to the Federal Bureau of Investigation (FBI), nearly 1.2 million violent crimes occurred in the United States in 2017. Violence includes assault, sexual assault, homicide, domestic violence, suicide, and child abuse. Compared with rates of violence in other industrialized countries, U.S. rates are unusually high in two areas: homicide and firearm-related deaths.

Assault

Assault is the use of physical force to inflict injury or death on another person. Most assaults occur during arguments or in connection with another crime, such as robbery. Poverty, urban settings, and the use of

alcohol and drugs are associated with higher rates of assault. Homicide victims are most likely to be male, between ages 19 and 24, and members of minority groups. Most homicides are committed with a firearm; the murderer and the victim usually know each other.

To protect yourself at home:

- Secure your home with good lighting and effective locks, preferably deadbolts. Make sure that all doors and windows are securely locked.
- Get a dog, or post "Beware of Dog" signs.
- Don't hide keys in obvious places, and don't give anyone the chance to duplicate your keys.
- Install a peephole in your front door. Don't open your door to people you don't know.
- If you or a family member owns a weapon, store it securely. Store guns and ammunition separately.
- If you are a woman living alone, use your initials rather than your full name on your door or buzzer. Don't use a greeting on your answering machine that implies you live alone or are not home.
- Teach everyone in the household how to get emergency assistance.
- Know your neighbors. Work out a system for alerting each other in case of an emergency.
- Establish a neighborhood watch program.

To protect yourself on the street:

- Avoid walking alone, especially at night. Stay where people can see and hear you.
- Walk on the outside of the sidewalk, facing traffic. Walk purposefully. Act alert and confident. If possible, keep at least two arm lengths between yourself and a stranger.
- Know where you are going. Appearing to be lost increases your vulnerability.
- Carry valuables in a fanny pack, pants pocket, or shoulder bag strapped diagonally across the chest.
- Always have your keys ready as you approach your vehicle or home.
- Carry a whistle to blow if you are attacked or harassed. If you feel threatened, run and/or yell. Go into a store or knock on the door of a home. If someone grabs you, yell for help.

To protect yourself in your car:

- Keep your car in good working condition, carry emergency supplies, and keep the gas tank at least half full.
- When driving, keep doors locked and windows rolled up at least three-quarters of the way.
- Park your car in well-lighted areas or parking garages, preferably those with an attendant or a security guard.
- Lock your car when you leave it, and check the interior before opening the door when you return.
- Don't pick up strangers. Don't stop for vehicles in distress; drive on and call for help.
- Note the location of emergency call boxes along highways and in public facilities. Carry a cell phone.
- If your car breaks down, raise the hood and tie a white cloth to the antenna or door handle. Wait in the car with the doors locked and windows rolled up. If someone approaches to offer help, open a window only a crack and ask the person to call the police or a towing service.

- When you stop at a light or stop sign, leave enough room to maneuver if you need an escape route.
- If you are involved in a minor automobile crash and you think you have been bumped intentionally, don't leave your car. Motion to the other driver to follow you to the nearest police station.
- If confronted by a person with a weapon, give up your car.

To protect yourself on public transportation:

- While waiting, stand in a populated, well-lighted area.
- Make sure that the bus, subway, or train is bound for your destination before you board it. Sit near the driver or conductor in a single seat or an outside seat.
- If you flag down a taxi, make sure it's from a legitimate service. When you reach your destination, ask the driver to wait until you are safely inside the building.

To protect yourself on campus:

- Make sure that door and window locks are secure and that halls and stairwells have adequate lighting.
- Don't give dorm or residence keys to anybody.
- Don't leave your door unlocked or allow strangers into your room.
- Avoid solitary late-night trips to the library or laundry room. Take advantage of on-campus escort services.
- Don't exercise outside alone at night. Don't take shortcuts across campus that are unfamiliar or seem unsafe.
- If security guards patrol the campus, know the areas they cover and stay where they can see or hear you.

Sexual Assault—Rape and Date Rape

The use of force and coercion in sexual relationships is one of the most serious problems in human interactions. The most extreme manifestation of sexual coercion—forcing a person to submit to another's sexual desires—is rape. Taking advantage of circumstances that render a person incapable of giving consent (such as when drunk) is also considered sexual assault or rape. Coerced sexual activity in which the victim knows or is dating the rapist is often referred to as date rape.

An estimated 700,000 females are raped annually in the United States, and some males—perhaps 10,000 annually—are raped each year by other males. Research shows that about 1 in 5 women and 1 in 71 men have experienced an attempted or completed rape. A study of college students also found that between 1 in 4 and 1 in 5 women experience a completed or attempted rape during their college years. Rape victims suffer both physical and psychological injury. The psychological pain can be substantial and long-lasting.

To protect yourself against rape:

- Follow the guidelines listed earlier for protecting yourself against assault.
- Trust your gut feeling. If you feel you are in danger, don't hesitate to run and scream.
- Think out in advance what you would do if you were threatened with rape. However, no one knows what he or she will do when scared to death. Trust that you will make the best decision at the time—whether to scream, run, fight, or give in to avoid being injured or killed.

To protect yourself against date rape:

- Believe in your right to control what you do. Set limits and communicate them clearly, firmly, and early. Be assertive; men often interpret passivity as permission.
- If you are unsure of a new acquaintance, go on a group date or double date. If possible, provide your own transportation.
- Remember that some men think flirtatious behavior or sexy clothing indicates an interest in having sex.
- Remember that alcohol and drugs interfere with judgment, perception, and communication about sex. In a bar or at a party, don't leave your drink unattended, and don't accept opened beverages; watch your drinks being poured. At a party or club, check on friends and ask them to check on you.
- Use the statement that has proved most effective in stopping date rape: "This is rape, and I'm calling the cops!"

If you are raped:

- Go to a safe place.
- Call the police. Tell them you were raped and give your location.
- Call someone you trust who can be with you and give support.
- Try to remember everything you can about your attacker and write it down.
- Don't wash or douche before the medical exam. Don't change your clothes, but bring a new set with you if you can.
- Be aware that at the hospital you will have a complete exam. Show the physician any bruises or scratches.
- Tell the police exactly what happened. Be honest and stick to your story.
- If you do not want to report the rape to the police, see a physician as soon as possible. Be sure you are checked for pregnancy and STIs.
- Contact an organization with skilled counselors so that you can talk about the experience. Look in the telephone directory under "Rape" or "Rape Crisis Center" for a hotline number.

Guidelines for men (pursuing women, but the same guidelines apply to men pursuing men):

- Be aware of social pressure. It's OK not to score.
- Understand that "No" means "No." No answer or no consent also means no. Stop making advances when your date says to stop. Remember that a person has the right to refuse sex.
- Don't assume that flirtatious behavior or sexy clothing means a woman is interested in having sex, that previous permission for sex applies to the current situation, or that your date's relationships with other men constitute sexual permission for you.
- Remember that alcohol and drugs interfere with judgment, perception, and communication about sex—both yours and another person's.

Guidelines for bystanders:

Everyone can help prevent sexual assaults. The Rape, Abuse, and Incest National Network (RAINN) recommends four strategies indicated by the acronym CARE for bystanders if they notice someone who looks at risk. Choose strategies that are appropriate for the situation, keep yourself and others safe, and act according to your comfort level:

- Create a distraction. Do what you can to interrupt a situation that doesn't seem right. A distraction can allow a person to leave a situation.

- Ask directly. Talk with a person who you think might be in trouble and make sure she or he gets to a safe place.
- Refer to an authority. Talk with a bartender, a security guard, or another employee about your concerns—for example, if someone is behaving aggressively.
- Enlist others. Ask another person for help or support. For example, ask someone who knows the person to check on her or him.

If appropriate, call 9-1-1. Visit the website for RAINN (https://www.rainn.org/safety-prevention) for additional suggestions on preventing sexual assault.

Stalking and Cyberstalking

Stalking is characterized by harassing behaviors such as following or spying on a person and making verbal, written, or implied threats. Cyberstalking, the use of electronic communications devices to stalk another person, is becoming more common. Although many cases are not reported, surveys have found that about 8% of internet users have been stalked online; rates are much higher among women ages 18–24. Cyberstalkers may send harassing or threatening e-mails or chat room messages to the victim, or they may encourage others to harass the victim by posting inflammatory messages and personal information on bulletin boards, chat rooms, or social media sites.

To protect yourself online:

- Never use your real name as an e-mail user name or chat room nickname. Select an age- and gender-neutral identity.
- Avoid filling out profiles for accounts related to e-mail use or chat room activities with information that could be used to identify you.
- Do not share personal information in public spaces anywhere online or give it to strangers.
- Learn how to filter unwanted e-mail messages.
- If you experience harassment online, do not respond to the harasser. Log off or surf elsewhere. Save all communications for evidence. If harassment continues, report it to the harasser's Internet service provider, your Internet service provider, and the local police.
- Don't agree to meet someone you've met online face-to-face unless you feel completely comfortable about it. Schedule a series of phone conversations first. Meet initially in a very public place and bring along a friend to increase your safety.

Coping After Terrorism, Mass Violence, or Natural Disasters

Trauma from natural disasters—for example, hurricanes, tornadoes, floods, and earthquakes—can be similar to trauma experienced from violent attacks. Whether episodes of mass violence such as occurred in New York 2001 and Boston 2013 or the multiple shootings that happen around the country each year, some people suffer direct physical harm and loss of loved ones. Many others experience emotional distress and are robbed of their sense of security.

Each person reacts differently to traumatic disaster, and it is normal to experience a variety of responses. Reactions may include disbelief and shock, fear, anger and resentment, anxiety about the future, difficulty concentrating or making decisions, mood swings, irritability, sadness and depression, panic, guilt, apathy, feelings of isolation or powerlessness, and many of the behavioral signs such as headaches or insomnia that are associated with excessive stress (see Chapter 10). Reactions may occur immediately or may be delayed until weeks or months after the event.

Taking positive steps can help you cope with powerful emotions. Consider the following strategies:

- Share your experiences and emotions with friends and family members. Be a supportive listener. Reassure children and encourage them to talk about what they are feeling.
- Take care of your mind and body. Choose a healthy diet, exercise regularly, get plenty of sleep, and practice relaxation techniques. Don't turn to unhealthy coping techniques such as using alcohol or other drugs.
- Take a break from media reports and images, and try not to develop nightmare scenarios for possible future events.
- Reestablish your routines at home, school, and work.
- Find ways to help others. Donating money, blood, food, clothes, or time can ease difficult emotions and give you a greater sense of control.

Everyone copes with tragedy in a different way and recovers at a different pace. If you feel overwhelmed by your emotions, seek professional help. Additional information about coping with terrorism and violence is available from the Federal Emergency Management Agency (www.fema.gov), the U.S. Department of Justice (www.usdoj.gov), and the National Mental Health Association (www.nmha.org).

Emergency Preparedness

Most prevention and coping activities related to terrorism, mass violence, and natural disasters occur at the federal, state, and community levels. However, one step you can take is to put together an emergency plan and kit for your family or household that can serve for any type of emergency or disaster.

Emergency Supplies Your kit of emergency supplies should include everything you'll need to make it on your own for at least three days. You'll need nonperishable food, water, first aid and sanitation supplies, a battery-powered radio, clothing, a flashlight, cash, keys, copies of important documents, and supplies for sleeping outdoors in any weather. Remember special-needs items for infants, seniors, and pets. Supplies for a basic emergency kit are listed in Figure A.2; add to your kit based on your family situation and the type of problems most likely to occur in your area.

You may want to create several kinds of emergency kits. The primary one would contain supplies for home use. Put together a smaller, lightweight version that you can take with you if you are forced to evacuate your residence. Smaller kits for your car and your workplace are also recommended.

A Family or Household Plan You and your family or household members should have a plan about where to meet and how to communicate. Choose at least two potential meeting places—one in your neighborhood and one or more in other areas. Your community may also have set locations for community shelters. Where you

Basic emergency supplies

Map of the area for locating evacuation routes or shelters	Signal flares	Shutoff wrench for gas and water supplies
Cash, coins, and credit cards	Fire extinguisher (small A-B-C type)	Shovel, hammer, pliers, screwdriver, and other tools
Copies of important documents stored in a watertight container	Whistle	Compass
	Ladder	Matches in a waterproof container
Emergency contact list and phone numbers	Tube tent and rope	Aluminum foil
Extra sets of house and car keys	Sleeping bags or warm blankets	Plastic storage containers, bucket
Flashlights or lightsticks	Foam pads, pillows, baby bed	Duct tape, utility knife, and scissors
Battery- or solar-powered radio	Complete change of warm clothing, footwear, outerwear (jacket or coat, long pants, long-sleeved shirt, sturdy shoes, hat, gloves, raingear, extra socks and underwear, sunglasses)	Paper, pens, pencils
Battery-powered alarm clock		Needles and thread
Extra batteries and bulbs		
Cell phone	Work gloves	

First aid kit

First aid manual	Insect repellent	Anti-diarrhea medication
Thermometer	Antibiotic ointment	Laxative
Scissors	Burn ointment	Antacid
Tweezers	Petroleum jelly or another lubricant	Activated charcoal (use if advised by Poison Control Center)
Safety pins, safety razor blades	Sterile adhesive bandages, several sizes	Potassium iodide (use following radiation exposure if advised by local health authorities)
Needle	Sterile rolled bandages and triangular bandages	
Latex or other sterile gloves	Cotton balls	Prescription medications and prescribed medical supplies
Sterile gauze pads	Eyewash solution	List of medications, dosages, and any allergies
Cleansing agents (soap, isopropyl alcohol, antiseptic towelettes)	Chemical heat and cold packs	Medicine dropper
Sunscreen	Aspirin or nonaspirin pain reliever	

Special needs items

Infant care needs (formula, bottles, diapers, powdered milk, diaper rash ointment)	Feminine hygiene supplies	Pet care supplies, including leash, pet carrier, copy of vaccination history, and tie-out stakes
	Denture needs	Other (list)
Books or toys	Hearing aid or wheelchair batteries; other special equipment	
Extra eyeglasses, contact lenses and supplies		

Food and related supplies

Manual (nonelectric) can opener	Eating utensils: mess kits, or paper cups and plates and utensils	Small cooking stove and cooking fuel (if food must be cooked)
Utility knife		
Paper towels	Plastic garbage bags and resealing bags	Water purification tablets

Water: Three-day-supply, at least 1 gallon of water per person per day, stored in plastic containers:

      Number of people: _____ x _1 gallon_ x _3 days_ = _____ total minimum gallons of water

Store additional water if you live in a hot climate or if your household includes infants, pregnant women, or people with special health needs. Don't forget to store water for pets. Containers can be sterilized by rinsing them with a diluted bleach solution (one part bleach to ten parts water). Replace your water supply every six months.

Food: At least a three-day supply of nonperishable foods—those requiring no refrigeration, preparation, or cooking and little or no water. Choose foods from the following list and add foods that members of your household will eat. Replace items in your food supply every six months.

Ready-to-eat canned meats, fruits, soups, and vegetables	Dried fruit	High-energy foods
	Nuts	Comfort/stress foods
Protein or fruit bars	Crackers	MREs (military rations)
Dry cereal or granola	Nonperishable pasteurized milk or powered milk	Infant formula and baby foods
Peanut butter	Coffee, tea, sodas	Pet foods
Sugar, salt, pepper		

Sanitation

Plastic garbage bags (and ties)	Personal hygiene items (toothbrush, shampoo, deodorant, comb, shaving cream, and so on)	Household chlorine bleach, disinfectant
Toilet paper		Powdered lime
Moist towelettes or hand soap	Plastic bucket with tight lid	Small shovel for digging latrine
Washcloth and towel		

For a clean air supply

Face masks or several layers of dense-weave cotton material (handkerchiefs, t-shirts, towels) that fit snugly over your nose and mouth.

Shelter-in-place supplies, to be used in an interior room to create a barrier between you and potentially contaminated air outside: Heavyweight plastic garbage bags or plastic sheeting; duct tape; scissors; and if possible, a portable air purifier with a HEPA filter.

Family emergency plan

Plan places where your family will meet; choose one location near your home and one outside your neighborhood.

      Local _____ Outside neighborhood _____

Have one local and one out-of-state contact person for family members to call if separated during a disaster. (It may be easier to make long-distance calls than local calls.)

      Local _____ Out-of-state _____

Figure A.2 Sample emergency preparedness kit and plan.

go may depend on the circumstances of the emergency situation. Use your common sense, and listen to the radio or television for instructions from emergency officials about whether to evacuate or stay in place. In addition, know all the transportation options in the vicinity of your home, school, and workplace; roadways and public transit may be affected, so a sturdy pair of walking shoes is a good item to keep in your emergency kit.

Everyone in the family or household should also have the same emergency contact person to call, preferably someone who lives outside the immediate area and won't be affected by the same local disaster. Local phone service may be significantly disrupted, so long-distance calls may be more likely to go through. Everyone should carry the relevant phone numbers and addresses at all times.

It is also important to check into the emergency plans at any location where you or family members spend time, including schools and workplaces. For each location, know the safest place to be for different types of emergencies—for example, near load-bearing interior walls during an earthquake or in the basement during a tornado. Also know how to turn off water, gas, and electricity in case of damaged utility lines; keep the needed tools next to the shutoff valves.

Other steps you can take to help prepare for emergencies include taking a first-aid class and setting up an emergency response group in your neighborhood, residential building, or office. Talk with your neighbors: Who has specialized equipment (for example, a power generator) or expertise that might help in a crisis? Do older or disabled neighbors have someone to help them? More complete information about emergency preparedness is available from local government agencies and from the following:

> American Academy of Pediatrics
>
> > (www.aap.org)
>
> American Red Cross
>
> > (www.redcross.org)
>
> Federal Emergency Management Agency
>
> > (www.fema.gov)
>
> U.S. Department of Homeland Security
>
> > (www.ready.gov)

PROVIDING EMERGENCY CARE

You can improve someone else's chances of surviving if you are prepared to provide emergency help. A course in first aid offered by the American Red Cross and on many college campuses can teach you to respond appropriately when someone needs help. Emergency rescue techniques can save the lives of people who have stopped breathing, who are choking, or whose hearts have stopped beating. Pulmonary resuscitation (also known as rescue breathing, artificial respiration, or mouth-to-mouth resuscitation) is used when a person is not breathing (refer back to Figure A.1). Cardiopulmonary resuscitation (CPR) is used when a pulse can't be found. Training is required before a person can perform CPR. Courses are offered by the American Red Cross and the American Heart Association.

When You Have to Provide Emergency Care Remain calm and act sensibly. The basic pattern for providing emergency care is *check-call-care:*

1. *Check the situation.* Make sure the scene is safe for both you and the injured person. Don't put yourself in danger; if you get hurt, too, you will be of little help to the injured person.

2. *Check the victim.* Conduct a quick head-to-toe examination. Assess the victim's signs and symptoms, such as level of responsiveness, pulse, and breathing rate. Look for bleeding and any indications of broken bones or paralysis.

3. *Call for help.* Call 9-1-1 or a local emergency number. Identify yourself and give as much information as you can about the condition of the victim and what happened.

4. *Care for the victim.* If the situation requires immediate action (for example, no pulse, shock), provide first aid if you are trained to do so (refer back to Figure A.1).

Selected Bibliography

Bren, L. 2005. Prevent your child from choking. *FDA Consumer,* September/ October.

Centers for Disease Control and Prevention. 2019. *Ten Leading Causes of Death and Injury* (https://www.cdc.gov/injury/wisqars/LeadingCauses.html).

Centers for Disease Control and Prevention. 2015. *Impaired Driving: Get the Facts. Injury Prevention and Control: Motor Vehicle Safety.* Atlanta, GA: Centers for Disease Control and Prevention.

Federal Bureau of Investigation. 2018. *Crime in the United States: 2017.* Washington, D.C.: U.S. Department of Justice.

National Highway Traffic Safety Administration. *Air Bags* (http://www.safercar.gov /Vehicle+Shoppers/Air+Bags/Side-Impact+Air+Bags).

National Highway Traffic Safety Administration. 2019. *Distracted Driving Overview* (https://www.nhtsa.gov/risky-driving/distracted-driving).

National Safety Council. 2017. *Cell Phone Distracted Driving* (http://www.nsc.org/learn /NSC-Initiatives/Pages/distracted-driving-problem-of-cell-phone-distracted-driving .aspx).

National Safety Council. 2017. *Injury Facts 2017 Edition.* Itasca, IL: National Safety Council.

Pew Research Center. 2017. *Online Harassment 2017* (https://www.pewinternet .org/2017/07/11/online-harassment-2017).

RAINN. 2019. *Your Role in Preventing Sexual Assault* (https://www.rainn.org/articles /your-role-preventing-sexual-assault).

U.S. Bureau of Labor Statistics. 2018. *Employer-Reported Workplace Injuries and Illnesses—2017* (https://www.bls.gov/news.release/archives/osh_11082018.htm).

U.S. Department of Health & Human Services, Office on Women's Health. 2018. *Stalking* (https://www.womenshealth.gov/relationships-and-safety/other-types /stalking).

U.S. Department of Homeland Security. 2014. *Ready America* (www.ready.gov).

Xu, J., et al. 2018. Deaths: Final data for 2016. *National Vital Statistics Reports* 67(5).

MONITORING YOUR PROGRESS

NAME _____ SECTION _____ DATE _____

As you completed the labs listed here, you entered the results in the Preprogram Assessment column of this appendix. Now that you have been involved in a fitness and wellness program for some time, do the labs again and enter your new results in the Postprogram Assessment column. You will probably notice improvement in several areas. Congratulations! If you are not satisfied with your progress thus far, refer to the tips for successful behavior change in Chapter 1 and throughout this book. Remember that fitness and wellness are forever. The time you invest now in developing a comprehensive, individualized program will pay off in a richer, more vital life in the years to come.

	Preprogram Assessment	Postprogram Assessment
LAB 2.3 Pedometer	Daily steps: _____	Daily steps: _____
LAB 3.1 Cardiorespiratory Endurance		
1-mile walk test	$\dot{V}O_{2max}$: _____ Rating: _____	$\dot{V}O_{2max}$: _____ Rating: _____
3-minute step test	$\dot{V}O_{2max}$: _____ Rating: _____	$\dot{V}O_{2max}$: _____ Rating: _____
1.5-mile run-walk test	$\dot{V}O_{2max}$: _____ Rating: _____	$\dot{V}O_{2max}$: _____ Rating: _____
Beep test	$\dot{V}O_{2max}$: _____ Rating: _____	$\dot{V}O_{2max}$: _____ Rating: _____
12-minute swim test	Rating: _____	Rating: _____
LAB 4.1 Muscular Strength		
1 RM bench press test (measured or predicted)	Weight: _____ lb Rating: _____	Weight: _____ lb Rating: _____
LAB 4.2 Muscular Endurance		
Curl-up test	Number: _____ Rating: _____	Number: _____ Rating: _____
Push-up test	Number: _____ Rating: _____	Number: _____ Rating: _____
Squat endurance test	Number: _____ Rating: _____	Number: _____ Rating: _____
LAB 5.1 Flexibility		
Sit-and-reach test	Score: _____ cm Rating: _____	Score: _____ cm Rating: _____
LAB 5.3 Low-Back Muscular Endurance		
Trunk flexor endurance test	Trunk flexor: _____ sec. Rating: _____	Trunk flexor: _____ sec. Rating: _____
Back extensor endurance test	Back extensor: _____ sec. Rating: _____	Back extensor: _____ sec. Rating: _____
Side bridge endurance test	Right: _____ sec. Rating: _____ Left: _____ sec. Rating: _____	Right: _____ sec. Rating: _____ Left: _____ sec. Rating: _____
Front plank test	Front plank: _____ sec. Rating: _____	Front plank: _____ sec. Rating: _____

	Preprogram Assessment	Postprogram Assessment
LAB 6.1 Body Composition		
Body mass index	BMI: _____ kg/m^2 Rating: _____	BMI: _____ kg/m^2 Rating: _____
Skinfold measurements (or other methods for determining percent body fat)	Sum of 3 skinfolds: _____ mm % body fat: _____ % Rating: _____	Sum of 3 skinfolds: _____ mm % body fat: _____ % Rating: _____
Waist circumference	Circumf.: _____ Rating: _____	Circumf.: _____ Rating: _____
Waist-to-hip ratio	Ratio: _____ Rating: _____	Ratio: _____ Rating: _____
LAB 8.1 Daily Diet		
Number of oz-eq of grains	Grains: _____ oz-eq	Grains: _____ oz-eq
Number of cups of vegetables	Vegetables: _____ cups	Vegetables: _____ cups
Number of cups of fruits	Fruits: _____ cups	Fruits: _____ cups
Number of cups of dairy	Dairy: _____ cups	Dairy: _____ cups
Number of oz-eq of protein foods	Protein foods: _____ oz-eq	Protein foods: _____ oz-eq
Number of tsp of oils	Oils: _____ tsp	Oils: _____ tsp
Number of g of solid fats	Solid fats: _____ g	Solid fats: _____ g
Number of g or tsp of added sugars	Added sugars: _____ g or tsp	Added sugars: _____ g or tsp
LAB 8.2 Dietary Analysis		
Percentage of calories	From protein: _____ %	From protein: _____ %
Percentage of calories	From fat: _____ %	From fat: _____ %
Percentage of calories	From saturated fat: _____ %	From saturated fat: _____ %
Percentage of calories	From carbohydrate: _____ %	From carbohydrate: _____ %
LAB 9.1 Daily Energy Needs	Daily energy needs: _____ cal/day	Daily energy needs: _____ cal/day
LAB 10.1 Identifying Stressors	Average weekly stress score: _____	Average weekly stress score: _____
LAB 11.1 Cardiovascular Health		
CVD risk assessment	Score: _____ Estimated risk: _____	Score: _____ Estimated risk: _____
Hostility assessment	Score: _____ Rating: _____	Score: _____ Rating: _____
LAB 12.1 Cancer Prevention		
Diet: Number of servings	Fruits/vegetables: _____	Fruits/vegetables: _____
Skin cancer	Score: _____ Risk: _____	Score: _____ Risk: _____

BEHAVIOR CHANGE WORKBOOK

This workbook is designed to take you step by step through a behavior change program. The first eight activities in the workbook will help you develop a successful plan—beginning with choosing a target behavior, moving through the planning steps described in Chapter 1, and completing and signing a behavior change contract. The final seven activities will help you work through common obstacles to behavior change and maximize your program's chances of success.

Part 1 Developing a Plan for Behavior Change and Completing a Contract

1. Choosing a Target Behavior
2. Gathering Information About Your Target Behavior
3. Monitoring Your Current Patterns of Behavior
4. Setting Goals
5. Examining Your Attitudes About Your Target Behavior
6. Choosing Rewards
7. Breaking Behavior Chains
8. Completing a Contract for Behavior Change

Part 2 Overcoming Obstacles to Behavior Change

9. Building Motivation and Commitment
10. Managing Your Time Successfully
11. Developing Realistic Self-Talk
12. Involving the People Around You
13. Dealing with Feelings
14. Overcoming Peer Pressure: Communicating Assertively
15. Maintaining Your Program over Time

ACTIVITY 1   CHOOSING A TARGET BEHAVIOR

Use your knowledge of yourself and the results of Lab 1.2 (Lifestyle Evaluation) to identify five behaviors that you could change to improve your level of wellness. Examples of target behaviors include smoking cigarettes, not exercising regularly, eating candy bars every night, not getting enough sleep, getting drunk frequently on weekends, and not wearing a safety belt when driving or riding in a car. List your five behaviors here.

1. _____
2. _____
3. _____
4. _____
5. _____

For successful behavior change, it's best to focus on one behavior at a time. Review your list of behaviors and select one to start with. Choose a behavior that is important to you and that you are strongly motivated to change. If this will be your first attempt at behavior change, start with a simple change, such as wearing your bicycle helmet regularly, before tackling a more difficult change, such as quitting smoking. Circle the behavior on your list that you've chosen to start with; this will be your target behavior throughout this workbook.

ACTIVITY 2   GATHERING INFORMATION ABOUT YOUR TARGET BEHAVIOR

Take a close look at what your target behavior means to your health, now and in the future. How is it affecting your level of wellness? What diseases or conditions does this behavior place you at risk for? What will changing this behavior mean to you? To evaluate your behavior, use information from this text, from the resources listed in the For Further Exploration section at the end of each chapter, and from other reliable sources.

Health behaviors have short-term and long-term benefits and costs associated with them. For example, in the short term, an inactive lifestyle allows for more time to play video games and hang out with friends but leaves a person less able to participate in recreational activities. In the long term, it increases the risk of cardiovascular disease, cancer, and premature death. Fill in the blanks below with the benefits and costs of continuing your current behavior and of changing to a new, healthier behavior. Pay close attention to the short-term benefits of the new behavior—these are an important motivating force behind successful behavior change programs.

Target (current) behavior _____

Benefits *Short-Term*   *Long-Term*

_____   _____

_____   _____

_____   _____

Costs *Short-Term*   *Long-Term*

_____   _____

_____   _____

_____   _____

New behavior _____

Benefits *Short-Term*   *Long-Term*

_____   _____

_____   _____

_____   _____

Costs *Short-Term*   *Long-Term*

_____   _____

_____   _____

_____   _____

ACTIVITY 3 MONITORING YOUR CURRENT PATTERNS OF BEHAVIOR

To develop a successful behavior change program, you need detailed information about your current behavior patterns. You can obtain this information by developing a system of record keeping geared toward your target behavior. Depending on your target behavior, you may want to monitor a single behavior, such as your diet, or you may want to keep daily activity records to determine how you could make time for exercise or another new behavior. Consider tracking factors such as the following:

- What the behavior was
- When and for how long it occurred
- Where it occurred
- What else you were doing at the time
- What other people you were with and how they influenced you
- What your thoughts and feelings were
- How strong your urge for the behavior was (for example, how hungry you were or how much you wanted to watch TV)

Figure 1.6 shows a sample log for tracking daily diet. Create a format for a sample daily log for monitoring the behavior patterns relating to your target behavior. Then use the log to monitor your behavior for a day. Evaluate your log as you use it. Ask yourself if you are tracking all the key factors that influence your behavior; make any necessary adjustments to the format of your log. Once you've developed an appropriate format, use a separate notebook, file, or app (your health journal) to keep records of your behavior for a week or two. These records will provide solid information about your behavior that will help you develop a successful behavior change program. Later activities in this workbook will ask you to analyze your records.

ACTIVITY 4 SETTING GOALS

For your behavior change program to succeed, you must set meaningful, realistic goals. In addition to an ultimate goal, set some intermediate goals—milestones that you can strive for on the way to your final objective. For example, if your overall goal is to run a 5K road race, an intermediate goal might be to successfully complete two weeks of your fitness program. If you set a final goal of eating seven servings of fruits and vegetables every day, an intermediate goal would be to increase your daily intake from three to four servings. List your intermediate and final goals here. Don't strive for immediate perfection. Allow an adequate amount of time to reach each of your goals. All your goals should be consistent with the SMART criteria described in Chapter 1.

Intermediate Goals   **Target Date**

_____   _____

_____   _____

_____   _____

_____   _____

_____   _____

Final Goals

_____   _____

ACTIVITY 5 EXAMINING YOUR ATTITUDES ABOUT YOUR TARGET BEHAVIOR

Your attitudes toward your target behavior can determine whether your behavior change program will be successful. Consider your attitudes carefully by completing the following statements about how you think and feel about your current behavior and your goal.

1. I like _____ because _____
            (current behavior)

_____

2. I don't like _____ because _____
                  (current behavior)

_____

3. I like _____ because _____
            (behavior goal)

_____

4. I don't like _____ because _____
                  (behavior goal)

_____

5. I don't _____ now because _____
              (behavior goal)

_____

6. I would be more likely to _____ if _____
                              (behavior goal)

_____

If your statements indicate that you have major reservations about changing your behavior, work to build your motivation and commitment before you begin your program. Look carefully at your objections to changing your behavior. How valid and important are they? What can you do to overcome them? Can you adopt any of the strategies you listed under statement 6? Review the facts about your current behavior and your goals.

ACTIVITY 6   CHOOSING REWARDS

Make a list of objects, activities, and events you can use as rewards for achieving the goals of your behavior change program. Rewards should be special, relatively inexpensive, and preferably unrelated to food or alcohol—for example, tickets to a ball game, a new piece of clothing, or a walk with a friend—whatever is meaningful for you. Write down a variety of rewards you can use when you reach milestones in your program and your final goal.

_____   _____

_____   _____

_____   _____

_____   _____

Many people also find it helpful to give themselves small rewards daily or weekly for sticking with their behavior change program. These could be things like a study break, a movie, or a Saturday morning bike ride. Make a list of rewards for maintaining your program in the short term.

_____   _____

_____   _____

_____   _____

_____   _____

And don't forget to congratulate yourself regularly during your behavior change program. Notice how much better you feel. Savor how far you've come and how you've gained control of your behavior.

ACTIVITY 7   BREAKING BEHAVIOR CHAINS

Use the records you collected about your target behavior in Activity 3 and in your health journal to identify what leads up to your target behavior and what follows it. By tracing these chains of events, you'll be able to identify points in the chain where you can make a change that will lead to your new behavior. The sample behavior chain on the next page shows a sequence of events for a person who wants to add exercise to her daily routine—but who winds up snacking and watching TV instead. By examining the chain carefully, you can identify ways to break it at every step. After you review the sample, go through the same process for a typical chain of events involving your target behavior. Use the blank behavior chain that follows the sample.

Some general strategies for breaking behavior chains include the following:

- *Control or eliminate environmental cues that provoke the behavior.* Stay out of the room where your television is located. Go out for an ice cream cone instead of keeping a half gallon of ice cream in your freezer.
- *Change behaviors or habits that are linked to your target behavior.* If you always smoke in your car when you drive to school, try taking public transportation instead.
- *Add new cues to your environment to trigger your new behavior.* Prepare easy-to-grab healthy snacks and carry them with you to class or work. Keep your exercise clothes and equipment in a visible location.

See also the suggestions in Chapter 1.

Chain of Events

Strategies for Breaking the Chain

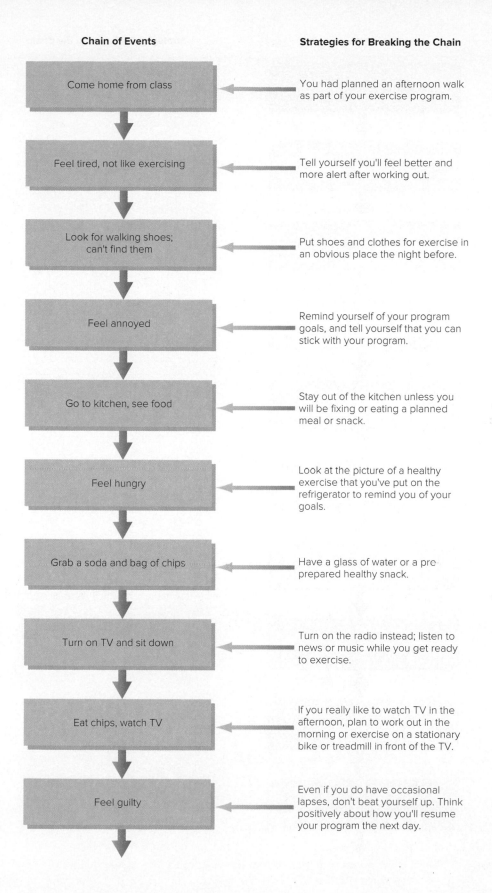

Chain of Events	Strategies for Breaking the Chain
Come home from class	You had planned an afternoon walk as part of your exercise program.
Feel tired, not like exercising	Tell yourself you'll feel better and more alert after working out.
Look for walking shoes; can't find them	Put shoes and clothes for exercise in an obvious place the night before.
Feel annoyed	Remind yourself of your program goals, and tell yourself that you can stick with your program.
Go to kitchen, see food	Stay out of the kitchen unless you will be fixing or eating a planned meal or snack.
Feel hungry	Look at the picture of a healthy exercise that you've put on the refrigerator to remind you of your goals.
Grab a soda and bag of chips	Have a glass of water or a pre-prepared healthy snack.
Turn on TV and sit down	Turn on the radio instead; listen to news or music while you get ready to exercise.
Eat chips, watch TV	If you really like to watch TV in the afternoon, plan to work out in the morning or exercise on a stationary bike or treadmill in front of the TV.
Feel guilty	Even if you do have occasional lapses, don't beat yourself up. Think positively about how you'll resume your program the next day.

Chain of Events

Strategies for Breaking the Chain

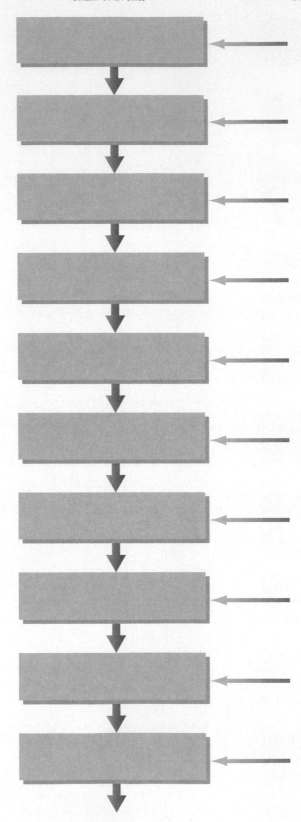

Your next step in creating a successful behavior change program is to complete and sign a behavior change contract. Your contract should include details of your program and indicate your commitment to changing your behavior. Use the information from previous activities in this workbook to complete the following contract. (If your target behavior relates to exercise, you may want to use the program plan and contract for a fitness program in Lab 7.1.)

1. I, _____ , agree to _____
                 (name)   (specify behavior you want to change)

   _____

2. I will begin on _____ and plan to reach my goal of _____
                (start date)   (specify final goal)

   _____ by _____ .

3. To reach my final goal, I have devised the following schedule of mini-goals. For each step in my program, I will give myself the reward listed.

(mini-goal 1)	(target date)	(reward)
(mini-goal 2)	(target date)	(reward)
(mini-goal 3)	(target date)	(reward)
(mini-goal 4)	(target date)	(reward)
(mini-goal 5)	(target date)	(reward)

   My overall reward for reaching my final goal will be _____

4. I have gathered and analyzed data on my target behavior and have identified the following strategies for changing my behavior: _____

   _____

   _____

5. I will use the following tools to monitor my progress toward reaching my final goal:

   _____
   (list any charts, graphs, or journals you plan to use)

   _____

   I sign this contract as an indication of my personal commitment to reach my goal.

   _____   _____
   (your signature)   (date)

   I have recruited a helper who will witness my contract and _____

   _____
   (list any way in which your helper will participate in your program)

   _____

   _____   _____
   (helper's signature)   (date)

Describe in detail any special strategies you will use to help change your behavior (refer to Activity 7).

Create a plan for any charts, graphs, or journals you will use to monitor your progress. The log format you developed in Activity 3 may be appropriate, or you may need to develop a more detailed or specific record-keeping system. Examples of journal formats are included in Labs 3.2, 4.3, 5.2, 8.1, and 10.1. You might also want to develop a graph to show your progress; posting such a graph in a prominent location can help keep your motivation strong and your program on track. Depending on your target behavior, you could graph the number of push-ups you can do, the number of servings of vegetables you eat each day, or your average daily stress level.

ACTIVITY 9 BUILDING MOTIVATION AND COMMITMENT

Complete the following checklist to determine whether you are motivated and committed to changing your behavior. Check the statements that are true for you.

_____ I feel responsible for my own behavior and capable of managing it.

_____ I am not easily discouraged.

_____ I enjoy setting goals and then working to achieve them.

_____ I am good at keeping promises to myself.

_____ I like having a structure and schedule for my activities.

_____ I view my new behavior as a necessity, not an optional activity.

_____ Compared with previous attempts to change my behavior, I am more motivated now.

_____ My goals are realistic.

_____ I have a positive mental picture of the new behavior.

_____ Considering the stresses in my life, I feel confident that I can stick to my program.

_____ I feel prepared for lapses and ups-and-downs in my behavior change program.

_____ I feel that my plan for behavior change is enjoyable.

_____ I feel comfortable telling other people about the change I am making in my behavior.

Did you check most of these statements? If not, you need to boost your motivation and commitment. Consider these strategies:

• Review the potential benefits of changing your behavior and the costs of not changing it (see Activity 2). Pay special attention to the short-term benefits of changing your behavior, including feelings of accomplishment and self-confidence. Post a list of these benefits in a prominent location.

• Visualize yourself achieving your goal and enjoying its benefits. For example, if you want to manage time more effectively, picture yourself as a confident, organized person who systematically tackles important tasks and sets aside time each day for relaxation, exercise, and friends. Practice this type of visualization regularly.

• Put aside obstacles and objections to change. Counter thoughts such as "I'll never have time to exercise" with thoughts like "Lots of other people do it, and so can I."

• Bombard yourself with propaganda. Take a class dealing with the change you want to make. Read books and watch videos on the subject. Post motivational phrases or pictures on your refrigerator, over your desk, or in a reminder smartphone app. Talk to people who have already made the change.

• Build up your confidence. Remind yourself of other goals you've achieved. At the end of each day, mentally review your good decisions and actions. See yourself as a capable person, as being in charge of your behavior.

List two strategies for boosting your motivation and commitment; choose from the list above, or develop your own. Try each strategy, and then describe how well it worked for you.

Strategy 1: _____

_____

How well it worked: _____

_____

Strategy 2: _____

_____

How well it worked: _____

_____

ACTIVITY 10 MANAGING YOUR TIME SUCCESSFULLY

"Too little time" is a common excuse for not exercising or engaging in other healthy behaviors. Learning to manage your time successfully is crucial if you are to maintain a wellness lifestyle. The first step is to examine how you are currently spending your time; use the following grid to track your activities.

Time	Activity	Time	Activity
6:00 A.M.		6:00 P.M.	
7:00 A.M.		7:00 P.M.	
8:00 A.M.		8:00 P.M.	
9:00 A.M.		9:00 P.M.	
10:00 A.M.		10:00 P.M.	
11:00 A.M.		11:00 P.M.	
12:00 P.M.		12:00 A.M.	
1:00 P.M.		1:00 A.M.	
2:00 P.M.		2:00 A.M.	
3:00 P.M.		3:00 A.M.	
4:00 P.M.		4:00 A.M.	
5:00 P.M.		5:00 A.M.	

Next, list each type of activity and the total time you engaged in it on a given day in the following chart (for example, sleeping, 7 hours; eating, 1.5 hours; studying, 3 hours; working, 3 hours). Take a close look at your list of activities. Successful time management is based on prioritization. Assign a priority to each of your activities according to how important it is to you: essential (A), somewhat important (B), or not important (C). Based on these priority rankings, make changes in your schedule by adding and subtracting hours from different categories of activities; enter a duration goal for each activity. Add your new activities to the list and assign a priority and duration goal to each.

Activity	Current Total Duration	Priority (A, B, or C)	Goal Total Duration

Prioritizing in this manner will involve trade-offs. For example, you may choose to reduce the amount of time you spend watching television, listening to music, and chatting on the telephone while you increase the amount of time spent sleeping, studying, and exercising. Don't feel that you have to miss out on anything you enjoy. You can get more from less time by focusing on what you are doing. Strategies for managing time more productively and creatively are described in Chapter 10.

ACTIVITY 11 DEVELOPING REALISTIC SELF-TALK

Self-talk is the ongoing internal dialogue you have with yourself throughout much of the day. Your thoughts can be accurate, positive, and supportive, or they can be exaggerated and negative. Self-talk is closely related to self-esteem and self-concept. Realistic self-talk can help maintain positive self-esteem, the belief that you are a good and competent person, worthy of friendship and love. A negative internal dialogue can reinforce negative self-esteem and can make behavior change difficult. Substituting realistic self-talk for negative self-talk can help you build and maintain self-esteem and cope better with the challenges in your life.

First, take a closer look at your current pattern of self-talk. Use your health journal to track self-talk, especially as it relates to your target behavior. Does any of your self-talk fall into the common patterns of distorted, negative self-talk shown in Chapter 10? If so, use the examples of realistic self-talk from Chapter 10 to develop more accurate and rational responses. Write your current negative thoughts in the left-hand column, and then record more realistic thoughts in the right-hand column.

Current Self-Talk about Target Behavior   **More Realistic Self-Talk**

_____   _____

_____   _____

_____   _____

_____   _____

Your behavior change program will be more successful if the people around you are supportive and involved—or at least are not sabotaging your efforts. Use your health journal to track how other people influence your target behavior and your efforts to change it. For example, do you always skip exercising when you're with certain people? Do you always drink or eat too much when you socialize with certain friends? Are friends and family members offering you enthusiastic support for your efforts to change your behavior, or do they make jokes about your program? Have they even noticed your efforts? Summarize the reactions of those around you in the chart here.

Target behavior _____

Person	Typical Effect on Target Behavior	Involvement in/Reaction to Program

It may be difficult to change the actions and reactions of the people who are close to you. For them to be involved in your program, you may need to develop new ways of interacting with them (for example, taking a walk rather than going out to dinner as a means of socializing). Most of your friends and family members will want to help you—if they know how. Ask for exactly the type of help or involvement you want. Do you want feedback, praise, or just cooperation? Would you like someone to witness your contract or to be involved more directly in your program? Do you want someone to stop sabotaging your efforts by inviting you to watch TV, eat rich desserts, and so on? Look for ways that the people who are close to you can share in your behavior change program. They can help to motivate you and to maintain your commitment to your program. Develop a way that each individual you listed above can become involved in your program in a positive way.

Person	Target Involvement in Behavior Change Program

Choose one person on your list to tackle first. Talk to that person about her or his current behavior and how you would like her or him to be involved in your behavior change program. Next, describe this person's reaction to your talk and her or his subsequent behavior. Did this individual become a positive participant in your behavior change program?

_____

_____

_____

_____

Long-standing habits are difficult to change in part because many of them represent ways people have developed to cope with certain feelings. For example, people may overeat when bored, skip their exercise sessions when frustrated, or drink alcoholic beverages when anxious. Developing new ways to deal with feelings can help improve the chance that a behavior change program will succeed.

Review the records on your target behavior that you kept in your health journal. Identify the feelings that are interfering with the success of your program, and develop new strategies for coping with them. Some common problematic feelings are listed here, along with one possible coping strategy for each. Put a check mark next to those that are influencing your target behavior, and fill in additional strategies. Add the other feelings that are significant roadblocks in your program to the bottom of the chart, along with coping strategies for each.

✓	Problem	Solution
	Stressed out	Go for a 10-minute walk.
	Anxious	Do one of the relaxation exercises described in Chapter 10.
	Bored	Call a friend for a chat.
	Tired	Take a 20-minute nap.
	Frustrated	Identify the source of the feeling and deal with it constructively.

Consider the following situations:

- Julia is trying to give up smoking; her friend Marie continues to offer her cigarettes whenever they are together.
- Emilio is planning to exercise in the morning; his roommates tell him he's being antisocial by not having breakfast with them.
- Tracy's boyfriend told her that in high school he once experimented with drugs and shared needles; she wants him to have an HIV test, but he says he's sure the people he shared needles with were not infected.

Peer pressure is the common ingredient in these situations. To successfully maintain your behavior change program, you must develop effective strategies for resisting peer pressure. Assertive communication is one such strategy. By communicating assertively—firmly, but not aggressively—you can stick with your program even in the face of pressure from others.

Review your health journal to determine how other people affect your target behavior. If you find that you often give in to peer pressure, try the following strategies for communicating more assertively:

- Collect your thoughts, and plan in advance what you will say. You might try out your response on a friend to get some feedback.
- State your case—how you feel and what you want—as clearly as you can.
- Use "I" messages—statements about how you feel—rather than "you" statements.
- Focus on the behavior rather than the person. Suggest a solution, such as asking the other person to change his or her behavior toward you. Avoid generalizations. Be specific about what you want.
- Make clear, constructive requests. Focus on your needs ("I would like . . .") rather than the mistakes of others ("You always . . .").
- Avoid blaming, accusing, and belittling. Treat others with the same respect you'd like to receive yourself.
- Ask for action ahead of time. Tell others what you would like to have happen; don't wait for them to do the wrong thing and then get angry at them.
- Ask for a response to what you have proposed. Wait for an answer and listen carefully to it. Try to understand other people's points of view, just as you would hope that others would understand yours.

With these strategies in mind, review your health journal and identify three instances in which peer pressure interfered with your behavior change program. For each instance, write out what you might have said to deal with the situation more assertively. (If you can't think of three situations from your experiences, choose one or more of the three scenarios described at the beginning of this activity.)

1. _____

_____

2. _____

_____

3. _____

_____

4. _____

_____

5. _____

_____

Assertive communication can help you achieve your behavior change goals in a direct way by helping you keep your program on track. It can also provide a boost for your self-image and increase your confidence in your ability to successfully manage your behavior.

If you maintain your new behavior for at least six months, you've reached the maintenance stage, and your chances of lifetime success are greatly increased. However, you may find yourself sliding back into old habits at some point. If this happens, there are some things you can do to help maintain your new behavior.

- Remind yourself of the goals of your program (list them here).

_____

_____

_____

_____

_____

- Pay attention to how your new pattern of behavior has improved your wellness status. List the major benefits of changing your behavior, both now and in the future.

_____

_____

_____

_____

_____

- Consider the things you enjoy most about your new pattern of behavior. List your favorite aspects.

_____

_____

_____

_____

_____

- Think of yourself as a problem solver. If something begins to interfere with your program, devise strategies for dealing with it. Take time out now to list things that have the potential to derail your program and develop possible coping mechanisms.

Problem	Solution
_____	_____
	_____
_____	_____
	_____
_____	_____

- Remember the basics of behavior change. If your program runs into trouble, go back to keeping records of your behavior to pinpoint problem areas. Make adjustments in your program to deal with new disruptions. Don't feel defeated if you lapse. The best thing you can do is renew your commitment and continue with your program.

INDEX

Page numbers followed by b indicate boxes; f, figures; (lab), laboratory activities; t, tables. **Boldface** page numbers indicate where terms are defined. Page numbers preceded by capitalized A or B indicate Appendixes. Page numbers preceded by capitalized W indicate Workbook.